CARDIOVASCULAR NUTRITION

STRATEGIES AND TOOLS FOR DISEASE MANAGEMENT AND PREVENTION

Penny Kris-Etherton, PhD, RD,
and Julie H. Burns, MS, RD, Editors

Brenda Eissenstat, MS, RD,
Associate Editor

THE AMERICAN DIETETIC ASSOCIATION

Design by Julie Anderson, Anderson Creative Services
Copyediting and indexing by Lynn Brown, Brown Editorial Service

Library of Congress Cataloging-in-Publication Data
Cardiovascular nutrition : strategies and tools for disease management and prevention / edited by Penny Kris-Etherton, Julie Burns.
p. cm.
Includes bibliographical references and index.
ISBN 0-88091-159-X
1. Cardiovascular system—Diseases—Nutrition aspects.
2. Cardiovascular system—Diseases—Diet therapy. I. Kris-Etherton, Penny. II. Burns, Julie.
[DNLM: 1. Cardiovascular Diseases—prevention & control.
2. Cardiovascular Diseases—diet therapy. 3. Diet. 4. Risk Factors. 5. Nutrition—education. WG 166 C2666 1997]
RC669.C2875 1998
616.1'0654—dc21
for Library of Congress 97-34401
CIP

10 9 8 7 6 5 4 3 2 1

CONTENTS

CONTRIBUTORS

Editors
Penny M. Kris-Etherton, PhD, RD
Nutrition Department
Pennsylvania State University
University Park, Pennsylvania

Julie H. Burns, MS, RD
SportFuel, Inc.
Western Springs, Illinois
Formerly Director of Research
Chicago Center for Clinical Research
Chicago, Illinois

Associate Editor
Brenda Eissenstat, MS, RD
Nutrition Department
Pennsylvania State University
University Park, Pennsylvania

Substantive Editors
Judith Dickson, MS
Eleanor Mayfield
Jennifer Scales
Science Editing
Rockville, Maryland

Contributing Authors
Cheryl Achterberg, PhD
Nutrition Department
Pennsylvania State University
University Park, Pennsylvania

Donna Alexander-Israel, PhD, RD
Preferred Nutrition Therapists
Richardson, Texas

Karen Balnicki, MS, RD
Nutrition Consultant
Oak Ridge, Tennessee

Michelle Berry, MS, RD
Research Nutritionist
Graduate School of Public Health
Department of Epidemiology
University of Pittsburgh
Pittsburgh, Pennsylvania

Julie H. Burns, MS, RD
SportFuel, Inc.
Western Springs, Illinois
Formerly Director of Research
Chicago Center for Clinical Research
Chicago, Illinois

Catherine Champagne, PhD, RD
Pennington Biomedical Research Center
Baton Rouge, Louisiana

Kristine L. Clark, PhD, RD
Director of Sports Nutrition
Pennsylvania State University
University Park, Pennsylvania

Michael Davidson, MD, FACC
Chicago Center for Clinical Research
Chicago, Illinois

Lynne DeMoor, MS, RD
Michigan Heart & Vascular Institute
Ann Arbor, Michigan

Karen Reznik Dolins, MS, RD
Nutrition Consultant
Scarsdale, New York

Lynn D. Dugan, MS, RD
Manager, Nutrition Communications
McDonald's Corporation
Oakbrook, Illinois

Brenda Eissenstat, MS, RD
Nutrition Department
Pennsylvania State University
University Park, Pennsylvania

Valerie Fishell, MS
Nutrition Department
Pennsylvania State University
University Park, Pennsylvania

Niki Gernhofer, MS, RD
Department of Community Health and Preventive Medicine
Northwestern University School of Medicine
Chicago, Illinois

Henry Ginsberg, MD
Director, Irving Center for Clinical Research
Columbia University
New York, New York

Wahida Karmally, MS, RD
Irving Center for Clinical Research
Columbia Presbyterian Medical Center
New York, New York

James J. Kenney, PhD, RD
Pritkin Longevity Center
Santa Monica, California

Kathryn Kolasa, PhD
Department of Family Medicine
East Carolina University
Greenville, North Carolina

Debra Krummel, PhD, RD
Department of Community Health and Preventive Medicine
West Virginia University
Morgantown, West Virginia

Donna Louie, BSN, RN
Cardiac Therapy Foundation of Mid-Peninsula
Palo Alto, California

Kevin C. Maki, MS
Chicago Center for Clinical Research
Chicago, Illinois

Arline McDonald, PhD
Chicago Center for Clinical Research
Chicago, Illinois

Jill Metz, PhD
Department of Medicine
Division of Nephrology, Hypertension, and Clinical Pharmacology
Oregon Health Sciences University
Portland, Oregon

John Milner, PhD
Nutrition Department
Pennsylvania State University
University Park, Pennsylvania

Kristen Moriarty, MS, RD
Nutrition Department
Pennsylvania State University
University Park, Pennsylvania

Natalie Partridge, MS, RD
Food and Nutrition Information Center
Beltsville, Maryland

Eileen Peters, MS, RD
Department of Community Health and Preventive Medicine
Northwestern University School of Medicine
Chicago, Illinois

Sharon Peterson, PhD, RD
Nutrition Education Consultant
Choices
Carterville, Illinois

Madeleine Sigman-Grant, PhD, RD
Nutrition Department
University of Nevada
Las Vegas, Nevada

Lori Silver-Kolodin, RD, MPH
The Mount Sinai Medical Center
New York, New York

Uma Srinath, MS
Formerly at Nutrition Department
Pennsylvania State University
University Park, Pennsylvania

Sharon Sugerman, MS, RD
Research Dietitian
Westat
Rockville, Maryland

Jill Upton-Stocki, MS, RD
Food and Nutritionist Specialist
Chicago Center for Clinical Research
Chicago, Illinois

Linda Van Horn, PhD, RD
Department of Community Health and Preventive Medicine
Northwestern University School of Medicine
Chicago, Illinois

Robin Wedell, RN, BSN
Cardiac Therapy Foundation of Mid-Peninsula
Palo Alto, California

Expert Reviewers

Jean Charles-Azure
Chief, Indian Health Service
Nutrition and Dietetics Training Program
Santa Fe, New Mexico
(Chapter 16)

Nancy E. Chronmiller, MMSc, RD
Nutrition Coordinator
Emory Clinic
Atlanta, Georgia

Ellen Coleman, MS, RD
Nutrition Consultant
Sport Clinic
Riverside, California
(Chapter 9)

Cindy Conroy, MA, RD
Iowa Heart Center
Des Moines, Iowa

Rachel Guthrie, MS, RD
Pitt Memorial Hospital Health Quest Program
Greenville, North Carolina
(Chapter 15)

Suzanne Jaax, MS, RD
Diet Modification Clinic
Methodist Hospital
Baylor College of Medicine
Houston, Texas

Carolyn J. Lackey, PhD, RD
North Carolina State University Cooperative Extension Service
Raleigh, North Carolina
(Chapter 15)

Mary McGhee, MS, RD
Clinical Nutritionist
Massachusetts General Hospital
Boston, Massachusetts

Suzanne Pelican, MS, RD
Indian Health Service
Nutrition and Dietetics Training Program
Santa Fe, New Mexico
(Chapter 16)

Lillian Sonnenberg, PhD, RD
Nutrition Services
Massachusetts General Hospital
Boston, Massachusetts

Neil Stone, MD
Distinguished Professor of Medicine
Northwestern University School of Medicine
Chicago, Illinois

Katherine Tate
Pitt Memorial Hospital Cardiac Rehabilitation Program
Greenville, North Carolina
(Chapter 15)

Elenora Zephier, RD, MPH
Chief, Nutrition and Dietetics Branch
Aberdeen Area Indian Health Service
Aberdeen, South Dakota
(Chapter 15)

ACKNOWLEDGMENTS

Our sincerest gratitude is extended to

Our husbands and children for their ever-present love, support, and patience, without which this work could not have been completed.

Our associate editor, Brenda Eissenstat, for her remarkable talents in editing and writing and for guiding countless tasks to closure throughout the duration of this project.

Our technical editor, Judith Dickson, for her superb assistance with the substantive editing of the chapters.

The contributing authors, for their tireless efforts and commitment to educating their colleagues to improve the health of Americans.

Our mentors and colleagues in cardiovascular nutrition and medicine for inspiring us and generously sharing their knowledge and passion for cardiovascular disease treatment and prevention.

The American Dietetic Association Publications Team, especially Cheryl Corbin, who guided us so well during the initiation of the project, and Betsy Hornick, who expertly steered us through its completion.

Penny Kris-Etherton
Julie H. Burns

FOREWORD

Despite an ever-increasing arsenal of potent lipid-lowering drugs, clinicians experienced in treating patients with coronary heart disease or those greatly at its risk have come to value the contributions of nutrition. This belief in the value of nutrition is based not on anecdotal experience, but on numerous studies that have critically examined the effects of various aspects of nutrition on atherosclerosis, thrombosis, and vessel wall reactivity. An increasing number of high-quality nutritional studies have recently appeared in major medical journals. Indeed, to emphasize the growing need by health care workers for detailed nutritional information, one of the premier journals of cardiovascular medicine, *Circulation*, began in 1996 to publish a series of reviews on nutritional subjects that relate to cardiovascular disease.

The importance of nutrition in the prevention and treatment of coronary heart disease is unquestioned. Crucial for patient care is that dietitians and nutritionists keep up to date with the rapidly expanding knowledge base in the area of diet and heart disease. This carefully compiled book translates the most recent key findings of laboratory experiments, metabolic ward studies, and clinical trials for practitioners charged with treating patients at risk for clinical sequelae of atherosclerotic vascular disease. Although this is a daunting task, *Cardiovascular Nutrition* handles it admirably.

What sets this book apart, however, is the wealth of practical information that it provides. There are numerous well-designed tools dietitians can use in practice. These will aid in assessing a patient's clinical condition, selecting an appropriate nutrition care plan, and determining follow-up activities, as well as in choosing effective evaluation strategies. Other tools are designed to assist in teaching patients about their clinical condition and ways to implement most effectively their prescribed diets. Most notably, the book provides gender-specific tables for determining coronary heart disease risk status. This allows a needed perspective on the potential benefits of risk factor intervention. Finally, the detailed treatment algorithms and medical nutrition therapy protocols should be quite useful in practice, especially in providing guidance for performing follow-up activities.

I believe this book will prove to be an important resource for physicians, dietitians, nurses, and exercise physiologists alike. It is a wonderful compendium of tools that are needed to provide the nutritional care our patients require for the prevention and treatment of coronary heart disease.

Neil J. Stone, MD
Professor of Clinical Medicine, Northwestern University School of Medicine
Distinguished Physician in Medicine, Northwestern Memorial Hospital
Chicago, Illinois

September 1997

INTRODUCTION

PENNY M. KRIS-ETHERTON, PHD, RD,
AND JULIE H. BURNS, MS, RD

Despite the considerable progress that has been made in decreasing cardiovascular disease (CVD) morbidity and mortality since the 1970s, it remains the leading cause of death in the United States. The costs associated with CVD are staggering, and are expected to reach $92 billion in 1997 because of both the direct medical care costs associated with treating this disease and the approximately $75 billion in indirect costs incurred. CVD affects not only individuals and their families, but our entire society (1).

Major risk factors, both modifiable and nonmodifiable, have been identified for CVD. Family history, age, and sex cannot be modified, but hypercholesterolemia, hypertension, cigarette smoking, overweight, physical inactivity, and a stressful lifestyle can be (2). Healthful lifestyle practices reduce CVD risk. Many studies have shown beneficial effects of risk factor modification on both the primary and secondary prevention of CVD. Although these intervention studies have targeted multiple risk factors and have included drug therapy, they nonetheless provide compelling evidence of the efficacy of risk factor management for the prevention and treatment of CVD (3-7). Lowering low-density lipoprotein (LDL) cholesterol levels has significant beneficial effects in low-risk patients and even greater effects in high-risk patients (8) and in patients with coronary artery disease (9).

The recent Cholesterol and Recurrent Event (CARE) Trial reported beneficial effects of cholesterol-lowering therapy in coronary artery disease patients who had only average cholesterol levels (10). In addition, lowering LDL cholesterol markedly (to below 100 mg/dL) reduced the progression of atherosclerosis in patients who had both bypass grafts because of atherosclerosis and thrombosis and an elevated LDL cholesterol level (11,12). A large body of strong and consistent evidence exists to recommend cholesterol-lowering therapy to prevent and treat CVD.

Diet is the cornerstone of preventing CVD. Diet, in conjunction with regular physical activity and other healthful lifestyle practices, favorably affects major risk factors for CVD. Healthful lifestyle practices that are embraced as a way of life can promote well-being and prevent CVD well into the golden years.

Diet is also a key component in the treatment of CVD. At the 1997 SCAN Symposium in St. Louis, Dr. Michael Davidson presented the ABCs of the treatment and prevention of CVD and noted that diet therapy is an integral part of many of these treatment modalities. The ABCs of treatment and prevention are

<u>A</u>spirin and ACE inhibitors
<u>B</u>eta blockers
<u>C</u>holesterol-lowering therapy
<u>D</u>iet
<u>E</u>xercise and vitamin <u>E</u>
<u>F</u>olate and other B vitamins (vitamins B-6 and B-12)
<u>G</u>lucose control

The enormous public health significance of CVD and the importance of diet in both the treatment and prevention of this disease inspired us to write this book. The first edition, entitled *Cardiovascular Disease: Nutrition for Prevention and Treatment,* was published by The American Dietetic Association in 1990 and was intended principally to deliver information to dietetic practitioners about CVD-nutrition relationships in order to provide rationale and support for relevant intervention activities. Since 1990 great strides have been made in the field, and many successful approaches and tools have been developed by and for dietetic practitioners. This second edition provides the latest information in a user-friendly format for dietitians and other health care professionals.

A recurring theme is the practical application of CVD intervention strategies that include both diet and physical activity. This book will be of great value to registered dietitians and other health care professionals who wish to implement current diet and physical activity guidelines in their clinical practice. Our intent is to help practitioners more effectively deliver preventative nutrition messages and medical nutrition therapy in an effort to reduce CVD morbidity and mortality.

The opening chapters provide information about our current understanding of CVD risk factor management and the basis for our current treatment decisions and prevention guidelines. Subsequent chapters provide state-of-the-art guidance on components of the nutrition care process, such as assessing nutritional status, prescribing medical nutrition therapy and exercise programs for both normal-weight and overweight individuals, and planning appropriate follow-up activities. Chapters that deal with special population groups and adherence provide tools for eliciting maximum compliance with the treatment plan in practice. Other chapters address such topics as effective grocery shopping, dining out, and functional foods, all of which are necessary for implementing a prescribed diet. The appendix on resources will help practitioners identify educational and instructional materials for updating their knowledge base and effectively teaching principles of medical nutrition therapy aimed at decreasing CVD risk.

All the information needed to assess individual patients, prescribe an appropriate diet, monitor the effectiveness of the treatment plan, and modify a plan if necessary are presented in this manual. It will assist registered dietitians in implementing CVD risk factor intervention programs that will decrease CVD morbidity and mortality in the United States and improve the health and well-being of society as a whole. We are hopeful that this book will make dietitians' jobs a little easier and enable them to realize many successful outcomes for their patients that are related to their nutrition care activities.

References

1. *American Heart Association Heart and Stroke Facts.* Dallas: American Heart Association; 1997.
2. *Second Report of the Expert Panel on Detection, Evaluation, and Treatment of High Blood Cholesterol in Adults.* Washington, DC: National Institutes of Health, National Heart, Lung, and Blood Institute; September 1993.
3. Lipid Research Clinics Program. The Lipid Research Clinics Coronary Primary Prevention Trial results. I. Reduction in incidence of coronary heart disease. *JAMA.* 1984;251:351-364.
4. Lipid Research Clinics Program. The Lipid Research Clinics Coronary Primary Prevention Trial results. II. The relationship of reduction in incidence of coronary heart disease to cholesterol lowering. *JAMA.* 1984;251:365-374.
5. Frick MH, Elo MO, Haapa K, et al. Helsinki Heart Study: primary-prevention trial with gemfibrozil in middle aged men with dyslipidemia. Safety of treatment, changes in risk factors, and incidence of coronary heart disease. *N Engl J Med.* 1987;317:1237-1245.
6. Manninen V, Tenkanen L, Koskinen P, et al. Joint effects of serum triglyceride and LDL cholesterol and HDL cholesterol concentrations on coronary heart disease risk in the Helsinki Heart Study: implications for treatment. *Circulation.* 1992;85:37-45.

7. Holme I. An analysis of randomized trials evaluating the effect of cholesterol reduction on total mortality and coronary heart disease incidence. *Circulation.* 1990;82:1916-1924.
8. West of Scotland Coronary Prevention Study: identification of high-risk groups and comparison with other cardiovascular intervention trials. *Lancet.* 1996;348:1339-1342.
9. Kjekshus J, Pedersen TR. Reducing the risk of coronary events: evidence from the Scandinavian Simvastatin Survival Study (4S). *Am J Cardiol.* 1995; 76:64C-68C.
10. Wilt TJ, Davis RR, Meyers DG, Rouleau JL, Sacks FM. Prevalence and correlates of symptomatic peripheral atherosclerosis in individuals with coronary heart disease and cholesterol levels less than 240 mg/dL: baseline results from the Cholesterol and Recurrent Events (CARE) Study. *Angiology.* 1996;47:533-541.
11. The Post Coronary Artery Bypass Graft Trial Investigators. The effects of aggressive lowering of low-density lipoprotein cholesterol levels and low-dose anticoagulation on obstructive changes in saphenous-vein coronary-artery bypass grafts. *N Engl J Med.* 1997;336:153-162.
12. Fuster V, Vorchheimer DA. Prevention of athersclerosis in coronary-artery bypass grafts. *N Engl J Med.* 1997;336:153-162. Editorial.

PART 1

INTRODUCTION

CHAPTER 1

Cardiovascular Risk Factors: Evaluation and Treatment Goals

Michael H. Davidson, MD, FACC, and Kevin C. Maki, MS

This chapter describes evaluation of cardiovascular risk factors and how the health care team and patient establish treatment goals.

Introduction

Atherosclerotic coronary heart disease (CHD) is the leading cause of mortality in the United States and other Western nations. However, during the past 40 years the age-adjusted incidence of CHD mortality declined approximately 40% (1,2). Although improved health care has played a role, this favorable trend is attributed primarily to lifestyle changes, particularly reduced cigarette use and dietary changes (1,2). In addition, several large, randomized intervention trials showed that treatment of CHD risk markers, such as hypertension and elevated low-density lipoprotein cholesterol (LDL-C) concentration, reduces fatal and nonfatal cardiovascular events (1,3).

Thus, compelling evidence supports the view that people at increased risk for CHD may be identified and that effective treatments are available to lower the risk of mortality and CHD events, such as myocardial infarction and revascularization procedures. Nevertheless, data from a number of sources have demonstrated that a large proportion of patients at high risk for CHD do not receive appropriate preventive care (4,5,6).

Improvements in the identification and treatment of cardiovascular risk factors will require an integrated approach involving input from disciplines including medicine, nutrition, nursing, exercise physiology, and behavioral science. An understanding of the atherosclerotic process and familiarity with the concepts of risk and risk factors are essential for appropriate decision making by all members of the health care team regarding clinical management of patients at risk for CHD.

Pathogenesis of Atherosclerosis

The atherosclerotic process can be broken down into three stages:

- formation of fatty streaks,
- transition to advanced lesions, and
- occurrence of acute coronary events.

Formation of Fatty Streaks

Studies in animal models and autopsies performed on young people who died from trauma show that the atherosclerotic process begins early in life (7). The first step in the development of an atherosclerotic plaque is the formation of a fatty streak. This earliest lesion appears to result from chronic minimal injury to the arterial endothelium, particularly at points of bifurcation or bending in an artery where shear forces from blood flow are greatest (3,8). In addition to local shear forces, other factors such as toxic chemicals from tobacco, high glucose and cholesterol concentrations, and infection may contribute to endothelial damage and dysfunction (3,8).

Endothelial dysfunction increases the entry of lipoprotein particles into the arterial wall. Of primary importance is the entry of LDL particles, which are subsequently consumed by cells known as macrophages. LDL particles in their native form are taken up via LDL receptors in a regulated fashion; that is, the ingestion of LDL particles will down-regulate the number of LDL receptors so that the cells do not become too full. However, if the LDL particles have been chemically modified in the artery wall (eg, oxidized, glycated, or complexed with antibodies), they are taken up via a different type of macrophage receptor, the "scavenger" receptor (8,9). This situation results in an unregulated form of LDL uptake in which the macrophages continue to ingest modified LDL particles, leading to the formation of lipid-engorged foam cells (8,9).

These foam cells remain trapped in the artery wall and may continue to take up modified LDL particles until they rupture.

The presence of modified LDL also stimulates the production of chemical attractants that help to recruit monocytes (a type of white blood cell) to the artery wall (9). Monocytes adhere to the artery wall and then migrate into the arterial intima (inner layer), where they are converted to macrophages. If sufficient quantities of modified LDL particles are present, the new macrophages may be converted to foam cells.

Transition to Advanced Lesions

Severe damage to the endothelial lining can expose the collagen tissue beneath to the circulating blood. Collagen acts as a potent platelet activator, resulting in platelet adherence to the damaged area. Activated platelets release platelet-derived growth factor, which causes arterial smooth muscle cells to proliferate and migrate from the media (middle layer) into the intima (8). Other growth factors released from macrophages or the endothelium may also contribute to this process (3,8). Eventually, fibrous connective tissue forms; advanced lesions are characterized by a connective tissue cap with a core of lipid-laden foam cells and smooth muscle (discussed in more detail in Chapter 3).

Acute Coronary Events

Acute coronary syndromes such as myocardial infarction or resting (unstable) angina pectoris most often result from disruption of the atherosclerotic plaque followed by thrombus formation (3,10). If the thrombus is large enough to severely impede blood flow, the area of the heart fed by that artery will become ischemic. If this lack of adequate blood supply continues long enough, the cells in the affected area will die, producing a myocardial infarction.

This necessarily simplified description of the atherosclerotic process provides some clues about the mechanisms through which risk factors exert their influence and suggests areas for possible intervention. For instance, chronic endothelial injury may be reduced or prevented by lowering elevated blood pressure and ceasing cigarette smoking. Reducing elevated concentrations of serum cholesterol may lessen the influx of LDL particles into the artery wall and reduce foam cell formation. Interventions that reduce the propensity toward platelet activation (eg, daily aspirin ingestion) may lower the risk of myocardial infarction by preventing the formation of an occlusive thrombus when an atherosclerotic plaque is disrupted.

Risk and Risk Factors

The term *risk* indicates the probability that a person will experience some event in the future. *Risk factors* are characteristics associated with an increased likelihood of developing a specific disease and may be laboratory measurements (eg, serum LDL-C), personal characteristics (eg, type A personality), or even sociological factors (eg, income and education). A statistical association indicates that the factor predicts the development of the disease and does not necessarily imply that a factor causes the disease. For example, a lower level of education is associated with a greater risk for CHD. It is unlikely, however, that lack of education directly causes atherosclerosis or acute coronary events. It is more plausible that educational achievement is associated with a variety of lifestyle factors, such as diet, smoking, chronic stress, and physical activity patterns, that may be more directly related to the disease process.

Some risk factors are amenable to modification whereas others are not. For example, high blood pressure can be treated with medication whereas family history of heart disease cannot be altered. Nevertheless, it is important to assess unmodifiable risk factors so that individuals displaying them may be targeted for more aggressive treatment of risk factors that can be altered.

As the number and severity of CHD risk factors increase, the associated increment in risk may be multiplicative. For example, in a middle-aged man, hypertension, high cholesterol, and cigarette smoking are individually associated with 3- to 4-fold increases in the probability of death from cardiovascular disease during the subsequent 12 years (2). However, if all three are present, the risk is increased by approximately 20-fold (Figure 1-1) (2).

Because CHD is multifactorial, an array of factors must be considered in estimating an individual patient's level of risk. This task is simplified with the Coronary Heart Disease Risk Factor Prediction Chart, created by investigators from the Framingham Heart Study (Table 1-1) (11). Using information such as a patient's sex, age, serum lipid profile (total and

FIGURE 1-1

Age-adjusted CHD mortality rate and relative risk of CHD death during 12-year follow-up, in relation to major CHD risk factors, in 342,815 men screened for the Multiple Risk Factor Intervention Trial.

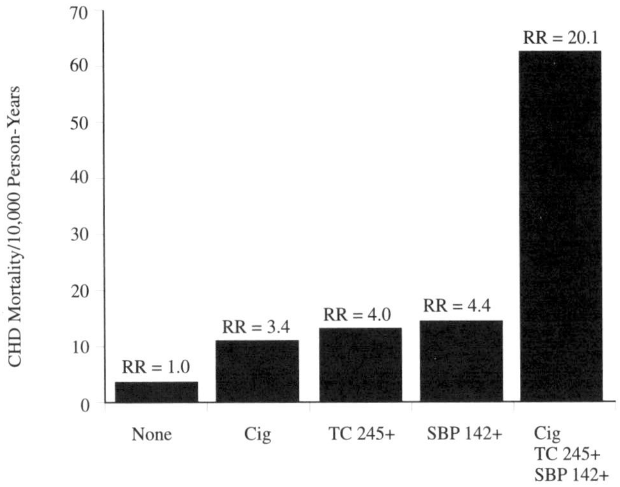

RR = relative risk, Cig = cigarette smoker, TC 245+ = total cholesterol ≥245 mg/dL, SBP = systolic blood pressure ≥142 mm Hg.

TABLE 1-1

Coronary Heart Disease Risk Factor Prediction Chart for Patients Without Known Artery Disease

Step 1 Find points for each risk factor:

Women				Men											
Age (yr)	**Pts**	**Age (yr)**	**Pts**	**Age (yr)**	**Pts**	**Age (yr)**	**Pts**	**HDL-C (mg/dL)**	**Pts**	**Total-C (mg/dL)**	**Pts**	**SBP (mm Hg)**	**Pts**	**Other**	**Pts***
30	-12	47–48	5	30	-2	57–59	13	25–26	7	139–151	-3	98–104	-2	Cigarettes	4
31	-11	49–50	6	31	-1	60–61	14	27–29	6	152–166	-2	105–112	-1	Diabetic (male)	3
32	-9	51–52	7	32–33	0	62–64	15	30–32	5	167–182	-1	113–120	0	Diabetic (female)	6
33	-8	53–55	8	34	1	65–67	16	33–35	4	183–199	0	121–129	1	ECG–LVH	9
34	-6	56–60	9	35–36	2	68–70	17	36–38	3	200–219	1	130–139	2		
35	-5	61–67	10	37–38	3	71–73	18	39–42	2	220–239	2	140–149	3		
36	-4	68–74	11	39	4	74	19	43–46	1	240–262	3	150–160	4		
37	-3			40–41	5			47–50	0	263–288	4	161–172	5		
38	-2			42–43	6			51–55	-1	289–315	5	173–185	6		
39	-3			44–45	7			56–60	-2	316–330	6				
40	0			46–47	8			61–66	-3						
41	1			48–49	9			67–73	-4						
42–43	2			50–51	10			74–80	-5						
44	3			52–54	11			81–87	-6						
45–46	4			55–56	12			88–96	-7						

Step 2 Sum points for all risk factors (subtract minus points from total):

_____ + _____ + _____ + _____ + _____ + _____ + _____ = _____
Age HDL-C Total-C SBP Smoker Diabetes ECG-LVH Point Total

Step 3 Look up risk corresponding to point total:

	Probability										
Pts	**5 yr**	**10 yr**	**Pts**	**5 yr**	**10 yr**	**Pts**	**5 yr**	**10 yr**	**Pts**	**5 yr**	**10 yr**
≤1	<1%	<2%	10	2%	6%	19	8%	16%	28	19%	33%
2	1%	2%	11	3%	6%	20	8%	18%	29	20%	36%
3	1%	2%	12	3%	7%	21	9%	19%	30	22%	38%
4	1%	2%	13	3%	8%	22	11%	21%	31	24%	40%
5	1%	3%	14	4%	9%	23	12%	23%	32	25%	42%
6	1%	3%	15	5%	10%	24	13%	25%			
7	1%	4%	16	5%	12%	25	14%	27%			
8	2%	4%	17	6%	13%	26	16%	29%			
9	2%	4%	18	7%	14%	27	17%	31%			

Step 4 Compare with average 10-year risk:

	Probability	
Age (yr)	**Women**	**Men**
30–34	<1%	3%
35–39	<1%	5%
40–44	2%	6%
45–49	5%	10%
50–54	8%	14%
55–59	12%	16%
60–64	13%	21%
65–69	9%	30%
70–74	12%	24%

*Zero points for each "no." ECG–LVH = electrocardiographic left ventricular hypertrophy; HDL-C = high-density lipoprotein cholesterol; pt = points; SBP = systolic blood pressure; Total-C = total cholesterol.

Source: Califf et al, Task Force 5, *J Am Coll Cardiol,* 1996. Reprinted with permission from the American College of Cardiology (*Journal of the American College of Cardiology,* 1996;27:1007-1012) (11).

HDL-C), systolic blood pressure, and smoking status and the presence of diabetes or electrocardiographic evidence of left ventricular hypertrophy (LVH), 5- and 10-year probabilities of developing the clinical manifestations of CHD can be estimated. For comparison, the chart also shows the average risk for a person of that age and sex. This tool was developed for individuals without known CHD; for those with previously diagnosed CHD, the level of risk is greater and other charts should be used (Tables 1-2 and 1-3).

Although the Framingham risk charts provide a reasonably accurate indication of a patient's risk status, considerable room exists for clinical judgment because not all of the potentially important CHD risk markers are included in these charts. Under some circumstances, additional information should be gathered and assessed in judging the aggressiveness with which risk factors should be managed. For example, health care providers commonly see patients with a strong family history of premature CHD or with a history of atherosclerotic disease whose score on the Framingham charts suggests average or below-average risk. In these cases, evaluation of some nontraditional risk markers such as blood fibrinogen, lipoprotein(a) [Lp(a)], and homocysteine concentrations (discussed below) may be justified; it may be reasonable to set more aggressive treatment goals for modifiable risk factors than would be suggested by the current guidelines.

TABLE 1-2

Risk of Coronary Artery Disease Event, Stroke, or Cerebrovascular Disease Death in Women with Existing Coronary Artery Disease

Age		Total-C	Points by HDL-C (mg/dL)									SBP	
(yr)	Points	(mg/dL)	25	30	35	40	45	50	60	70	80	(mm Hg)	Points
35	0	160	4	3	3	2	2	1	1	0	0	100	0
40	1	170	4	3	3	2	2	2	1	1	0	110	0
45	2	180	4	3	3	2	2	2	1	1	0	120	1
50	3	190	4	4	3	3	2	2	1	1	1	130	1
55	4	200	4	4	3	3	2	2	2	1	1	140	2
60	5	210	4	4	3	3	3	2	2	1	1	150	2
65	6	220	5	4	4	3	3	2	2	1	1	160	2
70	7	230	5	4	4	3	3	3	2	2	1	170	3
75	7	240	5	4	4	3	3	3	2	2	1	180	3
		250	5	4	4	4	3	3	2	2	1	190	3
		260	5	5	4	4	3	3	2	2	1	200	3
		270	5	5	4	4	3	3	2	2	2	210	4
Other	Pts	280	5	5	4	4	3	3	3	2	2	220	4
Diabetes	3	290	5	5	4	4	4	3	3	2	2	230	4
Smoking	3	300	6	5	4	4	4	3	3	2	2	240	4
												250	4

Total Points	2-yr Probability (%)	Average 2-yr Risk in Women with CVD: Age (yr)	Probability (%)
0	0	35–39	<1
2	1	40–44	<1
4	1	45–49	<1
6	1	50–54	4
8	2	55–59	6
10	4	60–64	8
12	6	65–69	12
14	10	70–74	12
16	15		
18	23		
20	35		
22	51		
24	68		
26	85		

CVD = cerebrovascular disease; other abbreviations as in Table 1-1.

Source: Califf et al, Task Force 5, *J Am Coll Cardiol,* 1996. Reprinted with permission from the American College of Cardiology (*Journal of the American College of Cardiology,* 1996;27:1007-1012) (11).

RISK FACTOR CATEGORIES

The 27th Bethesda Conference of the American College of Cardiology was convened to devise guidelines for matching the intensity of cardiovascular risk factor management with cardiovascular risk. A scheme was developed to classify risk factors into four categories according to the evidence available to support the effectiveness of treatment for reducing cardiovascular morbidity and mortality:

I. Risk factors for which interventions have been proven to reduce the incidence of cardiovascular disease events.
II. Risk factors for which interventions are likely, on the basis of current pathophysiologic understanding and on epidemiologic and clinical trial evidence, to reduce the incidence of cardiovascular disease events.
III. Risk factors clearly associated with an increase in cardiovascular disease risk that, if modified, might lower the incidence of cardiovascular disease events.
IV. Risk factors associated with increased risk but that cannot be modified or whose modification would be unlikely to change the incidence of cardiovascular disease events.

Table 1-4 summarizes the risk factors in categories I through IV as well as the evidence for their association with cardiovascular disease, the clinical usefulness of measuring the risk factor, and the responsiveness of the risk factor to therapy.

TABLE 1-3

Risk of Coronary Artery Disease Event, Stroke, or Cerebrovascular Disease Death in Men with Existing Coronary Artery Disease

Age (yr)	Points	Total-C (mg/dL)	Points by HDL-C (mg/dL) 25	30	35	40	45	50	60	70	80	SBP (mm Hg)	Points
35	0	160	6	5	4	4	3	2	1	1	0	100	0
40	1	170	6	5	5	4	3	3	2	1	0	110	1
45	1	180	7	6	5	4	4	3	2	1	1	120	1
50	2	190	7	6	5	4	4	3	2	2	1	130	2
55	2	200	7	6	5	5	4	4	3	2	1	140	2
60	3	210	7	6	6	5	4	4	3	2	1	150	3
65	3	220	8	7	6	5	5	4	3	2	2	160	3
70	4	230	8	7	6	5	5	4	3	3	2	170	4
75	4	240	8	7	6	6	5	4	4	3	2	180	4
		250	8	7	6	6	5	5	4	3	2	190	4
		260	8	7	7	6	5	5	4	3	2	200	5
		270	9	8	7	6	6	5	4	3	3	210	5
Other	Pts	280	9	8	7	6	6	5	4	4	3	220	5
Diabetes	1	290	9	8	7	7	6	5	4	4	3	230	6
		300	9	8	7	7	6	6	5	4	3	240	6
												250	6

Total Points	2-yr Probability (%)	Average 2-yr Risk in Men with CVD Age (yr)	Probability (%)
0	2	35–39	<1
2	2	40–44	8
4	3	45–49	10
6	5	50–54	11
8	7	55–59	12
10	10	60–64	12
12	14	65–69	14
14	20	70–74	14
16	28		
18	37		
20	49		
22	63		
24	77		

CVD = cerebrovascular disease; other abbreviations as in Table 1-1.

Source: Califf et al, Task Force 5, *J Am Coll Cardiol,* 1996. Reprinted with permission from the American College of Cardiology (*Journal of the American College of Cardiology,* 1996;27:1007-1012) (11).

Category I Risk Factors

Interventions focusing on the following risk factors have been proven to lower cardiovascular disease risk:

- cigarette smoking;
- high-saturated-fat, high-cholesterol diet;
- elevated low-density lipoprotein cholesterol;
- hypertension;
- left ventricular hypertrophy; and
- thrombogenic factors.

Cigarette Smoking. The evidence for cigarette smoking increasing coronary risk is overwhelming. An average smoker dies 3 years earlier than a nonsmoker and 10 to 15 years earlier if other major CHD risk factors are present (12). Cigarette smoking enhances endothelial damage, increases heart rate and blood pressure, lowers high-density lipoprotein cholesterol (HDL-C), and promotes thrombus formation (3,13). In surveys of physicians, cigarette smoking is routinely ranked as the most important risk factor for CHD (6). Observational evidence also supports the reduction of cardiovascular risk of those who quit smoking after a myocardial infarction compared with those who continue to smoke (14). The benefits of smoking cessation occur immediately, presumably because some of the risk attributable to smoking is mediated through its acute effects (eg, vasoconstriction and enhanced thrombogenicity) (1). After 1 year of abstinence, the exsmoker's CHD risk is reduced by 50% relative to those who continue to smoke (1).

TABLE 1-4

Cardiovascular Risk Factors: The Evidence Supporting Their Association with Disease, the Usefulness of Measuring Them, and Their Responsiveness to Intervention

	Evidence for Association with CVD		Clinical Measurement	Response to	
Risk Factor	Epidemiologic	Clinical Trials	Usefulness	Nonpharmacologic Therapy	Pharmacologic Therapy
Category I (risk factors for which interventions have been proven to lower CVD risk)					
Cigarette smoking	+++	++	+++	+++	++
LDL cholesterol	+++	+++	+++	++	+++
High-fat/cholesterol diet	+++	++	++	++	–
Hypertension	+++	+++ (stroke)	+++	+	+++
Left ventricular hypertrophy	+++	+	++	–	++
Thrombogenic factors	+++ (fibrinogen)	+++ (aspirin, warfarin)	+ (fibrinogen)	+	+++ (aspirin, warfarin)
Category II (risk factors for which interventions are likely to lower CVD risk)					
Diabetes mellitus	+++	+	+++	++	+++
Physical inactivity	+++	++	++	++	—
HDL cholesterol	+++	+	+++	++	+
Triglycerides; small, dense LDL	++	++	+++	++	+++
Obesity	+++	—	+++	++	+
Postmenopausal status (women)	+++	—	+++	—	+++
Category III (risk factors associated with increased CVD risk that, if modified, might lower risk)					
Psychosocial factors	++	+	+++	+	—
Lipoprotein(a)	+	—	+	—	+
Homocysteine	++	—	+	++	++
Oxidative stress	+	—	—	+	++
No alcohol consumption	+++	—	++	++	—
Category IV (risk factors associated with increased CVD risk which cannot be modified)					
Age	+++	—	+++	—	—
Male gender	+++	—	+++	—	—
Low socioeconomic status	+++	—	+++	—	—
Family history of early-onset CVD	+++	—	+++	—	—

CVD = cardiovascular disease; HDL = high-density lipoprotein; + = weak, somewhat consistent evidence; ++ = moderately strong, rather consistent evidence; +++ = very strong, consistent evidence; – = evidence poor or nonexistent.

Source: Califf et al, Task Force 5, *J Am Coll Cardiol,* 1996. Reprinted with permission from the American College of Cardiology (*Journal of the American College of Cardiology,* 1996;27:1007-1012) (11).

Despite the clearly demonstrated benefits of smoking cessation, most cigarette smokers are not provided adequate assistance in quitting. In fact, in a primary care setting, only 45% to 55% of patients who smoke report being given advice to quit smoking by their physician (6). Smoking status should be documented for every patient and guidance regarding smoking cessation should be incorporated into treatment plans. Family members who smoke should also be strongly encouraged to quit. Where appropriate, nicotine replacement and formal smoking cessation programs should be used.

High-saturated-fat, High-cholesterol Diet. Changing dietary patterns are considered to be a major factor contributing to the epidemic of CHD in the United States during the 20th century as well as to its decline since the 1960s. Dietary modification, along with increased energy expenditure through physical activity, is a central component in managing many of the major CHD risk factors. In general, dietary recommendations from the National Cholesterol Education Program (NCEP), the American Heart Association (AHA), the United States Department of Agriculture, and other organizations call for: limiting intake of saturated fat and cholesterol; reducing energy intake when necessary to maintain a desirable body weight; moderating sodium and alcohol intakes; and increasing consumption of fruits, vegetables, and whole grains. (Specific dietary guidelines are described in Chapter 6.)

Much of the attention to diet as it relates to CHD has traditionally focused on the effect of dietary fats and cholesterol on blood lipids. However, in recent years it has become clear that habitual dietary intake influences many other steps in the

TABLE 1-5

Initial Classification Based on Total Cholesterol and High Density Liopoprotein Cholesterol (HDL-C) Concentrations

Total cholesterol (mg/dL)	
<200	Desirable
200–239	Borderline-high
≥240	High
HDL-C (mg/dL)	
<35	Low HDL-C

Source: National Cholesterol Education Program Second Adult Treatment Panel, 1993 (16).

pathogenetic sequence leading to a coronary event (15). Much current research is focusing on elucidating the role of diet in propensity toward thrombosis, susceptibility to cardiac arrhythmias, and lipoprotein oxidation and other processes. Dietary recommendations are likely to be expanded and refined as we better understand the various mechanisms by which diet acts to promote and retard CHD.

Elevated Low-density Lipoprotein Cholesterol. In the fasting state, and in the absence of rare genetic disorders, total serum cholesterol consists of three major fractions: LDL-C, very-low-density lipoprotein cholesterol (VLDL-C), and HDL-C. Extensive epidemiologic, laboratory, and clinical trial data have shown that LDL-C is associated with the development of atherosclerosis. (See Chapter 3 for a thorough overview of lipoprotein metabolism.)

For screening purposes, the NCEP's Second Adult Treatment Panel (ATP II) recommends measuring total cholesterol and HDL-C (16). The initial classification for primary prevention is summarized in Table 1-5. People with total cholesterol less than 200 mg/dL and HDL-C of at least 35 mg/dL should be provided with general educational materials regarding lifestyle and advised to have a repeat check within 5 years. If the total cholesterol concentration is 200 mg/dL to 239 mg/dL and HDL-C is 35 mg/dL or greater, lipoprotein analysis is recommended if two or more CHD risk factors are present. If not, the subject may be provided with educational materials and advised to have a repeat check within 1 to 2 years.

For those with CHD or other atherosclerotic disease, high total cholesterol, low HDL-C, or multiple CHD risk factors, fasting lipoprotein analysis should be completed for the purpose of risk stratification. ATP II recommended different treatment goals based on three strata of CHD risk (Table 1-6). The factors considered by ATP II for risk stratification are positive family history (father or brother with definite myocardial infarction or sudden death before age 55, mother or sister with definite myocardial infarction or sudden death before age 65), age (male 45 or older, female 55 or older with premature menopause without estrogen replacement therapy), cigarette smoking, presence of diabetes mellitus, low HDL-C (less than 35 mg/dL), and hypertension. Elevated HDL-C (60 mg/dL or more) is considered a negative (protective) risk factor. Therefore, if a patient has a high HDL-C concentration, one risk factor should be subtracted from the risk factor total.

Table 1-6 summarizes the NCEP ATP II treatment recommendations and goals. Lifestyle modification (dietary change and regular exercise) is considered the first line of treatment for people with elevated LDL-C. If treatment goals are not achieved after an adequate trial of lifestyle modification, pharmacologic therapy should be considered. For

TABLE 1-6

Treatment Recommendations and Goals According to Risk Status

	LDL-C initiation level (mg/dL)	LDL-C goal (mg/dL)
Dietary therapy		
Without CHD[a] and with fewer than 2 risk factors	≥160	<160
Without CHD[a] and with 2 or more risk factors	≥130	<130
With known CHD[a]	>100	≤100
Drug treatment		
Without CHD[a] and with fewer than 2 risk factors	≥190[b]	<160
Without CHD[a] and with 2 or more risk factors	≥160	<130
With known CHD[a]	>130[c]	≤100

Source: National Cholesterol Education Program Second Adult Treatment Panel, 1993 (16).

CHD = coronary heart disease; LDL-C = low-density lipoprotein cholesterol.

[a]Includes patients with other atherosclerotic cardiovascular disease such as peripheral arterial occlusion or carotid atheroma.

[b]In men less than 35 years of age and premenopausal women with LDL-C levels of 190 mg/dL to 219 mg/dL, drug therapy should be delayed except in high-risk patients such as those with diabetes.

[c]In CHD patients with LDL-C levels of 100 mg/dL to 129 mg/dL, the physician should exercise clinical judgment in deciding whether to initiate drug treatment.

TABLE 1-7

Classification of Blood Pressure in Adults Age 18 Years or Older on the Basis of Two or More Readings on Two or More Occasions

Category[a]	Blood Pressure (mm Hg)	
	Systolic	Diastolic
Normal	<130	<85
High normal	130–139	85–89
Hypertension		
Stage I (mild)	140–159	90–99
Stage II (moderate)	160–179	100–109
Stage III (severe)	180–209	110–119
Stage IV (very severe)	>209	>119

Source: Fifth Joint National Commission on the Detection, Evaluation, and Treatment of High Blood Pressure, 1993 (17).

[a]The more severe classification is used if systolic and diastolic pressure categories do not agree.

patients with CHD or other atherosclerotic disease, drug treatment should be considered if the LDL-C concentration is 130 mg/dL or above. Clinical judgment should be exercised regarding pharmacologic therapy for CHD patients with LDL-C concentrations from 101 mg/dL to 129 mg/dL.

For people without CHD or other atherosclerotic disease who have two or more risk factors, the LDL-C concentration at which medication is recommended is 160 mg/dL or greater. For people who have fewer than two CHD risk factors, drug treatment should generally not be instituted unless the LDL-C concentration is 190 mg/dL or greater. However, it is recommended that a medication regime be delayed in men less than 35 years of age and premenopausal women with LDL-C values between 190 mg/dL and 220 mg/dL unless the patient is considered to be at particularly high risk because of diabetes mellitus, a strong family history, or other reasons.

Hypertension. Hypertension is an independent risk factor for both CHD and stroke (17). There is a continuous relationship between arterial pressure (systolic and diastolic) and cardiovascular risk. High blood pressure leads to enhanced endothelial cell damage and target-organ involvement including LVH, retinopathy, and renal insufficiency. In addition, hypertension is often associated with other risk factors, such as obesity, blood lipid abnormalities, insulin resistance, and glucose intolerance (18). Reducing blood pressure has been unequivocally shown to lower the incidence of stroke, CHD, and heart failure (17).

The Fifth Joint National Commission on the Detection, Evaluation, and Treatment of High Blood Pressure (JNC V) issued comprehensive guidelines for diagnosing and managing hypertension. Table 1-7 shows the classification of blood pressure by JNC V. As is the case for hypercholesterolemia, nonpharmacologic interventions should be the initial therapy unless the severity of the blood pressure elevation or end-organ damage necessitates immediate use of medication. Regardless, nonpharmacologic approaches should always be used as adjunctive therapy.

The treatment goal for hypertensive patients is to maintain a resting blood pressure of less than 140/90 mm Hg. However, the National High Blood Pressure Education Working Group on Hypertension in Diabetes report promotes a more aggressive blood pressure treatment goal of less than 130/85 mm Hg for patients with diabetes mellitus (19). If blood pressure remains above the treatment goal after 3 months of nonpharmacologic intervention, drug therapy should be initiated as outlined in the JNC V guidelines (17). The specific nonpharmacologic interventions recommended by the JNC V include weight loss where indicated, moderation of sodium and alcohol consumption, smoking cessation, and regular physical activity. In addition, the recommendations emphasize the importance of a balanced diet including intake of foods rich in potassium, magnesium, calcium, and dietary fiber.

Left Ventricular Hypertrophy. In the 1960s data were published indicating that evidence of LVH on an electrocardiogram was associated with a poor prognosis (20,21). The emergence of echocardiography as a relatively inexpensive diagnostic tool has allowed the use of this technique in epidemiologic studies. Results from several investigations showed that LVH prevalence is much greater than suggested by electrocardiography (21). The prevalence of LVH on echocardiograms was estimated to be as high as 10% to 20% for the general population and considerably higher for subgroups with predisposing factors such as hypertension, obesity, and advanced age. Echocardiographic evidence of LVH is associated with markedly increased risk for a variety of negative cardiovascular outcomes, including myocardial infarction, stroke, and congestive heart failure (21,22,23). The predictive power of LVH is apparent after adjustment for other risk markers, including the number and severity of atherosclerotic coronary vessels (22,23,24). This relationship is also robust, having been demonstrated in middle-aged and elderly men and women as well as in different racial and ethnic groups (21,22,23).

LVH develops in response to chronic pressure, volume overload, or a combination of both. Although elevated blood pressure is accepted as one of the primary determinants of

LVH, other factors contributing to its development include age, obesity, and probably dietary and other lifestyle factors. Unlike the other Category I risk factors, no large-scale trials have been conducted to demonstrate that treatment-induced regression of LVH reduces CHD risk. However, effective antihypertensive therapy will reduce left ventricular mass toward normal (1). Randomized clinical trials are currently underway to determine whether treatment of LVH (with or without resting hypertension) will improve outcomes. In the meantime, because of the marked increase in cardiovascular risk associated with LVH, its presence should serve as a signal to the health care team to aggressively manage the overall CHD risk factor profile, with particular emphasis on adequate control of blood pressure.

Thrombogenic Factors. The final event precipitating a myocardial infarction is usually the development of an intracoronary thrombosis (3,10). Alterations in several compounds related to coagulation and fibrinolysis were shown to be associated with an elevated risk for CHD (3,12). Notably, high circulating fibrinogen concentrations appear to increase CHD risk in a graded fashion (3,12). Plasminogen activator inhibitor-1, platelet aggregability, and factor VII, among others, were also linked to increased risk (3,12).

Antiplatelet therapy significantly reduces the incidence of cardiovascular events in men and women with a history of myocardial infarction (secondary prevention) and in men without such a history (primary prevention) (12,25). For example, the Physicians' Health Study showed that 325 mg of aspirin every other day reduced the incidence of myocardial infarction by 44% in middle-aged male physicians living in the United States (25). Although numerous trials have clearly demonstrated the benefits of antiplatelet therapy, data are not yet available that demonstrate that this risk reduction is associated with changes in specific aspects of platelet function. Daily intake of 80 mg to 325 mg of aspirin is recommended for patients who have experienced a cardiovascular event (6). Physicians may also recommend aspirin for some patients without a history of cardiovascular disease if the action is justified by the risk factor profile.

Category II Risk Factors

Interventions focusing on the following risk factors are likely to lower cardiovascular disease risk:

- diabetes mellitus,
- physical inactivity,
- low high-density lipoprotein cholesterol,
- obesity, and
- postmenopausal status without hormone replacement.

Diabetes Mellitus. In the United States 16 million people suffer from diabetes (26,27). Approximately 95% of all cases are Type 2, or noninsulin-dependent diabetes mellitus, whereas the remainder are Type 1, or insulin-dependent diabetes mellitus (26). (Note, however, that many people with Type 2 diabetes ultimately need insulin injections to control their blood glucose concentrations.) Nearly half of all people in the United States with Type 2 diabetes (approximately 7.5 million) are unaware that they have the condition (26,27). In fact, approximately 10% of all men and women older than age 50 have undiagnosed Type 2 diabetes (26,27).

Patients with diabetes mellitus have at least a threefold greater risk of CHD than does the general population (26,28), and the relative increase in CHD risk conferred by diabetes mellitus is greater for women than men. Thus, one of the most striking features of diabetes is that it eliminates the protection against CHD afforded by female gender (26). Although diabetes (Type 1 and Type 2) clearly increases CHD risk, the degree to which this is attributable to chronically elevated blood glucose concentrations is uncertain (29,30). People with diabetes, particularly those with Type 2 diabetes, are characterized by a cluster of metabolic alterations in addition to high blood glucose. This cluster includes insulin resistance; blood lipid abnormalities (high triglycerides; depressed HDL-C; and small, dense LDL particles); hypertension; elevated uric acid concentration; and central obesity (18,30,31). Furthermore, these metabolic disturbances are typically present for many years before the onset of frank hyperglycemia (31).

No large-scale clinical trial results are available to indicate that strict control of blood glucose concentration will reduce the macrovascular (primarily atherosclerotic) complications of diabetes (29,32). However, the Diabetes Control and Complications Trial recently showed that for patients with Type 1 diabetes mellitus, maintenance of near-normal levels of plasma glucose reduced the incidence of microvascular complications (retinopathy, neuropathy, and nephropathy) by 60% on average (26,33). American Diabetes Association guidelines for managing CHD risk factors in patients with diabetes emphasize adequate control of plasma glucose concentrations along with management of other cardiovascular risk factors (34). Data from recently published clinical studies suggest that people with diabetes benefit at least as much and perhaps more from risk-factor modification (antiplatelet therapy, control of hyperlipidemia, smoking cessation, and adequate management of hypertension) than do people without diabetes (34).

Because CHD has risk factors in common with Type 2 diabetes, people with one or more major CHD risk factors should generally have fasting plasma glucose measured as part of their CHD risk-factor evaluation (26,30). Values of 140 mg/dL or higher on two occasions are diagnostic for diabetes mellitus. Values of 115 mg/dL to 139 mg/dL are considered elevated and may need to be followed by a diagnostic oral glucose tolerance test to rule out Type 2 diabetes (26).

Physical Inactivity. A sedentary lifestyle and low cardiorespiratory fitness are each associated with a twofold or more increase in CHD risk (35). This relationship is based on more than 50 studies documenting that physical inactivity, low cardiorespiratory fitness, or both are associated with an increased incidence of negative cardiovascular events. Physical activity beneficially modifies many of the major CHD risk factors. Regular aerobic exercise reduces blood pressure, lowers triglyceride concentration, increases HDL-C, aids in weight control, and improves insulin sensitivity (36,37). Other potential benefits of exercise include increases in myocardial electrical stability and decreases in platelet aggregation and fibrinogen levels (36,37).

The frequency, intensity, and duration of exercise necessary to obtain cardiovascular benefit has not been clearly defined (35). Aerobic exercise such as walking, cycling, and swimming for 30 minutes to 60 minutes three to five times per week is generally considered optimal (36). More than five exercise sessions per week increase the risk of musculoskeletal injury, and there is no objective evidence of increased cardiovascular benefit (36). Aerobic exercise fewer than three times per week may offer benefit, but trials demonstrating weight loss and improved HDL-C generally used at least three weekly sessions. In addition, patients should be encouraged to supplement regular aerobic exercise with other types of background activity such as yard work, increased use of stairs rather than elevators, and parking the car at the far end of the parking lot (36). Guidelines from the Centers for Disease Control and Prevention and the American College of Sports Medicine for the general population recommend that every US adult accumulate 30 minutes or more of moderate-intensity physical activity on most—preferably all—days of the week (38).

Low High-density Lipoprotein Cholesterol. There is a strong inverse relationship between HDL-C concentrations and coronary events that is equal to the direct relationship between LDL-C concentrations and coronary events. For every 1 mg/dL decrease in HDL-C, the relative risk of a cardiovascular event increases by 2% to 3% (39). The difference in CHD rates between age-matched men and women may be largely explained by differences in HDL-C concentrations.

HDL-C has not achieved Category I risk status because of the lack of interventional data demonstrating that increasing HDL-C independently lowers CHD risk. Therapies that increase HDL-C also generally lower LDL-C, triglycerides, or both. Therefore, differentiating the effects of changes in the various lipids on CHD risk reduction has been difficult. In addition, the metabolisms of HDL-C and triglycerides are closely linked so that therapies that lower triglycerides typically increase HDL-C as well. Consensus regarding the benefits of therapies that raise HDL-C will require an interventional trial that differentiates the effects of HDL-C changes. However, clear and consistent data indicate that depressed HDL-C and an elevated ratio of total cholesterol to HDL-C (or LDL-C to HDL-C) are strong, independent risk factors for CHD. The NCEP's ATP II designated HDL-C concentration less than 35 mg/dL as "low" for the purpose of risk stratification; a value of 60 mg/dL or more is considered a negative (protective) risk factor.

HDL-C concentrations are significantly influenced by lifestyle factors. Cigarette smoking, obesity, and postmenopausal status are associated with lower HDL-C concentrations, whereas moderate alcohol consumption and aerobic exercise raise HDL-C concentrations (12). HDL-C concentrations are also strongly influenced by family history. Familial hypoalphalipoproteinemia is a dominant genetic disorder characterized by low HDL-C (less than 35 m/dL) and apolipoprotein A-I (the primary apolipoprotein associated with HDL particles). This genetic disorder is relatively common and is associated with a marked increase in CHD risk. For patients with low HDL-C, the general recommendations include weight loss, aerobic exercise, and control of concomitant triglyceride and LDL-C elevations. For postmenopausal women consideration should also be given to estrogen replacement therapy.

Obesity. Increased adiposity is associated with several other CHD risk factors, such as hypertension, sedentary lifestyle, glucose intolerance, low HDL-C concentration, and high triglyceride concentration (40). Obesity is a major health concern for the entire US population because of its association with increased morbidity and mortality from heart disease as well as diabetes and cancer. Moreover, the incidence of obesity in the United States has increased in recent years despite improvements in dietary fat intake and reductions in average blood cholesterol level (41,42). The prevalence of obesity now exceeds 30% for men and women in all of the major demographic strata (41).

Overall fat mass and regional distribution of body fat affect the degree to which obesity is associated with abnormalities in the metabolic cardiovascular risk profile. For a given fat mass, people with a primarily upper-body (android, or apple-shaped) fat distribution have a less favorable metabolic cardiovascular risk profile than do those with a more gluteofemoral (gynoid, or pear-shaped) fat storage pattern (40). In particular, excess deep abdominal fat (in contrast with subcutaneous abdominal fat) is associated with marked disturbances in lipoprotein and carbohydrate metabolism.

Unfortunately, anthropometric measures practical for use in a clinical setting do not clearly differentiate visceral from subcutaneous abdominal adiposity. Nevertheless, waist circumference is useful as a clinical indicator, representing a composite measure of total abdominal (visceral plus subcutaneous) adiposity (43). Insulin resistance and lipoprotein abnormalities become increasingly prevalent with elevated waist circumference (measured at the narrowest point), particularly when values exceed approximately 100 cm for men and women (43).

Although there is no direct evidence that fat loss decreases coronary events, reducing excess body weight is associated with improvements in blood pressure, blood lipid concentrations, insulin sensitivity, and other CHD risk markers (44). On the basis of this evidence, attempts to reduce excess body weight through moderate energy restriction and increased physical activity appear justified. However, it should be emphasized that long-term maintenance of weight loss has proven to be difficult and remains a source of frustration for both patients and clinicians. Moderate reduction in body weight (5 lb to 20 lb) is associated with substantial improvements in CHD risk factors even if a theoretically ideal body weight is not achieved (44). In men, a 10% weight loss reportedly had the effect of decreasing systolic blood pressure by 5.0 mm Hg, blood glucose by 2 mg/dL, and cholesterol by 11 mg/dL. In women the results were roughly half those seen in men. Therefore, reasonable individual weight-loss goals should be discussed with each patient, with emphasis placed on long-term maintenance.

Postmenopausal Status Without Hormone Replacement. Although CHD is the leading cause of death for both men and women, the increase in CHD with age in women lags about 10 years behind that in men and coincides with initiation of natural menopause. Menopause is associated with potentially proatherogenic changes in the blood lipid profile. LDL-C increases by approximately 20% to 30% whereas HDL-C declines by approximately 10% (45,46). These adverse lipoprotein changes are largely ameliorated by estrogen replacement therapy (47).

Observational studies suggest that long-term estrogen replacement confers an impressive 50% reduction in CHD incidence relative to women who have never used estrogen (48,49,50). The reduction in risk is even greater in women with preexisting CHD (1). However, because women who use estrogen may differ from those who do not in a number of respects (eg, access to health care, health practices, and socioeconomic status), the possibility of bias in these estimates cannot be ruled out.

The effects of estrogen on the lipid profile appear to account for only half of the reduction in CHD found in estrogen users (48). Therefore, other effects of estrogen are likely contributing to its cardioprotective influence. Possibilities include improvements in endothelial function, antioxidant properties of estrogens, favorable changes in mechanisms related to thrombogenesis, and enhanced sensitivity to insulin (48,49). Because unopposed estrogen increases the risk for endometrial cancer, a progestin is usually provided along with estrogen replacement for a woman with an intact uterus (49). Unfortunately, progestins tend to blunt or reverse some of the favorable effects of estrogens on CHD risk factors, particularly HDL-C (51). Progestins were not routinely prescribed until relatively recently and most of the available evidence for a protective influence of estrogen replacement on cardiovascular risk has been for unopposed estrogen preparations.

Because of the limitations inherent in observational study designs and uncertainties regarding the effects of progestins on the cardioprotective influence of estrogens, definitive conclusions regarding the benefits of estrogen-progestin replacement will have to await the results of ongoing prospective clinical trials, including the Women's Health Initiative (primary prevention) and the Heart and Estrogen Progesterone Replacement Study (secondary prevention).

Category III Risk Factors

Interventions focusing on the following risk factors may lower cardiovascular disease risk:

- psychosocial factors,
- elevated triglycerides,
- elevated lipoprotein(a),
- elevated homocysteine,
- oxidation and antioxidants, and
- alcoholic beverage consumption.

Psychosocial Factors. The influence of psychosocial factors—such as psychological stress and coronary-disease-prone behavior—on CHD risk have not been easy to quantify because of the difficulty in defining and measuring the relevant exposure variable. Considerable evidence links certain psychosocial factors with increased risk. The presence of major clinical depression after myocardial infarction is a powerful predictor of total mortality (1,12). Hostility and social isolation have also been associated with CHD incidence (12). A common thread that connects most psychosocial risk factors is the lack of perceived control combined with lack of adequate emotional support, either internal or external.

The mechanisms by which psychosocial variables may influence CHD risk are poorly understood and probably include direct effects via the neuroendocrine system as well as indirect actions, for example, by influencing compliance with therapeutic regimens. Intervention trials attempting to lower CHD incidence through interventions designed to reduce perceived stress or change coronary-disease-prone behavior have produced inconclusive results, although trends toward reduced mortality and improved adherence to medical therapies were noted (1,12).

Elevated Triglycerides. Circulating triglyceride concentration remains a widely misunderstood and controversial coronary risk factor. Increased triglyceride levels are associated with elevated CHD risk when considered in isolation, but triglyceride levels lose their predictive power when an adjustment is made for other risk factors, especially HDL-C (52). Elevated triglyceride levels are often associated with obesity, diabetes, hypertension, low HDL-C, and small, dense LDL particles (1). Thus, triglyceride concentration may not be directly responsible for increased risk but may be a marker for the presence of other metabolic disturbances.

As was the case for HDL-C, direct interventional data are lacking because therapies that lower triglycerides also increase HDL-C, decrease LDL-C, or do both. In addition, estrogen and alcohol consumption both raise triglycerides (and, paradoxically, HDL-C) but may reduce CHD risk. Patients with triglyceride concentrations greater than 1,000 mg/dL require therapy to reduce the risk of pancreatitis (16). For those with moderately high (250 mg/dL to 500 mg/dL) or high (500 mg/dL to 1,000 mg/dL) triglycerides, the recommended treatment goal is to lower the concentration to less than 200 mg/dL via nonpharmacologic measures if possible (16). Weight loss, increased physical activity, and moderation of alcohol consumption are often effective for reducing the triglyceride level (16,52). Generally, the decision to treat a borderline-high triglyceride concentration pharmacologically is driven by the presence of other risk factors, particularly elevated LDL-C and low HDL-C (52).

Elevated Lipoprotein(a). Lp(a) is an LDL-C particle with apolipoprotein(a) attached. Apolipoprotein(a) is a large protein structurally similar to plasminogen, an important contributor to clot lysis. Therefore, Lp(a), by interfering with the action of plasminogen, may impair fibrinolysis, perhaps favoring the formation of occlusive thrombi. An Lp(a) concentration greater than 30 mg/dL doubles the risk of CHD, although this has not been a universal finding (1). High Lp(a) concentrations may also increase the risk of bypass graft occlusion and reclosure of a coronary artery after angioplasty. Lp(a) appears to be genetically determined and mostly resistant to standard lipid-lowering therapies, possibly excepting niacin and estrogen-replacement therapies (1). Until effective therapeutic approaches are identified, elevated Lp(a) will remain a risk factor of uncertain importance. Some evidence suggests that Lp(a) loses its predictive power if LDL-C is maintained at a low level (53,54). Therefore, management of LDL-C in accordance with the NCEP ATP II guidelines is critical for patients with concomitant elevations in Lp(a).

Elevated Homocysteine. Heterozygosity for the enzyme disorder cystathionine synthase deficiency or inadequate intake of vitamins B-6, B-12, or folate causes elevated blood homocysteine concentrations in adults (55). Elevated homocysteine is associated with an increased risk for CHD and peripheral vascular disease and has a prevalence of approximately 10% in the general population (55). Normal plasma homocysteine concentration is below 10 μmol/L (55). Each 5 μmol/L increase above 10 μmol/L is associated with an increase in CHD risk of approximately 60% (55).

Screening for elevated homocysteine levels is not routine because of the expense and lack of data demonstrating its usefulness. Elevated homocysteine concentrations are effectively reduced by supplementation with B vitamins, especially folate but also vitamins B-6 and B-12 (55). Therefore, for patients with a history of premature heart disease or a strong family history of heart disease, screening or use of vitamin supplementation without screening may be a reasonable consideration. Definitive recommendations will have to await the completion of ongoing clinical trials. All patients should be encouraged to consume a balanced diet and maintain an adequate intake of whole grains, cereals, fruits, vegetables, and lean animal products that provide folate, B-6, and B-12.

Oxidation and Antioxidants. LDL-C oxidation is an important step in the atherosclerotic process. Antioxidants, especially vitamin E, increase LDL-C resistance to oxidation, and observational studies have shown that vitamin E protects against CHD. For example, data from the US Health Professionals Study and the US Nurses' Health Study suggest that the risk of a coronary event is approximately 35% to 40% lower in people who consume daily supplements containing at least 100 IU of supplemental vitamin E (56,57). In both of these studies, the greatest risk reduction was seen among supplement users consuming 100 IU to 249 IU of vitamin E per day for 2 or more years. An intake of 40 IU of vitamin E per day was the lowest amount that inhibited LDL oxidation; a dose-dependent effect was seen with up to 800 IU per day. Intakes of 200 IU to 400 IU of vitamin E per day decreased adhesion of platelets to vessel walls (58). Prevention of LDL oxidation and stabilization of platelet membranes are possible mechanisms by which vitamin E reduces CVD risk (59).

Vitamin E may play a pivotal role in the prevention of cardiovascular disease. The risk associated with daily vitamin E supplements of 200 IU to 600 IU appears to be small, but one intervention study reported an increased risk of hemorrhagic stroke (60). Although many questions remain unanswered and will require further investigation, the benefits from supplementation could be large.

Alcoholic Beverage Consumption. Although lack of alcohol consumption has been consistently linked with increased CHD risk, this is clearly a risk factor with a narrow risk-benefit ratio. Individuals who consume moderate amounts of alcohol (one to three drinks per day) have a 40% to 50% lower rate of CHD than do those who abstain (12). Greater alcohol intake is associated with increases in mortality from accidental death and liver cirrhosis. In addition, alcoholism is a major public health problem in the United States.

The protective influence of alcohol consumption may be secondary to increased HDL-C as well as reduced platelet and vascular reactivity (12). However, alcohol may also raise serum triglyceride concentrations and blood pressure in some patients. Thus, moderation of alcohol intake should be recommended for patients who consume more than two alcoholic drinks per day. Lower intakes may be prudent for some patients who have elevated triglyceride concentrations or blood pressure. There is a general consensus that because of the associated risks, people who abstain should not be advised to begin consuming alcohol to prevent CHD.

Category IV Risk Factors

Category IV includes major risk factors that, although useful for risk stratification, are not generally amenable to modification and thus are not targets for therapy. These include

- age,
- male sex,
- low socioeconomic status, and
- family history of early onset cardiovascular disease.

The association between these factors and CHD risk probably is partially mediated through other potentially modifiable risk markers.

OTHER RISK FACTORS

The list of CHD risk markers just given is far from all inclusive. Many other factors, numbering in the hundreds, have been found to predict coronary events, but the available data are not sufficient to warrant classification.

Summary

In general, the current US health care system offers excellent care for acute disorders, but the prevention of long-term chronic disease still requires considerable improvement. Several decades of research have provided much information about the importance of risk factors, the pathogenesis of atherosclerosis, and the benefits of risk-factor modification. This information has enabled health professionals to provide advice and treatments to significantly reduce cardiovascular morbidity and mortality. The challenge and opportunity is to effectively apply such information to benefit patient outcomes.

By using routinely collected clinical data, health care teams can ascertain an individual's cardiovascular risk status with reasonable accuracy, although considerable room exists for clinical judgment. Risk stratification is critical so that those at the highest risk receive the most intensive treatment efforts and the greatest expenditure of limited resources. A strategy of targeting treatment efforts toward CHD risk factors that are modifiable and for which benefits have been demonstrated (cigarette smoking, LDL-C, hypertension, left ventricular hypertrophy, and thrombogenic factors) will allow members of the health care team to offer high-quality, cost-effective preventive care. Nutrition professionals should play a prominent role in the risk management effort because diet influences many of the major risk factors and dietary modification represents an essential component of the overall treatment plan.

References

1. Forrester JS, Merz-Bairey CN, Bush TL, Cohn JN, Hunninghake DB, Parthasarathy S, Superko HR. 27th Bethesda Conference: matching the intensity of risk factor management with the hazard for coronary disease events. Task Force 4. Efficacy of risk factor management. *J Am Coll Cardiol.* 1996;27:991-1006.
2. Stamler J. Established major coronary risk factors. In: Elliott P, Marnot M, eds. *Coronary Heart Disease Epidemiology.* New York, NY: Oxford University Press; 1992:35-66.
3. Fuster V, Gotto AM, Libby P, Loscalzo J, McGill HC. 27th Bethesda Conference: matching the intensity of risk factor management with the hazard for coronary disease events. Task Force 1. Pathogenesis of coronary disease: the biologic role of risk factors. *J Am Coll Cardiol.* 1996;27:964-976.
4. Allen JK, Blumenthal RS. Coronary risk factors in women six months after coronary artery bypass grafting. *Am J Cardiol.* 1995;75:1092-1095.
5. DeBusk RF, Miller NH, Superko HR, Dennis CA, Thomas RJ, Lew HT, Berger WE 3rd, Heller RS, Romf J, Gee D. A case-management system for coronary risk factor modification after acute myocardial infarction. *Ann Intern Med.* 1994;120:721-729.
6. Pearson TA, McBride PE, Miller NH, Smith SC. Organization of preventive cardiology service. *J Am Coll Cardiol.* 1996;27:1039-1047.
7. Heald FP. Atherosclerosis during adolescence. *Med Clin North Am.* 1990;74(5):1321-1332.
8. Ross R. The pathogenesis of atherosclerosis—an update. *N Engl J Med.* 1986;314:488-500.
9. Steinberg D, Parthasarathy S, Carew TE, Khoo JC, Witztum JL. Beyond cholesterol: modifications of low density lipoprotein that increase its atherogenicity. *N Engl J Med.* 1989;320:915-923.
10. Schroeder AP, Falk E. Vulnerable and dangerous coronary plaques. *Atherosclerosis.* 1995;118 (suppl):S141-S149.
11. Califf RM, Armstrong PW, Carver JR, D'Agostino RB, Strauss WE. Task Force 5. Stratification of patients into high, medium, and low risk subgroups for purposes of risk factor management. *J Am Coll Cardiol.* 1996;27:1007-1019.
12. Pasternak RS, Grundy SM, Levy D, Thompson PD. Task Force 2 Spectrum of risk factors for coronary heart disease. *J Am Coll Cardiol.* 1996;27:978-990.
13. Stokes J, Rigotti NA. The health consequences of cigarette smoking and the internist's role in smoking cessation. *Adv Intern Med.* 1988;33:431-460.
14. Goldman L, Garber AM, Grover SA, Hlatky MA. Task Force 6. Cost effectiveness of assessment and management of risk factors. *J Am Coll Cardiol.* 1996;27:1020-1030.
15. Ulbright TLV, Southgate DAT. Coronary heart disease: seven dietary factors. *Lancet.* 1991;338:985-992.
16. National Cholesterol Education Program. *Second Report of the Expert Panel on Detection, Evaluation, and Treatment of High Blood Cholesterol in Adults (Adult Treatment Panel II).* Bethesda, Md: National Institutes of Health; 1993. NIH publication 93-3095.
17. JNC V. The fifth report of the Joint National Committee on Detection, Evaluation, and Treatment of High Blood Pressure. *Arch Intern Med.* 1993;153:154-183.
18. Reaven GM, Lithell H, Landsburg L. Hypertension and associated metabolic abnormalities: the role of insulin resistance and the sympathoadrenal system. *N Engl J Med.* 1996;334:374-381.
19. National High Blood Pressure Education Program. *Working Group Report on Primary Prevention of Hypertension.* Bethesda, MD: National Institutes of Health; 1993. NIH publication 93-2669.
20. Kannel WB. Epidemiologic insights into atherosclerotic cardiovascular disease—from the Framingham Study. In: Pollock ML, Schmidt DH, eds. *Heart Disease and Rehabilitation.* 2nd ed. Champaign, Ill: Human Kinetics; 1995.
21. Post WS, Levy S. New developments in the epidemiology of left ventricular hypertrophy: the Framingham Heart Study. *Curr Opin Cardiol.* 1994;9:534-541.
22. Cooper RS, Simmons BE, Castaner A, Santhanam V, Ghali J, Mar M. Left ventricular hypertrophy is associated with worse survival independent of ventricular function and number of coronary arteries severely narrowed. *Am J Cardiol.* 1990;65:441-445.
23. Levy D, Garrison RJ, Savage DD, Kannel WB, Castelli WP. Prognostic implications of echocardiographically determined left ventricular mass in the Framingham Heart Study. *N Engl J Med.* 1990;322:1561-1566.
24. Liao Y, Cooper RS, McGee DL, Mensah GA, Ghali JK. The relative effects of left ventricular hypertrophy, coronary artery disease, and ventricular dysfunction on survival among black adults. *JAMA.* 1995;273:1592-1597.
25. Manson JE, Tosteson H, Ridker PM, Satterfield S, Herbert P, O'Connor GT, Buring JE, Hennekens CH. The primary prevention of myocardial infarction. *N Engl J Med.* 1992;326(21):1406-1416.
26. American Diabetes Association. *Diabetes 1996 Vital Statistics.* Chicago, Ill: American Diabetes Association, Inc; 1996.
27. Harris MI. NIDDM: epidemiology and scope of the problem. *Diabetes Spectrum.* 1996;9:402-407.
28. Stamler J, Vaccaro O, Neaton JD, Wentworth D, for the Multiple

Risk Factor Intervention Trial Research Group. Diabetes, other risk factors, and 12-year cardiovascular mortality for men screened in the Multiple Risk Factor Intervention Trial. *Diabetes Care*. 1993;16:434-444.

29. Abraira C, Maki K. Does insulin treatment increase cardiovascular risk in NIDDM? *Clin Diabetes*. 1995;March/April:29-31.
30. Maki KC, Abraira C, Cooper RS. Arguments in favor of screening for diabetes during cardiac rehabilitation. *J Cardiopulmonary Rehabil*. 1995;15:97-102.
31. Haffner M, Stern MP, Hazuda HP, Mitchell BD, Patterson JK. Cardiovascular risk factors in confirmed prediabetic individuals: does the clock for coronary heart disease start clicking before the onset of clinical diabetes? *JAMA*. 1990;263:2893-2898.
32. Abraira C, Colwell JA, Nuttall FQ, Sawin CT, Nagel NJ, Comstock JP, Emanuele NV, Levin SR, Henderson W, Lee HS. Veterans Affairs Cooperative Study on glycemic control and complications in Type 2 diabetes (VA CSDM). Results of the feasibility trial. Veterans Affairs Cooperative Study in Type 2 Diabetes. *Diabetes Care*. 1995;18:1113-1123.
33. American Diabetes Association. *Medical Management of Non-Insulin-Dependent (Type II) Diabetes.* Chicago, Ill: American Diabetes Association; 1994.
34. American Diabetes Association. Clinical practice recommendations 1996. *Diabetes Care*. 1996;19(suppl 1):S1-S118.
35. Blair SN. Physical activity, fitness, and coronary heart disease. In: Bouchard C, Shephard RJ, Stephens T, eds. *Physical Activity, Fitness, and Health: International Proceedings and Consensus Statement.* Champaign, Ill: Human Kinetics; 1994:579-580.
36. American College of Sports Medicine. *ACSM Guidelines for Exercising Testing and Prescription.* 5th ed. Baltimore, Md: Williams and Wilkins; 1995.
37. Squires RW. Mechanisms by which exercise training may improve the clinical status of cardiac patients. In: Pollock ML, Schmidt DH, eds. *Heart Disease and Rehabilitation.* 3rd ed. Champaign, Ill: Human Kinetics; 1995:147-160.
38. Pate RR, Pratt M, Blair SN, Haskell WL, Macera CA, Bouchard C, Buchner D, Ettinger W, Heath GW, King AC. Physical activity and public health. A recommendation from the Center for Disease Control and Prevention and the American College of Sports Medicine. *JAMA*. 1995;273:402-407.
39. Gordon DJ, Probstfield JL, Garrison RJ, Neaton JD, Castelli WP, Knoke JD, Jacobs DR Jr, Bangdiwala S, Tyroler HA. High-density lipoprotein cholesterol and cardiovascular disease: four prospective American studies. *Circulation.* 1989;79:8-15.
40. Despres JP, Moorjani S, Lupien PJ, Tremblay A, Nadeau A, Bouchard C. Regional distribution of body fat, plasma lipoproteins, and cardiovascular disease. *Arteriosclerosis.* 1990;10:497-511.
41. Kuczmarski RJ, Flegal KM, Campbell SM, Johnson CL. Increasing prevalence of overweight among US adults. *JAMA*. 1994;272:205-211.
42. Johnson CL, Rifkind BM, Sempos CT, Carroll MD, Bachorik PS, Briefel RR, Gordon DJ, Burt VL, Brown CD, Lippel K. Declining serum total cholesterol level among US adults: the National Health and Nutrition Examination Surveys. *JAMA*. 1993;269:3002-3008.
43. Pouliot MC, Despres JP, Lemieux S, Moorjuni S, Bouchard C, Tremblay A, Nadeau A, Lupien PJ. Waist circumference and abdominal sagittal diameter: best simple anthropometric indexes of abdominal visceral adipose tissue accumulation and related cardiovascular risk in men and women. *Am J Cardiol*. 1994;73:460-468.
44. Franz M, Horton ES, Bantle JP, Beebe CA, Brunzell JD, Coulston AM, Henry RR, Hoogwenf BJ, Stacpoole PW. Nutrition principles for the management of diabetes and related complications. *Diabetes Care*. 1994;17:490-518.
45. Seed M, Crook D. Post-menopausal hormone replacement therapy, coronary heart disease, and plasma lipoproteins. *Lipidology*. 1994;5:48-58.
46. Stevenson JC, Crook D, Godsland IF. Influence of age and menopause on serum lipids and lipoprotein in healthy women. *Atherosclerosis*. 1993;98:83-90.
47. Walsh BW, Schiff I, Rosner B, Greenberg L, Ravnikar V, Sacks FM. Effects of postmenopausal estrogen replacement on the concentrations and metabolism of plasma lipoproteins. *N Engl J Med*. 1991;325:1196-1204.
48. Barrett-Connor E, Bush T. Estrogen and coronary heart disease in women. *JAMA*. 1991;265:1861-1867.
49. Bilezikan JP. Major issues regarding estrogen replacement therapy in postmenopausal women. *J Women's Health*. 1994;3:273-282.
50. Grady D, Rubin SM, Petitti DB, Fox CS, Black D, Ettinger B, Ernster VL, Cummings SR. Hormone therapy to prevent disease and prolong life in postmenopausal women. *Ann Intern Med*. 1992;117:1016-1037.
51. The Writing Group for the PEPI Trial. Effects of estrogen or estrogen/progestin regimens on heart disease risk factors in postmenopausal women. *JAMA*. 1995;273:199-208.
52. Triglyceride, high-density lipoprotein, and coronary heart disease. *NIH Consens Statement*. 1992;Feb. 26-28;10(2).
53. Baldassarre D, Tremoli E, Franceschini G, Michelagnoli S, Sirtori CR. Plasma lipoprotein(a) is an independent factor associated with carotid wall thickening in severely but not moderately hypercholesterolemic patients. *Stroke*. 1996;27:1044-1049.
54. Maher VM, Brown BG. Lipoprotein(a) and coronary heart disease. *Curr Opin Lipidol*. 1995;6:229-235.
55. Boushey CJ, Beresford SA, Omenn GS, Motulsky AG. A quantitative assessment of plasma homocysteine as a risk factor for vascular disease: probable benefits of increasing folic acid intakes. *JAMA*. 1995;274:1049-1057.
56. Rimm EB, Stampfer MJ, Ascherio A, Giovannicci E, Colditz GA, Willett WC. Vitamin E consumption and the risk of coronary heart disease in men. *N Engl J Med*. 1993;328:1450-1456.
57. Stampfer MJ, Hennekens CH, Manson JE, Colditz GA, Rosner B, Willett WC. Vitamin E consumption and the risk of coronary disease in women. *N Engl J Med*. 1993;328:1444-1449.
58. Steiner M. Vitamin E: more than an antioxidant. *Clin Cardiol*. 1993;16(suppl):16-18.
59. Weber P, Bendich A, Machlin LJ. Vitamin E and human health—rationale for determining recommended intake levels. *Int J Nutr.* (in press).
60. The Alpha-Tocopherol, Beta-Carotene Cancer Prevention Study Group. The effect of vitamin E and beta carotene on the incidence of lung cancer and other cancers in male smokers. *N Engl J Med*. 1994;330:1029-1035.

CHAPTER 2

Dyslipidemia and Hypertension: An Overview of Treatment

Arline McDonald, PhD; Kevin C. Maki, MS; and Michael H. Davidson, MD, FACC

The previous chapter summarizes treatment guidelines established by the National Cholesterol Education Program's (NCEP) Second Expert Panel on the Detection, Evaluation, and Treatment of High Blood Cholesterol in Adults (ATP II) (1). This chapter outlines strategies for achieving the NCEP treatment goals.

Dyslipidemias

The clinical management of dyslipidemia should be based on the underlying lipoprotein abnormality and the risk factor status of the patient. The various dyslipidemias generally fall into one of five categories:

- elevated low-density lipoprotein cholesterol (LDL-C),
- elevated very-low-density lipoprotein cholesterol (VLDL-C) and triglycerides,
- depressed high-density lipoprotein cholesterol (HDL-C),
- combined dyslipidemias (any combination of at least two of the preceding), and
- chylomicronemia.

The lipid pattern expressed will depend on an underlying genetic predisposition as well as a variety of environmental factors, particularly diet, excess body weight, and physical activity patterns. Optimal management will vary according to the specific abnormality present.

Effective therapy depends on long-term adherence to the treatment plan, which is one of the most challenging aspects of any intervention for control of blood lipids. For example, fewer than 50% of patients remain on lipid-lowering medication for more than 1 year. Thus, patients require information and guidance to minimize barriers to effective treatment. All members of the health care team play an important role in this regard.

Nonpharmacologic Therapies

Nonpharmacologic approaches to lipid management are recommended as the first line of treatment (1). Modification of lifestyle factors may have a dramatic influence in some patients, although the response varies considerably. The principal nonpharmacologic therapies that may have a clinically important influence on the serum lipid profile include

- NCEP Step I and Step II diets,
- loss of excess body weight,
- increased physical activity,
- smoking cessation,
- increased intake of water-soluble dietary fiber, and
- dietary n-3 fatty acid supplementation.

NCEP Step I and Step II Diets. The NCEP Step I and Step II diets are designed to progressively restrict intake of saturated fatty acids and cholesterol, the two dietary components most consistently linked to elevation of LDL-C. Both diets limit total fat intake to 30% or less of total calories. The Step I diet limits saturated fat consumption to 8% to 10% of calories and dietary cholesterol to no more than 300 mg/day. The Step II diet further restricts saturated fat (less than 7% of calories) and cholesterol intake (less than 200 mg/day). Typical LDL-C responses to these dietary modifications in free-living subjects are in the range of 3% to 10% for the Step I diet and 5% to 15% for the Step II diet (2,3). Similar total and LDL-C responses were reported recently in a large, multicenter intervention trial in 560 subjects having dyslipidemia, hypertension, diabetes, or a combination of these conditions who followed a Step I or a Step II prepared meal plan (4).

Loss of Excess Body Weight. In overweight subjects, weight loss lowers triglyceride and VLDL-C concentrations while raising HDL-C concentrations. The effects of weight loss on LDL-C are generally favorable but less dramatic than the effects on VLDL-C and triglycerides. Dattilo and Kris-Etherton (5) published a meta-analysis summarizing the results of studies evaluating the influence of weight loss on lipids and lipoproteins. They reported that an 11-lb weight loss is associated with a decline of approximately 10 mg/dL in total cholesterol, 40% of which is in the LDL fraction. Subjects with upper-body obesity have greater derangements in lipoprotein metabolism but may respond more favorably to weight reduction (6) (see Chapter 7).

Increased Physical Activity. An increase in physical activity reduces triglyceride and VLDL-C concentrations. LDL-C concentrations are usually not influenced by exercise training unless the training is accompanied by loss of excess body fat (7). HDL-C increases in a dose-dependent manner with increasing physical activity (7,8). The US Centers for Disease Control and Prevention recommend that all Americans accumulate 30 minutes or more of moderate-intensity physical activity on most days (9). A nonobese adult will burn approximately 200 kcal in 30 minutes of moderate intensity activity (eg, brisk walking).

Although diets high in carbohydrate and low in fat have beneficial effects on LDL-C, they may produce mild elevation of triglyceride and depression of HDL-C concentrations in serum. These potentially deleterious effects can be prevented or reversed by increasing physical activity and losing excess body fat, underlining the synergistic effects of these lifestyle interventions.

Smoking Cessation. Cigarette smoking is associated with elevations of triglyceride concentrations and depression of HDL-C concentrations in serum (10). These lipid abnormalities improve after smoking cessation. Thus, it is reasonable to suggest that the increased cardiovascular disease risk associated with cigarette smoking may be partly mediated through the effects of smoking on lipid metabolism, adding to the long list of reasons for emphasizing smoking cessation to patients.

Water-soluble Dietary Fiber Consumption. Certain water-soluble dietary fibers lower total cholesterol and LDL-C when consumed in sufficient quantities. Examples include fiber from psyllium husk, beta-glucan from oat and barley products, guar gum, and pectin. Glore and others (11) reviewed more than 70 clinical trials that assessed the effects of increased intake of water-soluble dietary fiber on serum lipids. Significant reductions in total cholesterol were noted in 88% of the studies reviewed. Most (75% or more) of the trials showed no effects on triglyceride or HDL-C concentrations, indicating that changes in total cholesterol result primarily from reductions in the LDL fraction.

Adding 6 g/day to 12 g/day of soluble fiber to an NCEP Step I or II diet usually produces additional LDL-C reductions of 5% to 15% (11,12). The favorable effects of soluble fiber on lipids have persisted in studies lasting 6 months or longer, suggesting the potential for long-term benefit (11,12). Soluble fiber intake appears to have a more pronounced effect when patients are following a diet higher in saturated fat and cholesterol (11,13,14,15). Accordingly, increased soluble fiber intake may help to counteract the influence of deteriorating dietary adherence that may occur through time.

Viscosity appears to be an important factor determining the effectiveness of dietary soluble fiber for reducing LDL-C. Highly viscous fibers consistently produce significant LDL-C reductions, whereas less viscous fibers (eg, acacia gum) have an inconsistent effect. Recommendations for increasing dietary fiber consumption for lipid management should be limited to fibers with proven efficacy (11) (discussed in more detail in Chapter 6).

n-3 Fatty Acids. Considerable attention has focused on the use of marine oils high in the n-3 fatty acids eicosapentaenoic acid (EPA) and docosahexaenoic acid (DHA) as a tool for managing dyslipidemia. At therapeutic doses (3 g or more of DHA and EPA), n-3 fatty acids lower serum triglycerides and VLDL-C (16,17). HDL-C and triglyceride concentrations are metabolically linked; thus, the triglyceride lowering in response to n-3 fatty acid supplementation is usually associated with a moderate elevation in HDL-C. The influence of n-3 fatty acids on LDL-C is variable. If these highly polyunsaturated fatty acids replace sources of dietary saturated fats, LDL-C may decline (16,17), but if no other changes in dietary fat intake occur, LDL-C may decline slightly, remain unchanged, or even increase (16,17) (discussed in more detail in Chapter 12).

The clinical significance of the LDL-C elevation produced by n-3 fatty acid intake is uncertain but cannot be assumed to be benign just because there are no definitive data. The increase in LDL-C is often accompanied by a similar or larger decline in VLDL-C, particularly in patients with hypertriglyceridemia. Thus, total circulating non-HDL-C (VLDL-C plus intermediate-density lipoprotein cholesterol plus LDL-C) concentration may not increase.

Two secondary prevention studies showed reduced cardiovascular mortality in subjects who received diets enriched with n-3 fatty acids (18,19). However, the quantity of n-3 fatty acids consumed in these trials was not sufficient to have clinically important effects on serum lipid profiles. Several mechanisms other than serum lipid changes may contribute to the apparent cardioprotective properties of n-3 fatty acids. Possibilities include reduced platelet aggregation, increased resistance to cardiac arrhythmia, and improved endothelial function (16,17).

Additional randomized clinical trials are needed to clearly define the risks and benefits of n-3 fatty acid supplementation for the management of hyperlipidemia. Until such data are available, the decision to use marine oil supplements is a matter of clinical judgment.

Pharmacologic Therapies

Several classes of pharmacologic agents with varying mechanisms of action are available for the management of dyslipidemia. These include

- hydroxymethyl glutaryl coenzyme A reductase inhibitors,
- bile acid sequestrants,
- fibric acid derivatives,
- niacin, and
- estrogen or estrogen-progestin replacement.

Hydroxymethyl Glutaryl Coenzyme A Reductase Inhibitors. The most commonly prescribed medications for the management of hypercholesterolemia are the hydroxymethyl glutaryl coenzyme A (HMG-CoA) reductase inhibitors, or statins (Table 2-1). These drugs are highly effective for reducing LDL-C and are well tolerated. The statins also raise HDL-C and lower triglyceride concentrations to a minor degree. They function by inhibiting the rate-limiting step in the synthesis of cholesterol by the liver. Randomized primary and secondary prevention trials showed reduced cardiovascular morbidity and mortality and reduced plaque progression when drugs in this class were used to lower elevated LDL-C (20).

The choice of which statin to use is based primarily on cost-effectiveness. Simvastatin and atorvastatin are the most potent agents in this class and should be used if LDL-C reductions of 30% or more are required. Atorvastatin seems to be distinctly more effective at reducing elevated triglycerides than are the other agents in this class and thus may be the best choice for patients having concomitant elevations in LDL-C and triglycerides (21).

Bile Acid Sequestrants. Bile acid sequestrants (cholestyramine and colestipol), also known as binding resins, lower LDL-C by reducing the reabsorption of bile acids in the intestinal tract. In turn, cholesterol is used to manufacture new bile acids in the liver, lowering the hepatic cholesterol content. The liver then increases LDL particle clearance from the blood, lowering the circulating LDL-C concentration. Because resins are not absorbed, they may be used in combination with other classes of medication to minimize the risk of drug-related side effects by enabling LDL-C to be controlled with lower doses of systemic medications. The usual dosage of cholestyramine is 4 g/day to 24 g/day and of colestipol is 5 g/day to 30 g/day.

Resins tend to produce a mild increase in triglyceride concentrations, making this class suboptimal for reducing LDL-C in patients with concomitant triglyceride elevation (greater than 200 mg/dL). Gastrointestinal side effects (gas, cramping, and changes in bowel patterns, usually constipation) are often associated with resin use, which may limit compliance. A psyllium bulking laxative (eg, Metamucil, Proctor & Gamble, Cincinnati, Ohio) may be used in conjunction with resin drugs, both to ease the gastrointestinal side effects and enhance the LDL-C response.

Fibric Acid Derivatives. Several fibric acid derivatives (fibrates) are available in Europe, but only one, gemfibrozil (Lopid, Parke-Davis, Morris Plains, NJ), has been approved for use in the United States. Fibrates are most useful for patients with hypertriglyceridemia, with or without concomitant LDL-C elevation or HDL-C reduction. The primary effects on the lipid profile are triglyceride reduction and HDL-C elevation. LDL-C is also typically reduced in response to fibrate treatment. However, LDL-C in some hypertriglyceridemic patients may increase, reflecting improved metabolism of VLDL particles (ie, increased conversion to LDL). Gemfibrozil is administered at a dose of 600 mg twice daily.

Niacin. Niacin (nicotinic acid) is a B vitamin that at pharmacologic doses (1 g/day to 6 g/day) dramatically affects the serum lipid profile. However, niacinamide, which has vitamin activity, is not active as a lipid-altering agent. Niacin lowers LDL-C and triglyceride concentrations while raising HDL-C concentration. Angiographic trials showed that niacin reduces the progression of atherosclerotic disease. In addition, the Coronary Drug Project investigators found that niacin reduced nonfatal myocardial infarction by 27% relative to placebo (22).

Nearly all patients experience an uncomfortable flushing sensation when they begin taking large doses of niacin. This side effect may limit compliance; thus, it is critical to discuss strategies with the patient for limiting the intensity and duration of niacin-induced flushing. These strategies include gradual dose titration, taking niacin with meals, and avoiding consumption of hot drinks near the dosing time. Taking an aspirin (or ibuprofen) tablet 30 minutes before taking niacin will also help to minimize flushing. Additional side effects include gastrointestinal upset, dry skin, and (rarely) liver toxicity and gout. Patients with diabetes or those who are at high risk for diabetes should generally not take high doses of niacin because its use is associated with the development of profound insulin resistance and may induce or worsen hyperglycemia (23,24).

Estrogen and Estrogen-progestin Replacement. The reduction in circulating estrogen concentration associated with menopause is associated with several potentially proatherogenic changes in the serum lipid profile, including elevation of LDL-C (10% to 25%) and depression of HDL-C (10% to 20%) (25). Fourfold more women 55 to 64 years of

TABLE 2-1

The Most Commonly Prescribed Medications for the Management of Hypercholesterolemia

Agents	Dosage
Fluvastatin (Lescol, Sandoz Pharmaceuticals Consumer Division, East Hanover, NJ)	10–40 mg nightly
Lovastatin (Mevacor, Merck & Co, Inc, West Point, PA)	10–80 mg nightly, or in divided doses
Pravastatin (Pravachol, Bristol-Myers Squibb Co, Princeton, NJ)	5–40 mg nightly
Simvastatin (Zocor, Merck & Co)	5–40 mg nightly
Atorvastatin (Lipitor, Parke-Davis, Morris Plains, NJ)	10–80 mg nightly

age than women 35 to 44 years of age are candidates for dietary intervention to lower LDL-C (52% compared with 13%, respectively), which underscores the potential public health impact of these lipid changes (26).

Oral estrogen-replacement therapy lowers LDL-C by approximately 15% and raises HDL-C and triglycerides by 10% to 20% (27,28,29). Other forms of estrogen delivery such as transdermal patches generally do not have as pronounced an effect on lipid profiles. The NCEP ATP II recommended that estrogen replacement be considered as a therapeutic option for management of hypercholesterolemia in postmenopausal women. However, unopposed estrogen is not recommended for women with an intact uterus because it increases the risk of uterine cancer (30). [Currently, about one-third of women in the United States have undergone hysterectomy by age 60 years (31).] Addition of a progestin reduces the risk of uterine cancer but also blunts the effects of estrogen on HDL-C (27). Moreover, because of the hypertriglyceridemic properties of oral estrogens, these treatments should be used with caution by women with elevated triglyceride concentrations (greater than 200 mg/dL).

The favorable effects of estrogen on LDL-C are not generally attenuated by the addition of a progestin (27). Therefore, estrogen replacement in conjunction with lifestyle modification may be reasonably expected to reduce LDL-C by 15% to 20%, making this an attractive treatment option for postmenopausal women with mild to moderate hypercholesterolemia.

Clinical Management of Dyslipidemia

Clinical management of dyslipidemia is based on the categories mentioned above:

- elevated LDL-C,
- elevated VLDL-C and triglycerides,
- depressed HDL-C,
- combined dyslipidemias, and
- chylomicronemia.

Elevated Low-density Lipoprotein Cholesterol. Isolated elevation of LDL-C is the most common lipid abnormality, and lifestyle modification is the suggested first-line therapy. This includes an adequate trial of dietary intervention (NCEP Step I and Step II diets), weight loss if the patient is overweight, and regular physical activity. Viscous water-soluble dietary fiber (eg, from oat bran, psyllium, and guar gum) may be a useful adjunct to a diet low in saturated fat and cholesterol. Nonpharmacologic interventions are often sufficient therapy if LDL-C is within 10% to 20% of the target level. HMG-CoA reductase inhibitors are the most commonly prescribed class of medication for this abnormality, although bile acid–binding resins and niacin may also be used. For postmenopausal women, hormone replacement therapy should also be considered.

Elevated Very-low-density Lipoprotein Cholesterol and Triglycerides. Isolated hypertriglyceridemia can result from a variety of causes, both genetic and environmental. Potentially modifiable factors contributing to triglyceride and VLDL-C elevation include obesity, poorly controlled diabetes mellitus, excessive alcohol consumption, and lack of regular physical activity. Control of these factors often has a marked effect. n-3 Fatty acids or marine oils may be useful for lowering elevated triglycerides in some situations (eg, combined with an agent to lower elevated LDL-C).

Drug therapy should be initiated for triglyceride reduction if the concentration remains greater than 400 mg/dL to 500 mg/dL after 6 months of lifestyle intervention. If the triglyceride concentration is greater than 1,000 mg/dL, drug therapy should be initiated sooner to prevent acute pancreatitis. Gemfibrozil is usually the first drug of choice for lowering triglyceride concentration. Niacin is also highly effective for both lowering the triglyceride concentration and raising HDL-C, is inexpensive, and may be purchased without a prescription. However, at therapeutic doses (1 g/day to 6 g/day) niacin has several side effects that limit its usefulness for some patients (24).

Depressed High-density Lipoprotein Cholesterol. Low HDL-C is often associated with hypertriglyceridemia. However, isolated low HDL-C is also a common disorder that confers increased risk for coronary artery disease. Weight loss and regular physical activity may raise HDL-C but are most effective for patients with concomitant triglyceride elevation. The best treatment approach for patients with isolated low HDL-C is uncertain. No large-scale clinical trials directly assessing and comparing different treatments have been completed. Aggressive programs for lowering LDL-C are generally recommended for such patients to improve the ratio of LDL-C to HDL-C (LDL-C:HDL-C), particularly for patients with coronary artery disease (1,32). Weight loss and increased physical activity may improve HDL-C concentration. However, isolated low HDL-C is often refractory to lifestyle interventions. Gemfibrozil or niacin may be used to raise HDL-C concentrations and improve LDL-C:HDL-C.

Combined Dyslipidemias. Combination dyslipidemias are often observed in clinical practice, and lifestyle modifications are the first line of treatment. The primary target for intervention is the LDL-C concentration; secondary goals include maintaining acceptable concentrations of triglycerides and HDL-C. Gemfibrozil and niacin may be particularly useful in these situations because they favorably influence all of the major serum lipid classes. Bile acid sequestrants and HMG-CoA reductase inhibitors primarily influence LDL-C concentration and are frequently not sufficient as monotherapies. However, atorvastatin appears to lower the triglyceride concentration more than do other HMG-CoA reductase inhibitors and thus may be particularly useful for patients with elevated LDL-C and triglycerides (21).

Chylomicronemia. Chylomicra carry triglyceride and cholesterol absorbed from the intestine. Normally these particles have been cleared from the blood after a 12-hour fast.

Although relatively rare, a number of familial and acquired conditions are associated with a reduced rate of chylomicron clearance, resulting in continued presence of chylomicra and marked hypertriglyceridemia in the fasting state (33).

A diet low in fat and cholesterol is essential for reducing the number of chylomicra entering the blood stream, and some patients respond well to consumption of a very low fat intake (less than 20% of energy from fat). Other nonpharmacologic strategies for management are identical to those for elevated VLDL-C and triglycerides, including alcohol restriction, adequate glycemic control in people with diabetes mellitus, weight loss, and increased physical activity. n-3 Fatty acid supplementation may be used when these measures are inadequate to maintain an acceptable triglyceride concentration (see Chapter 12). Pharmacologic therapies may be required if the triglyceride concentration cannot be maintained below 400 mg/dL to 500 mg/dL. Gemfibrozil, niacin, and progestins (in women) are effective for this purpose.

HYPERTENSION

The management of high blood pressure is a critical component of preventive strategies for reducing morbidity and mortality from cardiovascular disease. The strategies to manage high blood pressure include

- pharmacologic therapies,
- dietary intervention,
- weight reduction,
- moderate sodium restriction,
- moderation of alcohol intake, and
- increased intakes of calcium, potassium, and magnesium.

Uncontrolled blood pressure takes a toll on a number of organ systems, including not only the heart and blood vessels but also the brain, nerves, kidney, and retina. Normalization of both systolic and diastolic blood pressure has been associated with a substantial reduction in both morbidity and mortality (34). A decrease in the population mean systolic blood pressure of 2 mm Hg could be associated with a decline of 4% in coronary mortality, 6% in stroke mortality, and 3% in total mortality; a decrease in mean diastolic blood pressure of 5 mm Hg could be associated with a decline of 9% in coronary mortality, 14% in stroke mortality, and 7% in total mortality (34).

Blood pressure can be successfully normalized by either pharmacologic or nonpharmacologic means. Pharmacologic intervention uses one or more of five major types of antihypertensive medications. Nonpharmacologic intervention relies on modifications in diet, regular physical activity, and stress management. The most recent report of the Joint National Committee on Detection, Evaluation, and Treatment of High Blood Pressure (35) recommended nonpharmacologic intervention as the first step in the management of hypertension for individuals with mild or moderately elevated blood pressure (35).

Pharmacologic Therapies

Antihypertensive drugs are the most frequently prescribed class of medications in the United States (box). Each type of drug controls blood pressure through a different mechanism and may not be equally effective for all individuals, reflecting both the heterogeneity of the underlying pathology of the disease and the variability in individual responsiveness to a particular drug or combination of drugs. The effectiveness of antihypertensive medications in lowering blood pressure and maintaining it within clinically normal ranges was definitively established by several large-scale clinical trials (36,37,38,39,40,41,42).

Pharmacologic treatment of hypertension dramatically reduces the incidence of stroke, but the effects of antihypertensive therapy on coronary artery disease events in some large, randomized trials were less beneficial than expected on the basis of data from epidemiologic studies. This discordance was attributed in part to the metabolic derangements that commonly accompany the use of high doses of these drugs (43,44). Hypokalemia, hyperuricemia, hyperlipidemia, and hyperinsulinemia are the most common metabolic side effects reported, particularly with use of thiazide diuretics and beta-adrenergic blockers (45,46,47). These potentially adverse metabolic consequences of drug therapy are less pronounced at the lower doses more commonly used today.

Newer classes of antihypertensive medication (eg, angiotensin-converting enzyme (ACE) inhibitors, calcium channel blockers, and alpha-adrenergic blockers) have neutral or potentially favorable effects on lipid and carbohydrate metabolism (48,49). However, the most definitive data demonstrating reduced risk of morbidity and mortality comes from studies with beta-adrenergic blockers and diuretics (36,37,38,39,40,41,42). Many factors contribute to decisions influencing the choice of the appropriate antihypertensive treatment regimen, as summarized in the fifth report of the Joint National Committee on Detection, Evaluation, and Treatment of High Blood Pressure (35).

Dietary Intervention

Dietary intervention is the cornerstone of the nonpharmacologic approach to the treatment of hypertension (35). This approach also includes regular moderate physical activity

Types of Antihypertensive Drugs

Diuretics (thiazide, loop, or potassium sparing)

Antiadrenergic agents
(alpha- or beta-adrenergic blockers)

Vasodilators

Angiotensin-converting enzyme inhibitors

Calcium channel blockers

and stress management. The effect of dietary factors on blood pressure is supported by extensive research and documentation of the specific mechanisms involved and encompasses all aspects of blood pressure homeostasis. Blood pressure may be either favorably or adversely affected by dietary factors through effects on plasma volume and cardiac output; sympathetic nervous system activity and peripheral vascular resistance; concentrations of vasoactive prostacyclins, thromboxanes, and cytokines; and membrane ion transport activity.

Many of the adverse drug side effects associated with antihypertensive medications, such as hypokalemia, hyperlipidemia, and impaired glucose tolerance are responsive to dietary therapy involving losing weight, reducing fat and sodium intakes, and increasing potassium intake. The possibility of an adverse reaction developing and its responsiveness to dietary modification may depend on the particular drug and the dosage required for normalizing blood pressure. In general, at low dosages, calcium channel blockers and angiotensin-converting enzyme inhibitors are less likely to cause metabolic derangements than are diuretics and beta-adrenergic blockers (50).

The primary dietary modifications recommended for control of blood pressure are weight reduction, moderate sodium restriction, and moderation of alcohol intake. Attention to achieving sufficient intakes of calcium, potassium, and magnesium is also emphasized. In a multicenter clinical trial, a diet meeting these recommendations was given to subjects with hypertension, dyslipidemia, and/or diabetes and resulted in a decrease in systolic and diastolic blood pressure of 6.4 mm Hg and 4.2 mm Hg, respectively (4). Although not a primary focus of current intervention, recommendations to modify intakes of protein, n-3 fatty acids, and dietary fiber may be included in the future (51,52,53).

Weight Reduction

One of the strongest determinants of blood pressure is body weight. Body mass index and other correlates of obesity were found to be significantly associated with blood pressure (54). Overweight and obesity affect approximately 60% of all individuals with high blood pressure (55). More importantly from the standpoint of intervention effectiveness, reductions of body weight usually improve blood pressure control and may reduce or eliminate the need for medications (56,57).

Weight loss is a highly effective way to reduce blood pressure (57,58,59,60,61). Excess body weight is believed to impose a hemodynamic burden on the cardiovascular system that may elevate blood pressure because of the need to increase blood volume and cardiac output to perfuse excess body mass (62,63,64,65). Obesity is commonly associated with increases in both sympathetic activity and insulin resistance, which may adversely affect blood pressure through vascular effects caused by increased catecholamines and altered membrane sodium transport (66,67). Weight loss also lowers blood pressure by decreasing plasma renin activity (65).

Even without a sizable decrease in fat mass, restriction of energy intake may itself decrease blood pressure by reducing sympathetic activity and thus decreasing peripheral vascular resistance (65). In a practical sense, reduction in energy intake could also facilitate sodium restriction by limiting the amount of food consumed.

Weight loss goals for controlling blood pressure are consistent with those of achieving ideal body weight. However, even relatively small reductions in body weight could result in a favorable blood pressure response (56,60,61,65). For patients taking antihypertensive medications, the hypolipidemic effect of weight loss could offset the potential for raising serum lipid levels associated with some of these medications (47). Achieving and maintaining a weight loss of 10 lb or more improves the ability to maintain normalized blood pressure that results in either a reduced effective dosage of antihypertensive drugs or control of blood pressure without drugs (57,59,68).

Moderate Sodium Restriction

Moderate restriction of sodium intake is the oldest of the dietary approaches used for the nonpharmacologic control of blood pressure. The restriction of sodium intake has been recommended because elevated blood pressure is associated with sodium imbalances that are most likely the result of difficulty in renal handling of a sodium load (69). Whether a habitual diet high in sodium is responsible for this impairment in renal function or whether it is caused by a genetic lesion or other factors remains unresolved. In individuals with normal blood pressures, groups at highest risk for hypertension have the most difficulty excreting a sodium load. These groups include people older than 50, those with a positive family history of hypertension, and African Americans (70).

Limited data suggest that blood pressure responsiveness to sodium restriction may be related to plasma renin activity. Individuals with hypertension who do not have an appropriate response of the renin-angiotensin-aldosterone system with changes in sodium intake may benefit most from sodium restriction (71,72). Although it is currently impossible to predict every person who may respond favorably to sodium restriction with a reduction in blood pressure, it is reasonable to expect that most hypertensive individuals would benefit by a moderate restriction in sodium intake to no more than 100 mEq (approximately 2,000 mg) daily (73,74,75).

Restriction of sodium intake may be an especially important dietary intervention for people who do not need to lose weight. For subjects with hypertension participating in the Dietary Intervention Study of Hypertension, the success rate for maintaining blood pressure control without medications at week 56 of the study was highest for the nonoverweight group that reduced daily sodium intake to a mean of 97 mEq (74). Seventy-eight percent of the sodium-restricted nonoverweight group remained off medications, compared with 76% of the overweight group who lost an average of 10 lbs. Individuals having hypertension who were successful at moderately reducing their sodium intake were twice as likely to control their blood pressure without medication as were those who did not reduce their sodium intake (76).

Moderate sodium restriction may benefit all people with hypertension regardless of medication status by protecting against progression of the disease as manifested by development of left ventricular hypertrophy (77). Dietary sodium participates in the hypertrophic process independent of other determinants, possibly through mechanisms involving the renin-angiotensin system, sympathetic nervous system activity, and fluid-volume homeostasis. An average decrease of 5.4% in left ventricular mass was demonstrated in response to sodium restriction after 1 year in a group of subjects with hypertension who had been untreated for the 6 months before beginning the sodium-restricted diet (77).

Moderate sodium restriction may reduce the dosages of antihypertensive medications required to normalize blood pressure (78), thus decreasing the number and severity of dose-related side effects. Sodium restriction as an adjunct therapy with thiazide diuretics reduced potassium losses (60). Hypokalemia may develop from treatment with antihypertensive medications that promote sodium excretion, which is potentially dangerous because it can contribute to cardiac arrhythmias and promote the deterioration of glucose tolerance typically observed with potassium deficiency (79,80). Severe restriction of sodium intakes to less than 50 mEq (approximately 1,100 mg) is not recommended for patients taking antihypertensive medications, because at very low intakes of sodium, compensatory mechanisms involving the renin-angiotensin and sympathetic nervous systems may be stimulated (81).

Moderation of Alcohol Intake

Several large-scale observational studies showed an association between alcohol consumption and blood pressure (82,83,84,85,86). The prevalence of hypertension in a group of alcoholics whose mean daily alcohol consumption was greater than 80 g was reported to be as high as 55%, which is about twice the rate for the general population (87). Both systolic and diastolic blood pressures were significantly correlated with mean daily alcohol consumption over the previous 3 months and with the severity of withdrawal symptoms in this group of men and women (87). Furthermore, 78% (103 of 132) had normalized blood pressures when they were discharged after 7 days to 11 days of abstinence from alcohol. Blood pressure remained normal after 1 year in those who had abstained from alcohol. These observations, along with the epidemiologic data, have led to the speculation that there may be a specific type of hypertension—alcohol-induced hypertension—induced by chronic excess alcohol consumption. Sustained elevation in blood pressure resulting from heavy alcohol consumption has been estimated to explain about 3% to 12% of hypertension (depending on the diagnostic criteria used) (88).

Chronic excess consumption of alcohol can adversely affect blood pressure and blood pressure responsiveness to antihypertensive medications. The relationship between alcohol intake and blood pressure follows a curvilinear or J-shape pattern, with higher mortality found at the intake extremes (89). This pattern of mortality is the basis for the recommendation that, for alcohol consumers, an average of fewer than three alcoholic drinks be consumed per day to maintain compatibility with a good blood pressure response (90). A *drink* is defined as the alcohol equivalent of 4.5 fluid ounces of wine, 12 ounces of beer, or 1½ ounces of distilled liquors such as rum, bourbon, whiskey, gin, or vodka.

For many people, alcohol consumption habits are perhaps among the most difficult of behaviors to change. When weight control is a consideration, the elimination of alcohol as a contributor of empty calories is one approach that may encourage a change in consumption patterns. However, a small amount of alcohol in a dietary plan may promote better overall compliance.

Calcium, Potassium, and Magnesium

Diets rich in sources of calcium, potassium, and magnesium have been associated with favorable levels of blood pressure (91,92,93). The results of controlled clinical studies of the effects of individual supplements of these minerals on blood pressure confirmed the observations from the epidemiologic studies (94,95,96). More recently, impressive results were reported from the Dietary Approaches to Stop Hypertension study (97). In this multicenter study funded by the National Heart, Lung and Blood Institute, systolic and diastolic blood pressure were reduced by 11 mm Hg and 6 mm Hg, respectively, in hypertensive subjects in response to a diet rich in fruits, vegetables, and low-fat dairy products. These effects were attributed to relatively high amounts of dietary potassium (4.4 g/day), magnesium (480 mg/day), and calcium (1265 mg/day).

Several of these minerals may also be contributed by the water supply. In regions with "hard" water supplies that are rich in calcium and magnesium, mean blood pressures are lower than in regions with "soft" water supplies (98). Although additional amounts of both calcium and magnesium may be consumed by individuals living in regions having hard water, the contribution of drinking water to total daily calcium intake is proportionately much less than the contribution to total daily magnesium intake.

An interesting aspect of the association between blood pressure and intakes of potassium, calcium, and magnesium is that the metabolism of each of these minerals is interrelated with sodium metabolism. Urinary calcium excretion is more closely associated with dietary levels of sodium than are dietary levels of calcium (99). In fact, the association between sodium intake and blood pressure is strongest when calcium intake is low (100). The relationship between potassium and sodium metabolism appears to follow a pattern similar to that observed with calcium and sodium.

Potassium supplementation has a more pronounced effect on lowering blood pressure when sodium intake is high than when sodium intake is low (101). The urinary ratio of sodium to potassium also appears to be more closely associated with blood pressure response than is intake or excretion of either mineral alone (102). The interaction between sodium and magnesium is the least understood of the minerals examined.

Dietary modifications for management of hypertension should include an emphasis on foods rich in calcium, potassium, and magnesium in the diet plan. Increased intakes of these three minerals should augment the effectiveness of sodium restriction on blood pressure response. For individuals who are at ideal weights and are not responsive to sodium restriction, increased intakes of these minerals may provide an additional means for improving blood pressure response with or without medications.

SUMMARY

The control of blood pressure by dietary means offers an approach to the management of mild or moderate hypertension that may reduce or eliminate the need for medications and the development of adverse drug side effects that may accompany high dosages. As part of a nonpharmacologic approach to treatment of hypertension, weight control, moderate sodium restriction, and a moderation of alcohol intake included within a diet rich in food sources of calcium, potassium, and magnesium should maximize the risk-benefit ratio associated with normalization of blood pressure.

REFERENCES

1. National Cholesterol Education Program. *Second Report of the Expert Panel on Detection, Evaluation, and Treatment of High Blood Cholesterol in Adults.* Bethesda, Md: National Institutes of Health, 1993. NIH publication 93-3095.
2. Caggiula AW, Watson JE, Kuller LH, Olson MB, Milas NC, Berry M, Germanowski J. Cholesterol-lowering intervention program. *Arch Intern Med.* 1996;156:1205-1213.
3. Denke MA. Cholesterol-lowering diets. A review of the evidence. *Arch Intern Med.* 1995;155:17-26.
4. McCarron DA, Oparil S, Chait A, Haynes B, Kris-Etherton P, Stern JS, Resnick LM, Clark S, Moris CD, Hatton DC, Metz JA, McMahon M, Holcomb S, Snyder GW, Pi-Sunyer X. Nutritional management of cardiovascular risk factors. *Arch Intern Med.* 1997;157:169-177.
5. Dattilo AM, Kris-Etherton PM. Effects of weight reduction on blood lipids and lipoproteins: a meta-analysis. *Am J Clin Nutr.* 1992;56:320-328.
6. Despres JP. Dyslipidaemia and obesity. *Baillieres Clin Endocrinol Metab.* 1994;8:629-661.
7. Stefanick ML, Wood PD. Physical activity, lipid and lipoprotein metabolism, and lipid transport. In: Bouchard C, Shephard RJ, Stephens T, eds. *Physical Activity, Fitness, and Health, International Proceedings and Consensus Statement.* Champaign, Ill: Human Kinetics; 1994:417-431.
8. LaPorte RE, Adams LL, Savage DD, Brenes G, Dearwater S, Cook T. The spectrum of physical activity, cardiovascular disease, and health: an epidemiologic perspective. *Am J Epidemiol.* 1984;120:507-517.
9. Pate RR, Pratt M, Blair SN, Haskell WL, Macera CA, Bouchard C, Buchner D, Ettinger W, Heath GW, King AC. Physical activity and public health: a recommendation from the Centers for Disease Control and Prevention and the American College of Sports Medicine. *JAMA.* 1995;273:402-407.
10. Goldman L, Garber AM, Grover SA, Hlatky MA. Task Force 6. Cost effectiveness of assessment and management of risk factors. *JACC.* 1996;27:964-1047.
11. Glore SR, Treeck DV, Knehans AW, Guild M. Soluble fiber and serum lipids: a literature review. *J Am Diet Assoc.* 1994;94:425-436.
12. Jensen CD, Haskell W, Whittam JH. Long-term effects of water-soluble dietary fiber in the management of hypercholesterolemia in healthy men and women. *Am J Cardiol.* 1997;79:34-37.
13. Anderson JW, Zettwoch N, Feldman T, Tietyen-Clark J, Oeltgen P, Bishop CW. Cholesterol-lowering effects of psyllium hydrophilic mucilloid for hypercholesterolemic men. *Arch Intern Med.* 1988;148:292-296.
14. Bell LP, Hectorne K, Reynolds H, Balm TK, Hunninghake DB. Cholesterol-lowering effects of psyllium hydrophilic mucilloid. *JAMA.* 1989;261:3419-3423.
15. Bell LP, Hectorne K, Reynolds H, Hunninghake DB. Cholesterol-lowering effects of soluble-fiber cereals as part of a prudent diet for patients with mild to moderate hypercholesterolemia. *Am J Clin Nutr.* 1990;52:1020-1026.
16. Kinsella JE, Lokesh B, Stone RA. Dietary n-3 polyunsaturated fatty acids and amelioration of cardiovascular disease: possible mechanisms 1-3. *Am J Clin Nutr.* 1990;52:1-28.
17. Simopoulos AP. Omega-3 fatty acids in health and disease and in growth and development. *Am J Clin Nutr.* 1991;54:438-463.
18. Burr ML, Gilbert JF, Holliday RM, Elwood PC, Fehily AM, Rogers S, Sweetnam PM, Deadman NM. Effects of changes in fat, fish, and fibre intakes on death and myocardial reinfarction: Diet and Reinfarction Trial (DART). *Lancet.* 1989;334:757-761.
19. de Lorgeril M, Renaud S, Mamelle N, Salen P, Martin JL, Monjaud I, Guidollet J, Touboul P, Delaye J. Mediterranean alpha-linolenic acid-rich diet in secondary prevention of coronary heart disease. *Lancet.* 1994;343:1454-1459.
20. Kreisberg RA. Cholesterol-lowering and coronary atherosclerosis: good news and bad news. *Am J Med.* 1996;101:455-458.
21. Bakker-Arkema RG, Davidson MH, Goldstein RJ, Davignon J, Isaacsohn JL, Weiss SR, Keilson LM, Brown WV, Miller VT, Shurzinske LJ, Black DM. Efficacy and safety of a new HMG-CoA reductase inhibitor, atorvastatin, in patients with hypertriglyceridemia. *JAMA.* 1996;275:128-133.
22. The Coronary Drug Project Research Group. Clofibrate and niacin in coronary heart disease. *JAMA.* 1975;231:360-381.
23. Kahn SE, Beard JC, Schwartz MW, Ward WK, Ding HL, Bergman KN, Taborsky GJ Jr, Porte D Jr. Increased B-cell secretory capacity as mechanism for islet adaptation to nicotinic acid-induced insulin resistance. *Diabetes.* 1989;38:562-568.
24. Kreisberg RA. Niacin: a therapeutic dilemma "one man's drink is another's poison". *Am J Med.* 1994;97:313-316.
25. Stevenson JC, Crook D, Godsland IF. Influence of age and menopause on serum lipids and lipoproteins in healthy women. *Atherosclerosis.* 1993;98:83-90.
26. Sempos CT, Cleeman JI, Carroll MD, Johnson CL, Bachorik PS, Gordon DJ, Burt VL, Briefel RR, Brown CD, Lippel K.

Prevalence of high blood cholesterol among US adults. An update based on guidelines from the second report of the National Cholesterol Education Program Adult Treatment Panel. *JAMA*. 1993; 269:3009-3014.
27. The Writing Group for the PEPI Trial. Effects of estrogen or estrogen/progestin regimens on heart disease risk factors in postmenopausal women. *JAMA*. 1995; 273:199-208.
28. Sacks FM, Walsh BW. Sex hormones and lipoprotein metabolism. *Curr Opin Lipodol.* 1994;5:236-240.
29. Walsh BW, Schiff I, Rosner B, Greenberg L, Ravnikar V, Sacks FM. Effects of postmenopausal estrogen replacement on the concentrations and metabolism of plasma lipoproteins. *N Engl J Med*. 1991;325:1196-1204.
30. Grady D, Rubin SM, Petitti DB, Fox CS, Black D, Ettinger B, Ernster VL, Cummings SR. Hormone therapy to prevent disease and prolong life in postmenopausal women. *Ann Intern Med*. 1992;117:1016-1037.
31. Centers for Disease Control and Prevention. Hysterectomy prevalence and death rates for cervical cancer—United States, 1965–1988. *MMWR*. 1992;41:17-20.
32. Sniderman AD, Pedersen T, Kjekshus J. Putting low-density lipoproteins at center stage in atherogenesis. *Am J Cardiol*. 1997;79:64-67.
33. Chait A, Brunzell JD. Acquired hyperlipidemia (secondary dyslipoproteinemias). *Endocrinol Metab Clin North Am*. 1990;19:259-278.
34. Stamler J. Blood pressure and high blood pressure: aspects of risk. *Hypertension.* 1991;18(Suppl):I-95-I-107.
35. Joint National Committee on Detection, Evaluation, and Treatment of High Blood Pressure. The fifth report of the Joint National Committee on Detection, Evaluation, and Treatment of High Blood Pressure (JNC V). *Arch Intern Med*. 1993;153:154-183.
36. Veterans Administration Cooperative Study Group on Antihypertensive Agents. Effects of treatment on morbidity in hypertension, II: results in patients with diastolic blood pressure averaging 90-114 mm Hg. *JAMA*. 1970;213:1143-1152.
37. US Public Health Service Hospital Cooperative Study Group. Treatment of mild hypertension: results of a ten-year intervention trial. *Circ Res*. 1977;40 (suppl):I-98-I-105.
38. Hegleland A. Treatment of mild hypertension: a five year controlled drug trial: the Oslo Study. *Am J Med*. 1980;69:725-732.
39. Hypertension Detection and Follow-up Program Cooperative Group. Five-year findings of the Hypertension Detection and Follow-up Program, I: reduction in mortality of persons with high blood pressure, including mild hypertension. *JAMA*. 1979;242:2562-2571.
40. Management Committee of the Australian Therapeutic Trial in Mild Hypertension. The Australian Therapeutic Trial in Mild Hypertension: report by the Management Committee. *Lancet*. 1980;1:1260-1267.
41. Medical Research Council Working Party. MRC trial of treatment of mild hypertension: principal results. *BMJ*. 1985;291:97-104.
42. Multiple Risk Factor Intervention Trial Research Group. Mortality after 10.5 years for hypertensive patients in the Multiple Risk Factor Intervention Trial. *Circulation*. 1990;82:1616-1628.
43. Kaplan NM. The potential benefits of nonpharmacologic therapy. *Am J Hypertens*. 1990;3(5 Pt 1):425-427.
44. Kaplan NM. The case for low dose diuretic therapy. *Am J Hypertens*. 1991;4:970-971.
45. Grimm RH, Leon AS, Hunninghake DB, Lenz K, Hannan P, Blackburn H. Effect of thiazide diuretics on blood lipids and lipoproteins in mild hypertensive patients: a double-blind controlled trial. *Ann Intern Med*. 1981;94:7-11.
46. Lasser NL, Grandits G, Caggiula AW, Cutler JA, Briman RH Jr, Kuller LH, Sherwin RW, Stamler J. Effects of antihypertensive therapy on plasma lipids and lipoproteins in the Multiple Risk Factor Intervention Trial. *Am J Med*. 1984;76:117-121.
47. Weinberger MH. Antihypertensive therapy and lipids: evidence, mechanisms, and implications. *Arch Intern Med*. 1985;145:1102-1105.
48. Corry DB, Tuck ML. Glucose and insulin metabolism in hypertension. *Am J Nephrol*. 1996;16:223-236.
49. Madu EC, Reddy RC, Madu AN, Anyaogu C, Harris T, Fraker TD Jr. Review: the effects of antihypertensive agents on serum lipids. *Am J Med Sci*. 1996;312:76-84.
50. Alderman MH. Which antihypertensive drugs first—and why! *JAMA*. 1992;267:2786-2787.
51. Ascherio A, Hennekens C, Willett WC, Sacks F, Rosner B, Manson J, Witteman J, Stampfer MJ. Prospective study of nutritional factors, blood pressure, and hypertension among US women. *Hypertension*. 1996;27:1065-1072.
52. Obarzanek E, Velletri PA, Cutler JA. Dietary protein and blood pressure. *JAMA*. 1996;275:1598-1603.
53. Pietinen P. Dietary fat and blood pressure. *Ann Med*. 1994;26:465-468.
54. Stamler R, Stamler J, Riedlinger WF, Algera G, Roberts RJ. Weight and blood pressure: findings in hypertension screening of one million Americans. *JAMA*. 1978;240:1607-1610.
55. Tuck ML. Role of salt in the control of blood pressure in obesity and diabetes mellitus. *Hypertension*. 1991;17(Suppl I):1135-1142.
56. Heyden S, Borhani NO, Tyroler HA, Schneider KA, Langford HG, Hames CG, Hutchinson R, Oberman A. The relationship of weight change to changes in blood pressure, serum uric acid, cholesterol and glucose in the treatment of hypertension. *J Chronic Dis*. 1985;38:281-288.
57. Davis BR, Blaufox MD, Oberman A, Wassertheil-Smoller S, Zimbaldi N, Cutler JA, Kirchner K, Langford HG. Reduction in long-term antihypertensive medication requirements. Effects of weight reduction by dietary intervention in overweight persons with mild hypertension. *Arch Intern Med*. 1993;153:1773-1782.
58. Dustan HP, Weinsier RL. Treatment of obesity-associated hypertension. *Ann Epidemiol*. 1991;1:371-379.
59. Langford HG, Blaufox MD, Oberman A, Hawkins CM, Curb JD, Cutter GR, Wassertheil-Smoller S, Pressel S, Babcock C, Abernethy JD. Dietary therapy slows the return of hypertension after stopping prolonged medication. *JAMA*. 1985;253:657-664.
60. Langford HG, Davis BR, Blaufox D, Oberman A, Wassertheil-Smoller S, Hawkins M, Zimbaldi N. Effect of drug and diet treatment of mild hypertension on diastolic blood pressure. The TAIM Research Group. *Hypertension*. 1991;17:210-217.
61. Wassertheil-Smoller S, Langford HG, Blaufox MD, Oberman A, Hawkins M, Levine B, Cameron M, Babcock C, Pressel S, Caggiula A. Effective dietary intervention in hypertensives: sodium restriction and weight reduction. *J Am Diet Assoc*. 1985; 85:423-430.
62. Dustan HP, Tarazi RC, Mujais S. A comparison of hemodynamic and volume characteristics of obese and nonobese hypertensive patients. *Int J Obes*. 1981;5:19-25.
63. Reisin E, Frohlich ED, Messerli FH, Dreslinski GR, Dunn FG,

Jones MM, Batson HM Jr. Cardiovascular changes after weight reduction in obesity hypertension. *Ann Intern Med.* 1983;98:315-319.
64. Reisin E. Weight reduction in the management of hypertension: epidemiologic and mechanistic evidence. *Can J Physiol Pharmacol.* 1986;64:818-824.
65. Bunker CH, Wing RR, Mallinger AG, Becker DJ, Matthews KA, Kuller LH. Cross-sectional and longitudinal relationship of sodium-lithium countertransport to insulin, obesity, and blood pressure in healthy perimenopausal women. *J Hum Hypertens.* 1991;5:381-392.
66. Langford HG. Sodium-potassium interaction in hypertension and hypertensive cardiovascular disease. *Hypertension.* 1991;17(Suppl):I-155-I-157.
67. Weinsier RL, James LD, Darnell BE, Dustan HP, Birch R, Hunter GR. Obesity-related hypertension: evaluation of the separate effects of energy restriction and weight reduction on hemodynamic and neuroendocrine status. *Am J Med.* 1991;90:460-468.
68. Stamler R, Stamler J, Grimm R, Gosch FC, Elmer P, Dyer A, Berman R, Fishman J, Van Heel N, Civinelli J, McDonald A. Nutritional therapy for high blood pressure: final report of a four-year randomized controlled trial—the Hypertension Control Program. *JAMA.* 1987;257:1484-1491.
69. Guyton AC. The renal function: a key to understanding the pathogenesis of hypertension. *Hypertension.* 1987;10:11-17.
70. Luft FC, Rankin LI, Henry DP. Plasma and urinary norepinephrine values at extremes of sodium intake in normal man. *Hypertension.* 1979;1:261-266.
71. Sealey JE, Blumenfeld JD, Bell GM, Pecker MS, Sommers SC, Laragh JH. On the renal basis for essential hypertension: nephron heterogeneity with discordant renin secretion and sodium excretion causing a hypertensive vasoconstriction-volume relationship. *J Hypertens.* 1988;6:763-777.
72. Weinberger MH, Miller JZ, Luft FC, Grim FC, Fineberg NS. Definitions and characteristics of sodium sensitivity and blood pressure resistance. *Hypertension* 1986;8(II):127-134.
73. Andersson OK, Fagerberg B, Hedner T. Importance of dietary salt in the hemodynamic adjustment to weight reduction in obese hypertensive men. *Hypertension.* 1984;6:814-819.
74. Blaufox MD, Langford HG, Oberman A, Hawkins CM, Wassertheil-Smoller SW, Cutter GR. Effect of dietary change on the return of hypertension after withdrawal of prolonged antihypertensive therapy (DISH). Dietary Intervention Study of Hypertension. *J Hypertens.* 1984;2:S179-S181.
75. Wassertheil-Smoller S, Blaufox MD, Langford HG, Oberman A, Cutter G, Pressel S. Prediction of response to sodium intervention for blood pressure control. *J Hypertens.* 1986;4(Suppl):S343-S346.
76. Langford HG. Step-down therapy for hypertension: effect of weight reduction and sodium restriction on success. *Postgrad Med.* 1985;77:100-105, 108-110.
77. Jula AM, Karanko HM. Effects of left ventricular hypertrophy of long-term nonpharmacological treatment with sodium restriction in mild-to-moderate essential hypertension. *Circulation.* 1994;89:1023-1031.
78. Morgan TO, Myers JB. Hypertension treated by sodium restriction. *Med J Aust.* 1981;2:396-397.
79. Plavinik FL, Rodrigues CI, Zanella MT, Ribeiro AB. Hypokalemia, glucose intolerance, and hyperinsulinemia during diuretic therapy. *Hypertension.* 1992;19(2 Suppl):II26-29.
80. Thompson WG. An assault on old friends: thiazide diuretics under siege. *Am J Med Sci.* 1990;300:152-158.
81. MacGregor GA. The importance of the response of the renin-angiotensin system in determining blood pressure changes with sodium restriction. *Br J Clin Pharmacol.* 1987;23(Suppl 1):21S-26S.
82. Dyer AR, Stamler J, Paul O, Berkson DM, Lepper MH, McKean H, Shekelle RB, Lindberg HA, Garside D. Alcohol consumption, cardiovascular risk factors, and mortality in two Chicago epidemiological studies. *Circulation.* 1977;56:1067-1074.
83. Friedman GD, Klatsky AL, Siegelaub AB. Alcohol intake and hypertension. *Ann Intern Med.* 1983;98:846-849.
84. Harburg E, Ozgoren F, Hawthorne VM, Schork MA. Community norms of alcohol usage and blood pressure: Tecumseh, Mich: *Am J Public Health.* 1980;70:813-820.
85. Klatsky A, Friedman GD, Sieglaub MS, Gerard ME. Alcohol consumption and blood pressure: Kaiser-Permanente Multiphasic health examination data. *N Engl J Med.* 1977;296:1194-2000.
86. Klatsky AL, Friedman GD. The role of alcohol in the epidemiology of hypertension—is alcohol-associated hypertension a common preventable disease? *Ann Clin Res.* 1984;16(Suppl 43):89-96.
87. Saunders JB, Beevers DG, Paton A. Alcohol-induced hypertension. *Lancet.* 1981;2:653-656.
88. Larbi EB, Stamler J, Dyer A, Cooper R, Paul O, Shekelle RB, Lepper M. The population attributable risk of hypertension from heavy alcohol consumption. *Public Health Rep.* 1984;99:316-319.
89. Klatsky AL, Armstrong MA, Friedman GD. Risk of cardiovascular mortality in alcohol drinkers, ex-drinkers, and non-drinkers. *Am J Cardiol.* 1990;66:1237-1242.
90. Gillman MW, Cook NR, Evans DA, Rosner B, Hennekens CH. Relationship of alcohol intake with blood pressure in young adults. *Hypertension.* 1995;25:1106-1110.
91. Altura BM, Altura BT, Gebrewold A, Ising H, Gunther T. Magnesium deficiency and hypertension: correlation between magnesium-deficient diets and microcirculatory changes *in situ.* *Science.* 1984;223:1315-1317.
92. Cappuccio FP, MacGregor GA. Does potassium supplementation lower blood pressure? A metaanalysis of published trials. *J Hypertens.* 1991;9:465-473.
93. Resnick LM. The effects of sodium and calcium in clinical hypertension: mediating role of vitamin D metabolism. *Adv Second Messenger Phosphoprotein Res.* 1990;24:535-541.
94. MacGregor GA, Smith SJ, Markandu N, Banks RA, Sagnella GA. Moderate potassium supplementation in essential hypertension. *Lancet.* 1982;I:567-570.
95. McCarron DA, Morris CD. Blood pressure response to oral calcium in persons with mild to moderate hypertension. A randomized, double-blind, placebo-controlled, crossover trial. *Ann Intern Med.* 1985;103:825-831.
96. Motoyama T, Sano H, Fukuzaki H. Oral magnesium supplementation in patients with essential hypertension. *Hypertension.* 1989;13:227-232.
97. Appel LJ, Moore TJ, Obarzanek E, Vollmer WM, Svetkey LP, Sacks FM, Bray GA, Vogt TM, Cutler JA, Windhauser MM, Lin P, Karanja N. A clinical trial of the effects of dietary patterns on blood pressure. *N Engl J Med.* 1997;336:1117-1124.
98. Folsom AR, Prineas AJ. Drinking water composition and blood pressure: a review of the epidemiology. *Am J Epidemiol.* 1982;115:492-505.

99. Robinson BF. Sodium and calcium handling. In: Kaplan NM, Brenner BM, Laragh JH, eds. *The Kidney in Hypertension*. New York, NY: Raven Press; 1987:21-34.
100. Gruchow HW, Sobocinski KA, Barboriak JJ. Calcium intake and the relationship of dietary sodium and potassium to blood pressure. *Am J Clin Nutr.* 1988;48:1463-1470.
101. Skrabal F, Aubock J, Hortagl H. Low sodium/high potassium diet for prevention of hypertension: possible mechanisms of action. *Lancet.* 1985;2:895-900.
102. Zoccali C, Cumming AMM, Hutcheson MJ, Barnett P, Semple PF. Effects of potassium on sodium balance, renin, noradrenaline, and arterial pressure. *J Hypertens.* 1985;3:67-72.

PART 2

BACKGROUND AND ASSESSMENT

CHAPTER 3

Lipoprotein Metabolism and Atherosclerosis

Henry N. Ginsberg, MD

Detailed reviews of the pathology and cell biology of atherosclerosis are well beyond the scope and goals here (1-5). This chapter summarizes the concepts concerning the development of atherosclerotic lesions and focuses on the role of lipids and lipoproteins in this process.

Pathophysiology of Atherosclerosis

Despite a rapidly growing base of knowledge on the cell and molecular biology of the vessel wall, plasma lipids and lipoproteins still occupy the central, key role in atherogenesis. For this reason, a brief overview of lipoprotein transport is provided to set the stage for a review of atherogenesis. A more detailed description of abnormal lipid and lipoprotein metabolism follows.

Plasma cholesterol and triglycerides, two hydrophobic neutral lipids, are transported through the plasma in the core of lipoprotein particles (Figure 3-1, Table 3-1) (6,7). As shown in Figure 3-1, the polar lipids, triglyceride, and cholesteryl ester are in the core of the spherical particle, while the amphipathic components compose the surface. Chylomicrons, which are assembled in the small intestine, carry dietary triglycerides and cholesterol, whereas very-low-density lipoproteins (VLDLs), which are assembled in the liver, transport mainly endogenously derived core lipids.

In the plasma, chylomicrons and VLDLs lose their triglycerides after interacting with lipoprotein lipase at the vessel wall; they become, respectively, chylomicron remnants and VLDL remnants (the latter are also called intermediate-density lipoproteins). Chylomicrons and VLDLs can also be modified by the exchange of their core triglyceride for core cholesterol ester from high-density lipoproteins (HDLs) and low-density lipoproteins (LDLs) (8). Although the chylomicron remnant is, under normal conditions, almost quantitatively removed from plasma by the liver, VLDL remnants can be converted to LDL in addition to being taken up by the liver (9). Once LDL is formed, it can be removed from plasma by LDL receptors (Figure 3-2) (10,11).

Apoprotein B (apo B) is the major protein on chylomicrons, VLDLs, their remnants, and LDLs (12). The liver makes a full-length version of the polypeptide that is necessary for both the initial secretion of VLDL into the bloodstream and the removal of LDL via the LDL receptor. The intestine makes a shortened version of the protein. Although still required for chylomicron secretion into the circulation, this shortened version lacks the receptor-binding domain present in full-length apo B. All of the apo B–containing lipoproteins are potentially atherogenic if their metabolism is not regulated properly. In contrast, HDL, which has a very different protein—apo A-I—as its major protein, is antiatherogenic under most conditions (13,14).

Apo B–containing lipoproteins transport exogenously and endogenously derived lipids to peripheral tissues: triglycerides for energy use or storage and cholesterol for steroidogenesis and cell membrane structural integrity. To carry out their role, lipoproteins must be able to move across the endothelial covering of blood vessels and reach the extracellular space. LDL is the predominant lipoprotein passing through the endothelial layer, but there is evidence that both chylomicron and VLDL remnants can do so as well. Much of this transendothelial migration occurs in the capillaries, but some occurs in all vessels, including the large arteries. Present concepts of atherogenesis consider the passage of lipoproteins into the subendothelial space of larger arteries as the first critical step in the process.

During the brief contact with the endothelial cell barrier, lipoprotein may be modified (1,3,15,16). Modification may be in the form of oxidation of phospholipid, particularly phosphatidylcholine. Modified apo B–containing lipoproteins may be more liable to aggregate or to stick to extracellular matrix molecules in the subendothelial space. Alternatively, unmodified apo B lipoproteins may stick to matrix molecules in the subendothelial space, triggering interaction with overlying

FIGURE 3-1

Schematic representation of a cross section through a lipoprotein. From Ginsberg HN. Lipoprotein physiology and its relationship to atherogenesis. *Endocrinol Metab Clin North Am.* 1990;19(2):211. Reprinted with permission (7).

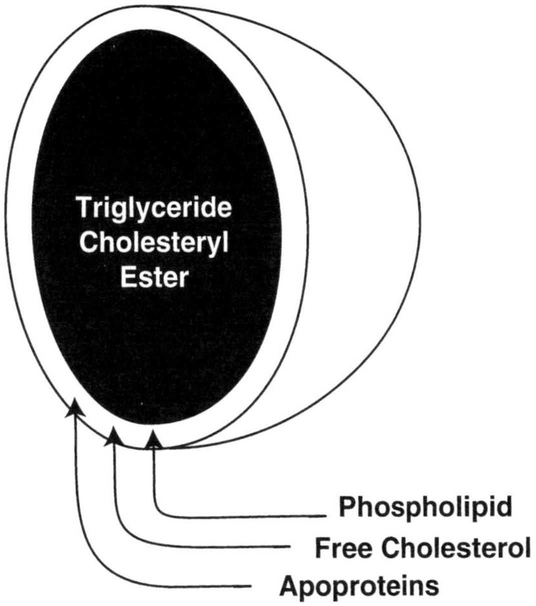

endothelial cells and subsequent modification of the lipoprotein. In either scheme, greater numbers of circulating lipoproteins will be associated by more infiltration and retention of apo B–containing lipoproteins.

Once modification and retention of apo B–containing lipoproteins occurs, signals to the endothelial cells result in the synthesis and display of several cell-adhesion molecules and monocyte chemotactic proteins and the secretion of monocyte colony stimulating factor. Together, these molecules stimulate the formation, sequestration, and transmigration of circulating monocytes at the site of retained subendothelial lipoproteins (4,17). When the monocytes enter the subendothelial space, they are activated and transformed into macrophages. These macrophages take up the modified lipoproteins through one or more receptors and develop into foam cells. They also secrete factors that can stimulate smooth muscle cell proliferation and migration. The monocyte-macrophages and the activated smooth muscle cells also begin to secrete extracellular matrix molecules. At this point, all of the components of the advanced lesion are in place and atherogenesis is well under way (Figure 3-3). In Figure 3-3 monocytes, the major precursor for foam cells in the fatty streak, are shown adhering to the endothelium and then penetrating to the subendothelial space. Oxidized LDL can directly stimulate this by virtue of its lysolecithin content, and lightly oxidized LDL (MM-LDL) can stimulate indirectly by increasing the release of MCP-1 from endothelial cells. Oxidized LDL is a ligand for the scavenger receptor that is expressed as the monocyte differentiates to a tissue macrophage, and this leads to the accumulation of lipids in the developing foam cells. This monocyte/macrophage differentiation can be facilitated by the release of macrophage-colony stimulating factor (M-CSF) from endothelial cells under the influence of MM-LDL. Finally, oxidized LDL can induce endothelial damage and thus facilitate the atherogenic process by allowing entry of elements from the blood and by allowing adherence of platelets (18).

HDLs appear to protect against atherosclerosis (13,14,19). Two major hypotheses have been presented to explain the negative association of HDL cholesterol (HDL-C) levels with atherosclerotic cardiovascular disease. First, there is a large body of data indicating a role for HDL in the reverse transport of cholesterol from tissues throughout the body back to the liver (19,20). Because the apo B–containing lipoproteins, particularly LDL, are thought to deliver several hundred milligrams of cholesterol to peripheral tissues daily, there must be some mechanism to balance that delivery system; HDL is thought to be the vehicle for such balance. Small, cholesterol-poor HDLs (either spherical or disc-like) are good acceptors of membrane-free cholesterol in the extracellular space.

FIGURE 3-2A

Schematic depicting the transport of exogenously derived lipids from the intestine to peripheral tissues and liver via the chylomicron system, as well as the cyclic movement of several apoproteins between HDL and chylomicrons. From Ginsberg HN. Lipoprotein physiology and its relationship to atherogenesis. *Endocrinol Metab Clin North Am.* 1990;19(2):211. Reprinted with permission (7).

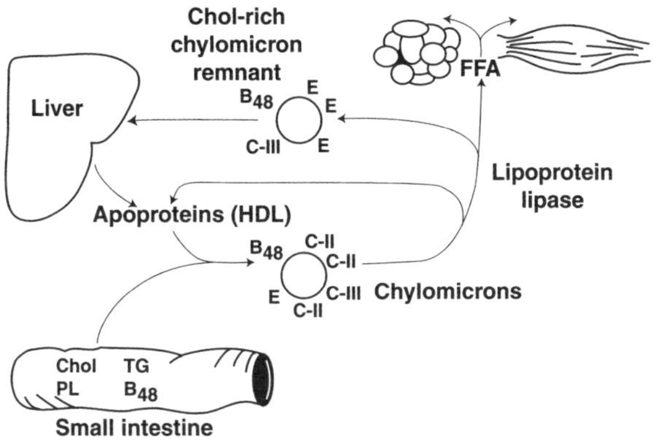

FIGURE 3-2B

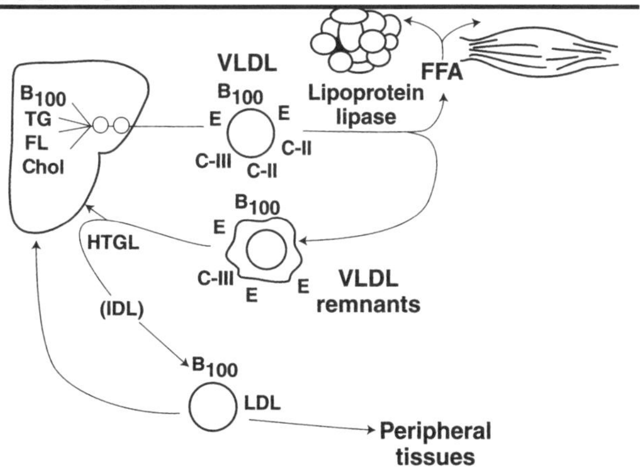

FIGURE 3-3

A schematic outline of the oxidative modification hypothesis showing the several ways in which oxidized low-density lipoprotein (OX-LDL) is potentially more atherogenic than native LDL. LDL = low-density lipoprotein; Ox = oxidized. From Steinberg D. Antioxidants and atherosclerosis: a current assessment. *Circulation*. 1991;84:1420-1425. Reprinted with permission (18).

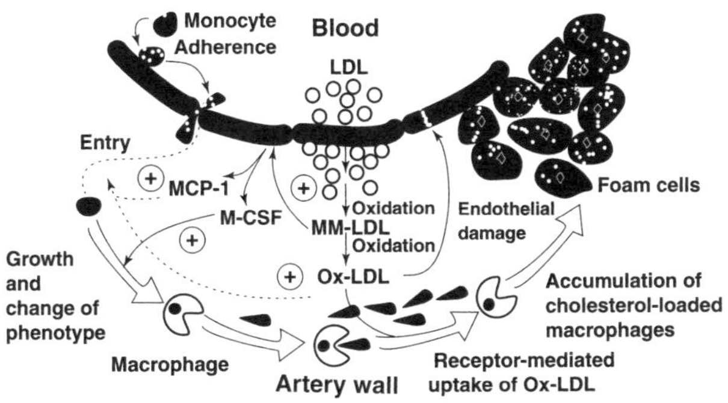

HDL particles enriched in free cholesterol can then be modified by the enzyme lecithin cholesterol acyl transferase, which esterifies the free cholesterol with linoleate from lecithin. The cholesterol ester moves from the surface of the lipoprotein to the core (because of its hydrophobicity), allowing more free cholesterol to be adsorbed onto the surface and resulting in particle enlargement. As HDLs become enriched in cholesterol ester, they become significant vehicles for delivering esters to the liver for conversion to bile acids or excretion as biliary cholesterol.

How this final step in the reverse cholesterol transport pathway is achieved is unclear: Either HDLs deliver the cholesterol esters themselves via selective uptake (21) or endocytosis of the entire HDL particle occurs or they transfer the cholesterol esters to triglyceride-rich VLDLs or chylomicrons via cholesterol ester transfer proteins (22). The latter transfer, which is bimolecular with a triglyceride going to HDL, can be followed by uptake of the chylomicron or VLDL remnant by the liver (Figure 3-4). Free cholesterol is accepted from peripheral tissues by HDL_3, and after esterification may be transferred to apo B-100 lipoproteins. Cholesteryl ester may also be delivered directly to the liver by HDL itself, either by "docking" or by internalization. The significance of each of the three possible transport systems for cholesterol in overall reverse cholesterol transport is unknown (6).

The second potential antiatherogenic activity of HDL relates to its role as an antioxidant or antiaggregant in the vessel wall (23,24,25), although fewer data are available to support this activity. Additionally, apo A-I directly protects LDL against oxidative modification in vitro; apo A-I infusions into swine had an antiatherogenic effect even though plasma HDL concentrations showed no measurable change. This will be an exciting area to watch.

PATHOPHYSIOLOGY OF DYSLIPIDEMIA

As stated earlier, despite the complexity of the atherosclerotic process and the multicomponent nature of advanced lesions, the key initiator of atherogenesis appears to be the presence of increased amounts of retained and modified lipoproteins in the subendothelial space. The latter is a direct consequence of increased quantities of atherogenic lipoproteins in the circulation. It is, therefore, important to understand the pathophysiology of the various dyslipidemias. The following discussion presents some details of the genetic and molecular basis of various dyslipidemias grouped by clinical relevance (Table 3-2):

- isolated hypercholesterolemia,
- hypertriglyceridemia,
- hypertriglyceridemia with hypercholesterolemia, and
- reduced high-density lipoprotein cholesterol.

Isolated Hypercholesterolemia

Elevated concentrations of plasma total cholesterol in a fasting state are usually associated with increased concentrations of plasma LDL-C because LDL carries about 65% to 75% of total plasma cholesterol. If plasma triglyceride concentrations are markedly increased, however, VLDL-C, which is usually 5% to 10% of total plasma cholesterol, may as a result be great enough to elevate total plasma cholesterol concentrations even when LDL-C concentrations are normal. VLDL-C may also be a major component of total cholesterol in dysbetalipoproteinemic subjects (with the apo E2/2 phenotype). The rare patient with significantly elevated HDL-C may also appear to have moderately increased total plasma cholesterol.

Elevations of LDL-C can result from single gene defects, polygenic disorders, and environmental effects on lipoprotein metabolism. Familial hypercholesterolemia,

FIGURE 3-4

Simplified representation of HDL metabolism and the role of HDL in reverse cholesterol transport. From Ginsberg HN. Lipoprotein physiology and its relationship to atherogenesis. *Endocrinol Metab Clin North Am*. 1990;19(2):211. Reprinted with permission (7).

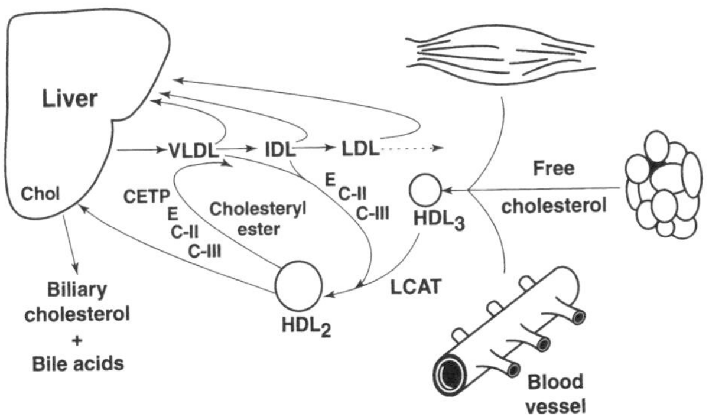

TABLE 3-1

Physical and Chemical Characteristics of the Major Lipoprotein Classes

Lipoprotein	Density (g/dL)	Molecular weight	Diameter (nm)	Lipid (%)[a]		
				Triglyceride	Cholesterol	Phospholipid
Chylomicrons	0.95	~400×10^6	75–1200	80–95	2–7	3–9
VLDL	0.95–1.006	$10\text{-}80 \times 10^6$	30–80	55–80	5–15	10–20
IDL	1.006–1.019	$5\text{-}10 \times 10^6$	25–35	20–50	20–40	15–25
LDL	1.029–1.063	2.3×10^6	18–25	5–15	40–50	20–25
HDL	1.063–1.21	$1.7\text{-}3.6 \times 10^5$	5–12	5–10	15–25	20–30

[a]Percent composition of lipids: apolipoproteins make up the rest.
VLDL = very-low-density lipoprotein; IDL = intermediate-density lipoprotein; LDL = low-density lipoprotein; HDL = high-density lipoprotein.

which occurs in the heterozygous form in approximately 1 of 300 to 500 individuals, is associated with mutations in the gene for the LDL receptor (10). In people with familial hypercholesterolemia, plasma total cholesterol and LDL-C concentrations are increased at birth and remain so throughout life.

Adults heterozygous for familial hypercholesterolemia have total cholesterol levels that range from 300 to 500 mg/dL when untreated, and both tendon xanthomas and premature atherosclerosis with coronary artery disease are common. Plasma triglyceride concentrations are usually normal whereas HDL-C concentrations may be normal or reduced. Metabolic studies showed decreased fractional clearance of LDL apo B in subjects with familial hypercholesterolemia, consistent with reduced numbers of LDL receptors, although increased production of LDL was also

TABLE 3-2

Characteristics of Common Hyperlipidemias

Type	Plasma lipid levels (mg/dL)	Lipoproteins elevated	Clinical signs
Isolated hypercholesterolemia			
Familial hypercholesterolemia:			
Heterozygotes	Total Chol = 300–500	LDL	Usually develop xanthomas in adulthood and vascular disease at 30–50 years of age
Homozygotes	Total Chol = 400–800	LDL	Usually develop xanthomas and vascular disease in childhood
Polygenic hypercholesterolemia	Total Chol = 225–350	LDL	Usually asymptomatic until vascular disease develops; no xanthomas
Isolated hypertriglyceridemia			
Mild	TG = 250–750 (plasma may be cloudy)	VLDL	Asymptomatic; may be associated with increased risk of vascular disease
Severe	TG > 750 (plasma may be milky)	Chylomicrons, VLDL	May be asymptomatic; may be associated with pancreatitis, abdominal pain, hepatosplenomegaly
Hypertriglyceridemia and hypercholesterolemia			
Combined hyperlipidemia	TG = 250–750 Total Chol = 250–500	VLDL LDL	Usually asymptomatic until vascular disease develops; familial form may also be present as isolated high TG or as isolated high LDL cholesterol
Dysbetalipoproteinemia	TG = 250–500 Total Chol = 250–500	VLDL, IDL (LDL normal)	Usually asymptomatic until vascular disease develops; may have palmar or tuboeruptive xanthoma

Chol = cholesterol; LDL = low-density lipoprotein; TG = triglyceride; VLDL = very-low-density lipoprotein; IDL = intermediate-density lipoprotein.

observed (26). The latter may result from more efficient conversion of VLDL to LDL in familial hypercholesterolemia patients concomitant with reduced LDL receptor function and reduced VLDL remnant removal from plasma. However, increased assembly and secretion of VLDL (or more dense apo B–containing lipoproteins) may be concomitant with defective hepatic catabolism of circulating LDL. In any event, markedly elevated levels of LDL-C are the hallmark of familial hypercholesterolemia and are associated with the increased risk for coronary artery disease in these patients. The homozygous form of familial hypercholesterolemia occurs in 1 of 1 million individuals and is associated with plasma cholesterol levels >500 mg/dL, large tendon and planar xanthomas, and very aggressive, premature coronary artery disease.

A second single gene disorder causing significant LDL-C elevations involves a mutation in apo B in the region of the protein associated with binding to the LDL receptor. This disorder has been linked to defective catabolism of LDL in vivo and to hypercholesterolemia that is transmitted in an autosomal dominant fashion (27). Isolated elevations of LDL-C also have been found in subjects with familial combined hyperlipidemia (28).

Polygenic causes of hypercholesterolemia, which are likely to interact with environmental effects on lipoprotein metabolism, are much more common than familial hypercholesterolemia. Most evidence indicates that both overproduction and reduced fractional catabolism of LDL play significant roles in the pathophysiology of this disorder. Production and fractional catabolism are probably affected by dietary saturated fat and cholesterol consumption, age, and level of physical activity. Plasma total cholesterol values are in the range of from 250 mg/dL to 350 mg/dL, plasma triglyceride and HDL cholesterol values are usually normal, and tendon xanthomas are not present. As genes related to regulation of cholesterol metabolism are identified, some of the "polygenic" forms of hypercholesterolemia probably will be found to result from the interaction of two or three specific genes.

Hypertriglyceridemia

Elevated levels of fasting plasma triglycerides in the range of 250 mg/dL to 750 mg/dL are generally associated with increased concentrations only of VLDL triglycerides. When VLDL triglyceride concentrations are markedly elevated (regardless of etiology), or when lipoprotein lipase is either significantly reduced or totally deficient, chylomicron triglycerides may also be present, even after a 14-hour fast. Elevations in plasma triglycerides most often are associated with the synthesis and secretion of excessive quantities of VLDL triglyceride by the liver (29). Hepatic triglyceride synthesis is regulated by substrate flow (particularly the availability of free fatty acids), energy status (particularly the glycogen stores in the liver), and hormonal status (particularly the balance between insulin and glucagon). Obesity, excessive consumption of simple sugars and saturated fats, inactivity, alcohol consumption, and glucose intolerance or diabetes mellitus have been commonly associated with hypertriglyceridemia.

Although no single gene disorder associated with increased hepatic synthesis of triglycerides has been identified, some recent studies have suggested a link between abnormal bile acid metabolism and overproduction of triglycerides in some subjects with hypertriglyceridemia. It is believed that in this group of disorders, sometimes referred to as primary hypertriglyceridemia, only triglyceride synthesis is increased and the liver secretes a normal number of large, triglyceride-enriched VLDL particles. The secretion of a normal number of VLDL particles limits the rate of production of LDL particles, and these subjects may not be at increased risk for coincident elevations of LDL-C. However, subjects with familial combined hyperlipidemia can present with isolated hypertriglyceridemia.

The degree of hypertriglyceridemia present in any individual also depends on the quantity and activity of the two key triglyceride hydrolases: lipoprotein lipase and hepatic lipase. Most data suggest that lipoprotein lipase activity is normal in most subjects with moderate hypertriglyceridemia (250 mg/dL to 500 mg/dL) but may be reduced in more severely affected individuals (having levels greater than 750 mg/dL). However, several recent studies suggested that heterozygosity for lipoprotein lipase deficiency, as a result of specific mutations, can occur in approximately 5% to 10% of the hypertriglyceridemic population (30,31,32). As noted earlier, when VLDL triglyceride concentrations are markedly elevated (greater than 1,000 mg/dL), otherwise normal lipoprotein lipase may be either saturated or actually consumed, so that the patient is relatively deficient in the enzyme during the postprandial period. Chylomicron triglycerides may then add to the hypertriglyceridemia in such patients. If lipoprotein lipase is totally deficient, plasma triglyceride concentrations greater than 2,000 mg/dL are common, with both chylomicrons and VLDL significantly contributing to the hyperlipidemia.

Hepatic lipase activity is frequently elevated in hypertriglyceridemic patients and the meaning of this association is unclear, although it may be relevant to the reduced HDL-C levels found in this condition. Hepatic lipase deficiency is rare in humans and results in defective final catabolism, abnormal remodeling of small VLDLs and intermediate-density lipoproteins, or both (33,34).

Hypertriglyceridemia with Hypercholesterolemia

Hypertriglyceridemia can also occur in two phenotypes in association with hypercholesterolemia. In the first, called *combined hyperlipidemia,* both total plasma triglycerides and LDL-C concentrations are elevated compared with age- and sex-matched controls (28). Although it is likely that a variety of combinations of regulatory defects in lipid metabolism account for a significant number of individuals with this phenotype, a familial form of combined hyperlipidemia

(FCHL) has been identified in which patients may have combined hyperlipidemia, only hypertriglyceridemia, or only elevated LDL-C concentrations. In the familial disorder, which appears to be transmitted as an autosomal dominant gene (35,36), the diagnosis must rest on the presentation of combined hyperlipidemia or the presence of various lipid phenotypes in first-degree family members along with either isolated hypertriglyceridemia or isolated LDL-C elevation in the patient.

Familial Combined Hyperlipidemia. FCHL appears to be associated with secretion of increased numbers of VLDL particles (as determined by the flux of VLDL apo B) (37,38). Hence, individuals with FCHL are predisposed to high levels of plasma VLDL triglycerides if they synthesize triglycerides at an increased rate. Once these individuals assemble and secrete increased numbers of large, triglyceride-rich VLDLs, their plasma triglyceride concentrations depend on their ability to hydrolyze VLDL triglycerides with lipoprotein lipase and, to a lesser degree, hepatic lipase.

The ability to hydrolyze VLDL triglycerides also regulates the generation of LDLs in plasma. Thus, subjects with FCHL who had very high VLDL triglyceride concentrations (and were not able to efficiently catabolize VLDLs) might have normal or reduced numbers of LDL particles in the circulation and thus a normal LDL-C concentration. If these same individuals were able to efficiently catabolize the increased numbers of VLDL particles that were entering their plasma, they would generate increased numbers of LDL particles and have both hypertriglyceridemia and a high LDL-C level. Subjects with FCHL who synthesized only normal quantities of triglycerides and secreted increased numbers of VLDLs carrying normal triglyceride loads would generate increased numbers of LDL particles and have elevated plasma LDL-C concentrations only.

FCHL may occur in as many as 1 in 50 to 1 in 100 Americans and is the most common familial lipid disorder found in survivors of myocardial infarction (28). A link was found between combined hyperlipidemia and insulin resistance (39,40). The pathophysiologic basis for this link has not been elucidated, although increased free fatty acid flux to the liver, which is common in individuals with insulin resistance, could stimulate the secretion of VLDLs.

Dysbetalipoproteinemia. The second disorder in which elevations of both plasma triglycerides and cholesterol can occur is dysbetalipoproteinemia. In this rare disorder affecting 1 in 10,000 people, mutations in the gene for apo E result in synthesis of defective forms of this apolipoprotein. Because apo E appears to play crucial roles in the catabolism of chylomicron and VLDL remnants (41), subjects with defective apo E accumulate these cholesterol ester–enriched remnant lipoproteins in their plasma. Hence, both VLDL triglyceride and VLDL-C concentrations are elevated, and chylomicron remnants are present in fasting plasma from dysbetalipoproteinemic subjects. LDL-C concentrations are not elevated in this disorder. Of interest is that 1 in 100 people are homozygous for the mutant apo E form (the apo E2 isoform); 99% of these homozygous subjects have normal plasma triglyceride and cholesterol concentrations and reduced LDL-C concentrations (possibly resulting from their inability to process VLDLs normally). Thus, a second defect in lipid metabolism must be present in the 1 in 10,000 individuals with the clinically relevant entity, dysbetalipoproteinemia.

Reduced High-density Lipoprotein Cholesterol

Low concentrations of HDL-C are most often seen in patients with coexistent hypertriglyceridemia, although primary hypoalphalipoproteinemia has been identified in both individuals and families (42). The pathophysiologic basis of reduced HDL-C concentrations is not well defined and is probably complex (22,43). The relationship between hypertriglyceridemia and low HDL concentrations probably results from the transfer of cholesterol ester from the core of HDL to VLDL mediated by cholesterol ester transfer protein; the shift of surface components, particularly phospholipids and apolipoproteins C-II and C-III, from HDL to VLDL; and the increased fractional catabolism of the cholesterol ester-poor, surface-poor HDL that results from the first two processes. The complexity of the situation is highlighted by the failure of HDL concentrations to normalize when fasting plasma triglycerides are significantly reduced in most patients who present initially with hypertriglyceridemia and low HDL-C concentrations.

Primary hypoalphalipoproteinemia refers to the state when HDL-C concentrations are markedly reduced but plasma triglyceride concentrations are normal. Although this disorder certainly exists, many subjects who present with this phenotype have had hypertriglyceridemia in the past or have an older (or more obese) first-degree relative who has both low HDL and increased triglyceride concentrations. Hence, carefully conducted family studies and long-term follow-up may be necessary to identify individuals who truly have primary reductions in HDL-C. The basis for such reductions is unknown except for extremely rare situations in which genetic mutations in the area of the apo A-I gene have been described (44,45). Other rare disorders in which HDL-C is severely reduced include Tangiers' disease and lecithin cholesterol acyl transferase deficiency.

SUMMARY

Atherosclerotic cardiovascular disease is the number one cause of death in Western nations and is rapidly becoming a prominent cause of death in economically underdeveloped countries as well. In this review the abnormalities of lipoprotein transport have been linked to the atherogenic process and common lipid phenotypes have been used as examples of atherogenic disorders of lipoprotein metabolism.

Many of the key genes that either alone or, more commonly, in combination result in abnormalities of lipid transport and increased risk of atherosclerosis will be identified in the next several years. These new findings should allow for better dietary and pharmacological approaches to lipid disorders, leading in turn to further reductions in morbidity and mortality from cardiovascular disease.

REFERENCES

1. Steinberg D, Parthasarathy S, Carew TE, Khoo JC, Witztum JL. Beyond cholesterol: Modifications of low density lipoprotein that increase its atherogenicity. *N Engl J Med.* 1989;320:915-924.
2. Ross R. Cell biology of atherosclerosis. *Annu Rev Physiol.* 1995;57:791-804.
3. Berliner JA, Navab M, Fogelman AM, Frank JS, Demer LL, Edwards PA, Watson AD, Louis AJ. Atherosclerosis: basic mechanisms. Oxidation, inflammation, and genetics. *Circulation.* 1995;91:1488-1496.
4. Gimbrone MA Jr, Cybulsky MI, Kume N, Collins T, Resnick N. Vascular endothelium. An integrator of pathophysiological stimuli in atherogenesis. *Ann N Y Acad Sci.* 1995;748:122-132.
5. Clinton SK, Libby P. Cytokines and growth factors in atherogenesis. *Arch Pathol Lab Med.* 1992;116:1292-1300.
6. Gotto AM Jr , Pownall HJ, Havel RJ. Introduction to the plasma lipoproteins. *Methods Enzymol.* 1986;128:3-41.
7. Ginsberg HN. Lipoprotein physiology and its relationship to atherogenesis. *Endocrinol Metab Clin North Am.* 1990;19:211-228.
8. Tall AR. Plasma lipid transfer proteins. *J Lipid Res.* 1986; 27:361-367.
9. Ginsberg HN. Lipoprotein metabolism and its relationship to atherosclerosis. *Med Clin North Am.* 1994;78:1-20.
10. Brown MS, Goldstein JL. How LDL receptors influence cholesterol and atherosclerosis. *Sci Am.* 1984;251:58-66.
11. Brown MS, Herz J, Kowal RC, Goldstein JL. The low-density lipoprotein receptor-related protein: double agent or decoy? *Curr Opin Lipidol.* 1991;2:65-72.
12. Young SG. Recent progress in understanding apolipoprotein B. *Circulation.* 1990;82:1574-1594.
13. Miller GJ, Miller NE. Plasma high density lipoprotein concentration and development of ischaemic heart disease. *Lancet.* 1975;I:16-19.
14. Miller NE, Thelle DS, Forde OH, Mjos OD. The Tromso heart study. High density lipoprotein and coronary heart disease: a prospective case control study. *Lancet.* 1977;8019:965-968.
15. Parthasarathy S, Steinberg D, Witztum JL. The role of oxidized low-density lipoproteins in the pathogenesis of atherosclerosis. *Annu Rev Med.* 1992;43:219-225.
16. Steinberg D. Modified forms of low-density lipoprotein and atherosclerosis. *J Intern Med.* 1993;233:227-232.
17. Cybulsky MI, Gimbrone MA Jr. Endothelial expression of a mononuclear leukocyte adhesion molecule during atherogenesis. *Science.* 1991;251:788-791.
18. Steinberg D. Antioxidants and atherosclerosis. A current assessment. *Circulation.* 1991;84:1420-1425 (from Figure 3-3).
19. Reichl D, Miller NE. Pathophysiology of reverse cholesterol transport. Insights from inherited disorders of lipoprotein metabolism. *Arteriosclerosis.*1989;9:785-797.
20. Glosmet JA. The plasma lecithin: cholesterol acyltransferase reaction. *J Lipid Res.* 1968;9:155-167.
21. Pitmann RC, Knecht TP, Rosenbaum MS, Taylor CA Jr. A non-endocytic mechanism for the selective uptake of high density lipoprotein-associated cholesterol esters. *J Biol Chem.* 1987;262:2443-2451.
22. Tall AR. Plasma high density lipoproteins. Metabolism and relationship to atherogenesis. *J Clin Invest.* 1990;86:379-384.
23. Decossin C, Tailleux A, Fruchart JC, Fievet C. Prevention of in vitro low-density lipoprotein oxidation by an albumin-containing Lp A-I subfraction. *Biochim Biophys Acta.* 1995;1255:31-38.
24. Kunitake ST, Jarvis MR, Hamilton RL, Kane JP. Binding of transition metals by apolipoprotein A-I-containing plasma lipoproteins: inhibition of oxidation of low density lipoproteins. *Proc Natl Acad Sci USA.* 1992;89:6993-6997.
25. Plump AS. Human apolipoprotein A-I. *Proc Natl Acad Sci USA.* 1994;91:9607-9611.
26. Demant T, Carlson LA, Holmquist L, Karpe F, Nilsson-Ehle P, Packard CJ, Shepard J. Lipoprotein metabolism in hepatic lipase deficiency: studies on the turnover of apolipoprotein B and on the effect of hepatic lipase on high density lipoprotein. *J Lipid Res.* 1988;29:1603-1611.
27. Innerarity TL, Mahley RW, Weisgraber KH, Bersot TP, Krauss RM, Vega GL, Grundy SM, Friedl W, Davignon J, McCarthy BJ. Familial defective apolipoprotein B-100: A mutation of apolipoprotein B that causes hypercholesterolemia. *J Lipid Res.* 1990;31:1337-1349.
28. Goldstein JL, Schrott HG, Hazzard WR, Bierman EL, Motulsky AG. Hyperlipidemia in coronary heart disease: II. Genetic analysis in 176 families and delineation of a new inherited disorder, combined hyperlipidemia. *J Clin Invest.* 1973;52:1544-1568.
29. Ginsberg HN. Very low density lipoprotein metabolism in diabetes mellitus. *Diabetes Metab Rev.* 1987;3:571-589.
30. Reymer PW, Gagne E, Groenemeyer BE, Zhang H, Forsyth I, Jansen H, et al. A lipoprotein lipase mutation (Asn291Ser) is associated with reduced HDL cholesterol levels in premature atherosclerosis. *Nat Genet.* 1995;10:6-7.
31. Mailly F, Tugrul Y, Reymer PWA, Bruin T, Seed M, Groenemeyer BF, et al. A common variant in the gene for lipoprotein lipase (Asp9-Asn). Functional implications and prevalence in normal and hyperlipidemic subjects. *Arterioscler Thromb Vasc Biol.* 1995;15:468-478.
32. Minnich A, Kessling A, Roy M, Giry C, DeLangavant G, Lavigne J, Lussier-Cacan S, Davignon J. Prevalence of alleles encoding defective lipoprotein lipase in hypertriglyceridemic patients of French Canadian descent. *J Lipid Res.* 1995;36:117-124.
33. Goldberg L, Le N, Paterniti J, Ginsberg H, Brown WV. Effect of acute inhibition of hepatic triglyceride lipase on very low density lipoprotein metabolism in the cynomolgus monkey. *J Clin Invest.* 1982;70:1184-1192.
34. Breckenridge WC, Little JA, Steiner G, Chow A, Poapst M. Hypertriglyceridemia associated with deficiency of apolipoprotein C-II. *N Engl J Med.* 1978;298:1265-1273.
35. Austin MA. Genetic and environmental influences on LDL subclass phenotypes. *Clin Genet.* 1994;46:64-70.
36. Jarvik GP, Brunzell JD, Austin MA, Krauss RM, Motulsky AG, Wijsman E. Genetic predictors of FCHL in four large pedigrees. Influence of ApoB level major locus predicted genotype and LDL subclass phenotype. *Arterioscler Thromb.* 1994;14:1687-1694.
37. Teng B, Sniderman AD, Soular AK, Thompson GR. Metabolic basis of hyperapobetalipoproteinemia: turnover of apolipoprotein B in low density lipoprotein and its precursors and subfractions compared with normal and familial hypercholesterolemia. *J Clin Invest.* 1986;77:663-672.
38. Arad Y, Ramakrishnan R, Ginsberg HN. Lovastatin therapy reduces low density lipoprotein apo B levels in subjects with com-

bined hyperlipidemia by reducing the production of apo B-containing lipoproteins: implications for the pathophysiology of apo B production. *J Lipid Res.* 1990;31:567-582.

39. Reaven GM. Role of insulin resistance in human disease. *Diabetes.* 1988;37:1595-1607.
40. Reaven GM. Syndrome X: 6 years later. *J Intern Med.* 1994; 236(S736):13-22.
41. Mahley RW. Apolipoprotein E: cholesterol transport protein with expanding role in cell biology. *Science.* 1988;240:622-630.
42. Ginsberg HN, Ngai C, Wang X, Ramakrishnan R. Increased production rates of low density lipoproteins are common in individuals with low plasma levels of high density lipoprotein cholesterol, independent of plasma triglyceride concentrations. *Arterioscler Thromb Vasc Biol.* 1993;13:842-851.
43. Horowitz BS, Goldberg IJ, Merab J, Vanni T, Ramakrishnan R, Ginsberg HN. Increased plasma and renal clearance of an exchangeable pool of apolipoprotein A-I in subjects with low levels of high density lipoprotein cholesterol. *J Clin Invest.* 1993;91:1743-1752.
44. Norum RA, Forte TM, Alaupovic P, Ginsberg HN. Clinical syndrome and lipid metabolism in hereditary deficiency of apolipoproteins A-I and C-III, variant I. In: Angel A, Frohlich J, eds. *Lipoprotein Deficiency Syndromes.* New York, NY: Plenum Publishing, 1986.
45. Norum RA, Lakier JB, Goldstein S, Angel A, Goldberg RB, Block WD, Noffze DK, Dolphin PJ, Edelglass J, Bogorad DD, Alaupovic P. Familial deficiency of apolipoproteins AI and CIII and precocious coronary-artery disease. *N Engl J Med.* 1982;306:1513-1519.

CHAPTER 4

Dietary Assessment for Cardiovascular Disease Risk Determination and Treatment

Sharon Bridges Sugerman, MS, RD, FADA;
Brenda Eissenstat, MS, RD; and Uma Srinith, MS

The evaluation of an individual's dietary intake is an integral part of a complete nutritional assessment. It is critical to understanding the needs of the patient and formulating an appropriate treatment plan but can be the most difficult and frustrating part of the nutrition assessment.

The Role of Dietary Assessment in Cardiovascular Disease

The components of a comprehensive nutrition assessment include

- dietary assessment,
- biochemical data,
- clinical examination and pertinent history,
- anthropometric data, and
- psychosocial data.

Although dietitians frequently gather and evaluate many components of a nutrition assessment, the dietary assessment especially benefits from the expertise and judgment of a dietitian. (See Table 4-1 for examples of relevant nutrition assessment questions.)

The dietary assessment can take many forms but is designed to elucidate the knowledge, attitudes, and practices of the client.

- Knowledge: What does the client know about the foods he or she eats and the effect of diet on health?
- Attitude: How does the client feel about making dietary changes? What degree of commitment does the client exhibit? What barriers may hinder the client's good intentions?
- Practices: What is the client actually eating?

In addition, the dietary assessment can include subjective information about special diets; weight changes; activity levels; food aversions, intolerances, and allergies; and gastrointestinal function. Success in obtaining the needed information depends on the willingness and ability of the client to provide information and on the training and expertise of the person administering the assessment.

The dietitian can use the information obtained to

- determine baseline data and the degree of risk reduction that can be reasonably expected from dietary changes;
- plan the nutrition intervention: learn patient's preferences and needs, establish goals and priorities to meet the most urgent objectives, establish a time line to meet specific objectives because all objectives may not be immediately attainable, and identify and positively reinforce healthful behaviors;
- monitor the client's progress: ensure that nutrition intervention is appropriate and identify new nutrition concerns; and
- evaluate the outcome and success of the intervention: did the patient's risk profile change? Were goals met within a reasonable time? Would a different intervention produce better results, be more cost effective, or take less time?

Regardless of the objectives of the assessment, it is essential to understand the strengths and limitations of the various techniques and be prepared to make adjustments to fit the situation.

Considerations in Choosing an Assessment Technique

The following ought to be considered when an assessment technique is chosen:

- type of information needed,
- type of information that the client can provide,
- the assessment as a teaching tool,
- dietitian- vs client-administered assessment,
- time limitations,
- technology vs cost, and
- needs of special populations.

TABLE 4-1

Important Information Needed in Addition to the Dietary Assessment for a Complete Nutrition Assessment

Meals	**Financial Issues**
Where meals are eaten	Financial resources
Number of meals eaten at home	Food budget
Who prepares home meals	Employment status or occupation
Who shops	Food stamp availability (if Medicaid)
Who the person eats with	
Psychosocial Measures	**Restaurant Related**
Food used to deal with negative emotions	What person orders at restaurant
Food linked to social events	Types of restaurants used
Binge eating	
Presence or absence of social support	
Living arrangements	**Diet Related**
Other behavioral measures related to eating	Current or past therapeutic diets
	Past experience with changing diet
	Level of comprehension
Food Habits	Current compliance with cardiovascular disease risk-reduction diet
Types or brands of fat used at home	
Salt habits	**Other**
Food allergies or intolerance	Marital status
Strong food aversions	Height and weight
Food preferences	Weight history
Proportion convenience, home cooked, restaurant meals	Medical history
Label reading	Family history
Ability to evaluate nutrients in unlabeled food	Medications, food-medicine interaction risk
Appetite	Literacy level and education
Use of supplements	Culture, religion, ethnicity
Problems chewing and swallowing	Travel
	Disease acceptance
	Exercise or physical activity
	Smoking habits
	Alcohol use

Source: Compiled from the results of a survey of experienced cardiovascular disease dietitians.

Type of Information

The objective of the diet assessment influences the scope and detail of the information collected and in large part also determines the kind of instrument needed. Patients with or at high risk for cardiovascular disease (CVD) need counseling and education. During the initial interview, a thorough dietary evaluation is appropriate for guiding the design of effective and acceptable changes to reduce risk. Patients in a cardiac rehabilitation setting who are being seen for follow-up or reevaluation may benefit from a brief assessment that targets specific areas of concern and evaluates the appropriateness of current dietary practices. Quick, easy screening tools may be needed to identify high-risk individuals within the community and can be brief instruments or standardized, less time-intensive instruments, such as food frequency questionnaires (FFQs). Research applications require a much greater degree of precision, accuracy, and reliability in analysis of intake. A thorough discussion of considerations and methodologies for research applications can be found in articles by Wheeler and Buzzard (1) and Kant (2).

The chief nutrients of concern to clinicians caring for cardiac patients and individuals at high risk of disease used to be cholesterol, fatty acids, and sodium. However, a recent comprehensive review of the literature suggested that indexes of overall dietary quality, rather than individual nutrients or foods, may be more related to risk of chronic disease (2). The potential role of antioxidant vitamins, phytochemicals, and folate as independent risk factors for CVD is presently of great interest to researchers.

Type of Information the Client Can Provide

The validity of the assessment also depends on the accuracy of the information the client can provide. Assessment methods have been categorized by some researchers as either retrospective or prospective. Retrospective assessments (ie, 24-hour food recall and FFQ) require the patient or caregiver to remember the foods eaten. Many people have difficulty remembering what they ate or conceptualizing frequency of consumption. The prospective assessment (ie, food diary) involves record keeping concurrent with intake. This type of assessment requires higher literacy and increased commitment. These methods are discussed in detail later in this chapter. The client's ability to provide accurate information is a critical factor in selecting an assessment tool.

The Assessment as a Teaching Tool

Often the assessment can serve two purposes: identifying current food choices and identifying healthful alternatives. An assessment with dual purposes can be especially useful when it is self-administered by someone without easy access to a dietitian. Health fairs, worksite pamphlets, and newspaper articles are examples of instances in which the dual purposes of the assessment are especially valuable. Dietitians can also use assessments to help clients identify healthful alternatives to their present diet or, during follow-up, to compare present and past behaviors. In a nutrition class participants can compare personal evaluations with recommended goals or guidelines. Problematic areas identified by the assessment can then be used as topics for group discussion.

Dietitian- vs Client-administered Assessment

Dietary assessments designed to be self-administered need to be clear and unambiguous. Without the benefit of a dietitian to explain confusing terminology, the information recorded may be inconsistent and an invalid representation of the client's intake. The self-administered assessment must be designed to reflect the unique characteristics of the population for which it is intended. These characteristics should reflect the client's literacy level, degree of commitment, ability to remember foods eaten, regional food preferences, seasonal foods, ability to estimate size of food portions or frequency of use, and understanding of food preparation and ingredients, as well as others (3). Preparing a user-friendly questionnaire can be difficult but expedient when the dietitian is working with many people.

The skilled dietitian can administer an assessment while clarifying statements and asking probing questions to elicit more complete responses (see Food Records in this chapter). The disadvantage, however, is the time required for a personal interview. An alternative that is often more time efficient combines the self-administered assessment with follow-up clarification by the dietitian.

Time Limitations

Time can be a factor not only in administering the assessment but also in evaluating the information. Quick, nutrient- or behavior-specific instruments may require only 10 minutes to 20 minutes to complete and evaluate. A multinutrient evaluation of a 4-day food record will take considerably longer and will depend on the ability of the analyst and use of computer programs. Multiple-day food records also require an extensive time commitment by the client both to learn how to record and measure portions and to complete the food record.

Technology vs Cost

The use of technology can be time efficient, allowing the calculation of multiple nutrients rarely possible within a reasonable time if done by hand. However, an accurate, precise evaluation of the diet is a time-intensive, expensive undertaking. The client must be willing and able to record or recall food intake in great detail. Despite the attractiveness of most computer reports, the assessment is only as good as the data collected, the accuracy of the database, and the coding ability of the analyst.

Computerized dietary analysis software is continually changing. Acquiring a computer system generally represents a significant investment of dollars and training time. The choice of software should reflect available resources (staff, time, and money) and expected needs; considerations in choosing software include

- which nutrient component to use (eg, macronutrients, fatty acids, or antioxidants);
- whether to sort nutrients by item, meal, day, or multiple-day average;
- whether to evaluate nutrients relative to a variety of standards (eg, *Recommended Dietary Allowances, US Dietary Guidelines for Americans,* National Cholesterol Education Program);
- how to report nutrients (per kilogram of body weight or per 1,000 kcal);
- whether to give nutrient percentages from macronutrients, food groups, or food items;
- how to rank sources of macro- and micronutrients;
- whether to use nutrient ratios (eg, polyunsaturated to saturated fat or calcium to phosphorus);
- whether to use measures of overall dietary quality (eg, Index of Nutritional Quality); and
- whether to use such features as calculation of food-group frequencies and food exchanges, personalized dietary reports with text editing, menu planning and recipe evaluation, and physical activity or weight maintenance plans.

Computerized diet analysis programs vary also in the quality of each program's database and operating features. Lee, Nieman, and Rainwater (4) provide a review of eight microcomputer dietary analysis programs. Appendix 1 describes special features of a variety of assessment programs selected for their innovative features, frequent use in peer-reviewed research publications, or availability through US government agencies. The appendix also contains contact information for the Food and Nutrition Information Center (FNIC) of the National Agricultural Library of the US Department of Agriculture (USDA). FNIC maintains a list of nutrient analysis and clinical nutrition programs along with ordering information.

Another source of information is the newsletter *Byting In,* which presents bimonthly updates on issues relating to nutrition and computers and publishes a biannual software buyer's guide. Factors to consider when evaluating a nutrient database are presented in Box 4-1 (5,6). Before software is purchased, it is advisable to thoroughly research the options available, and ease of learning and of use.

Needs of Special Populations

Assessment techniques often have to be adapted to fit the special needs of an individual or group. Populations with strong regional, ethnic, or seasonal food habits are rarely represented accurately by FFQs. To adequately assess dietary intake, dietitians should know as much as possible about the population. (See Chapter 16 for suggestions for working with various ethnic populations, older adults, and lower-literacy individuals, including how to conduct meaningful nutrition assessments, and see Appendix 1 for a list of assessment tools and techniques specifically designed for special populations.) Visual assessment tools, discussed later in this chapter, can be valuable when working with clients when language is a barrier.

Accurately assessing the diet of children and adolescents can be problematic. Often children may be old enough to choose foods independently but have difficulty reporting what or how much they ate (7,8). Dietary assessment information obtained from parents or an adult caregiver is usually accurate for meals but often excludes foods eaten outside the view of adults (9,10). A dietary assessment with children should include a consensus review of the diet with the child and a responsible adult. Even young children may be consuming foods without parents' knowledge.

Domel et al (11) reported that children's recall of food eaten was enhanced by appearance (how the food looked on the plate: its color, shape, or consistency), familiarity, association (with other food items or activities during the meal or day, being hungry, or a food-related illness), and preference (whether the food was liked or disliked). Probing questions may be more informative if associated with ways in which children remember (eg, "Before you had cake at the party, did you eat or drink anything?").

Working with adolescents involves additional considerations. During this period of increasing independence from parents, more food choices are made away from home. Regular meals may be less frequent and snacking may become the major source of nutrients. Adolescents are often able to record the foods they have eaten, with minimal assistance from parents on portion sizes, recipes, brand names, and food preparation methods. Keeping the interest of adolescents can be difficult if the purpose of the assessment is not made relevant to them. Because they are usually interested in anything that will help them look better or be more fit, presenting nutrition as a means toward that end may be beneficial. Chapter 10 discusses additional considerations for CVD risk reduction in children and adolescents.

METHODS FOR COLLECTING AND EVALUATING DIETARY DATA

Many methods exist for collecting and evaluating dietary data, including

BOX 4-1 Factors to Consider in Evaluating Nutrition Software

- Will the program run on your computer? For example, a program written for Windows 95 will not run on a computer equipped with Windows 3.0 as its operating system.
- If you use computer networking, will the software run on a networked computer and under the networking software you are using?
- Do you have enough RAM and hard disk space to support the program?
- Is your monitor's resolution adequate to display the graphics?
- Do you have a CD-ROM drive, if required?
- Is the program documentation easy to use?
- Do the reports generated give you the information you need (for example, diabetic exchanges, percentage of energy from saturated fat)?
- Where does the information for the nutrient database come from?
- What type of quality control does the database have?
- Is the number of database entries inflated by duplicate entries or discontinued foods?
- Do you agree with the calculations used to determine calories required or activity factors?
- Is the software up-to-date? Does it use the most current nutrient data, the food pyramid, or the latest diabetic exchange system?

Source: Adapted with permission from references Sugerman (5) and Grossbauer (6).

- 24-hour food recalls,
- multiple-day food records,
- diet histories,
- food frequency questionnaires,
- brief instruments,
- tools for assessing special nutrients,
- visual assessment tools, and
- informal assessment tools.

Twenty-four-hour Food Recalls

A recall of food intake can be for any length of time but usually covers 24 hours. The recall can be self-administered or obtained by interview. Although one 24-hour record does not accurately represent a person's usual or habitual intake, it can provide a clinically useful overview of the diet if the day is representative. If the previous day was atypical, the participant can be asked to recall or record an earlier typical day or describe in what manner the day was different from usual.

A self-administered assessment form with explicit directions can be used but is less likely to capture the complete intake. Bingham et al (12) recommended that the interview occur in a quiet place, with the review of the food intake moving sequentially through the day beginning with the first food or drink. An interview period from midnight to midnight was used for all participants in the third National Health and Nutrition Examination Survey (NHANES III) (13). This time period can be especially useful for night workers, students, and those who routinely stay up late. Recommended memory aids include graduated measuring tools; two- and three-dimensional food models; household cups, glasses, bowls, and spoons; and a ruler. An experienced interviewer assists by using nonleading prompts to help the person remember, inquiring, for example, whether the day was a workday or leisure day, with whom the day was spent, or where the person traveled. Box 4-2 contains a checklist of items frequently omitted from 24-hour recalls. Frank et al (14) used prompts with schoolchildren that linked the recall with food-related activities, such as parties, sports events, and club meetings.

Large food intakes are frequently underestimated by the recall method and small intakes are often overestimated (15). An analysis of almost 12,000 recalls reported by participants in NHANES II suggested that 31% of respondents significantly underestimated 24-hour intake (16). Those at greatest risk for underreporting were less well educated, heavier, female, and younger.

Food Records

Food records, or diaries, allow for estimates of foods actually consumed during a specific time, usually 1 to 7 days. The multiple-day food record may be the most valid of the usual dietary intake measures (17). The strengths of the food record are that clients can be instructed about record keeping, which minimizes recording errors, and errors of recall are reduced because foods are recorded soon after being eaten. Potential limitations of food records are that recording requires greater literacy skill, time is required to learn how to keep the record and actually record foods, the act of recording can influence the dietary choices of some people, and the time and cost to analyze the record can be substantial.

Food records can be useful in establishing an initial working relationship with a client. Reviewing the foods eaten and associated activities can provide valuable insight into the client's lifestyle. The food record can serve also as a teaching tool, enabling the dietitian and client to focus on current food intake, areas appropriate for behavior change, and problem solving. Positive behaviors can also be identified and reinforced.

BOX 4-2 Final Checklist: Items Often Omitted from 24-Hour Recalls

Interviewer's Sample Script

The foods you have described will help us work together to improve your health. Consequently, I would like to make sure our record is as complete as possible. Here are some foods and drinks that other people often forget to mention. I'll read them now.

- Crackers, breads, rolls, tortillas
- Hot or cold cereals
- Cheese added as a topping on vegetables or on a sandwich
- Chips, candy, nuts, seeds
- Fruit eaten with meals or as a snack
- Coffee, tea, soft drinks, juices
- Beer, wine cocktails, brandy, any other drinks made with liquor

Can you think of anything else you ate or drank yesterday that we have not mentioned?

Source: Adapted from *NHANES III Dietary Interviewer's Manual* (13).

Although the multiple-day food record can validly represent dietary intake, time constraints often obligate practitioners to use abbreviated versions. An informal survey of cardiovascular dietitians in clinical practice found that because of time and resource constraints, the dietitians analyzed only 1 day's diet record per client. Unfortunately, analysis of a 1-day diet record is not a reliable indicator of actual usual intake. (The actual average number of days required to estimate true average intake with statistical confidence for an individual ranges from 27 for energy to 390 for Vitamin A [18].) Seven- to 9-day records estimate an individual's usual nutrient intake to within 10%. In clinical practice, it is preferable to evaluate at least 3 or 4 days of records, including 1 weekend day, because intake often varies from weekdays to weekends (19).

Preparing Participants to Keep Food Records. Complete record-keeping instructions will help reduce the most common problem associated with food records: the recording of incomplete or inaccurate information. A letter of instruction can be sent with a sample record and the record-keeping form (see model letter and sample record in Box 4-3). Alternatively, the nutritionist and client can meet and discuss the instructions before record keeping begins. Whichever method is selected, the need for accurate, detailed information on the following must be emphasized:

- What was eaten? (Name food as specifically as possible; include brand name if applicable.)
- How much was eaten? (Measure or use models to estimate size, eg, ounces, cups, and teaspoons.)
- How was it prepared (eg, broiled, baked, or fried)?
- Were any condiments added at the table (eg, ketchup, salad dressing, or steak sauce)?
- Were any ingredients added while cooking (eg, oil, breading, or sauce)?

The food record form should contain prompts for the details needed and adequate space for the client to write the information clearly. Clients should be encouraged to inquire about preparation method, food ingredients, and fats used in preparation of foods eaten away from home. A set of standardized two-dimensional drawings of food can accompany the recording forms to help clients accurately estimate serving sizes when measuring is not feasible (refer to Visual Assessment Tools in this chapter). Video instruction has also been used to train research study participants in record keeping (a training video available at a nominal cost from Professional Nutrition Systems, Inc, is listed in Appendix 1).

Evaluating the Food Record. When the client returns the food record, the dietitian should review it and ask for clarification as needed to ensure that the record is accurate and complete. Attention to detail by both the client and the dietitian can greatly affect the outcome. Table 4-2 shows the influence on energy, fat, and sodium documentation of including fats and salts used in preparation as reported by the client. For this example, not only does the careful probing for fat and salt used in preparation identify problematic levels of both nutrients, it also illustrates how small amounts of added fat throughout the day produce a total energy excess that could lead to obesity. If meals are being prepared for the client, it can be helpful to verify food preparation with the person doing the cooking.

The evaluation of the food record can range from describing the intake of food relative to food groups in the Food Guide Pyramid to calculating energy, nutrients, and other food components. Most detailed nutrient analyses are now done with computer programs, but manual computations can be done with use of the USDA's *Composition of Foods, Raw, Processed and Prepared* (Handbook No. 8) (20).

When the specific information required by computer programs is incomplete, a table of standardized assumptions can be used to more accurately calculate the fat content of a diet. Table 4-3 lists suggested default serving sizes for added fats, which are based on standards used for national studies, such as NHANES III. Most nutrient databases require the individual entering data to know how much extra fat should be added (an exception is the Nutrient Data System; see Appendix 1). Diet diaries can also be evaluated by an established data analysis center. Costs for such a service vary; some centers charge an additional fee to train staff (see Appendix 1).

Another innovative option for dietary data collection currently under development is the Nutrition Evaluation Scale System (NESSy), a user-friendly computerized data collection and analysis system in which individuals weigh and code their food on their own (21). In validation studies, energy intake was found to be within 5% of the reference standard.

The Three-Day Cholesterol Control Reporter is a machine-scannable, standardized 3-day food record (see Nutrition Scientific in Appendix 1). Users are given a booklet picturing standard portions of a number of common foods with blanks to write in the number of portions of that food eaten on days 1, 2, and 3. Users can also record their food preparation and nonstandard foods consumed. Use of such an instrument significantly reduces coding and data entry time. The booklet can then be sent to the vendor for data entry.

Food Record Scoring Systems. Use of a food-scoring system allows food records to be analyzed more quickly. The Food Record Rating System (FRR) was developed as a counseling and self-monitoring tool for the Multiple Risk Factor Intervention Trial (22). The goal of the FRR is to enable a patient to self-monitor the degree of atherogenicity of the current diet and evaluate improvement. The blood cholesterol raising or lowering effect is measured with each food's B score, as determined by the equation developed by Keys, Anderson, and Grande (23):

$$B = 0.475(SFA - [0.5 \times PUFA]) + (0.2 \times Chol)$$

where SFA is grams of saturated fatty acids, PUFA is grams

BOX 4-3 Food Record and Model Letter of Instructions to Client

Dear ______________________________

Please find enclosed a diet record to complete before your next appointment with the dietitian. The information you provide is important for the dietitian and other health professionals to have when planning appropriate goals and therapy to improve your health. Some people feel they should try to eat especially well on their food record days, but it would be more helpful to you if you eat during the time period you keep the record as you usually would. The following instructions will help you provide a complete and accurate record of the foods you eat and beverages you drink. Please follow them closely.

Begin keeping your food record at least 4 days before your scheduled appointment on . Record all foods and beverages consumed for three days: 2 weekdays and 1 weekend day if possible. Begin the day at midnight one day and end it at midnight the next day to include any late night eating or drinking.

Write down everything you eat and drink all day and evening, including alcohol. Be specific about how the food was prepared and any ingredients added in preparation or at the table.

When possible, measure or weigh your food, or use the enclosed food pictures to help estimate the amount you ate or drank.

Please write down brand names and gram or ounce weights of commercially prepared foods, if you have that information. It is often helpful to bring in the nutrition labels from products you eat when you return the food record.

Include vitamin pills and nutritional supplements you take. For these products, bring in the bottles, packages, or labels to ensure accuracy in your diet record.

If you eat food from a restaurant or fast-food or carryout restaurant, please include the name and phone number of the establishment on your food record. Indicate on your record whether you ate the complete serving. Most servings are a standard size. Your waiter can find out the size of your serving and how it was prepared (eg, type of cooking fat). This information will help make your report more accurate and meaningful.

Skip a line between each new meal or snack time. Take as much space as you need to record everything that seems relevant. If later you realize you left something out and that page is full, put the correct date on a later page and fill in the information you omitted.

If you have any questions, please call the dietitian at ____________________. Thank you.

Sample Food Record

Food Record Day 1 Date: February 25 Day of week: Wednesday

Time	Item	Amount	Preparation Method/Comments
	List food or drink here.	Specify: tsp, oz, Tbsp, cups, g, etc.	Describe how food was prepared or any other relevant comments
7 am	Kellogg's corn flakes[a]	1½ cup	At home
	Reduced-fat milk	8 oz	Left half in bowl
	Cantaloupe	¼ melon	
	Sugar on cereal	2 tsp	
1 pm	Joe's Deli, Chicago		338-2311
	Tuna fish sandwich:		
	Whole-wheat bread	2 slices	Part whole-wheat
	Tuna salad	½ cup	Made with real mayonnaise
	Mayonnaise	1 Tbsp	
	Tomato slices	3 medium	
	Shredded lettuce	1/3 cup	
	French fries	20 fries, thick type	
	Pepsi[b]—not diet	12-oz can	Decaf
5:30 pm	Tom's Bar, Oak Park		848-3269
	Miller lite beer[c]	2 12-oz cans	
	Tortilla chips	2 cups	
	Red salsa	½ cup	
8 pm	Stouffer's Swedish[d] Meatballs w/noodles	9½ oz	Finished all
	Rye bread	2 slices, thin	
	Margarine	2 tsp	Promise light, unsalted
11 pm	Oreos double stuffed[e]	4 cookies	
	Reduced-fat milk	8-oz glass	

[a] Kellogg's Company, Battle Creek MI, 49016
[b] Pepsi-Cola, Pepsico Inc. Somers, NY 10589
[c] Miller Brewing Company Inc, Milwaukee, WI
[d] Nestlé Frozen Food Company, Solon, OH 44139
[e] Nabisco, East Hanover, NJ 07956

TABLE 4-2

The Effect of Detailed Probing About Added Energy Sources, Fat, and Salt on Nutrient Estimates

		Calories	Total fat (g)	Sodium (mg)
Foods listed by patient as "everything I ate"				
Breakfast:	2 slices toast	133	1.8	269
	scrambled eggs	164	13.5	141
	1 slice cheese	80	4.7	304
	small glass orange juice	70	0.1	2
Lunch:	bologna sandwich	313	17.8	848
	3 chocolate chip cookies	139	6.4	95
	1 glass fruit drink	116	0	44
Dinner:	1 bowl salad	11	0.2	7
	baked chicken, 2 pieces	190	9.9	64
	½ cup green peas	62	0.2	70
	¾ cup rice	154	0.3	1
	large glass fruit drink	139	0	52
	strawberry shortcake	191	1.1	16
Snack:	3 cups homemade popcorn with oil	212	14.6	1
	1 can cola	152	0	15
Totals:		2126	69.9[a]	1929
Food actually eaten[b]				
Breakfast:	2 slices toast & margarine	167	5.6	320
	2 eggs scrambled in margarine	215	16.3	674
	1 slice American cheese	80	6.6	304
	5 fl oz orange juice	70	0.1	2
Lunch:	bologna sandwich with lettuce and mayonnaise	361	22.6	908
	3 chocolate chip cookies	139	6.4	95
	10 fl oz fruit drink	116	0	44
Dinner:	1.5 cup lettuce salad & Italian dressing	45	3.7	65
	baked chicken, 2 pieces with crumb coating	402	23.7	839
	½ cup green peas, salted with margarine	79	2.1	266
	¾ cup rice cooked in salted water with margarine	204	6.1	510
	12 fl oz fruit drink	139	0	52
	1 3-inch spongecake with sweetened strawberries and frozen topping	229	4.2	19
Snack:	3 cups homemade popcorn with oil, salted, topped with margarine	364	31.7	568
	1 can cola	152	0	15
Totals:		2765	129[c]	4756

[a] 29.6% of energy.

[b] Nutrient values calculated using Nutrition Data System Version 2.6, University of Minnesota, defaults when patient does not know amounts of fat and salt used.

[c] 42% of energy.

of polyunsaturated fatty acids, and Chol is milligrams of cholesterol. For example, the B score for a 100-g serving of beef bologna would be calculated as follows:

$$\text{Bologna B} = 0.475\ (12.11 - [0.5 \times 0.9]) + (0.2 \times 15) = 8.5$$

The FRR score is the sum of all the B scores for the foods listed in the diet record. The B value is based only on the type of foods eaten, not actual nutrient intake, and it is not adjusted for energy differences. A low score is desirable, and polyunsaturated fatty acids in the diet lower the score. Foods of similar composition are grouped together by content of saturated fatty acids, polyunsaturated fatty acids, and cholesterol. Newer fat-modified foods have not been categorized consistently.

The Cholesterol Saturated Fat Index (CSI) places a numeric value on the relative atherogenicity of foods; it is calculated from a regression equation that weights the effects of cholesterol and saturated fat on the plasma cholesterol concentration (24). CSI can be used to evaluate a day's food intake for its atherogenicity and to help plan low-fat diets. A pocket-sized self-monitoring scorecard based on the CSI was recently developed (25). The CSI for an individual consuming a diet of 40% of energy from fat, 14% of energy from saturated fat (21 g), and 400 mg cholesterol, with a daily intake of 2,000 kcal, is calculated as follows:

$$\text{CSI} = (1.01 \times \text{g saturated fat}) + (0.05 \times \text{mg Chol})$$

$$\text{CSI} = (1.01 \times 21) + (0.05 \times 400) = 41$$

TABLE 4-3

Standardized Assumptions for Serving Sizes and Added Fat in Foods

Item		Standard
Salad dressing		½ Tbsp/cup of lettuce salad
Margarine or butter on bread		1½ tsp/slice as spread or used for grilling (as in a grilled cheese sandwich)
Margarine or butter on English muffin		2 tsp fat/whole muffin
Margarine or butter on mashed potatoes		1 tsp fat/½ cup mashed potatoes
Gravy on mashed potatoes		4 Tbsp gravy/cup mashed potatoes
Cheese, sour cream, salsa, or guacamole on Tex-Mex food or chili		1 Tbsp/taco or 1 Tbsp/cup of "mixed dish" like a casserole
Olives on Tex-Mex food or chili		½ Tbsp/item or cup
Main dish salads on sandwiches		⅓ cup salad (ham, tuna)/sandwich
Meat, poultry, or cheese on sandwich		3 oz total weight meat & cheese (standard) 6 oz total weight meat & cheese (deli)
Sauce on meat, chicken, or fish (any type)		½ Tbsp/oz meat
Sauce on vegetables		4 Tbsp/cup vegetable
Chinese foods (stir-fry with oil)	Light or low-fat	½ tsp/cup
	Regular	1 tsp/cup
	Greasy or oily	2 tsp/cup (add 50% more if main ingredient is breaded and fried)
Fat on a pasta or rice dish		1 tsp/½ cup
Cheese on a pasta or rice dish		1 Tbsp/cup
Milk or cream in cereal		½ cup/cup hot or cold cereal
Milk, cream, or cream substitute (liquid) in coffee or tea		1 Tbsp/6 fl oz
Whipped topping on pudding, gelatin, or sundae		2 Tbsp/½ cup serving
Salt added at table		125 mg/"medium-sized" serving of food
Soy sauce packet		1 tsp soy sauce/packet

Source: Adapted from *NHANES III Dietary Interviewer's Manual* (13).

The Ratio of Ingested Saturated Fat and Cholesterol to Calories (RISCC) is a computer-aided nutritional analysis program that is based on CSI (26). RISCC is best used to document dietary compliance for research purposes when diets contain different amounts of polyunsaturated fatty acids, many fat-modified foods, or foods for which nutrient values are obtained from food labels. A low RISCC score is desirable. For example, the daily RISCC score for the person used in the previous example would be

$$\text{RISCC} = (1.01 \times \text{g SFA}) + (0.05 \times \text{mg Chol})/(\text{kcal}/1{,}000)$$

$$\text{RISCC} = (1.01 \times 21 \text{ g SFA}) + (0.05 \times 400 \text{ mg Chol})/(2{,}000/1{,}000) = 20.5$$

Table 4-4 compares FRR, CSI, and RISCC daily goal scores for step I and step II diets at three energy levels. The RISCC score appears to be somewhat better than the FRR score for distinguishing among National Cholesterol Education Program (NCEP) step I, NCEP step II, and non-NCEP diets and identifying the risk for diets that partially meet NCEP criteria (ie, meet some but not all of the criteria for total fat, saturated fat, and cholesterol). FRR and RISCC calculations require the same amount of a client's time, but calculation of the RISCC score requires computer-aided data analysis, thus increasing professional costs. None of the three calculations takes monounsaturated fatty acids into account.

TABLE 4-4

Comparison of FRR, CSI, and RISCC Daily Goal Scores for Step I and Step II Diets at Three Energy Levels

	FRR		CSI		RISCC	
Energy (kcal)	Step I	Step II	Step I	Step II	Step I	Step II
1200	63	41	22	19	18.3	15.8
2000	65	44	37	26	18.5	13.0
2800	67	47	49	32	17.5	11.4

FRR= Food Record Rating System; CSI = Cholesterol Saturated Fat Index; RISCC = Ratio of Ingested Saturated Fat and Cholesterol to Calories.

Diet History

Diet history refers to any dietary assessment that requires the subject to report about past diet and is often used synonymously for FFQ (see below). However, the diet history was designed to determine a client's usual intake over a specified period of time. As first envisioned by Burke (27), the diet history was a combination of a 3-day diet record, a food frequency checklist, and an interview that included a 24-hour recall and questions about the usual eating pattern such as, "What do you usually have for lunch?" Combining techniques allowed the dietitian to cross check responses and cover total intake.

Box 4-4 provides an example of a multiple-component diet history. The process is time consuming and requires a client who is observant of food intakes. Other researchers have developed improved diet history methods that expand the food frequency list to characterize foods in greater detail (eg, preparation methods, combination foods, and details of food consumed at each meal) (28,29). (In practice, provide ample writing space.)

Food Frequency Questionnaires

FFQs usually consist of two parts: a list of foods or food groups and a set of response options for reporting the usual frequency of consumption of each food or food group for a specific period. Some FFQs conduct a comprehensive nutrient intake survey (30,31), whereas others limit their scope to just a few nutrients, such as fat and cholesterol (32,33). FFQs sometimes ask about preparation details (34). The amount of detail asked about methods of food preparation, serving size, and use of ingredients in combination foods can vary. FFQs can circumvent recent changes in diet that are caused by illness or behavior change because they ask for general descriptions of prior food intake. FFQs can often be self-administered, which requires less time than when they are interviewer-administered. Food frequency responses can also be used to rank individuals according to their usual consumption of foods or food groups.

Unquantified FFQs ask about the number of servings or units of food but not the amounts. An unquantified questionnaire is being used for NHANES III (35). Semiquantitative FFQs ask about portion size (eg, "How often do you consume a medium, 3-oz serving of meat?"). Completely quantified FFQs ask open-ended questions (eg, "When you consume that food, how much do you eat?") or present a choice of small, medium, large, and extra-large servings, with the medium serving amount specified (1). Picture cards can be used to help people better identify their usual serving size (36). When portion-size estimates are included, FFQs can be used to rank individuals according to nutrient intake.

Food lists are usually developed by examining the leading food sources for the target population (as identified by food record or recall surveys) and the nutrients of interest (eg, energy, fat, calcium, and carotenoids). Food lists may be brief and contain general categories of food (eg, vegetables) or may contain more specific categories (eg, fruits and vegetables, side dishes, and main courses). FFQs have become the dietary data collection method of choice for epidemiologic studies investigating the link between diet and disease risk, especially for cancer, because costs of data collection and processing and the respondent burden are usually much lower for FFQs than for multiple diet records or recalls. Some FFQs can be optically scanned (31,33,37), reducing both data entry cost and processing time. An interactive FFQ is available on CD-ROM (see Nutrition DISCovery, 1995, in Appendix 1) (38).

A major limitation of the food frequency method is that details of dietary intake that may significantly affect the nutrient profile are often not measured. For example, FFQs may not accommodate the many low-fat, low-cholesterol versions of traditional high-fat, high-cholesterol foods. Inaccuracies result from an incomplete listing of possible foods, and FFQs need to be modified to reflect cultural or regional food preferences. Important questions have been raised about the cognitive demands of FFQs for memory and for mathematical computations. FFQs require long-term memory and assume that a standard pattern of dietary intake exists. Inaccuracies are common, especially when frequency of consumption and serving size are estimated. As a result, FFQs are not as accurate as recalls or records. Adjustments can be made, however, to address some of these concerns (Table 4-5).

If a clinician's goal is to quickly assess regular intake from the various food groups, a brief, nonquantified FFQ may be adequate. FFQs are especially useful for identifying foods that are used irregularly, but recalls or food records more accurately describe specific foods and amounts eaten.

Brief Instruments

For clinicians, brief instruments may be the quickest, most practical method for giving patients immediate, useful feedback. Commonly used assessment methods such as diet records, 24-hour recalls, and detailed FFQs are lengthy and time consuming. Brief dietary assessment instruments focus on a few foods and nutrients targeted to reduce hyperlipidemia or on behaviors thought to characterize diets associated with high CVD risk. They can be quickly and easily administered and are useful in a variety of settings, such as health fairs, community-wide interventions, clinics, and doctors' offices. They may be quantitative, nonquantitative (similar to FFQs), or behavioral. Box 4-5 contains an example of a brief questionnaire, the Current Dietary Practices Questionnaire, used in CVD research at Baylor University to evaluate compliance with NCEP step I guidelines.

A well-known FFQ-type brief questionnaire is MEDFICTS (meat, eggs, dairy, fried foods, in-baked goods, convenience foods, table fats, snacks), which was developed for NCEP (Box 4-6) (39). MEDFICTS was designed to assess adherence to NCEP step I and step II diets. Frequency of intake and portion sizes of foods that are major and common contributors of fat, saturated fat, and

BOX 4-4 Diet History: Nutrition History Form, Food Intake Record, and Usual Daily Intake

NUTRITION HISTORY FORM

NAME ______________________________ DATE ______________________

OCCUPATION ______________________________

HEIGHT _______ ' _______ "

To be completed by dietitian

PRESENT WEIGHT ___________

GOAL WEIGHT ________ BMI _______

1. How would you generally describe your eating habits? Good ☐ Fair ☐ Poor ☐
2. Has your appetite changed recently? Yes ☐ No ☐
3. How many times a day do you eat? _______
4. How long does it usually take to complete a meal? ______________________
5. When you chew your food, do you: take your time? __________ Or chew a few times, then swallow? __________
6. Do you use a straw to drink beverages? Yes ☐ No ☐
7. Do you chew gum? Yes ☐ No ☐
8. Number of carbonated beverages daily _______
9. Number of caffeine beverages daily (coffee, regular colas, tea)
   ______cups of coffee (regular)
   ______cans of cola (regular, diet, other caffeine-containing sodas, ie, Mellow Yellow, Mountain Dew)
   ______cups of tea (regular)
10. Do you have dentures? Yes ☐ No ☐
11. Do you have any problems chewing? Yes ☐ No ☐
12. Do you take any vitamin/mineral supplements? ______________________
13. List any foods that you do NOT tolerate: ______________________
14. Are you now or have you ever followed any special diet? ___________ If so, what type of diet? ______________________
15. How often do you eat out? ________ times per week. What type of restaurants? ______________________

FOOD INTAKE RECORD

Please indicate which foods you eat.

Food Type	Less Than Once a Week	Not Daily, But at Least Once a Week	Daily
Milk, yogurt			
Cheese			
Red meat			
Poultry			
Fish			
Eggs			
Mixed dishes			
Dried beans, legumes			
Peanut butter			
Nuts			
Breads, cereal			
Potatoes, pasta, rice			
Fruits, juices			
Vegetables			
Margarine, butter			
Cooking oil			
Sour cream, salad dressing			
Ice cream			
Cookies, cake, pie			
Candy			
Soft drink			
Coffee			
Tea, iced tea			
Alcohol			

Describe your usual daily eating pattern (include amount eaten)

Time	Meal	Food/Method of Preparation	Amount Eaten	Calculation (For RD)
	Breakfast			
	Snack			
	Lunch			
	Dinner			
	Snack			

Source: Reprinted with permission from *Medical Nutrition Therapy Across the Continuum of Care.* Chicago, Ill: The American Dietetic Association; 1996.

TABLE 4-5

Problems Frequently Encountered in Food Frequency Questionnaires (FFQs) and Possible Solutions to Increase Accuracy

Problem	Solution
Seasonal foods	Limit the FFQ to 1-3 months
Estimating intake of similar foods (lists of fruits, vegetables, or breads)	Ask "global questions" at onset of questionnaire: "In a typical week, how often do you eat fruit, not counting juices?" "In a typical week, how often do you eat vegetables, not counting green salad and potatoes?"
Quantifying a specific nutrient such as fat	Ask questions such as "In a typical week, how often do you cook with butter, margarine, or oil?" "Do you add other fats for seasoning?" "What type of fat do you use?" "In a typical week, how often do you season foods at the table with butter, margarine, gravy, or oil?"
Cultural or regional foods	Identify common foods of the ethnic group or population. Modify FFQ to include these foods. Ask, "Are there any other foods you eat regularly that were not listed?"
Combination foods—does not report grilled cheese sandwiches when asked about bread and cheese separately	Ask, "Are there any other combination foods, such as sandwiches, soups, or casseroles, you eat regularly that were not separately listed?"
Difficulty estimating portion sizes	Use visual assessment aids: food models or two-dimensional paper models, measuring cups, spoons, common glasses, bowls, and plates of different sizes; compare to common items: a deck of cards (3 oz portion), a golf ball (1 oz portion).
Modified foods or foods for a special diet	Ask, "Do you eat any special, modified, or "diet" foods such as foods with fat or sugar substitutes, nutrient supplements, or beverages?"

cholesterol are recorded quickly. Attention to portion size is important for successful adherence to step I and step II diets. The MEDFICTS food list includes a broad spectrum of food selections in an easy-to-follow table format. MEDFICTS scores were validated against recent 3-day diet records and correlated highly with percentage of energy from fat, saturated fat, and dietary cholesterol (40). MEDFICTS can be quickly completed by clients while they wait in a doctor's office or lipid clinic and can be an effective nutrition education tool when reviewed with a dietitian.

Rate Your Plate, developed by the Pawtucket Heart Health Program, is an eating pattern assessment and educational tool designed for use at cholesterol screenings and educational programs. The primary focus of the questionnaire is identifying food components that affect blood cholesterol. Rate Your Plate was originally designed as a qualitative educational tool rather than a quantitative tool to measure actual dietary intake. However, a strong correlation was found between the Rate Your Plate score and dietary fats, especially saturated fat, estimated by the Willett semiquantitative FFQ (also known as the Harvard semiquantitative FFQ; see Appendix 1 for additional information). The Rate Your Plate questionnaire appears in Box 4-7.

The Food Habits Questionnaire is a 20-item questionnaire that measures dietary patterns related to selecting a low-fat, high-fiber diet during the previous 3-month period (41). The questionnaire is based on anthropological work by Bennett (42) and Jerome (43) and is more behavioral in scope than typical for FFQs. It assesses five behaviors associated with adherence to a low-fat diet:

- modification of meat preparation to reduce fat,
- avoidance of fat as a seasoning,
- replacement of high-fat foods with low-fat alternatives,
- substitution of specially made lower-fat alternatives for high-fat foods, and
- replacement of high-fat foods with fruits or vegetables.

Fat and fiber factor scores can both be calculated. The questionnaire can be adapted for use with ethnic and regional populations and can be self-administered. Questions were raised about its validity with a less-educated male population in Canada, the arrangement of questions within the behavior subscales, and aspects of the questionnaire that were prone to misinterpretation (44). Administering the Food Habits Questionnaire to a client would likely reduce any confusion associated with the questions or scoring.

Table 4-6 presents information about a few of the many other brief instruments developed for use in assessing CVD risk in various settings and populations. Although brief dietary instruments have many applications, they are not without limitations. They are a viable alternative to more

BOX 4-5 **Current Dietary Practices Questionnaire**

CURRENT DIETARY PRACTICES

Please read through the following list. Place a check in the column that reflects your current eating habits. (Use column 3 only if you never eat that particular food.)

	1 Yes	2 No	3 Never eat this food
Vegetables and Fruits			
Eat 3 to 5 servings of vegetables daily (½ c cooked or 1 c raw equals one serving)	☐	☐	☐
Eat 2 to 4 servings of fruit daily (1 medium piece or ½ c canned equals one serving)	☐	☐	☐
Use avocados and olives in small amounts, less than once per week	☐	☐	☐
Milk Products			
Use only skim, ½%, or 1% milk	☐	☐	☐
Use only nonfat or low-fat cheese (<10% fat or no more than 2 to 6 g fat per oz)	☐	☐	☐
Use only nonfat, 1%, or 2% cottage cheese	☐	☐	☐
Use frozen yogurt, sherbet, sorbets, Popsicles, or ice milk in place of ice cream	☐	☐	☐
Avoid nondairy substitutes (coffee creamer, whipped topping, frozen desserts) made from coconut or palm oil	☐	☐	☐
Breads, Cereals, Pasta, and Starchy Vegetables			
Eat only low-fat breads and rolls (white, wheat, rye, french)	☐	☐	☐
Eat only low-fat crackers (saltines, melba toast, flatbread)	☐	☐	☐
Use margarine, herbs, or lemon juice to season pasta and starchy vegetables instead of cream or cheese sauces	☐	☐	☐
Meat, Poultry, Seafood, Eggs, Dried Beans, and Peas			
Eat only lean cuts of beef, pork, lamb, and veal. Examples include chuck, flank, round, and extra-lean ground beef (15% fat or less)	☐	☐	☐
Eat no more than 6 oz total of meat, poultry, fish, and shellfish per day	☐	☐	☐
Avoid high-fat luncheon meats, hotdogs, sausages, and bacon (includes poultry hot dogs and sausage)	☐	☐	☐
Trim all fat from meat and remove skin from poultry before cooking	☐	☐	☐
Eat seafood or poultry more often than red meat	☐	☐	☐
Eat fish at least 2 times per week	☐	☐	☐
Limit intake of liver and other organ meats to once a month or less	☐	☐	☐
Eat no more than 3 egg yolks per week	☐	☐	☐
Eat one or more meatless meals per day	☐	☐	☐
Fats and Oils			
In place of butter use only tub or liquid margarine that lists water or liquid vegetable oil such as safflower, canola, corn, or soybean as the first ingredient	☐	☐	☐

	1 Yes	2 No	3 Never eat this food
Use olive, canola, safflower, sunflower, corn, soybean, or cottonseed oil in place of lard or shortening	☐	☐	☐
Use no more than 6 to 8 tsp of margarine or oil per day	☐	☐	☐
Use salad dressings and mayonnaise made with liquid vegetable oils (fat-free salad dressings are also good choices) in place of those made with real cheese or cream	☐	☐	☐
Use nuts, nut butter, and seeds in moderation (1 serving = 1 tsp)	☐	☐	☐
Avoid seasoning with bacon, salt pork, suet, and ham hocks	☐	☐	☐
Avoid products containing palm oil, palm kernel oil, coconut oil, shortening, lard, beef tallow, or meat fat (may include commercially prepared cookies, crackers, mixes, and granola cereals)	☐	☐	☐
Eat chocolate candy in moderation (1 to 2 times a week)	☐	☐	☐
Snacks			
Avoid high-fat snacks like potato chips, corn chips, cheese puffs, bagel chips, and cheese balls	☐	☐	☐
Use lower-fat snacks like pretzels, unbuttered popcorn, hard bread sticks, and lower-fat crackers	☐	☐	☐
Limit high-fat commercial baked goods (such as doughnuts, sweet rolls, cakes, pies, and pastries) to once a week or less	☐	☐	☐
Use ingredients lower in saturated fat or cholesterol (margarine, vegetable oil, 1% or skim milk, egg substitute) in homemade baked goods	☐	☐	☐
Eat low-fat commercial products such as angel food cake, graham crackers, ginger snaps, vanilla wafers, and fig bars	☐	☐	☐

HOW DID YOUR DIET RATE?

To rate your score, add the number of boxes you checked in Columns 1 and 3. Compare your score to the chart below.

Number of Checkmarks in Columns 1 and 3	Rating
27–33 (100% compliance)	Heart Smart! Congratulations. You are following a diet low in cholesterol, total fat, and saturated fat, which helps you to decrease your risk of heart disease.
24–26 (80% compliance)	Good Start! Set goals to improve compliance in specific areas of your diet.
23 or less (70% compliance)	Be aware! A diet high in cholesterol and fat increases your risk of heart disease. Discuss with a dietitian the guidelines for following a Step I, NCEP, low-fat, low-cholesterol program.

Source: Used with permission from Professional Nutrition Systems, 1993.

c = cup; NCEP = National Cholesterol Education Program.

BOX 4-6 **MEDFICTS Assessment Tool**

In each food category for both Group 1 and Group 2 foods check one square from the "Weekly Consumption" column (number of servings eaten per week) and then check one square from the "Serving Size" column (size of the serving). If you check Rarely/Never, do not check a serving size square. See bottom of next page for score.

Food Category	Weekly Consumption				Serving Size			Score
Meats ■ • Recommended amount per day: 6 oz (equal in size to 2 decks of playing cards). • Base your estimate on the food you consume most often. • Beef and lamb selections are trimmed to ⅛" fat.	Rarely/ never	3 or less	4 or more		Small < 6 oz/d 1 pt	Average 6 oz/d 2 pts	Large > 6 oz/d 3 pts	
1. 10 g or more total fat in 3 oz cooked portion								
Beef—Ground beef, Ribs, Steak (T-bone, Flank, Porterhouse, Tenderloin), Chuck blade roast, Brisket, Meatloaf (w/ground beef), Corned beef **Processed meats**— ¼ lb burger or lg sandwich, Bacon, Lunch meat, Sausage/knockwurst, Hot dogs, Ham (bone-end), Ground turkey **Other meats, Poultry, Seafood**—Pork chops (center loin), Pork roast (Blade, Boston, Sirloin), Pork spareribs, Ground pork, Lamb chops, Lamb (ribs), Organ meats*, Chicken w/ skin, Eel, Mackerel, Pompano	☐	☐ 3 pts	☐ 7 pts		× ☐ 1 pt	☐ 2 pts	☐ 3 pts	
2. Less than 10 g total fat in 3 oz cooked portion								
Lean beef—Round steak (Eye of round, Top round), Sirloin**, Tip and bottom round**, Chuck arm pot roast**, Top loin** **Low-fat processed meats**—Low-fat lunch meat, Canadian bacon, "Lean" fast food sandwich, Boneless ham. **Other meats, Poultry, Seafood**—Chicken, Turkey (w/o skin)§, most Seafood*, Lamb leg shank, Pork tenderloin, Sirloin top loin, Veal cutlets, Sirloin, Shoulder, Ground veal, Venison, Veal chops and Ribs**, Lamb (whole leg, loin, fore-shank, sirloin)**	☐	☐	☐		× ☐	☐ 6 pts†	☐	
Eggs ■ Weekly consumption is the number of times you eat eggs each week					Check the number of eggs eaten each time			
1. Whole eggs, Yolks	☐	☐ 3 pts	☐ 7 pts		≤1 × ☐ 1 pt	2 ☐ 2 pts	≥3 ☐ 3 pts	
2. Egg whites, Egg substitutes (½ c = 2 eggs)	☐	☐	☐		× ☐	☐	☐	
Dairy ■								
Milk—Average serving 1 cup 1. Whole milk, 2% milk, 2% buttermilk, Yogurt (whole milk)	☐	☐ 3 pts	☐ 7 pts		× ☐ 1 pt	☐ 2 pts	☐ 3 pts	

MEDFICTS Assessment Tool, continued

2. Skim milk, 1% milk, Skim buttermilk, Yogurt (nonfat, low-fat)	☐	☐	☐		×	☐	☐	☐
Cheese—Average serving 1 oz								
1. Cream cheese, Cheddar, Monterey Jack, Colby, Swiss, American processed, Blue cheese, Regular cottage cheese (½ c), and Ricotta (¼ c)	☐	☐ 3 pts	☐ 7 pts		×	☐ 1 pt	☐ 2 pts	☐ 3 pts
2. Low-fat and fat-free cheeses, Skim milk mozzarella, String cheese, Low-fat, Skim milk & Fat-free cottage cheese (½ c) and Ricotta (¼ c)	☐	☐	☐		×	☐	☐	☐
Frozen Desserts—Average serving = ½ c								
1. Ice cream, Milk shakes	☐	☐ 3 pts	☐ 7 pts		×	☐ 1 pt	☐ 2 pts	☐ 3 pts
2. Ice milk, Frozen yogurt	☐	☐	☐		×	☐	☐	☐
Frying Foods ■ Average servings: see below. This section refers to method of preparation for vegetables and meat.								
1. French fries, Fried vegetables ½ c), Fried chicken, fish, meat (3 oz)	☐	☐ 3 pts	☐ 7 pts		×	☐ 1 pt	☐ 2 pts	☐ 3 pts
2. Vegetables, not deep fried (½ c), Meat, Poultry, or Fish—prepared by baking, broiling, grilling, poaching, roasting, stewing: (3 oz)	☐	☐	☐		×	☐	☐	☐
In Baked Goods ■ Average serving size: 1 serving								
1. Doughnuts, Biscuits, Butter rolls, Muffins, Croissants, Sweet rolls, Danish, Cakes, Pies, Coffee cakes, Cookies	☐	☐ 3 pts	☐ 7 pts		×	☐ 1 pt	☐ 2 pts	☐ 3 pts
2. Fruit bars, Low-fat cookies/cakes/pastries, Angel food cake, Homemade baked goods with vegetable oils, breads, bagels	☐	☐	☐		×	☐	☐	☐
Convenience Foods ■								
1. Canned, Packaged, or Frozen dinners: eg, Pizza (1 slice), Macaroni & cheese (1 c), Pot pie (1), Cream soups (1 c), Potato, rice & pasta dishes with cream/cheese sauces (½ c)	☐	☐ 3 pts	☐ 7 pts		×	☐ 1 pt	☐ 2 pts	☐ 3 pts
2. Diet/Reduced-calorie or reduced-fat dinners (1 dinner), Potato, rice, and pasta dishes without cream/cheese sauces (½ c)	☐	☐	☐		×	☐	☐	☐
Table Fats ■ **Average serving: 1 Tbsp**								
1. Butter, Stick margarine; Regular salad dressing; Mayonnaise, Sour cream: 2 Tbsp	☐	☐ 3 pts	☐ 7 pts		×	☐ 1 pt	☐ 2 pts	☐ 3 pts
2. Diet and tub margarine, Low-fat and fat-free salad dressings, Low-fat and fat-free mayonnaise	☐	☐	☐		×	☐	☐	☐
Snacks ■								
1. Chips (potato, corn, taco), Cheese puffs, Snack mix, Nuts (1 oz), Regular crackers (½ oz), Candy (milk chocolate, caramel, coconut) (about 1½ oz), Regular popcorn (3 c)	☐	☐ 3 pts	☐ 7 pts		×	☐ 1 pt	☐ 2 pts	☐ 3 pts
2. Pretzels, Fat-free chips (1 oz), Low-fat crackers (½ oz), Fruit, Fruit rolls, Licorice, Hard candy (1 med piece), Bread sticks (1-2 pc), Air-popped or low-fat popcorn (3 c)	☐	☐	☐		×	☐	☐	☐

MEDFICTS Assessment Tool, continued

Total from page 1 ____________
Total from page 2 ____________
FINAL SCORE ____________

† Score 6 pts if this square is checked.
§ All parts not listed in group 1 have < 10 g total fat.
* Organ meats, shrimp, abalone, and squid are low in fat but high in cholesterol.
**Only lean cuts with all visible fat trimmed. If not trimmed of all visible fat, score as if in Group 1.

To Score: For each food category, multiply points in weekly consumption box by points in serving size square and record total in score column. If group 2 foods are checked, no points are scored (except for Group 2 meats, large serving = 6 pts).

Example:

	☐	☐ 3 pts	☑ 7 pts		× ☐ 1 pt	☐ 2 pts	☑ 3 pts	21

Add score on page 1 and page 2 to get final score.

Key:
≥ 70 Need to make some dietary changes
40–70 Step I Diet
< 40 Step II Diet

Source: Adapted from NIH Publication 94-2920 (39).

lengthy instruments when the goal is health screening or assessing perceived behavior change rather than quantifying level of nutrient intake or linking diet to disease. They cannot measure changes in nutrient intake or make associations between diet and disease. To be effective, brief instruments must adequately include the target population's significant nutrient contributors.

Specific food behaviors found, by use of a brief instrument, to correlate with dietary intake in one study may not correlate similarly in another population or in the same population at another time. For example, concerns were recently raised about an excessive emphasis on fat avoidance as a strategy for increased nutritional health (53). Excess weight itself is a major factor in maintaining hyperlipidemia and hypertriglyceridemia, and very-low-fat, high-carbohydrate diets may aggravate these conditions, especially in CVD patients with non-insulin-dependent diabetes mellitus. A common assumption is that excess energy comes from excess fat (54), but if the excess energy comes from sugared cereals, sweetened beverages, fat-free baked goods that are high in sugar, or alcohol, a fat-oriented brief instrument may not be useful in helping the counselor and patient identify the most effective areas for dietary change.

Many tools for collecting and evaluating dietary information are available. Table 4-7 summarizes the applications, advantages, and disadvantages of the major techniques discussed here.

Assessing Special Nutrients

Fatty Acids. The results of studies of the relationship between CVD and *trans* fatty acids, monounsaturated fatty acids, and n-3 fatty acids remain inconclusive. Some studies report protective effects associated with monounsaturated and n-3 fatty acids (55,56,57,58), whereas others have found no association (see Chapter 12). Similarly, research on the relationship among *trans* fatty acids and total serum cholesterol, low-density lipoprotein cholesterol (LDL-C), and high-density lipoprotein cholesterol (HDL-C) requires additional controlled clinical studies.

Individuals interested in assessing the fatty acid content of foods are referred to provisional tables on the n-3 fatty acid content of selected foods (Box 4-8) (59). The USDA's Special Purpose Table 1 contains analytical data on the fat and fatty acid content of foods containing *trans* fatty acids (60). Box 4-9 contains the fat and *trans* fatty acid content of selected foods.

Alcohol. Alcohol raises both plasma triglyceride and HDL-C levels. However, because of the added health risks of excessive alcohol intake, it is not recommended as a means of raising HDL-C (61). Alcohol intake is often difficult to assess accurately. People who consume a lot of alcohol frequently underreport intake, whereas people who consume very little forget to report intake. An alcohol assessment questionnaire appears in Box 4-10.

Sodium. In addition to weight loss, reducing sodium intake is an effective nonpharmacologic way to reduce hypertension in some individuals, especially for those older than age 50, those with a positive family history of hypertension, and African Americans. Several 1-day food records or recalls will provide a reasonable estimate of intake for population groups. A sodium assessment instrument appears in Box 4-11. For FFQ purposes, a standard serving has been identified as 125 mg per medium serving of food (see Appendix 1, HHHQ DIETSYS).

BOX 4-7 **Rate Your Plate Dietary Assessment Tool**

Food Group:	Column 1: 1 point	Column 2: 2 points	Column 3: 3 points	POINTS
MEAT, FISH, AND POULTRY, ETC.				
Meats such as beef, pork, lamb, veal	*Usually eat:* high-fat cuts such as regular hamburger, spareribs, sausage, hot dogs (all kinds).	*Usually eat:* lean cuts such as pork (loin, leg); veal (most cuts); and beef (round, sirloin, extra lean hamburger).	*Always eat:* lean cuts or rarely eat meat.	
Organ meats such as liver, brain, kidney	*Usually eat:* 1-2 times a week.	*Usually eat:* 1-2 times a month.	*Rarely or never eat.*	
Chicken, turkey	*Usually:* cook with skin and eat skin.	*Usually:* cook with skin but discard before eating.	*Usually:* cook without skin.	
Seafood	*Rarely or never eat.*	*Usually eat:* 1 serving or less a week.	*Usually eat:* 2 servings or more a week.	
Breakfast and luncheon meats	*Usually eat:* high-fat varieties such as bologna, sausage, salami, bacon.	*Usually eat:* lean varieties such as Canadian bacon, turkey breast, roast beef, ham.	*Always eat:* lean varieties, or *rarely eat* breakfast and luncheon meats.	
Serving sizes of cooked meat, poultry, seafood, organ, breakfast and luncheon meats	*Usually eat:* large servings (7 oz or more).	*Usually eat:* medium servings (4-6 oz).	*Usually eat:* small servings (3 oz or less).	
Split peas, lentils, dried beans such as kidney, lima, garbanzo	*Rarely or never eat.*	*Usually eat:* at least twice a month.	*Usually eat:* once a week or more.	
Eggs	*Usually eat:* 7 or more a week.	*Usually eat:* 5–6 a week.	*Usually eat:* 4 or less a week or use cholesterol-free egg substitute.	
DAIRY PRODUCTS				
Milk	*Usually use:* whole milk or *never use* milk at all.	*Usually use:* 2% low-fat milk.	*Usually use:* 1% low-fat or skim milk.	
Cheese such as cheddar, American, and Swiss (1 serving = 1 oz)	*Often eat* cheese.	*Sometimes eat* cheese.	*Rarely eat:* cheese or do eat low-fat or calorie-reduced cheese.	
Frozen dairy desserts (1 serving = ½ cup)	*Often eat* ice cream.	*Sometimes eat* ice cream.	*Rarely eat:* ice cream or do eat ice milk, frozen low-fat yogurt, or sherbet.	
			Total, Page 1	

Food Group:	Column 1: 1 point	Column 2: 2 points	Column 3: 3 points	POINTS
FATS, OILS, SWEETS, AND SNACKS				
Fats, oils (for cooking and eating)	*Usually use:* butter, butter blends, shortening and/or lard.	*Usually use:* margarine and/or vegetable oil.	*Always use:* margarine and/or vegetable oil.	
Food preparation	*Usually eat* deep-fried foods.	*Sometimes eat* deep-fried foods.	*Usually eat:* foods cooked by other methods such as baking, steaming, broiling, etc.	
Snacks	*Often eat:* chips, nuts, crackers.	*Sometimes eat:* chips, nuts, crackers.	*Usually eat:* fruit, low-fat crackers, plain popcorn, pretzels.	
Sweets such as donuts, cookies, cakes, pies, sweet rolls, chocolate	*Often eat* sweets.	*Sometimes eat* sweets.	*Rarely or never eat.*	
BREADS, CEREALS, AND PASTA				
Breads, cereals, and pasta (1 serving = 1 slice or ½ cup)	*Rarely or never eat.*	*Usually eat:* 5 servings or less a day.	*Usually eat:* 6 servings or more a day.	
Whole grain products such as whole wheat bread, brown rice, oatmeal, other high-fiber cereal	*Rarely or never eat.*	*Sometimes eat.*	*Usually eat.*	
FRUITS AND VEGETABLES				
Fruits and vegetables (1 serving = 1 piece or ½ cup)	*Rarely or never eat.*	*Usually eat:* 4 servings or less a day.	*Usually eat* 5 or more a day.	
			Total, Page 2	

If Your Score Is: Page 1 total ______ + Page 2 total ______ = Total _______

18–28 There are *many* ways you can make your eating pattern more heart healthy.
29–41 There are *some* ways you can make your eating pattern more heart healthy.
42–54 You are making *many* heart healthy choices.

Goal Setting: To improve my blood cholesterol reading, the first change I will make in my eating pattern is:

____

____

By the time I get my follow-up cholesterol reading, I will make the following changes:

1. ____

2. ____

Changes in eating patterns do not happen overnight. If you find your score in column one, make changes in your eating pattern that move you gradually to column 2 and finally to column 3.
Changes made over time are more likely to become changes you can live with for a lifetime!
Date:____________________

Source: Rate Your Plate (© 1988) is reprinted with permission from Division of Health Education, Memorial Hospital of Rhode Island.

TABLE 4-6

Brief Instruments Used in Cardiovascular Health Screening, Clinical Practice, and Research

Instrument and citation	Description	Administration	Comments
MEDFICTS (40) (Box 4-6)	A well-known FFQ developed for NCEP, designed to assess adherence to Step I and Step II diets	Best information obtained if dietitian administered; can be self-administered, 15–20 min	Can be an effective nutrition education tool when reviewed with a dietitian, correlated highly with % energy from fat, saturated fat, and cholesterol
Current Dietary Practices Questionnaire (Box 4-5)	A quick questionnaire to estimate fat, saturated fat, and cholesterol	Self-administered, 10 min	Easy for self-administration
Food Habits Questionnaire (41)	20-item questionnaire, measures dietary patterns related to a low-fat, high-fiber diet in last 3-months	Can be self-administered or dietitian-administered	Assesses 5 behaviors associated with adherence to a low-fat diet; can be adapted for use with ethnic and regional populations
Block Fat Screener (34,45,46)	15-item semiquantitative FFQ for leading sources of fat; ranks low- or high-fat eaters;	Self-administered, 10 min	Developed from general population data; missing three major Hispanic food sources
Dietary Risk Assessment (32,47)	Brief FFQ, Food for Heart program, literacy level grade 5 to 6, developed for low-income patients in the Southern United States	Interviewer nonnutritionist, 10-15 min	Ranks by dietary atherogenic risk, significant correlation with Keys score; coordinated with set of low-literacy educational materials
Diet Habit Survey (48)	32-item eating behavior test, developed with white, middle-class population; fat scoring based on CSI, + score (low fat, high fiber) associated with 5-year reduction in total serum cholesterol	Self-administered, 30 min; review and scoring by RD, 5 min	Strong test–retest reliability; moderate correlation with 24-hour recall; also evaluates salt and restaurant habits
Eating Pattern Assessment Tool (49)[a]	Weekly FFQ with serving sizes; 2 parts; used in primary care setting; measures compliance with NCEP step I and II diets; developed with primarily white employed population in Minnesota	Self-administered	Good for repeat measures of change over time; useful for screening large numbers of people (work site, health fairs)
Fat Intake Scale (50)[b]	12-item questionnaire that assesses intake of foods high in fat, saturated fat, and cholesterol; used to screen subjects for further intervention; also used as a follow-up quick assessment and counseling tool	Self-administered and self-scored in a few minutes	Compared favorably with 4-day food records for validity; good test-retest reliability; uses metric measures
Quick Check (QC) Programs (33,51)	Developed for health risk screening; 4 instruments: Quick Check for fat, QC for saturated fat, QC for fat and coronary risk, QC for diet progress	Interviewer nonnutritionist; can be coded by bar code scanner (5 to 10 min) or data entry clerk	QC fat and coronary risk is available in Spanish with some adjustments to food items; QC diet progress has many low-fat choices and is the best of the four QC programs for examining dietary change

Instrument and citation	Description	Administration	Comments
"CLIP" Food Log[c]	Cholesterol Lowering Intervention Program, teaching and assessment tool	Users tally food intake for one week; a quick review reveals the main source of cholesterol and saturated fat	Based on the MRFIT Food Record Rating system
Food Scoring Tool[d]	Assesses dietary adherence to a cholesterol-lowering diet		
Rate Your Plate (52) (Box 4-7)	An eating pattern assessment and educational tool used at cholesterol-screening and education programs	Can be self-administered; provides immediate feedback to participants	Provides qualitative information related to food choices, especially fat, saturated fat, and cholesterol content of foods; Spanish and Portuguese versions have been developed

FFQ = food frequency questionnaire; CSI = Cholesterol Saturated Fat Index; NCEP = National Cholesterol Education Program; MRFIT = Multiple Risk Factor Intervention Trial.

[a] The Eating Pattern Assessment Tool (50 forms for $25) is available from: PBNP Materials Coordinator, University of Minnesota, Box 192, UMHC, Minneapolis, MN 55455.

[b] The Fat Intake Scale is available on the Internet (http://weber.u.washington.edu/~retz) or order Document No. 05383 (2-page photocopy) from NAPS c/o Microfiche Publication, PO Box 3513, Grand Central Station, New York, NY 10163-3513. Remit with your order, not under separate cover, $7.75 in US funds on a US bank only. Outside the US and Canada, add postage of $4.50. There is a $15 invoicing charge for all orders filled before payment.

[c] The "CLIP" Food Log is available from the Nutrition Center, University of Pittsburgh, Graduate School of Public Health, Keystone Building, Suite 510, Pittsburgh, PA 15213.

[d] The food scoring tool is available from Dr. C.C. Tagney, Department of Clinical Nutrition, Rush-Presbyterian-St. Luke's Medical Center, 1742 West Harrison 502SSH, Chicago, IL 60612.

Carotenoid Antioxidants. Researchers can use the USDA-National Cancer Institute (NCI) Carotenoid Food Composition Data Base to obtain standardized estimated values derived from analytical data for alpha and beta carotene, lutein plus zeaxanthin, cryptoxanthin, and lycopene for a wide range of fruits, vegetables, and prepared foods (62,63). These differ somewhat from the carotenoid values that are part of the database of the NCI HHHQ DIETSYS. (See Appendix 1 for further information.)

Visual Assessment Tools

Accuracy in self-reports of intakes is improved by the use of measuring devices, food models, or photographs. Visual aids are practical tools that increase the accuracy of portion-size reporting by patients using food records or recalls and can act as cues to help improve recall. Drawings of two-dimensional food models can be either abstract (eg, mounds, squares, and circles) or realistic (eg, pizza wedges, bread slices, and pictures of meat). Two-dimensional models typically require a higher level of abstract and spatial thinking than do three-dimensional models. They are especially good for use with persons used to measuring and quantifying and, when provided in advance, for telephone surveys (64). An assortment of common household plates, glasses, bowls, and measuring spoons can be useful for verifying serving sizes when a dietitian reviews a food record with a client. Comparing a serving of food to a common object, such as a deck of cards (approximately 3 oz meat) or a golf ball (approximately 1 oz) can also help the patient approximate serving sizes. Table 4-8 provides additional examples.

A picture-sort method was developed by Kumanyika et al (36) to administer the NCI FFQ to older adults. Nutrient intakes recorded with the use of this method were comparable with estimates based on 24-hour recalls and were similar to those reported for conventionally administered FFQs. The picture-sort format reportedly was more enjoyable for clients than was the conventional FFQ list of foods and may be helpful for clients with limited literacy or English language skills.

Informal Assessment Techniques

Because the keeping of food records requires literacy, it is not always a feasible choice. Alternatives can be explored with a population unwilling or unable to keep written records, such as poorly educated individuals, recent immigrants, children, some elderly people, people with learning disabilities, or people who are very busy. Alternatives include the use of a tape recorder, telephone interviews, intermittent 24-hour recalls, and review of itemized supermarket tapes. A brief FFQ or usual-behavior measure may be used with any of these techniques to increase the accuracy of information collected. Telephone interviews can be an effective means of assessment when the client is notified in advance and provided with instructions and paper food models (65) but may not be possible with people in unstable housing situations.

A problem frequently noticed when individuals record

TABLE 4-7

Summary of Dietary Intake Assessment Methods

Applications	Advantages	Disadvantages
Thorough diet history		
Provides clinician with best clues to potential barriers and avenues for positive change	Most comprehensive and accurate; provides detailed information on long-term food intake and preparation methods	Most time- and labor-intensive; should be administered by a trained dietitian; nutrient intake estimates are relative, not absolute; may be difficult for individuals, especially those who do not have regular eating patterns
Analyzed food records or successive 24-hour recalls		
Collects information about individual diet patterns; can evaluate criteria such as percent of energy from fat and saturated fat or grams of fiber	High degree of accuracy if patient is trained to keep record and dietitian verifies entries and checks for omissions	Record keeping may influence intake; training to weigh and measure food is time consuming and difficult for some patients; requires a minimum of 3 collection days; usually not feasible for large populations; requires extensive time to clarify and evaluate data
Food scoring system as a way of evaluating diet records (1-3 days)		
Provides immediate feedback to client and increases effectiveness of dietary counseling; used in MRFIT[a] as scoring and teaching tool to change fat intake	Quick and easy method to estimate intake; administered by dietitian or client; based on food record and therefore has fewer recall errors	Same concerns as food records with the exception of data evaluation (see above) and, if self-administered, client must be trained in scoring method
24-hour food recall		
A useful starting point for discussion of dietary concerns; use to compare with a "typical" day, to provide feedback on patient's choices, and to discuss alternatives when needed	Quicker and easier than 3-day food record; most appropriate when assessing average dietary intake of many people	Limited by constraints of memory; major incidence of underreporting across all populations; takes a minimum of 20-40 minutes to collect quality recalls, depending on the complexity of the diet; multiple recalls have same disadvantages as food records (see above)
Food frequency questionnaire (FFQ)		
Can provide a quick overview of the client's typical dietary pattern; if global questions are asked about overall use of fruits and vegetables and type of fat used in cooking, obvious excesses or shortfalls can be identified	Can define current and past intake (past month, past 3 months, or past year); can be mailed and self-administered in some populations	Limited by constraints of memory and patient's ability to "average out" variable intake; actual intake is not identified; nutrient intakes are relative, not absolute; unquantified FFQs make portion size assumptions that may not be valid; can be difficult for people with irregular or seasonal eating patterns to describe diet; may need to be modified for special populations; can take an hour or more for the interviewer to administer an extensive FFQ
Brief questionnaires		
Best used for health screening and counseling; quickly identifies habits to focus on as first steps of change to reduce fat intake and increase fiber, fruit, and vegetable intake	Very quick, inexpensive, and easy to administer	Measures are not quantitatively meaningful; often focus on limited nutrients; cannot assess entire diet; excessive focus on dietary fat reduction and inadequate attention to total calorie intake or overall diet quality; standard instruments may need to be modified for special populations

[a]MRFIT = Multiple Risk Factor Intervention Trial.

BOX 4-8 **Fat, n-3 Fatty Acids, and Cholesterol Content of Selected Foods (100-g Raw Edible Portion)**

	Fat (g)	n-3 Fatty acids (g)[a]	Cholesterol (mg)
Fish			
Anchovy, European	4.8	1.4	—[b]
Bass, striped	2.3	0.8	80
Bluefish	6.5	1.2	59
Carp	5.6	0.3	67
Catfish, channel	4.3	0.3	58
Cod, Atlantic	0.7	0.3	43
Cod, Pacific	0.6	0.2	37
Flounder, unspecified	1.0	0.2	46
Haddock	0.7	0.2	63
Halibut, Pacific	2.3	0.4	32
Herring, Atlantic	9.0	1.6	60
Herring, Pacific	13.9	1.7	77
Mackerel, Atlantic	13.9	2.5	80
Mullet, unspecified	4.4	1.1	34
Ocean perch	1.6	0.2	42
Pike, walleye	1.2	0.3	86
Pompano, Florida	9.5	0.6	50
Sablefish	15.3	1.4	49
Salmon, Atlantic	5.4	1.2	—
Salmon, chinook	10.4	1.4	—
Salmon, pink	3.4	1.0	—
Salmon, sockeye	8.6	1.2	—
Sardines, in sardine oil[c]	15.5	21.1	—
Shark	1.9	0.5	44
Snapper, red	1.2	0.2	—
Sole	1.2	0.1	50
Sturgeon	3.3	0.3	—
Swordfish	2.1	0.2	39
Trout, brook	2.7	0.4	68
Trout, lake	9.7	1.6	48
Trout, rainbow	3.4	0.5	57
Tuna	2.5	0.5	54
Crustaceans			
Crab, Alaska king	0.8	0.3	—
Crab, Dungeness	1.0	0.3	59
Crayfish, unspecified	1.4	0.1	158
Lobster, northern	0.9	0.2	95
Shrimp, unspecified	1.1	0.3	147
Mollusks			
Abalone, New Zealand	1.0	Trace	—
Clam, hard shell	0.6	Trace	31
Clam, littleneck	0.8	Trace	—
Mussel, blue	2.2	0.5	38
Octopus, common	1.0	0.2	—
Oyster, Pacific	2.3	0.6	—
Scallop, unspecified	0.8	0.2	45
Squid, unspecified	1.1	0.3	—
Fish oils			
Cod liver oil	100.0	18.5	570
Herring oil	100.0	11.4	766
MaxEPA[c]	100.0	29.4	600
Salmon oil	100.0	19.9	485
Other sources			
Broccoli	0.4	0.1	0
Butternuts, dried	57.0	8.7	0
Soybeans, green	21.3	3.2	0
Soybean oil	100.0	6.8	0
Strawberries	0.4	0.1	0
Beans, common, dry	1.5	0.6	0
Walnuts, black	56.6	3.3	0

	Fat (g)	n-3 Fatty acids (g)[a]	Cholesterol (mg)
Walnut oil	100.0	10.4	0
Beef, ground	27.0	0.2	85
Butter	81.1	1.2	219
Chicken, broiler fryers	14.8	0.1	90
Lamb, leg	17.6	0.3	71
Pork bacon	57.5	0.8	67

[a] 20:5 plus 22:6.

[b] Dashes indicate a lack of reliable cholesterol data at the present time.

[c] Hall Labs, Portland, OR 97219; Jones Medical Industries, St Louis, MO 63146; Miller Pharmaceutical Group, West Chicago, IL 60185; Moore HL. Drug Exchange, New Britain, CT 06050; Nature Made Vitamins, Los Angeles, CA 91331; The Rexall Group, Ft Lauderdale, FL 33334; Rugby Labs, Rockville Centre, NY 11570; Schein Pharmaceutical, Port Washington, NY 11050; and Sundown Vitamins, Ft Lauderdale, FL 33334

Source: From Hepburn FN, Exler J, Weihrauch JL. Sources of omega-3 fatty acids in seafood, *J Am Diet Assoc.* 1986;86:788-793, and from USDA publication HNIS/PT-103. For additional information, see King I, Childs M, Dorsett C, Ostrander JG, Monsen ER. Shellfish: proximate composition, minerals, fatty acids and sterols. *J Am Diet Assoc.* 1990;90:677-685.

BOX 4-9 ***Fatty Acid Data Selected from Special Purpose Table No. 1: Fat and Fatty Acid Content of Selected Foods Containing Trans-Fatty Acids***

Food Name	Fat added*	Total Poly (g/100 g)	Total MFA (g/100 g)	Total SFA (g/100 g)	Total *trans* (g/100 g)	Trans Fatty Acid (%)
Baked products						
Biscuits, mix	hVeg	1.57	8.54	3.81	3.18	22.85
Biscuits, plain refrig	hSoy	0.83	7.54	2.76	4.06	36.46
Bread, cracked wheat	hSoy, hVeg, SoyL	1.23	2.44	1.31	0.99	19.98
Bread, rye	hSoy, hVeg	0.98	1.24	0.72	0.14	4.82
Bread, white com	hSoy, M/D, B	1.50	2.00	1.02	0.71	15.61
Bread, white com	hSoyO, M/D	0.55	0.42	0.25	0.11	9.24
Cake, pound com	hSoyO, CotO, M/D	2.50	12.51	4.29	5.43	28.13
Cake, pound com	M/D	0.24	0.84	0.34	0.40	28.27
Cookies, choc chip	hSoyO	2.06	14.05	7.89	5.84	24.31
Cookies, choc chip	hVeg	1.33	9.42	10.60	4.00	18.74
Cookies, van sandwich	hSoyO, hCotO	1.18	13.47	4.19	7.09	37.65
Crackers, saltine	L, hSoyO, hCotO	1.77	6.78	4.47	1.51	11.63
Crackers, saltine	hSoyO	0.71	7.27	1.95	3.96	39.92
Crackers, std snack	hVeg	2.44	15.01	3.24	8.18	39.52
Donut, cake-type	Unknown	3.11	14.03	6.51	6.91	29.22
Donut, cake-type	hVeg, beef	1.53	5.93	6.73	0.54	3.81
Rolls, hamburger	SoyO, CotO	2.53	0.92	0.75	0.09	2.15
Rolls, hamburger	hSoyO, M/D	0.96	2.87	1.18	1.29	25.63
Breakfast cereal						
RTE corn and oat	NFA	0.42	0.72	0.58	0.34	19.64
RTE corn and oat	hCotO, hSoyO, M/D	0.29	1.96	0.83	1.24	40.32
RTE corn flakes	hSunO	0.22	0.77	0.16	0.15	12.97
RTE crisp rice	hSunO	0.46	1.51	0.67	0.84	31.58
RTE wheat, bran	hSunO, CocO	0.66	1.50	2.42	0.19	4.15
Dairy products						
Cheese food, Am p/proc	NAF	0.89	6.57	14.62	0.77	3.49
Cheese spread, p/proc	NAF	0.79	5.21	13.88	0.48	2.41
Cheese, Am p/proc	NAF	1.09	7.65	19.36	0.74	2.64
Cheese, cheddar	NAF	1.50	8.18	24.79	0.87	2.54
Milk, whole	NA	0.14	0.86	2.14	0.09	2.79
Yogurt, low-fat, plain	NAF	0.06	0.35	0.95	0.03	2.08
Fast foods						
Milk shake, choc	NA	0.01	0.04	0.12	0.01	3.18
Potato fries, brand a	animalF	0.77	5.58	7.40	1.00	7.25
Potato fries, brand a	VegO	1.44	9.97	4.64	5.22	32.51

Fats and oils						
Lard, brand a	L	14.73	42.50	38.21	1.56	1.64
Marg, stick, brand a	h&lCornO,CanO	11.44	41.92	9.40	17.31	27.58
Marg, stick, brand a	h&lSoyO	16.12	47.45	15.10	25.06	31.86
Marg, tub, brand a	h&lCornO,CanO	19.60	35.73	9.21	11.30	17.52
Marg tub, brand c	hCornO	18.42	13.52	6.61	3.05	7.91
Mayo, brand a	h&lSoyO	41.91	22.86	11.43	3.40	4.46
Salad dressing, French	SoyO	23.50	8.54	5.97	0.27	0.72
Salad dressing, Italian	Soy&OliveO	10.91	6.56	3.53	0.19	0.91
Salad dressing, ranch	hSoy	19.10	15.44	6.90	3.71	8.95
Salad dressing, ranch lc	hSoyO	0.91	0.91	0.36	0.30	13.80
Shortening, brand a	hSoyO, CotO	28.29	42.56	24.75	21.26	22.24
Shortening, brand a	hVegO	5.79	39.36	27.57	12.98	13.99
Shortening, brand c	hMeat&VegO	4.03	47.38	44.19	10.68	11.17
Spread, ex lt	h&lCornO	15.67	14.73	6.72	5.66	15.24
Vegetable oil, brand a	CanO	27.14	61.97	6.48	0.22	0.23
Vegetable oil, brand c	SunO	67.08	16.32	12.20	0.48	0.50
Vegetable oil, brand e	OliveO	9.34	70.72	15.54	0.09	0.09
Meat						
Beef, ground, 20.8% ck	NAF	0.52	7.77	7.23	0.70	4.48
Beef ground, 22.1% ck	NAF	0.50	9.42	8.26	1.04	5.71
Poultry						
Chicken, broiler fat	NAF	12.62	32.13	20.19	0.75	1.15
Chicken, broiler skin	NAF	6.19	15.50	9.54	0.37	1.20
Turkey breast, raw	NAF	0.46	0.53	0.54	0.04	2.30
Turkey, ground a, raw	NAF	1.81	2.64	2.03	0.17	2.55
Turkey, ground b, raw	NAF	1.67	2.63	1.98	0.32	5.15
Sausages and lunchmeat						
Bologna, beef	NAF	0.90	14.83	12.11	1.52	5.48
Bologna, pork	NAF	3.02	13.81	9.92	0.21	0.78
Frankfurter, beef	NAF	0.88	13.91	11.87	0.99	3.71
Frankfurter, pork & beef	NAF	2.92	13.50	9.41	0.18	0.70
Snacks						
Granola bar, chewy	hVegO	1.11	5.58	4.30	1.96	17.88
Popcorn, microwave	hSoyO	3.16	14.99	5.97	7.65	31.74
Popcorn, low-fat	hSoyO	1.50	6.33	2.56	3.16	30.37
Potato chips, brand a	VegO	10.05	19.55	6.23	10.64	29.71
Potato chips, brand b	CotO	19.52	5.97	9.36	0.31	0.90
Potato chips, brand c	VegO	12.84	13.85	10.73	3.95	10.54
Tortilla chips, brand a	VegO	6.00	14.01	3.57	4.12	17.48
Sweets						
Candy, milk choc	CocoaB	1.23	12.08	17.65	0.10	0.31
Frostings, choc	hVegO	1.91	9.96	5.79	3.52	19.91
Frozen dessert, van	Milkfat	0.51	3.16	7.98	0.44	3.76

[a] Fatty acid profiles of similar food items may vary considerably as a result of the type of fat added.

Total Poly = total polyunsaturated fatty acids; Total Mono = total monounsaturated fatty acids; Total SFA = total saturated fatty acids; FA, fatty acids.

Food name abbreviations: refrig = refrigerated; choc = chocolate; van = vanilla; RTE = ready to eat; Am = American; p/proc = pasteurized/processed; Marg = margarine; lc = low calorie; ex lt = extra light; ck = cooked.

Fat added abbreviations: hVeg = hydrogenated vegetable shortening (may contain soybean oil and/or cottonseed oil and coconut oil); hSoy = hydrogenated soybean oil; h = hydrogenated oil; h&l = hydrogenated and liquid oil; SoyL = soy lecithin (emulsifier); M/D = mono- and diacylglycerols; B = butter; L = lard; beef = beef fat; hMeat = hydrogenated meat fat (not specified); animalF = probably animal fat; CanO = canola oil; CocO = coconut oil; CornO = corn oil; CotO = cottonseed oil; OliveO = olive oil; SoyO = soybean oil; SunO = sunflower oil; VegO = vegetable oil (may contain one or more of the following: cottonseed, corn, canola, palm, peanut, soybean); CocoaB = Cocoa butter; NA = not available; NAF = no added fat.

Source: Adapted from Exler J, Lemar L, Smith J. *Fat and Fatty Acid Content of Selected Foods Containing Trans-Fatty Acids. Special Purpose Table No. 1.* Riverdale, Md: US Department of Agriculture, ARS NDL; 1996. (Complete table available from USDA ARS Nutrient Data Laboratory, 4700 River Road, Unit 89, Riverdale, MD 20737, (301) 734-8491, or from http://www.nal.usda.gov/fnic/foodcomp/data/other/other.html.)

BOX 4-10 **Alcohol Assessment Questionnaire**

1. During the past three months, have you consumed any beer, wine, or hard liquor? *(Circle all that apply.)*

IF YOU DRANK BEER:

2. During the past three months, on average, how many days per week or per month did you drink *beer?*
_____ days per week or _____ days per month
3. About how many fluid ounces of beer did you usually drink on each day you drank?
___________ fluid ounces
4. Would you say your consumption of beer varies by season of the year?
☐ Yes ☐ No
(If no, go to question 6.)
5. In what season(s) of the year do you usually drink the most beer? (Circle all that apply.)
Spring Fall Summer Winter

IF YOU DRANK WINE:

6. During the past three months, on average, how many days per week or per month did you drink wine?
_____ days per week or ____ days per month
7. About how many fluid ounces of wine did you usually drink on each day you drank?
____________fluid ounces
8. Would you say your consumption of wine varies by season of the year?
☐ Yes ☐ No
(If no, go to question 10.)
9. In what season(s) of the year do you usually drink the most wine? (Circle all that apply.)
Spring Fall Summer Winter

IF YOU DRANK HARD LIQUOR:

10. During the past three months, on average, how many days per week or per month did you drink hard liquor?
_____ days per week or _____ days per month
11. About how many fluid ounces of hard liquor did you usually drink on each day you drank?
___________ fluid ounces
12. Would you say your consumption of hard liquor varies by season of the year?
☐ Yes ☐ No
(If no, go to question 14.)
13. In what season(s) of the year do you usually drink the most hard liquor? (Circle all that apply.)
Spring Fall Summer Winter

IF YOU DRINK ANY ALCOHOLIC BEVERAGES:

14. On what days of the week do you usually consume alcoholic beverages? (Circle all that apply.)
Monday Tuesday Wednesday Thursday Friday Saturday Sunday

Note to dietitians: More than two alcoholic drinks (24 oz beer, 8 oz wine, or 2 shots hard liquor) per day is not recommended.

Source: Adapted from US Department of Agriculture. *Nationwide food consumption survey.* Hyattsville, Md: US Department of Agriculture; 1987:16-17.

BOX 4-11 Sodium Assessment Questionnaire

Instructions: Check the box under the number of servings that corresponds to the average intake for each food group. Record the corresponding points in the last column and total to obtain the sodium score.

Section I

This section measures food on a *daily* basis.

Food Groups	Serving size	Servings per day	Servings per day	Servings per day	Servings per day	Pts
Dairy foods:						
Milk (skim, 2%, whole, chocolate)	½ cup					
Yogurt	½ cup	5+	3-4	2	0-1	
Nonfat dry milk	2 Tbsp (⅛ cup)	☐	☐	☐	☐	
Evaporated milk	¼ cup	15 pts	11 pts	6 pts	2 pts	
Meat eaten at restaurant or at home:						
Beef, pork, lamb, or venison	2 oz					
Chicken, turkey, or other poultry	2 oz					
Fish (fresh or frozen)	2 oz	6+	4-5	2-3	0-1	
Crab, lobster, scallops, shrimp,		☐	☐	☐	☐	
clams, or oysters	2 oz	16 pts	12 pts	7 pts	2 pts	
Eggs	2					
(Processed meat and fast foods will be counted separately)						
Breads and cereals:						
Bread	1 slice					
Dinner roll	1 small					
Bagel or kaiser roll	½					
Doughnut, muffin, biscuit, or pancake	1 small	7+	5-6	3-4	0-2	
Tortilla or taco shell	2 shells	☐	☐	☐	☐	
Dry cereal	¾ cup	61 pts	48 pts	30 pts	9 pts	
Cooked cereal (cooked with salt)	½ cup					
Noodle, pasta, macaroni, or spaghetti (with salt)	⅓ cup					
Grains, cereal, and pasta cooked *without* salt:						
Cooked cereal (no salt added)	½ cup					
Pasta (no salt added)	½ cup	7+	5-6	3-4	0-2	
Wheat germ	½ Tbsp	☐	☐	☐	☐	
White rice	½ cup	0 pts	0 pts	0 pts	0 pts	
Brown rice	¼ cup					
Vegetables:						
Tossed salad	1 cup					
Raw vegetables	1 cup					
Cooked vegetables	½ cup	6+	4-5	2-3	0-1	
Tomato	1 small	☐	☐	☐	☐	
Low-sodium canned vegetables		5 pts	4 pts	2 pts	1 pt	
or tomato sauce	½ cup					
(potato will be counted separately)						
Canned vegetables	½ cup	6+	4-5	2-3	0-1	
Tomato sauce or spaghetti sauce	½ cup	☐	☐	☐	☐	
		46 pts	34 pts	19 pts	4 pts	
Fruits:						
Fresh fruits (whole grapefruit or banana count as 2 servings)	1 small					
Canned fruits	½ cup	6+	4-5	2-3	0-1	
Fruit juice	½ cup	☐	☐	☐	☐	
Dried fruits (raisins, dates, figs,		1 pt	1 pt	0 pts	0 pts	
or prunes)	2 Tbsp (⅛ cup)					

BOX 4-11 Sodium Assessment Questionnaire, continued

Food Groups	Serving size	Servings per day	Servings per week	Servings per week	Servings per week	Pts
Fats and oils:						
Butter or margarine (salted)	1 Tbsp	6+	4-5	2-3	0-1	
Mayonnaise	1 Tbsp	☐	☐	☐	☐	
Salad dressing (regular or low-cal)	1 Tbsp	33 pts	30 pts	14 pts	3 pts	
(do not count low-sodium products)						
Beverages:						
Coffee or tea	1 cup (8 oz)	3	2	1	0	
Beer	12 oz	☐	☐	☐	☐	
Wine	4 oz	1 pt	0 pts	0 pts	0 pts	
				Section I point total		

Section II

This section measures food on a *weekly* basis.

Food Groups	Serving size	Servings per day	Servings per week	Servings per week	Servings per week	Pts
Cheeses:						
Cheddar, colby, Swiss, provolone, mozzarella, or other natural cheese	1 oz	1+	5-6	3-4	0-2	
Cottage cheese	¼ cup	☐	☐	☐	☐	
Cream cheese	2 oz (4 Tbsp)	9 pts	7 pts	5 pts	2 pts	
Parmesan, grated	2 Tbsp					
Convenience foods:						
Soups (canned or prepared from powder mix)	1 cup					
Macaroni and cheese	1 cup					
Ready-to-serve products (eg, beef		1+	5-6	3-4	0-2	
and vegetable stew, chili, ravioli,		☐	☐	☐	☐	
or spaghetti with meat sauce)	1 cup	43 pts	34 pts	22 pts	6 pts	
Frozen dinners	1 dinner					
Ramen noodles (oriental noodles)	1 pkg					
Fast foods:						
Hamburger or cheeseburger	1 burger					
Fish or chicken sandwich	1 sandwich					
Pizza	⅛ of lg	1+	5-6	3-4	0-2	
Hoagies	4 in.	☐	☐	☐	☐	
Fried chicken	1 thigh	30 pts	24 pts	15 pts	5 pts	
Chicken nuggets	6 nuggets					
Taco or burrito	1					
Processed meat/processed cheese:						
Luncheon meat	1 oz					
Hot dog or sausage	1 (6 in)					
Bacon	1 slice	1+	5-6	3-4	0-2	
Tuna or salmon (canned)	1 oz	☐	☐	☐	☐	
Sardines (canned)	2 med	15 pts	12 pts	8 pts	3 pts	
American or processed cheese	1 oz					
Cheese spread	1 oz (2 Tbsp)					
Snacks:						
Snack crackers	10					
Corn chips or Doritos	10	1+	5-6	3-4	0-2	
Popcorn, salted	2 cups	☐	☐	☐	☐	
Pretzels	½ oz (10 small)	7 pts	5 pts	3 pts	1 pt	

BOX 4-11 Sodium Assessment Questionnaire, continued

Food Groups	Serving size	Servings per day	Servings per week	Servings per week	Servings per week	Pts
Milk-based desserts and drinks:						
Ice cream	1 cup					
Ice milk, soft serve	½ cup	1+	5-6	3-4	0-2	
Custard or pudding	½ cup	☐	☐	☐	☐	
Milkshake or malted milk	½ cup	4 pts	3 pts	2 pts	1 pt	
Eggnog	½ cup					
Sorbet	1 cup					
Potatoes:						
Baked potato	½ potato	1+	5-6	3-4	0-2	
Mashed potato (low sodium)	½ cup	☐	☐	☐	☐	
Hash browns (low sodium)	½ cup	0 pts	0 pts	0 pts	0 pts	
French fries (with no salt added)	10 fries					
Potato items with salt added:						
Mashed potato (with salt added)	½ cup	1+	5-6	3-4	0-2	
Hash browns (with salt added)	½ cup	☐	☐	☐	☐	
French fries	10 fries	9 pts	7 pts	4 pts	2 pts	
Potato chips	1 oz (10 chips)					
Potato salad, potatoes au gratin, or scalloped potatoes	½ cup					
Legumes, beans, nuts, and peanut butter:						
Lentils (cooked w/o salt)	¼ cup					
Beans, cooked w/o salt (ie, kidney beans, lima beans, pinto beans)	¼ cup	1+	5-6	3-4	0-2	
		☐	☐	☐	☐	
Split peas (cooked)	¼ cup	0 pts	0 pts	0 pts	0 pts	
Unsalted nuts (almonds, cashews, peanuts)	1 oz (⅛ cup)					
Low-sodium peanut butter	1 Tbsp					
Salted beans, nuts, and peanut butter:						
Beans, cooked with salt or canned	¼ cup	1+	5-6	3-4	0-2	
Nuts, salted	1 oz	☐	☐	☐	☐	
Peanut butter	1 Tbsp	5 pts	4 pts	2 pts	1 pt	
Seasonings, spices, and sauces:						
Bacon bits	½ cup					
Steak sauce, barbecue sauce, or catsup	1 Tbsp	1+	5-6	3-4	0-2	
Chili sauce	1 Tbsp	☐	☐	☐	☐	
Seasonings with salt	⅛ tsp	7 pts	5 pts	3 pts	1 pt	
Soy sauce	½ tsp					
Gravy	2 Tbsp					
Miscellaneous:						
Molasses	1 tsp					
Brown sugar	1 Tbsp	1+	5-6	3-4	0-2	
Apple butter	1 Tbsp	☐	☐	☐	☐	
Chocolate candy	2 (1-in sq)	0 pts	0 pts	0 pts	0 pts	
Hershey kisses	3 pieces					
					Section II point total	

____________ + ____________ = ____________

Section I Section II Total Sodium Score[a]

[a]If sodium score is >100, dietary modifications should be considered.

BOX 4-11 Sodium Assessment Questionnaire, continued

Section III

This section refers to use of added salt.

1. How often do you, or the person who prepares your food, add salt during cooking?	Always	Sometimes	Seldom	Never	Uncertain
2. How often do you use salt at the table?	Always	Sometimes	Seldom	Never	Uncertain

Source: Chan, Chi Yee (unpublished data).

food intake is that the act of recording often influences their selection of foods and portion sizes. Some clients may also have erratic eating habits that do not show up on a 24-hour recall or 1-day food record. If the client's diet appears too good to be true, it may be useful to ask for an example of an erratic day when the client did not eat properly. Be aware of cognitive messages the client may express when relating the "bad day." Feelings of guilt or shame associated with eating particular foods may indicate disordered eating behavior. (See Chapter 7 for a discussion on assessing disordered eating behavior.)

There are many creative ways of assessing diet that are informal but effective. For example, while clients are waiting for their appointment, ask them to write down what they ate yesterday and circle the foods they believe should be

TABLE 4-8

What's in a Serving?

Food	Looks like...	Estimated serving size
Lean meat, fish, poultry	a deck of cards, bar of soap, or audiocassette	3 oz
Peanut butter[a]	a ping pong ball	2 Tbsp
Cheese[a]	3 dominoes, ½ cup grated	1½ oz
	a thumb or golf ball	1 oz
Cooked rice, pasta, cereal, or vegetables	an ice cream scoop, fist, or racquet ball	½ cup
Fresh whole fruit	a baseball	½ cup or medium-sized fruit
Muffin	a baseball	1 medium
Raw vegetables		
Carrots	12 sticks (stick = 4" × ½")	½ cup
	7 packaged, peeled baby carrots	½ cup
Cucumbers (2" x 7½")	8 slices (⅛" thick)	½ cup
Lettuce, leaf and romaine	2 large leaves	½ cup
Tomatoes, medium	4 slices (¼" thick)	½ cup
Tomatoes, cherry	8	½ cup
Raw fruit		
Grapefruit	½ softball, 2 fruits/lb	½ medium grapefruit
Cantaloupe	small melon, 5½" diameter	¼ melon
Grapes	15 grapes	½ cup

Source: Used with permission from Jaqueline Nugent, RD.

[a] Potentially high-fat choices, limit amount of peanut butter, choose low-fat or nonfat cheese.

changed to improve their health. This quick 24-hour recall can provide information about the client's diet, belief system about food, and knowledge of nutrition. Dietitians should be encouraged to explore and share creative alternatives for assessing dietary intakes.

CONCLUSION

Each of the different dietary assessment techniques discussed has limitations. Some techniques depend on the accuracy of the client's memory; others may require extended amounts of time or expense or sacrifice accuracy for speed. Although it is possible to recognize when clients have difficulty remembering food intake, it is difficult to anticipate suppressions or distortions of memory. It is not uncommon for clients to modify their food record on the basis of a sense of what should be reported.

Despite the inherent limitations of currently available techniques, the valuable information obtained by the dietary assessment is critical to planning all medical therapies for the treatment or prevention of CVD. The validity and accuracy of the methods available will undoubtedly improve as researchers and practitioners continue to develop and test various assessment tools and share them with colleagues.

Acknowledgment

We acknowledge the contributions of Carol Ballew, Jolene Held, Phyllis Stumbo, Pao-Hwa Lin, and the many skilled cardiovascular clinicians who responded to our dietary assessment practice survey: Debra Drewke, Christine Palumbo, Fran Oppenheimer, C Oehme Soule, Jill Stocki, Ilene Kroscher, Jan Kristensen, Diane Petruska, Suzanne Jaax, Lynne Scott, Daniele Branchi, and several more who answered anonymously.

REFERENCES

1. Wheeler ML, Buzzard IM. How to report dietary assessment data. *J Am Diet Assoc.* 1994;94:1255-1256.
2. Kant AK. Indexes of overall diet quality: a review. *J Am Diet Assoc.* 1996;96:785-791.
3. Subar AF, Thompson FE, Smith AF, Jobe JB, Ziegler RG, Potischman N, Schatzkin A, Hartman A, Swanson C, Kruse L, Hayes RB, Lewis DR, Harlan LC. Improving food frequency questionnaires: a qualitative approach using cognitive interviewing. *J Am Diet Assoc.* 1995;95:781-788.
4. Lee RD, Nieman DC, Rainwater M. Comparison of eight microcomputer dietary analysis programs with the USDA Nutrient Data Base for Standard Reference. *J Am Diet Assoc.* 1995;95:858-867.
5. Sugerman S. What makes a software package worth buying? *Byting In.* 1996;7:1,3.
6. Grossbauer S. The numbers game. *Byting In.* 1996;7:3.
7. Baranowski T, Dworkin R, Henske JC, Clearman DR, Dunn JK, Nader PR, Hooks PC. The accuracy of children's self-reports of diet: Family Health Project. *J Am Diet Assoc.* 1986;86:1381-1385.
8. Peterson LA, Carlgren G. Measuring children's diets: evaluation of dietary assessment techniques in infancy and childhood. *Int J Epidemiol.* 1984;13:506-517.
9. Baranowski T, Sprague D, Baranowski JH, Harrison JA. Accuracy of maternal dietary recall for preschool children. *J Am Diet Assoc.* 1991;91:669-674.
10. Davidson FR, Hayek LE, Altschul AM. Towards accurate assessment of children's food consumption. *Ecol Food Nutr.* 1986;18:309-317.
11. Domel SB, Thompson WO, Baranowski T, Smith AF. How children remember what they have eaten. *J Am Diet Assoc.* 1994;94:1267-1272.
12. Bingham SA, Nelson M, Paul AA, Haraldsdottir J, Loken EB, Van Staveren WJ. Methods for data collection at an individual level. In: Cameron ME, Van Staveren WJ, eds. *Manual on Methodology for Food Consumption Studies.* New York, NY: Oxford University Press; 1988:53-106.
13. *NHANES III Dietary Interviewer's Manual.* Rockville, Md: Westat, Inc; 1992.
14. Frank G, Berenson GS, Schilling PE, Moore MC. Adapting the 24-hr recall for epidemiologic studies of school children. *J Am Diet Assoc.* 1977;71:26-31.
15. Gutherie HA. Selection and quantification of typical food portions by young adults. *J Am Diet Assoc.* 1984;84:1440.
16. Klesges RC, Eck LH, Ray JW. Who underreports dietary intake in a dietary recall? Evidence from the second National Health and Nutrition Examination Survey. *J Consult Clin Psychol.* 1995;63:438-444.
17. Block G. A review of validations of dietary assessment methods. *Am J Epidemiol.* 1982;114:492-505.
18. Basiotis PP, Welsh SO, Cronin FJ, Kelsay JL, Mertz W. Number of days of food intake: records required to estimate individual and group nutrient intakes with defined confidence. *J Nutr.* 1987;117:1638-1641.
19. Jackson B, Dujovne CA, DeCoursey S, Beyer P, Brown EF, Hassanein K. Methods to assess relative reliability of diet records: minimum records for monitoring lipid and calorie intake. *J Am Diet Assoc.* 1986;86:1531-1535.
20. Watt BK, Merrill AL. *Composition of Foods, Raw, Processed and Prepared.* Washington, DC: US Dept of Agriculture; 1963. Agriculture Handbook No. 8, rev.
21. Kretsch MJ, Fong AKH. Validity and reproducibility of a new computerized dietary assessment method: effects of gender and educational level. *Nutr Res.* 1993;13:133-146.
22. Remmell PS, Gordor DD, Hall Y, Tillotson JL. Assessing dietary adherence in the Multiple Risk Factor Intervention Trial (MRFIT). *J Am Diet Assoc.* 1980;76:351-356.
23. Keys A, Anderson J, Grande F. Serum cholesterol response to changes in the diet. *Metabolism.* 1965;14:747-787.
24. Connor SL, Gustafson JR, Artaud-Wild SM, Classick-Kohn CJ, Connor WE. The cholesterol-saturated fat index for coronary pre-

vention: background, use, and a comprehensive table of foods. *J Am Diet Assoc.* 1989;89:807-816.

25. Mitchell DT, Korslund MK, Brewer BK, Novascone MA. Development and validation of the Cholesterol-Saturated Fat Index (CSI) scorecard: a dietary self-monitoring tool. *J Am Diet Assoc.* 1996;96:132-136.
26. Harris WS, Held SJ, Dujovne CA. Comparison of two scoring systems used to monitor diets in outpatient clinical trials. *J Cardiovasc Risk.* 1995;2:359-365.
27. Burke BS. The dietary history as a tool in research. *J Am Diet Assoc.* 1947;23:1041-1046.
28. McDonald A, Van Horn L, Slattery M, Hilner J, Bragg C, Caan B, Jacobs O Jr, Liu K, Hubert H, Geruhofer N, Betz E, Havlik D. The CARDIA dietary history: development, implementation and evaluation. *J Am Diet Assoc.* 1991;91:1104-1112.
29. Kohlmeier L. Gaps in dietary assessment methodology: meal vs list-based methods. *Am J Clin Nutr.* 1994;59(suppl):175S-179S.
30. Block G, Hartman AM, Dresser CM, Carroll MD, Gannon J, Gardner L. A data-based approach to diet questionnaire design and testing. *Am J Epidemiol.* 1986;124:453-469.
31. Willett WC, Reynolds RD, Cottrell-Hoehner S, Sampson L, Browne ML. Validation of a semi-quantitative food frequency questionnaire: comparison with a 1-year diet record. *J Am Diet Assoc.* 1987;87:43-47.
32. Ammerman AS, Haines PS, DeVellis RF, Strogatz DS, Keyserling TC, Simpson RJ, Siscovik DJ. A brief dietary assessment to guide cholesterol reduction in low-income individuals: design and validation. *J Am Diet Assoc.* 1991;91:1385-1390.
33. Schaefer D, Selzer RH, Rosenfield F, Darnall J, Blankenhorn DH. Quick Check for Fat: a bar-coded food frequency analysis to accompany blood cholesterol screening. *Nutr Metab CVD.* 1992; 2:174-177.
34. Thompson FE, Byer T. Dietary assessment resource manual. *J Nutr.* 1994;124S:2296S-2298S.
35. US Dept of Health and Human Services. *National Health and Nutrition Examination Survey III Data Collection Forms.* Hyattsville, Md: Public Health Service, Centers for Disease Control, National Center for Health Statistics; 1990.
36. Kumanyika S, Tell GS, Fried L, Martel J, Chinchilli VM. Picture-sort method for administering a food frequency questionnaire to older adults. *J Am Diet Assoc.* 1996;96:137-144.
37. Block G, Thompson FE, Hartman AM, Larkin FA, Guire KE. Comparisons of two dietary questionnaires validated against multiple dietary records collected during a 1-year period. *J Am Diet Assoc.* 1992;92:686-693.
38. Sumner NE, Keller B, Diamond L. Nutrition DISCovery personalized diet assessment program. *J Nutr Educ.* 1996;28:47C.
39. *Step by Step: Eating to Lower Your High Blood Cholesterol.* Bethesda, Md: US Dept of Health and Human Services; 1994. NIH Publication 94-2920.
40. Srinath U, Shacklock F, Scott LW, Jaax S, Kris-Etherton PM. Development of MEDFICTS. *J Am Diet Assoc.* 1993;93:A-105. Abstract.
41. Kristal AR, Shattuck AL, Henry HJ. Patterns of dietary behavior associated with selecting diets low in fat: reliability and validity of a behavioral approach to dietary assessment. *J Am Diet Assoc.* 1990;90:214-230.
42. Bennett JW, Food and culture in Southern Illinois. *Am Sociol Rev.* 1942;7:645-660.
43. Jerome NW. On determining food patterns of urban dwellers in contemporary United States society. In: Arnott MI, ed. *Gastronomy, the Anthropology of Food Habits.* Paris: Mouton Publishers; 1976:91-111.
44. Birkett NJ, Boulet J. Validation of a food habits questionnaire: poor performance in male manual laborers. *J Am Diet Assoc.* 1995;95:558-563.
45. Block G, Clifford C, Naughton MD, Henderson M, McAdams M. A brief dietary screen for high fat intake. *J Nutr Educ.* 1989;21:199-207.
46. Coates RJ, Serdula MK, Byers T, Mokdad A, Jewell S, Leonard SB, Ritenbaugh C, Newcomb P, Mares-Perlman J, Chavez N, Block G. A brief telephone-administered food frequency questionnaire can be useful for surveillance of dietary fat intakes. *J Nutr.* 1995;125:1473-1483.
47. Ammerman AS, DeVellis BM, Haines PS, Keyserling TC, Carey TS, DeVellis RF, Simpson RJ Jr. Nutrition education for cardiovascular disease prevention among low-income populations: description and pilot evaluation of a physician-based model (DRA). *Patient Educ Couns.* 1992;19:5-18.
48. Connor SL, Gustafson JR, Sexton G, Becker N, Artaud-Wild S, Connor WE. The Diet Habit Survey: a new method of dietary assessment that relates to plasma cholesterol changes. *J Am Diet Assoc.* 1992;92:41-47.
49. Peters JR, Quiter ES, Brekke ML, Admire J, Brekke MJ, Mullis RM, Hunninghake DB. The Eating Pattern Assessment Tool (EPAT): a simple instrument for assessing dietary fat and cholesterol intake. *J Am Diet Assoc.* 1994;94:1008-1013.
50. Retzlaff BM, Dowdy AA, Walden MS, Bovbjerg VE, Knopp RH. The Northwest Lipid Research Clinic Fat Intake Scale: validation and utility. *Am J Public Health.* 1997;87:181-185.
51. Selzer RH, Dubois-Blowers L, Darnall J, Azen SP, Blankenhorn DH. Fat and cholesterol intake of attendees at two national USA cardiovascular annual meetings. *Am J Cardiol.* 1991;67:1090-1096.
52. Gans KM, Sundaram SG, McPhillips JB, Hixson ML, Linnan L, Carleton RA. Rate Your Plate: An eating pattern assessment and educational tool used at cholesterol screening and education programs. *J Nutr Ed.* 1993;25:29-36.
53. Allred JB, Too much of a good thing? *J Am Diet Assoc.* 1995;95:417-418.
54. Franz MJ, Horton ES, Bantle JP, Beebe CA, Brunzell JD, Coulston A, Henry RR, Hoogwerf BJ, Stacpoole PW. Nutrition principles for the management of diabetes and related complications. *Diabetes Care.* 1994;17:490-518.
55. Jonnalagadda SS, Mustad VA, Champagne C, Kris-Etherton PM. Margarine and plasma cholesterol: a perspective for dietitians on *trans* fatty acids in the diet. *Perspect Appl Nutr.* 1995;3:9-15.
56. Mattson FH, Grundy SM. Comparison of dietary saturated, monounsaturated, and polyunsaturated fatty acids on plasma lipids and lipoproteins in man. *J Lipid Res.* 1985;26:194-202.

57. Garg A, Bonanome A, Grundy SM, Zhang ZJ, Unger RH. Comparison of a high-carbohydrate diet with a high mono-unsaturated fat diet in patients with non-insulin-dependent diabetes mellitus. *N Engl J Med.* 1988;319:829-864.
58. Herold PM, Kinsella JE. Fish oil consumption and decreased risk of cardiovascular disease: a comparison of findings from animal and human feeding trials. *Am J Clin Nutr.* 1986;43:566-598.
59. Hepburn FN, Exler J, Weihrauch JL. Provisional tables on the content of omega-3 fatty acids and other fat components of selected foods. *J Am Diet Assoc.* 1986;86:788-793.
60. Exler J, Lemer L, Smith J. *Special Purpose Table No. 1.* Riverdale, Md: USDA Nutrient Data Laboratory; 1996.
61. NIH Consensus Development Panel on Triglyceride, High-Density Lipoprotein, and Coronary Heart Disease. Triglyceride, high-density lipoprotein, and coronary heart disease. *JAMA.* 1993;269:505-510.
62. Chug-Ahuja JK, Holden JM, Forman M, Mangels AR, Beecher GR, Lanza E. The development and application of a carotenoid database for fruits, vegetables, and selected multicomponent foods. *J Am Diet Assoc.* 1993;93:318-323.
63. Mangels AR, Holden JM, Beecher GR, Forman M, Lanza E. The carotenoid content of fruits and vegetables: an evaluation of analytical data. *J Am Diet Assoc.* 1993;93:284-296.
64. Posner BM, Borman CL, Morgan JL, Borden WS, Ohls JC. The validity of a telephone-administered 24 hour dietary recall methodology. *Am J Clin Nutr.* 1982;36:546-553.
65. Posner BM, Martin-Munley SS, Smigelski C, Cupples LA, Cobb JL, Schaefer E, Miller DR, D'Agostino RB. Comparison of techniques for estimating nutrient intake: the Framingham Study. *Epidemiology.* 1992;3:171-177.

PART 3

MANAGEMENT

CHAPTER 5

Treatment Algorithms for Patients with Cardiovascular Disease

Donna Alexander-Israel, PhD, RD

To increase the likelihood that patients receive high-quality medical nutrition therapy (MNT) at a reasonable cost, treatment algorithms were developed by the American Dietetic Association (ADA) and the American Heart Association for treating patients with hyperlipidemia, hypertension, and cardiovascular disease (CVD). ADA also developed treatment algorithms for related conditions and diseases (ie, weight management and diabetes [both insulin-dependent and non-insulin-dependent]) as well as other conditions.

American Dietetic Association Algorithms

In 1996 and 1997, ADA published patient protocols for the medical nutrition management of disease states (1, 2). The algorithm for each disease state contains a patient protocol; an expected-outcomes documentation form; appropriate tools; and a guide indicating the expected number of interventions, length of contact time between interventions, cost-per-charge log, and references.

In the protocols, clinical outcomes (blood lipids, weight, and body mass index) and behavioral outcomes (dietary intake, knowledge, etc.) have expected results and associated goals. Patients following the protocols will have clinical goals determined by the physician and behavioral goals agreed on with the dietitian. Clinical outcomes for hypertension, overweight and obesity, and diabetes include blood pressure, body weight, and serum glucose, respectively. Behavioral outcomes include planning diets and meals, using healthful cooking techniques, participating in an exercise program, and quitting smoking.

The MNT protocols for hyperlipidemia (Box 5-1), hypertension (Box 5-2), weight management (Box 5-3), and diabetes (Boxes 5-4 and 5-5) include guidelines for the number and length of sessions, assessment procedures, intervention strategies, and goals.

The algorithm for hyperlipidemia will be used to illustrate the implementation of the MNT protocol. Three sessions spaced 3 to 4 weeks apart are recommended. Blood lipid outcomes are assessed at baseline and after 3 months. Behavioral outcomes are assessed at baseline and after the two intervention sessions. When low-density lipoprotein cholesterol (LDL-C) level is the primary goal of therapy, the timeline is as follows. If LDL-C goals are met after adherence to the step I diet (ie, diet behavioral goals have also been met), then quarterly follow-up is recommended for the first year and biannual follow-up thereafter to assess and reinforce continued adherence. If LDL-C goals are not met after 3 months of nutrition therapy, the patient is instructed on the step II diet and diet adherence is evaluated monthly. Alternative or more aggressive diets are often begun after 4 to 6 weeks of a step I diet if lipid goals are not attained. Six months of dietary intervention with good adherence is recommended for most patients before drug therapy is begun (3). Drug therapy may be started sooner for patients with very high LDL-C levels, CVD, or both. When lipid-lowering drugs are used, a step II diet still should be followed to enhance drug efficacy.

American Heart Association Algorithms

Treatment guidelines for comprehensive risk reduction in patients with coronary and other vascular diseases were recently published by the American Heart Association (3). Figures 5-1 and 5-2 present treatment algorithms for individuals without coronary heart disease (CHD) or other atherosclerotic disease and patients diagnosed with CHD. Diet is a key component of both treatment algorithms. A step I diet is recommended for individuals without CHD—as is recommended for the American public in general; depending on risk factor status and LDL-C level, a step II diet may be prescribed. For patients with CHD or other atherosclerotic disease, a step II diet is prescribed initially. Both algorithms provide guidelines for drug therapy.

Box 5-6 presents a guide to comprehensive risk reduction for patients with coronary and other vascular disease. Diet is an important component of lipid management. Other important nonpharmacologic components include physical activity and weight management.

SUMMARY

Implementation of effective MNT depends on the use of standardized treatment protocols. The algorithms presented in this chapter are intended to be used as guidelines so that the highest quality health care possible for hyperlipidemia, hypertension, weight management, and diabetes is the result. These algorithms should enable health care to be delivered in an economically efficient manner. Use of these treatment algorithms will improve the quality of dietetic practice in the United States and could benefit the health of many Americans.

BOX 5-1 Hyperlipidemia Expected Outcomes

Setting: Ambulatory Care (Adult 18+ years old)
Number of sessions: 3

No. of interventions	Length of contact	Time between interventions	Cost/charge
1	60 minutes	3-4 weeks	
2	30 minutes	3-4 weeks	
3	30 minutes	as prescribed by PCP; recheck lab in 3 months	

Outcome assessment factors	Baseline	Evaluation of intervention		Expected outcome	Ideal/goal value
	Intervention				
	1	2	3		
Clinical Outcomes					
• Biochemical parameters (measure <30 days prior to nutrition session) Lipid profile (blood chol, trig, LDL-C, HDL-C)	√		√	Chol ↓ 20% Trig ↓ or no change LDL-C ↓ HDL-C ↑ or no change Ratio TC/HDL ↓ or no change	Chol <200 mg/dL Fasting trig <250 mg/dL LDL-C <130 mg/dL (no CHD) LDL-C <100 mg/dL (w/CHD) HDL-C >35 mg/dL Ratio TC/HDL <4.5
• Anthropometrics Weight, height, & BMI	√	√	√	↓, ↑, or maintain as appropriate	Within reasonable body weight
• Clinical signs and symptoms	√		√	As appropriate: ↓ in retinal deposit ↓ shortness of breath ↓ in angina	
Behavioral Outcomes*					MNT Goal Fat and cholesterol consumed follow nutrition prescription, eg, <20% total fat, 10% MUFA
• Food/meal planning	√	√	√	• Limits foods ↑ in chol, total fat, & saturated fat • Uses monounsaturated fat as preferred fat	
• Food label reading			√	• Accurately reads food label	
• Knowledge of soluble fiber			√	• Increases intake of foods ↑ in soluble fiber	
• Recipe modification			√	• Modifies recipes to ↓ total fat/saturated fat	
• Food preparation			√	• Uses low-fat cooking techniques	
• Dining out		√	√	• Selects appropriately from restaurant menu	
• Simple sugar and alcohol intake	√	√	√	• Limits per nutrition prescription, if applicable	
• Exercise pattern	√	√	√	• Participates in aerobic activity 3x/wk, 45-min sessions	
• Smoking	√	√	√	• Verbalizes importance of smoking cessation	
• Potential food/drug interaction	√	√	√	• Verbalizes potential food/drug interaction	

* Session in which behavioral topics are covered may vary according to patient's readiness, skills, resources, and need for lifestyle changes.

PCP = primary care physician

Reprinted with permission from *Medical Nutrition Therapy Across the Continuum of Care* (Chicago: American Dietetic Association; 1996).

BOX 5-2 Hypertension Expected Outcomes

Setting: Ambulatory Care (Adult 18+ years old)
Number of sessions: 3

No. of interventions	Length of contact	Time between interventions	Cost/charge
1	60 minutes	3-4 weeks	
2	30 minutes	3-4 weeks	
3	30 minutes	as prescribed by PCP	

Outcome assessment factors	Baseline	Evaluation of intervention		Expected outcome	Ideal/goal value
	Intervention				
	1	2	3		
Clinical Outcomes					
• Biochemical parameters (measure < 30 days prior to nutrition session)				Blood pressure within normal limit If patient on medication, decrease or eliminate medication dosage	Blood pressure: Systolic <140 mm Hg Diastolic <90 mm Hg
Blood pressure	√	√	√		
Lipid profile (blood chol, trig, LDL-C, HDL-C)	√			Recheck lipid profile (session 3), if elevated	Chol <200 mg/dL Fasting trig <250 mg/dL LDL-C <130 mg/dL (no CHD) LDL-C <100 mg/dL HDL-C >35 mg/dL
• Anthropometrics Weight, height, & BMI	√	√	√	↓, ↑, or maintain weight as appropriate	Within reasonable body weight or 10 lb weight loss
• Clinical signs and symptoms	√	√	√	As appropriate: ↓ angina ↓ shortness of breath ↓ edema ↓ headaches ↓ palpitations	
Behavioral Outcomes*					MNT Goal Follow nutrition prescription, eg, appropriate meal pattern (caloric restriction if appropriate), <2300 mg sodium, calcium and magnesium to meet RDA, adequate potassium intake, if appropriate
• Food/meal planning	√	√	√	• Restricts calories, as appropriate • Limits foods ↑ in sodium • Consumes RDA for calcium and magnesium • Maintains/increases intake of foods ↑ in potassium, if applicable	
• Alcohol intake	√	√	√	• Limits alcohol to 2 drinks/day	
• Food label reading		√	√	• Accurately reads food labels	
• Recipe modification		√	√	• Modifies recipes to ↓ salt, sodium, and fat	
• Food preparation		√	√	• Uses low-sodium and low-fat cooking techniques	
• Dining out	√	√	√	• Selects appropriately from restaurant menu	
• Knowledge of potential food/drug interaction	√	√	√	• Verbalizes potential food/drug interaction	
• Exercise	√	√	√	• Participates in aerobic activity 3x/wk, 45-min sessions	
• Smoking	√	√	√	• Verbalizes importance of smoking cessation	

* Session in which behavioral topics are covered may vary according to patient's readiness, skills, resources, and need for lifestyle changes.

PCP = primary care physician

Reprinted with permission from *Medical Nutrition Therapy Across the Continuum of Care* (Chicago: American Dietetic Association; 1996).

BOX 5-3 Weight Management Nutrition Progress Notes

Weight Management — Adults
Other Diagnosis ______________________________

Outcomes of Medical Nutrition Therapy (MNT)

Patient's Name ______________________________
Medical Record # ______________________________
DOB ______________ Gender ______________
Ethnic Background (Optional) ______________
Referring Physician ______________

Expected outcome	Intervention provided to meet goal (Intervention = self-management training plus patient verbalizes/demonstrates)				Goal reached (Check indicates goal reached)			
Date Session	____ 1 (60 min)	____ 2 (30 min)	____ 3 (30 min)	____ 4 (30 min)	____ 1	____ 2	____ 3	____ 4
Clinical Outcomes					Value	Value	Value	Value
Serum glucose					____mg/dL			____mg/dL
Glycohemoglobin (Hemoglobin A_1c)					____%			____%
Cholesterol					____mg/dL			____mg/dL
Chol/HDL ratio					____			____
LDL/HDL ratio					____			____
Triglycerides					____mg/dL			____mg/dL
TSH					____mU/liter			____mU/liter
Resin uptake test T-3					____mcg/dL			____mcg/dL
Thyroxine T-4					____%			____%
Blood pressure					____/____	____/____	____/____	____/____
Height____Weight_____					____lb	____lb	____lb	____lb
BMI______					____kg/m^2	____kg/m^2	____kg/m^2	____kg/m^2
Body fat composition					____%		____%	____%
Waist to hip ratio					____		____	____
Waist circumference					____"		____"	____"
MNT Goal Adhere to appropriate meal pattern, increase or maintain adequate hydration and adhere to physical activity plan to maintain or decrease weight, body fat, and risk factors					____kcal ____g CHO ____g fat ____meals ____snacks ____fluids ____fiber	____kcal ____g CHO ____g fat ____meals ____snacks ____fluids ____fiber	____kcal ____g CHO ____g fat ____meals ____snacks ____fluids ____fiber	____kcal ____g CHO ____g fat ____meals ____snacks ____fluids ____fiber
Behavioral Outcomes • Eats meals/snacks at appropriate times • Chooses foods & amounts/meal pattern • Accurately reads food labels • Modifies recipes to ↓ total fat/saturated fat and sugar • Uses healthy cooking techniques • Selects appropriately from menu								
• Participates in aerobic/anaerobic activity per physical activity prescription					____x/wk ____min	____x/wk ____min	____x/wk ____min	____x/wk ____min
• Verbalizes importance of smoking cessation					____ppd	____ppd	____ppd	____ppd
• Modifies medication/food for activity/lifestyle • Increases appetite control • Verbalizes food/drug interaction Drug______________					____dose	____dose	____dose	____dose
Overall Compliance Potential								
• Comprehension					E G P	E G P	E G P	E G P
• Receptivity					E G P	E G P	E G P	E G P
• Adherence					E G P	E G P	E G P	E G P

E=excellent, G=good, P=poor

Reprinted with permission from *Medical Nutrition Therapy Across the Continuum of Care* (Chicago: American Dietetic Association; 1996).

BOX 5-4 NIDDM Nutrition Progress Notes

Non-Insulin-Dependent Diabetes Mellitus
Other Diagnosis ______________________

Outcomes of Medical Nutrition Therapy (MNT)

Patient's Name ______________________
Medical Record # ______________________
DOB ____________ Gender ____________
Ethnic Background (Optional) ______________
Referring Physician ______________

Expected outcome	Intervention provided to meet goal (Intervention = self-management training plus patient verbalizes/demonstrates)				Goal reached (Check indicates goal reached)			
Date	____	____	____	____	____	____	____	____
Session	1 (60 min)	2 (30 min)	3 (30 min)	4 (30 min)	1	2	3	4
Clinical Outcomes					Value	Value	Value	Value
Serum glucose					____mg/dL		____mg/dL	____mg/dL
HbA_1C					____%		____%	____%
SMBG, % in target range					____%		____%	____%
Cholesterol					____mg/dL		____mg/dL	____mg/dL
LDL-C					____mg/dL		____mg/dL	____mg/dL
HDL-C					____mg/dL		____mg/dL	____mg/dL
Triglycerides					____mg/dL		____mg/dL	____mg/dL
Blood pressure					____/____		____/____	____/____
Ketone/protein					____/____		____/____	____/____
Microalbumin					____mg/24h		____mg/24h	____mg/24h
Height____Weight_____					____lb	____lb	____lb	____lb
BMI_____					____kg/m²	____kg/m²	____kg/m²	____kg/m²
Hypo/hyperglycemic episode					___/___x/mo	___/___x/mo	___/___x/mo	___/___x/mo
Urination					____x/day	____x/day	____x/day	____x/day
↑ energy					+ /–	+ /–	+ /–	+ /–
Improved visual acuity								
MNT Goal Adhere to appropriate meal pattern, exercise, and medication treatment plan to maintain blood glucose and lipids within normal limits					____Cal ____g CHO ____g fat ____meals ____snacks	____Cal ____g CHO ____g fat ____meals ____snacks	____Cal ____g CHO ____g fat ____meals ____snacks	____Cal ____g CHO ____g fat ____meals ____snacks
Behavioral Outcomes								
• Eats meals/snacks at appropriate times								
• Chooses food & amounts per meal plan								
• Verbalizes sick day management skills								
• Accurately reads food labels								
• Modifies recipes to ↓ total fat/saturated fat and sugar								
• Uses healthy cooking techniques								
• Selects appropriately from restaurant menu								
• Participates in aerobic activity per exercise prescription					____x/wk ____min	____x/wk ____min	____x/wk ____min	____x/wk ____min
• Verbalizes importance of smoking cessation					____ppd	____ppd	____ppd	____ppd
• Modifies medication/food for activity/lifestyle								
• Verbalizes potential food/drug interaction Drug ____________ ____________ ____________					____dose	____dose	____dose	____dose
Overall Compliance Potential								
• Comprehension					E G P	E G P	E G P	E G P
• Receptivity					E G P	E G P	E G P	E G P
• Adherence					E G P	E G P	E G P	E G P

E=excellent, G=good, P=poor

Reprinted with permission from *Medical Nutrition Therapy Across the Continuum of Care* (Chicago: American Dietetic Association; 1996).

BOX 5-5 IDDM Nutrition Progress Notes

Insulin-Dependent Diabetes Mellitus	Patient's Name ____________________
Initial Continuing Intensive	Medical Record # ____________________
Other Diagnosis ____________________	DOB ____________ Gender ____________
	Ethnic Background (Optional) ____________________
Outcomes of Medical Nutrition Therapy (MNT)	Referring Physician ____________________

Expected outcome	Intervention provided to meet goal (Intervention = self-management training plus patient verbalizes/demonstrates)				Goal reached (Check indicates goal reached)			
Date Session	____ 1 (60 min)	____ 2 (30 min)	____ 3 (30 min)	____ 4 (30 min)	________ 1	________ 2	________ 3	________ 4
Clinical Outcomes					Value	Value	Value	Value
Serum glucose					____mg/dL		____mg/dL	____mg/dL
HbA_1C					____%		____%	____%
Cholesterol					____mg/dL		____mg/dL	____mg/dL
LDL-C					____mg/dL		____mg/dL	____mg/dL
HDL-C					____mg/dL		____mg/dL	____mg/dL
Triglycerides					____mg/dL		____mg/dL	____mg/dL
Ketone/protein					____/____		____/____	____/____
Microalbumin					____mg/24h	____mg/24h	____mg/24h	____mg/24h
Blood pressure					____/____	____/____	____/____	____/____
Height ____Weight____					____lb	____lb	____lb	____lb
Hypo/hyperglycemic episode					____x/mo	____x/mo	____x/mo	____x/mo
Urination					____x/day	____x/day	____x/day	____x/day
↑ energy					+ /–	+ /–	+ /–	+ /–
Improved visual acuity								
MNT Goal Adhere to appropriate meal pattern, exercise, and medication treatment plan to maintain blood glucose and lipids within normal limits					____Cal ____g CHO ____meals ____snacks	____Cal ____g CHO ____meals ____snacks	____Cal ____g CHO ____meals ____snacks	____Cal ____g CHO ____meals ____snacks
Behavioral Outcomes								
• Eats meals/snacks at appropriate times								
• Chooses foods & amounts per meal pattern								
• Verbalizes sick day management skills								
• Accurately reads food labels								
• Modifies recipes to ↓ total fat/saturated fat and sugar								
• Uses healthy cooking techniques								
• Selects appropriately from menu					____x/wk	____x/wk	____x/wk	____x/wk
• Participates in aerobic activity per exercise prescription					____min	____min	____min	____min
• Verbalizes importance of smoking cessation					____ppd	____ppd	____ppd	____ppd
• Modifies insulin/food for activity/lifestyle								
• Verbalizes food/drug interaction								
Drug ____________					____dose	____dose	____dose	____dose
____________					____dose	____dose	____dose	____dose
____________					____dose	____dose	____dose	____dose
Overall Compliance Potential								
• Comprehension					E G P	E G P	E G P	E G P
• Receptivity					E G P	E G P	E G P	E G P
• Adherence					E G P	E G P	E G P	E G P

E=excellent, G=good, P=poor

Reprinted with permission from *Medical Nutrition Therapy Across the Continuum of Care* (Chicago: American Dietetic Association; 1996).

FIGURE 5-1

No CHD or other atherosclerotic disease

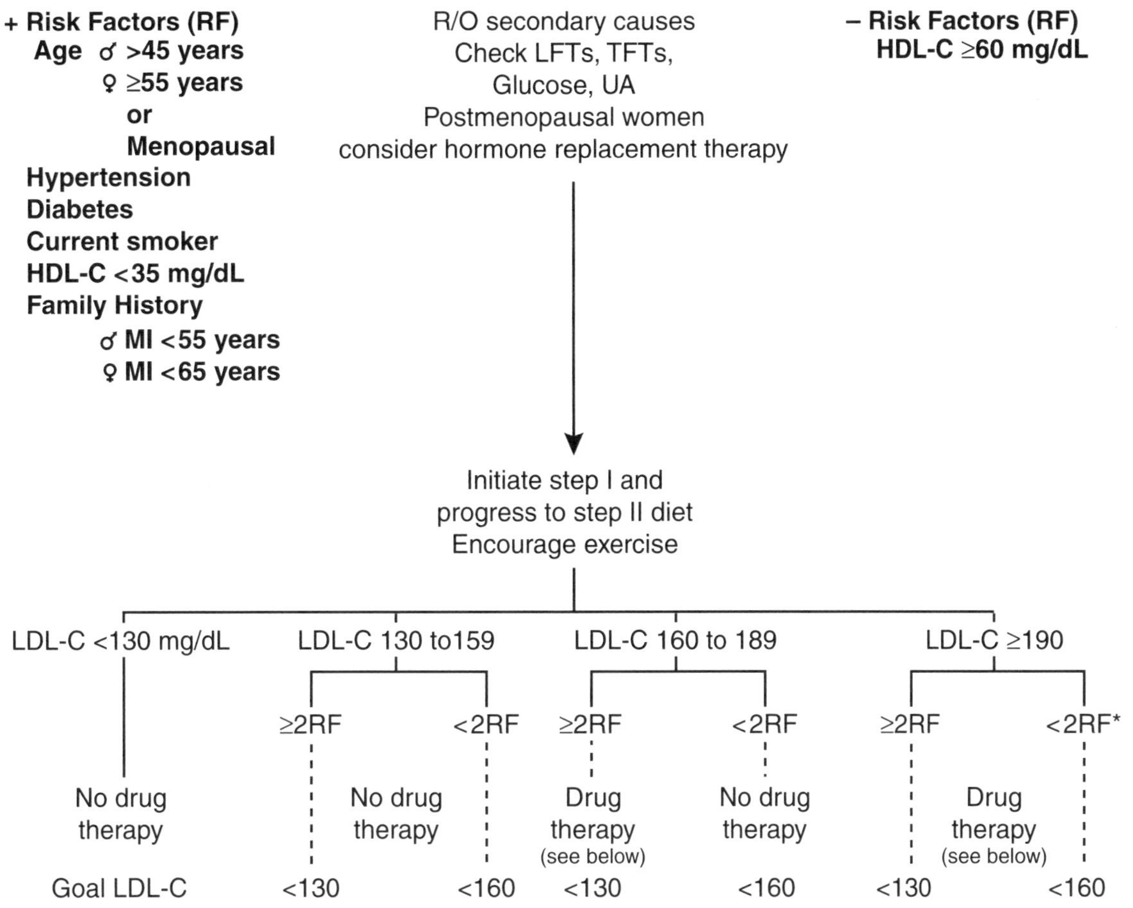

DRUG THERAPY AFTER DIETARY THERAPY		
↑ LDL	HDL <35†	TG >200†
Resin	Niacin	Niacin
Statin	Statin	Statin
Niacin	Gemfibrozil	Gemfibrozil

*Consider LDL >220 as cut-off for drug therapy in:
♂ <35 years
♀ premenopausal

†Drugs only in high-risk patients.
If TG persistently >500 after dietary therapy and optimization of glucose control, initiate niacin or gemfibrozil to prevent pancreatitis.

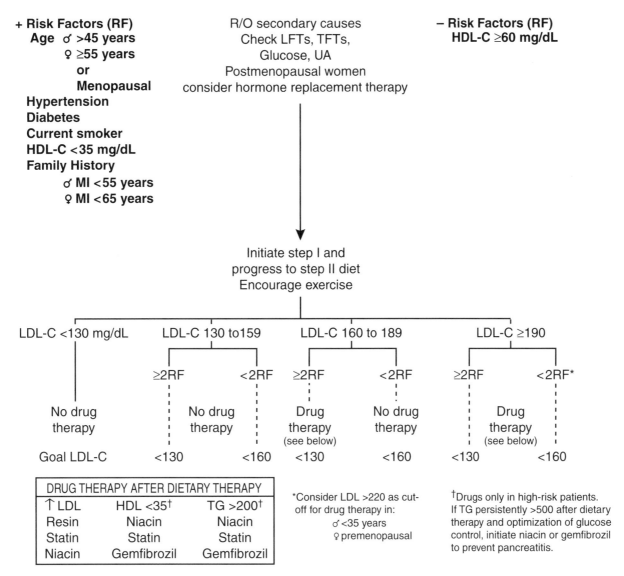

LFT=liver function tests; TFT=thyroid function tests

FIGURE 5-2

CHD or other atherosclerotic disease

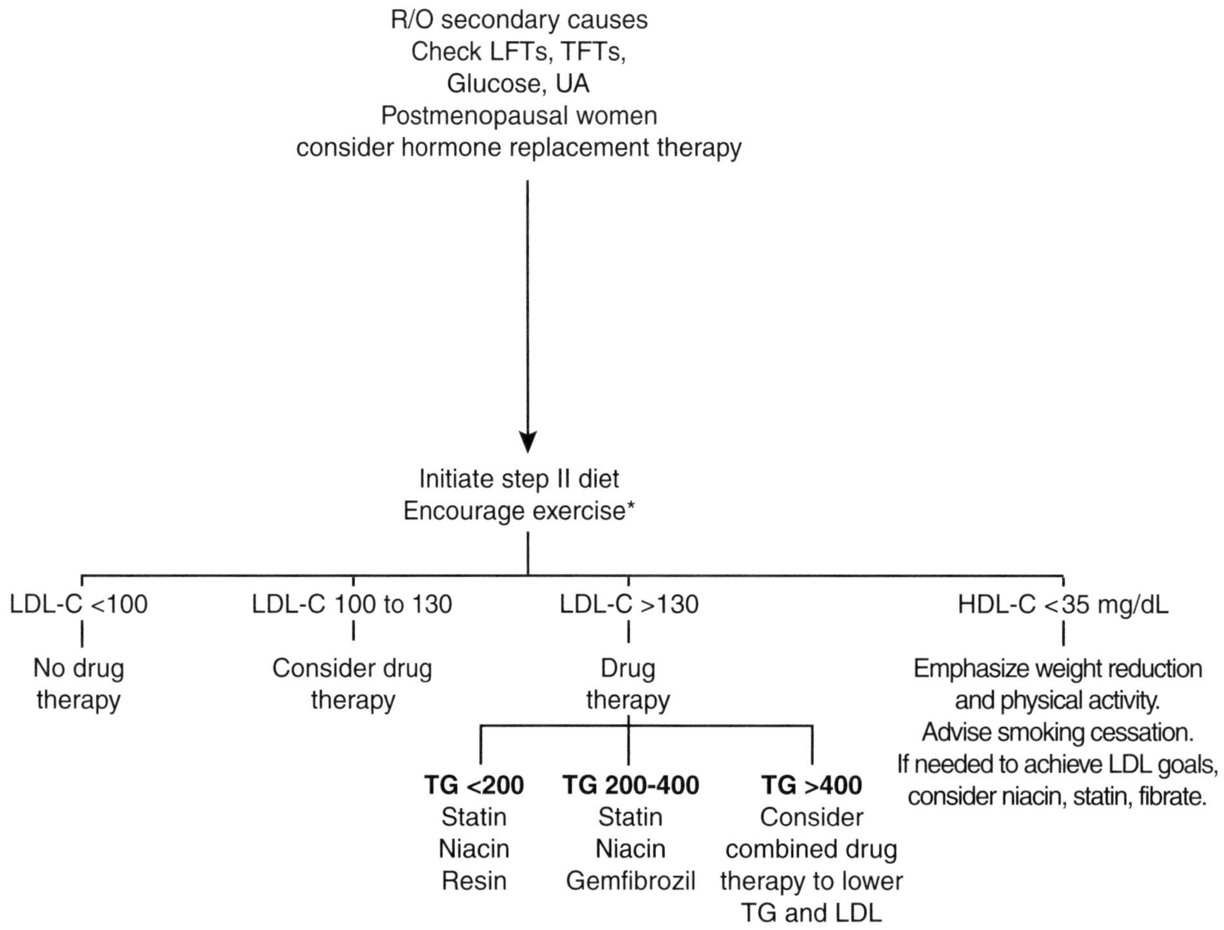

MEDICATIONS	DOSAGE	SIDE EFFECTS	LAB TEST
Statins[1]	lovastatin 10–80 mg qd pravastatin 10–40 mg qd simvastatin 5-40 mg qd fluvastatin 20-40 mg qd	myopathy, hepatitis	LFTs
Niacin[2]	1.5–3 g/day (bid or tid) (titrate up)	flushing, hepatitis	LFTs, glucose, uric acid
Resins[3]	cholestyr. 4–12 g bid colestipol 5–15 g bid	↑ TG, GI distress	none
Gemfibrozil[4]	600 mg bid	GI distress, cholelithiasis, myopathy	LFTs

***GOAL: LDL-C ≤100**
Secondary goals: HDL-C ≥35
TG <200
If goal is not achieved,
consider combination therapy.

[1]Use with caution in combination with gemfibrozil, niacin, cyclosporin, and erythromycin.
[2]Contraindications: Hx peptic ulcer disease, liver disease, gout, diabetes.
[3]Do not use in patients with high TG. Associated with decreased absorption of some drugs.
[4]Contraindication: renal failure. Lower dose in renal insufficiency. Follow PT in patients on warfarin.

LFT=liver function tests; TFT=thyroid function tests

Reproduced with permission from *Comprehensive Risk Reduction in Patients with Coronary and Other Vascular Disease.* Copyright 1996 the American Heart Association.

BOX 5-6 **Guide to Comprehensive Risk Reduction for Patients with Coronary and Other Vascular Disease**

<table>
<tr><td>RISK INTERVENTION</td><td colspan="5">RECOMMENDATIONS</td></tr>
<tr><td>Smoking:
<u>Goal</u>
Complete cessation</td><td colspan="5">Strongly encourage patient and family to stop smoking.
Provide counseling, nicotine replacement, and formal cessation programs as appropriate.</td></tr>
<tr><td rowspan="6">Lipid management:

<u>Primary Goal</u>
LDL<100 mg/dL

<u>Secondary Goal</u>
HDL >35 mg/dL;
TG <200 mg/dL</td><td colspan="5">Start AHA step II diet in all patients: ≤30% fat, <7% saturated fat, <200 mg/day cholesterol.
Assess fasting lipid profile. In post-MI patients, lipid profile may take 4 to 6 weeks to stabilize.
Add drug therapy according to the following guide:</td></tr>
<tr><td rowspan="5">LDL <100 mg/dL

No drug therapy</td><td colspan="2">LDL 100 to 130 mg/dL

Consider adding drug therapy to diet, as follows:</td><td>LDL >130 mg/dL

Add drug therapy to diet, as follows:</td><td rowspan="5">HDL <35 mg/dL

Emphasize weight management and physical activity. Advise smoking cessation. If needed to achieve LDL goals, consider niacin, statin, fibrate.</td></tr>
<tr><td colspan="3">Suggested drug therapy</td></tr>
<tr><td>TG <200 mg/dL</td><td>TG 200 to 400 mg/dL</td><td>TG >400 mg/dL</td></tr>
<tr><td>Statin
Resin
Niacin</td><td>Statin
Niacin</td><td>Consider combining drug therapy (niacin, fibrate, statin)</td></tr>
<tr><td colspan="3">If LDL goal not achieved, consider combination therapy.</td></tr>
<tr><td>Physical activity:
<u>Minimum Goal</u>
30 minutes 3 to 4 times per week</td><td colspan="5">Assess risk, preferably with exercise test, to guide prescription. Encourage minimum of 30 to 60 minutes of moderate-intensity activity 3 to 4 times weekly (walking, jogging, cycling, or other aerobic activity) supplemented by an increase in daily lifestyle activities (e.g., walking breaks at work, using stairs, gardening, household work). Maximum benefit 5 to 6 hours a week. Advise medically supervised programs for moderate- to high-risk patients.</td></tr>
<tr><td>Weight management:</td><td colspan="5">Start intensive diet and appropriate physical activity intervention, as outlined above, in patients >120% of ideal weight for height. Particularly emphasize need for weight loss in patients with hypertension, elevated triglycerides, low HDL, or elevated glucose levels.</td></tr>
<tr><td>Antiplatelet agents/ anticoagulants:</td><td colspan="5">Start aspirin 80 to 325 mg/day if not contraindicated. Manage warfarin to international normalized ratio = 2 to 3.5 for post-MI patients not able to take aspirin.</td></tr>
<tr><td>ACE inhibitors post-MI:</td><td colspan="5">Start early post-MI in stable high-risk patients (anterior MI, previous MI, Killip class II [S_3 gallop, rales, radiographic CHF]). Continue indefinitely for all with LV dysfunction (ejection fraction ≤40%) or symptoms of failure. Use as needed to manage blood pressure or symptoms in all other patients.</td></tr>
<tr><td>Beta-blockers:</td><td colspan="5">Start in high-risk post-MI patients (arrhythmia, LV dysfunction, inducible ischemia) at 5 to 28 days. Continue 6 months minimum. Observe usual contraindications. Use as needed to manage angina, rhythm, or blood pressure in all other patients.</td></tr>
<tr><td>Estrogen:</td><td colspan="5">Consider estrogen replacement therapy in all post-menopausal women. Individualize recommendation consistent with other health risks.</td></tr>
<tr><td>Blood pressure control:
<u>Goal</u>
≤140/90 mm Hg</td><td colspan="5">Initiate lifestyle modification-weight control, physical activity, alcohol moderation, and moderate sodium restriction in all patients with blood pressure >140 mm Hg systolic or 90 mm Hg diastolic. Add blood pressure medication, individualized to other patient requirements and characteristics (i.e., age, race, need for drugs with specific benefits) if blood pressure is not less than 140 mm Hg systolic or 90 mm Hg diastolic in 3 months or if initial blood pressure is >160 mm Hg systolic or 100 mm Hg diastolic.</td></tr>
</table>

ACE indicates angiotensin-converting enzyme; MI, myocardial infarction; TG, triglycerides; and LV, left ventricular.

E=excellent, G=good, P=poor

Reproduced with permission from *Comprehensive Risk Reduction in Patients with Coronary and Other Vascular Disease.* Copyright 1996 the American Heart Association.

REFERENCES

1. American Dietetic Association. *Medical Nutrition Therapy Across the Continuum of Care: Patient Protocols.* Chicago, Ill: ADA; 1996.
2. American Dietetic Association. *Medical Nutrition Therapy Across the Continuum of Care: Client Protocols. Supplement 1.* Chicago, Ill: ADA; 1997.
3. American Heart Association. *Comprehensive Risk Reduction in Patients with Coronary and Other Vascular Disease.* Dallas, Tex: AHA; 1996.

CHAPTER 6

Medical Nutrition Therapy for Cardiovascular Disease and Associated Risk Factors: Specific Diets for Prevention and Treatment

Debra Krummel, PhD, RD; Michelle Berry, MS, RD; and Kristin Moriarty, MS, RD

The American Heart Association (AHA) and the National Cholesterol Education Program (NCEP) promote diet therapy, now called medical nutrition therapy, as the first line of treatment for hypercholesterolemia (1,2). The two diets recommended for the prevention and treatment of hypercholesterolemia are the step I and step II diets. These diets focus on progressively lowering saturated fatty acids (SFAs) and cholesterol at an energy level that facilitates optimal weight management. Other modifications to cholesterol-lowering diets can be made (for example, restricting sodium and alcohol intakes, emphasizing monounsaturated fatty acids [MUFAs] and n-3 fatty acids, and adding fiber) and these are indicated for some patient subgroups as discussed below. All cardiac patients are candidates for medical nutrition therapy.

Treatment Guidelines for Diet Intervention

Many dietary variables affect cardiovascular disease (CVD) risk factors. The goal of medical nutrition therapy is to find the optimal combination of variables that will achieve blood lipid and other physiological goals (3). Practitioners can use a variety of dietary combinations to manage CVD risk factors. The step I and step II diets are recommended as the first level of intervention for patients with hypercholesterolemia. If response to these diets is inadequate, alternative diets such as a very-low-fat diet should be tried with motivated patients before dietary intervention alone is dismissed. For some patients, such as those with genetic hyperlipidemia or established coronary disease, a more restrictive diet is recommended at the outset (2,4). Likewise, for patients who have appreciable elevations in triglycerides in response to a step I or step II diet, a diet high in MUFAs and low in SFAs and cholesterol may be preferred. Overall, nutrition intervention goals are formulated to facilitate lifelong changes in eating and activity behaviors to promote an optimal risk factor status.

According to current estimates, candidates for dietary intervention total 29% of the US population (5); this value increases to more than 50% in the subgroup of men and women older than 55 years. However, according to the Cholesterol Awareness Survey, only 20% of adults have tried to follow an NCEP step I diet on their own (6). In 1990, physicians and other health professionals recommended dietary intervention for less than 10% of their patients (6).

Medical nutrition therapy is indicated for patients with dyslipidemia, hypertension, excess body weight, and diabetes (7). NCEP has developed guidelines for treatment based on the low-density lipoprotein cholesterol (LDL-C) level, the number of risk factors, and the presence or absence of CVD. Clinical and behavioral outcomes, concomitant goals, and algorithm schematics are presented and discussed in Chapter 5.

Specific Diets

The following diets will be discussed in detail in the chapter:

- step I and step II diets,
- very-low-fat, high-carbohydrate diets,
- high-monounsaturated-fatty-acid diet,
- high-soluble-fiber diet,
- vegetarian diets,
- sodium-restricted diets, and
- cardiac diet.

Step I and Step II Diets

Many Americans older than 2 years will benefit from the step I and step II diets, especially individuals at high risk for CVD, individuals with blood cholesterol levels greater than 200 mg/dL, and individuals taking lipid-lowering medication.

TABLE 6-1

The Step I and Step II Diets

Nutrient	Step I Diet	Step II Diet
Total fat	≤ 30% of energy	Same as step I
Saturated fatty acids	8%-10% of total calories	< 7% of total calories
Polyunsaturated fatty acids	Up to 10% of total calories	Same as step I
Monounsaturated fatty acids	Up to 15% of total calories	Same as step I
Carbohydrate	≥ 55% of total calories	Same as step I
Protein	~ 15% of total calories	Same as step I
Cholesterol	< 300 mg	< 200 mg
Total calories	To achieve and maintain desirable body weight	Same as step I

From: Second Report of the Expert Panel on Detection, Evaluation, and Treatment of High Blood Cholesterol in Adults. National Cholesterol Education Program. National Institutes of Health, National Heart, Lung, and Blood Institute, NIH publication 93-3095, 1993.

Description. The step I diet contains 30% or less of energy from fat, with 8% to 10% from SFAs and less than 300 mg cholesterol (Table 6-1). Polyunsaturated fatty acids (PUFAs) should not exceed 10% of total energy, and MUFAs provide the remaining energy from fat (up to 15%). Carbohydrate is 55% of energy; the amount will vary depending on protein and fat intakes. Energy intake is set to achieve or maintain optimal body weight. Goals for total fat and SFAs are shown in Table 6-2. The step II diet further limits SFAs (to less than 7% of energy) and cholesterol (to less than 200 mg/day). With sufficient planning, both diets can be nutritionally adequate. Fiber-rich foods are encouraged to achieve an intake of 25-30 grams a day. Although levels of n-3 fatty acids are also not specifically addressed, encouraging increased fish consumption is advisable (see Chapter 12 for complete discussion of functional foods). For sodium, the NCEP supports the National High Blood Pressure Education Program (NHBPEP) recommendation that persons with hypertension consume less than 6 g of sodium chloride per day (less than 2,300 mg sodium/day) (8). To meet the sodium recommendation, intake of many processed foods, foods prepared outside the home, and discretionary salt must be limited (see the discussion about sodium below).

The step I diet should be considered the starting point for any medical nutrition therapy for the management of CVD risk factors. Other indicated modifications, such as sodium restriction, can be added to the step I goals. Although fat-modified products may help patients achieve the step I and step II goals, dietitians should emphasize basic staple foods (ie, whole grains, vegetables, lean meats, fish and poultry, nonfat dairy products, and fruits) (Table 6-3). With

TABLE 6-2

Total Fat and Saturated Fatty Acid Goals for Step I, Step II, Very-Low-Fat, and High-MUFA Diets

	Step I[1]		Step II[2]		Very-Low-Fat[3]		High-MUFA[4]	
	Total (g)	SFA (g)	Total (g)	SFA (g)	Total (g)	SFA (g)	Total (g)	SFA (g)
1,200	40	12	40	8	27	8	47	12
1,400	47	14	47	9	31	9	54	14
1,500	50	15	50	10	33	10	58	15
1,600	53	16	53	11	36	11	62	16
1,800	60	18	60	12	40	12	70	18
2,000	67	20	67	13	44	13	78	20
2,200	73	22	73	15	49	15	86	22
2,400	80	24	80	16	53	16	93	24
2,600	87	26	87	17	58	17	101	26
2,800	93	28	93	19	62	19	109	28
3,000	100	30	100	20	67	20	117	30
3,200	107	32	107	21	71	21	124	32

[1] Total fat = 30% of calories; SFA = 9% of calories.
[2] Total fat = 30% of calories; SFA = 6% of calories.
[3] Total fat = 20% of calories; SFA = 6% of calories.
[4] Total fat = 35% of calories; SFA = 9% of calories.

the step I diet, no food groups are omitted, although lower-fat and lean choices are emphasized. Some higher-fat choices can be included in small portions, and a variety of foods should be eaten to ensure that the diet is nutritionally adequate.

The knowledge required to follow a step I or II diet is extensive. Knowledge about the relationship between diet and disease can help motivate a patient to make changes, and some knowledge about fats, cholesterol, and fiber is essential for success. For example, a patient must be able to

TABLE 6-3

Food Group Plan for the Step I and II Diets

Food Group	Number of Servings	Serving Size	Some Suggested Foods
Vegetables	3-5	1 cup leafy/raw	Leafy greens, lettuce
		½ cup other	Corn, peas, green beans, broccoli, carrots, cabbage, celery, tomato, spinach, squash, bok choy, mushrooms, eggplant, collard and mustard greens
		¾ cup juice	Tomato juice, vegetable juice
Fruits	2-4	1 piece fruit ½ cup diced fruit	Orange, apple, applesauce, pear, banana, grapes, grapefruit, tangerine, plum, peach, strawberries and other berries, melons, kiwi, papaya, mango, lychee
		¾ cup juice	Orange juice, apple juice, grapefruit juice, grape juice, prune juice
Breads, cereals, pasta, grains, dry beans, peas, potatoes, and rice	6-11	1 slice	Wheat, rye, or enriched breads/rolls, corn and flour tortillas
		½ bun, bagel, muffin	English muffin, bagel, muffin, cornbread
		1 oz. dry cereal	Wheat, corn, oat, rice, bran cereal, or mixed grain cereal
		½ cup cooked cereal	Oatmeal, cream of wheat, grits
		½ cup dry beans or peas	Kidney beans, lentils, split peas, black-eyed peas
		½ cup potatoes	Potato, sweet potato
		½ cup rice, noodles, barley, or other grains	Pasta, rice, macaroni, barley, tabbouli
		½ cup bean curd	Tofu
Nonfat/low-fat dairy products	2-3	1 cup skim, 1% milk	Low/nonfat yogurt, skim milk, 1% milk, buttermilk
		1 oz low-fat, fat-free cheese	Low-fat cheeses
Lean meat, poultry and fish		≤ 6 oz/day step I diet ≤ 5 oz/day step II diet	Lean and extra lean cuts of meat, fish and skinless poultry, such as: sirloin, round steak, skinless chicken, haddock, cod
Fats and oils	≤ 6-8 *	1 tsp soft margarine 1 TBSP salad dressing	Soft or liquid margarine, vegetable oils
		1 oz nuts	Walnuts, peanuts, almonds, pecans
Eggs		≤ 4 yolks/week step I diet ≤ 2 yolks/week step II diet	Used in preparation of baked products
Sweets and snack foods		In moderation	Cookies, fortune cookies, pudding, bread pudding, rice pudding, angel food cake, frozen yogurt, candy, punch, carbonated beverages Low-fat crackers and popcorn, pretzels, fat-free chips, rice cakes

* Includes fats and oils used in preparation, also salad dressings and nuts.

Adapted from: Second Report of the Expert Panel on Detection, Evaluation, and Treatment of High Blood Cholesterol in Adults. National Cholesterol Education Program. National Institutes of Health, National Heart, Lung, and Blood Institute, NIH publication 93-3095, 1993.

TABLE 6-4

Exchanges for Step I Diets [1]

	Step I Diet (~30% Energy from Fat)[2]						Step I Diet (~25% Energy from Fat)[2]					
Kcals	Strch	Pro	Veg	Frt	Milk[3]	Fat	Strch	Pro	Veg	Frt	Milk	Fat
1,200	6	4	2	3	1	5	6	4	2	4	1	4
1,400	7	5	3	3	1	6	7	5	3	4	1	5
1,500	8	5	3	3	1	7	7	5	3	4	2	5
1,600	8	5	3	3	2	7	8	6	3	4	2	5
1,800	9	6	3	4	2	8	9	6	3	5	2	6
2,000	10	6	4	4	2	10	10	6	4	6	2	7
2,200	10	6	4	5	3	11	10	6	4	7	3	8
2,400	11	6	5	6	3	12	11	6	4	8	3	10
2,600	12	6	5	7	3	14	12	6	5	9	3	11
2,800	12	6	5	8	4	15	12	6	5	10	4	12
3,000	13	6	5	9	4	16	13	6	6	11	4	13
3,200	14	6	5	10	4	18	14	6	7	12	4	14

[1] Where Strch = starch exchanges; Pro = lean meat exchanges (<4 egg yolks/week); Veg = vegetable exchanges; Frt = fruit exchanges; Milk = nonfat milk exchanges; Fat = fat exchanges.

[2] Both step I diets have <10% energy from saturated fat and <300 mg cholesterol.

[3] Check adequacy of calcium—diet may need to be supplemented.

find the amounts of fat, saturated fat, cholesterol, and fiber in foods (eg, label-reading skills) to be able to follow a low-fat, high-fiber diet. Knowledge about how the different types of fat and fiber affect the body is not essential for behavior change but can be helpful in promoting compliance in some patients. Conversely, some patients find such technical information confusing and may be less likely to adopt a regime they perceive as too complicated. Behavioral strategies and factors related to promoting adherence are discussed in Chapter 13. Depending on the education level and motivation of the patient, a variety of methods can be used to teach step I and step II concepts. Either a food-group (Table 6-3) or an exchange approach (Tables 6-4 and 6-5) can be used. Patients can also be taught to count grams of fat, grams of SFA, milligrams of cholesterol, and calories. For patients requiring a more simplified approach, the Food Guide Pyramid can be used with an emphasis on lower-fat choices (9). Step I and step II menus for different cuisines can be developed using the Ethnic and Regional Food Practices Series books (see Appendix 1), or by custom tailoring exchange lists with preferred foods. For more information about diets for various ethnic groups see Chapter 16.

TABLE 6-5

Exchanges for Step II Diets [1]

	Step II Diet (~27% Energy from Fat)[2]						Step II Diet (~22% Energy from Fat)[2]					
Kcals	Strch	Pro	Veg	Frt	Milk	Fat	Strch	Pro	Veg	Frt	Milk	Fat
1,200	6	4	3	3	1	5	6	4	3	4	1	3
1,400	7	4	3	4	1	6	7	5	3	5	1	4
1,500	8	5	3	4	1	6	7	5	3	5	2	4
1,600	8	5	3	4	2	6	8	6	3	5	2	4
1,800	9	6	4	4	2	7	9	6	3	6	2	5
2,000	10	6	4	5	2	8	10	6	4	7	2	6
2,200	11	6	5	5	3	9	10	6	4	8	3	7
2,400	12	6	5	6	3	11	11	6	5	9	3	8
2,600	13	6	5	7	3	12	12	6	6	10	3	9
2,800	14	6	5	7	4	13	12	6	6	11	4	10
3,000	15	6	6	8	4	14	13	6	7	12	4	11
3,200	16	6	7	9	4	15	14	6	8	13	4	12

[1] Where Strch = starch exchanges; Pro = lean meat exchanges (<2 egg yolks/week); Veg = vegetable exchanges; Frt = fruit exchanges; Milk = nonfat milk exchanges; Fat = fat exchanges.

[2] Both step II diets have <7% energy from saturated fat and <200 mg cholesterol.

Background. The effects of diet on blood lipids have been studied for more than 30 years. It is now known that diet plays a critical role in the management of blood lipids and CVD prevention (10). In the 1970s there was a specific therapeutic diet for treatment of each type of hyperlipoproteinemia (11). This was followed by AHA recommending a three-phase approach to managing hyperlipidemia through sequential reductions in total fat, SFAs, and cholesterol. In 1988, the AHA and NCEP simplified the diet recommendations to the step I and step II diets for lowering blood cholesterol (12). Today, these diets continue to be recommended both by AHA (13) and by the NCEP Adult Treatment Panel II for treatment of elevated LDL-C levels (2).

Rationale. Dietary SFAs, cholesterol, and excess body weight have the greatest impact on blood lipid lipoprotein levels. Furthermore, intakes of energy, total fat, SFAs, and cholesterol have been directly related to atherosclerotic disease progression independent of blood lipid levels; this is probably due to negative effects on coagulation factors (14,15). Reducing SFAs, cholesterol, and body weight can improve lipid profiles, promote disease regression, and thereby decrease CVD risk (16). Therefore, targeted behaviors for CVD risk reduction are diet modification, weight management, and regular physical activity.

Advantages and Disadvantages. One major advantage of the step I diet is that it is generally appropriate and desirable for the whole family except children younger than 2 years, which eliminates the need for separate foods or meals for the patient trying to adhere to the diet. Some patients need to make only a few simple changes to adhere to a step I diet. For example, using low-fat cooking methods, lean meat and nonfat dairy choices, and fat-modified products often is enough to meet step I goals. Foods needed to comply with both step I and step II diets are readily available in most supermarkets. Although the step I goals should not be that difficult to achieve, many patients have problems adhering to a step I diet. For these patients and for patients trying to follow a step II diet, the NCEP report strongly recommends referral to a registered dietitian.

Very-low-fat, High-carbohydrate Diets

The population most likely to benefit from very-low-fat, high-carbohydrate diets is patients with diagnosed CVD and high-risk patients with genetic hyperlipidemia (familial hypercholesterolemia).

Description. Goals for fat and SFA intakes for very-low-fat diets are shown in Table 6-2. Very-low-fat diets usually provide at least 65% of energy from carbohydrates. Depending on the calorie level, up to 6 oz of lean meats, poultry, and fish can be incorporated daily into this diet (Table 6-6). Low-fat grains, legumes, vegetables, and fruits are emphasized.

Background. The terms *low-fat diet* and *very-low-fat diet* are usually used somewhat loosely because no formal definitions exist. As used here, a very-low-fat diet contains less than 20% of energy from fat. Examples are the AHA Phase III diet (13) and Connors' New American Diet (17). Diets containing less than 10% of energy from fat, such as the Pritikin Diet (18) and Dean Ornish's Reversal Diet (19), are usually some form of a vegetarian diet (discussed later in this chapter). The Pritikin diet is an exception because it allows 3½ oz of very lean meat, poultry, or fish each day. A comparison of these diets with the step I diet is shown in Table 6-7.

TABLE 6-6

Exchanges for Very-low-fat Diets [1]

	Very-low-fat Diet (~16% Energy from Fat)[2]						Very-low-fat Diet (~12% Energy from Fat)[2]					
Kcals	Strch	Pro	Veg	Frt	Milk	Fat[3]	Strch	Pro	Veg	Frt	Milk	Fat[3]
1,200	5	3	4	3	3	3	6	3	5	3	2	2
1,400	6	3	4	4	3	3	7	3	5	4	3	2
1,500	7	3	5	4	3	3	8	3	5	4	3	2
1,600	8	4	5	4	3	3	8	4	5	4	3	2
1,800	9	4	6	4	3	4	9	4	6	5	3	3
2,000	10	5	6	5	3	4	10	5	6	5	4	3
2,200	11	5	6	5	4	5	12	5	7	5	4	3
2,400	12	5	7	6	4	6	13	6	7	6	4	3
2,600	14	6	7	6	4	6	15	6	7	7	4	3
2,800	16	6	7	6	4	7	16	6	8	7	4	4
3,000	17	6	7	7	4	8	18	6	9	7	4	5
3,200	18	6	7	8	4	9	20	6	9	8	4	5

[1] Where Strch = starch exchanges; Pro = lean meat exchanges (<4 egg yolks/week); Veg = vegetable exchanges; Frt = fruit exchanges; Milk = nonfat milk exchanges; Fat = fat exchanges.

[2] Both very-low-fat diets have <7% energy from saturated fat and <200 mg cholesterol.

[3] Fat choices must be from MUFA and PUFA lists only; no SFA choices are allowed to meet SFA goal.

TABLE 6-7

Comparison of Low-Fat Diets

	Step I Diet [1]	New American Diet [2]	Reversal Diet [3]
Fat (% calories)	30	20	10
Saturated fat (% calories)	8-10	5	2
Monounsaturated fat (% calories)	13	8	4
Polyunsaturated fat (% calories)	7	7	4
Cholesterol, mg/day	<300	100	25
Carbohydrate (% calories)	55	65	75
Dietary fiber, grams	20-35	45-60	60-90
Protein, (% of calories)	15	15	15

[1] *Second Report of the Expert Panel on Detection, Evaluation, and Treatment of High Blood Cholesterol in Adults.* National Cholesterol Education Program. National Institutes of Health, National Heart, Lung, and Blood Institute, NIH Publication No. 93-3095, 1993.

[2] Connor SL, Connor WE (17).

[3] Ornish D (19).

Very-low-fat diets have been recommended because with these diets maximal reductions in cholesterol-raising nutrients (SFAs and cholesterol) can be achieved. Furthermore, these diets facilitate energy restriction and weight reduction. In observational studies total fat intake was correlated with coronary heart disease incidence (20) and the number of advanced lesions seen in patients at autopsy (21). Although these observations have led some clinicians to advocate very-low-fat diets, the use of these diets remains controversial. Most authorities believe there is insufficient evidence to recommend consumption of these diets for the general public. However, for patients with hyperlipidemia, very-low-fat diets have been recommended for more than a decade (13).

Rationale. Several lines of evidence suggest that lower-fat diets may be advantageous for preventing CVD. Populations, such as the Chinese, whose traditional diets are high in carbohydrate and low in SFAs have much lower rates of coronary heart disease than do populations consuming high-SFA diets (22). In angiographic studies, higher-fat diets are associated with new atherosclerotic lesions (23), which may be due to the increased postprandial lipemia, chylomicron remnants, and LDL-C levels seen with consumption of high-fat diets. Support for very-low-fat diets for CVD patients has come from intervention studies. Diets low in SFAs and cholesterol with 20% or less of energy from fat, combined with an exercise program or stress management techniques, slowed progression of CVD and promoted regression in intervention patients compared with usual-care patients (24,25).

Advantages and Disadvantages. The major advantage of a very-low-fat diet is that some patients will be able to achieve lipid goals and avoid drug therapy and, possibly, bypass surgery. Also, patients may accrue other health benefits from a high intake of fruits and vegetables. However, there are two disadvantages to a very-low-fat diet. First, long-term maintenance can be difficult and requires motivation and both cognitive and behavior shaping skills (see Chapter 13). The ability to maintain a diet with less than 20% of energy from fat requires intensive intervention, long-term follow-up, and a high level of patient motivation and commitment because major lifestyle changes are required. Two-thirds of women at risk for breast cancer were able to maintain a very-low-fat diet for 2 years with multiple group-intervention sessions led by a registered dietitian over an 18-month period (26). In the Family Heart Study population, only 11% of the sample were able to both decrease their intake of SFAs and cholesterol and increase their intake of complex carbohydrate after 5 years (27). In a culture and environment where high-fat foods are plentiful, compliance to very-low-fat diets is challenging.

A second disadvantage of very-low-fat diets is that the improvement in blood lipids is often accompanied by a decrease in high-density lipoprotein cholesterol (HDL-C) and an increase in triglycerides. Because populations that consume these diets have both a low HDL-C level and a low incidence of coronary heart disease, some scientists believe that this decrease is not detrimental to risk. Accumulating evidence indicates that some very-low-fat diets can worsen glucose tolerance and the lipid profile in patients with non-insulin-dependent diabetes mellitus (Type 2 diabetes) and hypertriglyceridemia (28). Consequently, the use of very-low-fat diets may be contraindicated in some of these patients.

High-monounsaturated-fatty-acid Diet

The population most likely to benefit from a high-monounsaturated-fatty-acid diet includes individuals who have a strong Mediterranean ethnic eating style; individuals who have hypertriglyceridemia or low HDL-C (such as patients with Syndrome X), Type 2 diabetes and dyslipidemia, or familial combined hyperlipidemia; and individuals who find adherence to a 30% fat diet difficult or impossible.

Description. Primary sources of MUFAs include olive oil, olives, canola oil, nuts, seeds, avocado, and special varieties of oils from plants genetically selected to be high in oleic acid (high-oleic safflower and sunflower oils). In the high-MUFA diet at least 15% of total energy is from MUFAs. In addition,

BOX 6-1 ***SFA, MUFA, and PUFA Fat Exchanges***

SFA Exchange = 5g total fat, 3g SFA, 1g MUFA, 1g PUFA

Bacon, cooked		1 slice (20 slices/lb)
Bacon, grease		1 tsp
Butter:	stick	1 tsp
	whipped	2 tsp
	reduced-fat	1 Tbsp
Chitterlings, boiled		1 Tbsp
Coconut, sweetened, shredded		2 Tbsp
Cream, half and half		2 Tbsp
Cream cheese:	regular	1 Tbsp (½ oz)
	reduced-fat	2 Tbsp (1 oz)
Shortening or lard		1 tsp
Sour cream:	regular	2 Tbsp
	reduced-fat	3 Tbsp

MUFA Exchange = 5g total fat, 1g SFA, 3g MUFA, 1g PUFA

Avocado, medium		1/8 (1 oz)
Oil (canola, olive, peanut)		1 tsp
Olives:	ripe (black)	8 large
	green, stuffed*	10 large
Nuts:	almonds, cashews	6 nuts
	mixed (50% peanuts)	6 nuts
	peanuts	10 nuts
	pecans	4 halves
Peanut butter, smooth or crunchy		1 Tbsp
Tahini paste		2 tsp

PUFA Exchange = 5g total fat, 1g SFA, 1g MUFA, 3g PUFA

Margarine:	stick, tub or squeeze	1 tsp
	lower-fat (30-50% vegetable oil)	1 Tbsp
Mayonnaise:	regular	1 tsp
	reduced-fat	1 Tbsp
Nuts:	walnuts, English	4 halves
Oil (corn, safflower, soybean)		1 tsp
Salad dressing:	regular*	1 Tbsp
	reduced-fat*	2 Tbsp
Miracle Whip Salad Dressing®:	regular	2 tsp
	reduced-fat	1 Tbsp
Seeds:	pumpkin, sunflower	1 Tbsp

* = 400 mg or more of sodium per exchange.

Adapted from: Exchange Lists for Weight Management. American Diabetes Association, Inc, and The American Dietetic Association, 1995.

SFA and PUFA intakes are maintained at 10% or less and energy is adjusted to maintain ideal body weight. A total fat intake of 35% or less of energy is recommended; however, higher fat intakes may be justified on an individual basis. To achieve a high-MUFA diet (15% of energy) with 35% or less of energy from fat at an energy intake of 2,000 kcal/day, one of the following would need to be consumed daily: 2 tablespoons of olive oil, 1 medium avocado, or 2 oz of peanuts or almonds (29). The fat distribution of exchanges (Box 6-1) and exchanges for high-MUFA diets (Table 6-8) illustrate how to incorporate MUFAs at 15% of energy intake. Table 6-8 represents exchanges needed to meet goals of ~35% total fat and ~9% saturated fat. If a lower level of SFA is desired (ie, to meet step II goals), animal protein sources will need to be eliminated from the diet. This results from the accumulation of SFA from MUFA exhanges (1 g SFA/MUFA exchange). Thus, Table 6-8 does not necessarily represent the Mediterranean diet depicted in Figure 6-1.

If the Mediterranean diet is desired, the Mediterranean diet pyramid (Figure 6-1) can be used to convey the types, amounts, and relative proportions of foods recommended to approximate this traditional eating style. As described by

TABLE 6-8

Exchanges for High-MUFA Diets[1]

High-MUFA Diet (~9% Energy as SFA)[2]						
Kcals	**Strch**	**Pro**[3]	**Veg**	**Frt**	**Milk**	**Fat MUFA**
1,200	4	2	3	2	2	8
1,400	5	2	3	3	2	9
1,500	5	2	4	3	2	10
1,600	6	2	4	3	2	11
1,800	7	3	4	3	2	12
2,000	8	3	5	3	2	14
2,200	9	3	5	3	3	15
2,400	9	3	6	4	3	17
2,600	10	3	6	5	3	19
2,800	11	4	6	5	3	20
3,000	12	4	7	6	3	21
3,200	13	4	8	6	3	231

[1] Where Strch = starch exchanges; Pro = lean meat exchanges; Veg = vegetable exchanges; Frt = fruit exchanges; Milk = nonfat milk exchanges; Fat (MUFA) = MUFA fat exchanges.

[2] High-MUFA diets have ~35% energy from fat, ~20% MUFA and <300 mg cholesterol.

[3] Up to 6 egg yolks a week can be included in the high-MUFA diet if nonfat milk exchanges are used.

Willett, Sacks, Trichopoulou, Drescher, Ferro-Luzzi, Helsing, and Trichopouos (30), the diet is

> characterized by abundant plant foods (fruit, vegetables, breads, other forms of cereals, potatoes, beans, nuts, and seeds), fresh fruit as the typical daily dessert, olive oil as the principal source of fat, dairy products (principally cheese and yogurt), and fish and poultry consumed in low to moderate amounts, zero to four eggs consumed weekly, red meat consumed sparingly, and wine consumed in low to moderate amounts, normally with meals…moderation in wine consumption is defined as one to two glasses per day for men [5 oz per glass]…for women, moderation…is defined as one glass per day…butter should be used only in small amounts or on special occasions, and olive oil should replace—not be added to—other sources of dietary fat.

Background. When SFAs are decreased in the diet, the energy that they supplied must be replaced for patients to maintain their weight. SFAs can be replaced with carbohydrate or other types of fatty acids. For years, PUFAs were recommended as replacement energy to lower LDL-C because MUFAs were believed to be neutral (ie, to have no effect on blood cholesterol levels when compared with carbohydrates). However, MUFAs have more recently been found to have about the same cholesterol-lowering effect as PUFAs when they replace SFAs in the diet (31).

High intakes of PUFAs can decrease both LDL-C and HDL-C levels. High-fat diets that are high in MUFAs and low in SFAs (total fat at 33% to 50% of energy, MUFAs at 17% to 33% of energy, and SFAs at less than 7% of energy) decrease LDL-C and increase HDL-C compared with low-fat diets (30% or less of energy from fat). This has led to the use of high-MUFA diets for individuals with low HDL-C or high triglyceride levels to prevent further reductions in HDL-C and increases in triglycerides that occur in response to a low-fat diet. However, when diets contain less than 30% of energy from fat, with 15% as MUFA, HDL-C levels are decreased or unchanged (32-34). Thus, the positive HDL-C response appears to occur only with higher total fat and MUFA intakes. An additional benefit to a high-MUFA diet (as compared with a high-PUFA diet) is reduced oxidative modification of LDL-C assessed in vitro (34).

Because patients with Type 2 diabetes can have dyslipidemia that worsens with a high-carbohydrate intake, there is interest in high-MUFA diets for the management of hypertriglyceridemia in these patients (29). Some studies showed that people with Type 2 diabetes have a more favorable triglyceride response to a high-MUFA diet than to a low-fat, high-carbohydrate diet (35,36). Other studies did not observe any lipid differences of high-MUFA versus high-carbohydrate diets in patients with Type 2 diabetes (37,38).

A good example of a high-MUFA, low-SFA intake is the Mediterranean diet, named for the Mediterranean region (Greece, parts of Italy and France, Lebanon, Morocco, Portugal, Spain, Syria, Tunisia, and Turkey), where olive

FIGURE 6-1

The Mediterranean diet pyramid: a cultural model for healthy eating. The Mediterranean diet pyramid, along with an extensive set of explanatory notes, is available in the form of a large, three-color poster. To receive a copy, send a check for $8 per poster to Oldways Preservation & Exchange Trust, 25 First Street, Cambridge, MA 02141. Telephone (617) 621-3000; fax (617) 621-1230.

Reprinted with permission of Oldways Preservation and Exchange Trust.

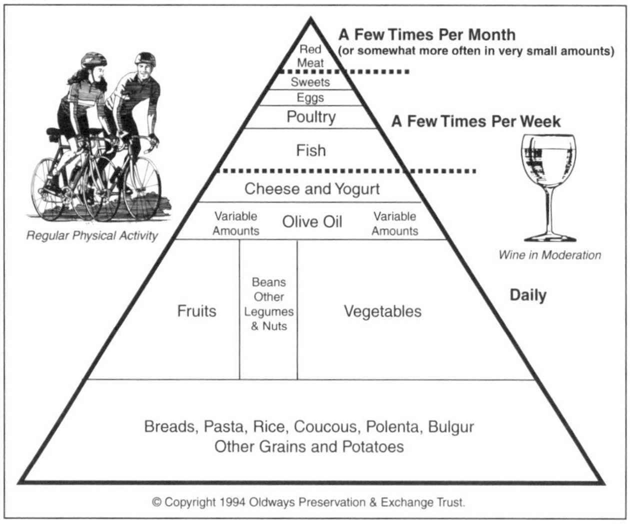

cultivation predominates and the intake of olive oil is high. In these areas, olive oil (74% MUFAs) has been consumed as the predominant source of fat for thousands of years. Overall, the Mediterranean eating pattern has been associated with a high life expectancy and low rates of CVD, certain cancers, and other diet-related chronic diseases (39).

In addition to the MUFA content, other factors (fiber, antioxidants, and various phytochemicals present in the fresh and minimally processed foods most often consumed) may be responsible for the health benefits attributed to the Mediterranean diet. Two additional factors associated with Mediterranean lifestyles—high levels of physical activity and maintenance of lean body weight—also play a role in disease prevention. Sociocultural factors include a high degree of social support in preparing, sharing, and enjoying meals; lengthy meals that provide time for relaxation; and after-lunch siestas that provide relief from daily stress. Although the diet is high in MUFAs, the benefits of the Mediterranean eating style may be due to an overall lifestyle that is conducive to cardiovascular health.

Rationale. The high-MUFA diet is often higher in total fat than recommended for the step I diet but low in SFAs. This low SFA intake results in the reduction in LDL-C reported in patients who adopt this diet.

At higher levels of fat consumption, MUFAs (primarily as oleic acid) are considered to be preferable to PUFAs (primarily as linoleic acid) because they are less likely to be oxidized in LDL-C and may contribute to maintaining higher levels of HDL-C. High MUFA intake from olive oil has been typical of Mediterranean areas for thousands of years with no evidence of harm, whereas long-term effects of a high PUFA intake are unknown.

In patients with diabetes, the high-MUFA diet provides a way to decrease SFAs and cholesterol without a corresponding increase in carbohydrate levels. High-carbohydrate, very-low-fat diets may exacerbate hypertriglyceridemia in some individuals similarly to the situation for patients with diabetes. Blood glucose control should be the first step taken to reduce elevated triglycerides along with other standard recommendations (reduce weight, decrease alcohol intake, and increase physical activity). A moderate-carbohydrate (50% of energy), high-MUFA diet may also improve triglyceride response.

Advantages and Disadvantages. A high proportion of MUFAs can be integrated into any of the other lipid-lowering diets simply by emphasizing high-MUFA oils and foods that are low in SFA. Many standard patient-education materials and exchange lists can easily be adapted to reflect high-MUFA food sources (Table 6-8). For individuals who have difficulty adhering to lower-fat diets, high-MUFA intakes offer a viable alternative. The high-MUFA diet is nutritionally adequate when a variety of food choices are made. Higher levels of HDL-C are observed with a high-MUFA, high-fat diet, so the diet may be of particular benefit to those with low HDL-C levels. Conversely, a disadvantage of the high-MUFA diets is that the higher fat content may make energy control challenging and, hence, weight management difficult in patients trying to lose or maintain weight.

High-soluble-fiber Diet

The population most likely to benefit from a diet high in soluble fiber includes anyone with hypercholesterolemia, especially anyone with a low intake of dietary fiber, and individuals with Type 2 diabetes and dyslipidemia.

Description. A high soluble-fiber intake is adjunctive to the dietary goals of the step I and step II diets. An adequate amount of dietary soluble fiber can be achieved with three servings of both fruits and vegetables, six or more servings of whole-grain products, and one serving of beans daily (40). The total and soluble fiber content of some common foods is shown in Table 6-9. Patients can be given the step I or step II goals or basic tip sheets for increasing fiber intake (such as shown in Box 6-2). Patients are advised to increase their fiber intake slowly. Dietary fiber intake should be assessed as part of the baseline diet assessment and should be increased in increments of 5 to 10 g/week; this increase should be accompanied by adequate fluid intake (8 to 12 glasses per day). Exchanges for high-fiber diets are similar to the American Dietetic Association exchanges except the starch group only contains breads, grains, and crackers (Table 6-10) (40); the cereal group only includes high-fiber choices; and there is an exchange group for beans.

Background. A number of studies since the 1970s have linked low intakes of dietary fiber to obesity, diabetes, and CVD. Fiber intake is also believed to facilitate weight loss and long-term maintenance because high-fiber foods tend to be low in fat, take longer to eat, increase fullness, and possibly suppress appetite by decreasing insulin concentrations (40).

Today several national nutrition guidelines promote the benefits of high fiber intakes for optimal health, including the National Cancer Institute 5-A-Day Program and the US Department of Agriculture Food Guide Pyramid (9,42). The amount of fiber currently recommended for healthy adults is 20 to 35 g/day or 10 to 13 g fiber/1,000 kcal consumed (40). Higher intakes (25 to 30 g/1,000 kcal) have been used to treat patients with diabetes (43). Until further research is available, a minimum intake of 20 g/day and a maximum intake of 60 g/day are considered feasible, well tolerated, and safe (44).

Fiber is classified according to its solubility in water. Insoluble fiber does not dissolve in water and is found in foods such as wheat bran, whole grains, and vegetables. Insoluble fiber promotes normal laxation and colonic function. Recent epidemiologic studies reported an inverse association between total dietary fiber and ischemic heart disease mortality and myocardial infarction (45,46). Rimm, Acherio, Giovannucci, Spiegelman, Stampfer, and Willett (46) reported that diets high in fiber, especially from cereal

TABLE 6-9

Fiber and Soluble Fiber Content of Common Foods

		Total Fiber (g)	Soluble Fiber (g)
Cereals			
Oat bran	½ cup	7.24	3.58
Oatmeal	½ cup dry	4.29	1.98
Oatmeal, instant	1 packet	3.09	1.43
Bran flakes	¾ cup	5.30	0.51
Raisin bran	1 cup	5.30	1.35
Whole-wheat bread	1 slice	1.96	0.34
Fruits			
Apple	1 medium	3.73	0.97
Banana	1 medium	2.74	0.68
Peaches, canned	½ cup	1.76	0.79
Pears, canned	½ cup	1.64	0.16
Prunes, dried	4	2.39	1.28
Orange	1 medium	3.14	1.83
Vegetables			
Broccoli, cooked	½ cup	2.76	1.38
Carrots, raw	1 medium	2.16	1.08
Corn, canned	½ cup	1.64	0.16
Potato, baked, w/skin	1 small	2.21	0.92
Black beans	½ cup	6.46	2.18
Garbanzo beans	½ cup	4.35	1.31
Kidney beans	½ cup	5.66	2.83
Lentils	½ cup	7.82	0.59
Split peas	½ cup	8.13	1.08

From: Minnesota Nutrition Data System, version 2.9. Nutrition Coordinating Center, University of Minnesota, Minneapolis, MN.

BOX 6-2 Tips for Adding Fiber to the Diet

- Choose fresh fruits rather than canned fruits or juices.
- Choose whole-grain breads.
- Leave the skins on fruits such as apples, pears, and peaches.
- Leave the skins on vegetables such as potatoes, squash, and carrots.
- Have a salad every day.
- When mashing potatoes, leave the skin on.
- Use brown rice rather than white rice.
- Use oats as a filler in casseroles, meat loaf, or salmon patties.
- Use whole-grain flours for baking.
- Use oats or oat bran as a thickening agent for sauces.
- Use high-fiber cereal daily.
- Choose raw vegetables and fresh fruits for snacks.
- Use whole-wheat pasta.
- Eat beans and peas often.
- Have a serving of dried beans or peas daily.
- Blenderize oats and use in cooking and baking.
- Eat foods in their most naturally occurring state.

From: Anderson JW (41).

but also from vegetables and fruit, significantly reduce coronary heart disease risk. Soluble fiber is soluble in water and affects blood lipid levels. Total cholesterol and LDL-C were significantly lowered in most soluble-fiber studies whereas HDL-C and triglycerides were unchanged (47).

The amount of soluble fiber necessary to lower blood cholesterol is shown in Table 6-11. For these sources of soluble fiber, the lipid-lowering effect is dose dependent. Overall, the average cholesterol lowering of a blood-cholesterol-lowering diet (ie, a step I diet) with soluble fiber was 11%. For LDL-C, a greater response was seen in hypercholesterolemic subjects (14% reduction) than in normolipemic subjects (10% reduction) (47). Soluble fiber from two servings of oats increased the cholesterol-lowering effect of a fat-modified diet by 2% to 3% (48) or 4% (49).

The addition of as little as 3 g of soluble fiber from oat products may result in modest reductions (5 to 6 mg/dL) in total cholesterol (48). Three grams of soluble fiber are equivalent to one large bowl of ready-to-eat oat bran cereal or three packets of instant oatmeal (oat bran has approximately twice the amount of soluble fiber of oatmeal).

Daily consumption of 6 to 10 g of soluble fiber is recommended for patients with hyperlipidemia (40). A 1:3 ratio of soluble to insoluble fiber is recommended. Dietary intake of appropriate foods is considered the most acceptable and safe approach to increasing soluble fiber consumption. Excellent food sources of soluble fiber include oats, legumes, beans, and dried peas. Fruits, vegetables, and barley are sources of both soluble and insoluble fiber. Fiber supplements made from pectin, guar gum, locust bean gum, and psyllium husks provide another source; however, viscosity, taste characteristics, and gastrointestinal side effects may be deterrents to their long-term use. The bulk laxative Metamucil (Procter & Gamble, Cincinnati, Ohio), which contains psyllium seed husks, has been used clinically in patients with hypercholesterolemia to reduce LDL-C by approximately 8% (1 teaspoon 3 times per day with meals provides approximately 10 g of soluble fiber) (50).

Rationale. Possible mechanisms for the cholesterol-lowering properties of soluble fiber include depletion of the bile acid pool (the fibers bind bile acids), which removes cholesterol from serum for bile acid synthesis and pool replenishment; inhibition of hepatic cholesterol synthesis by short-chain fatty acids that are produced by the colonic fermentation of soluble fiber; increased LDL-C catabolism; and replacement of dietary saturated fat and cholesterol with lower-fat choices that are concomitantly higher in soluble fiber (47).

Glore, Van Treeck, Knehans, and Guild (47) reviewed 77 studies on soluble fiber and found that 69 (88%) reported

TABLE 6-10

Exchanges for High-Fiber Diets

Exchange and Serving Size	Energy (kcal)	Protein (g)	Fat (g)	CHO (g)	Fiber (g)
Nonfat milk (1 cup)	90	8	0	12	0
Vegetables (½ cup)	25	1	0	5	2
Beans (½ cup)	95	7	0	17	5
Lean meat (1 oz)	55	7	3	0	0
Cereals[1] (1 oz)	90	3	0	20	4
Starches[2] (½ cup or 1 slice)	70	2	0	15	2
Fruits (½ cup)	60	0	0	15	2.5
Fats (1 tsp)	45	0	5	0	0

[1] Cereal exchanges include cold and hot cereals.

[2] Starch exchanges include breads, muffins, crackers, pasta, rice, and starchy vegetables.

From: Anderson JW, Smith BM, Gustafson NJ (40).

TABLE 6-11

Fiber Intake and Blood Cholesterol Changes

Food Source	Type of Fiber	Dry Weight (g/day)	Total Cholesterol (% change)
Fruits	Pectin	35	–13
Guar	Gum	20	–13
Beans[1]	Legumes	125	–13
Oatmeal[1]	Oats	100	–16
Wheat	Cellulose	15	0
Vegetables	Lignin	12	0

[1] Data based on hyperlipemic subjects (all others based on normolipemic subjects).

Adapted from: Kris-Etherton PM, Krummel D, Russell ME, Dreon D, Mackey S, Borchers J, Wood PD (10).

BOX 6-3 Prevention of Flatulence with Increasing Dietary Fiber

It can take a few months for the GI tract to adapt to high-fiber foods or a vegetarian eating style. The following tips may help to reduce intestinal gas during the transition to a diet high in fruit, vegetables, bran, whole grains, and/or beans.

- Increase the intake of raw and high-fiber foods gradually (5-10 g increments).
- Keep quantities small until GI tolerance improves.
- Drink sufficient fluid—at least 8-12 glasses a day—because higher fiber intakes increase fluid needs. Note: Beverages with caffeine or alcohol don't count because they increase fluid loss.
- Foods that are cooked or canned may be better tolerated than raw or fresh ones. Fruits, vegetables, or beans that are mashed, blenderized, or pureed may also be easier to digest—mix or blend them into baked goods, sauces, and other foods.
- Rinse canned beans before using. Boil and then soak dry beans for 4 hours; drain the soak water and replace it with fresh water for cooking.
- Maintain regular exercise.
- If needed, consult your doctor or pharmacist for special products that decrease the production of intestinal gas. Examples include Beano™, BeSure™, and Flatulex™—experiment with different types to find the brand that suits you best.

significant reductions in total cholesterol, 41 of 49 (84%) reported significant reductions in LDL-C, 43 of 57 (75%) reported no change in HDL-C, and 50 of 58 (86%) reported no change in triglyceride levels. Although the sources and amounts of soluble fiber varied, the authors concluded that most evidence points to significant lowering of total and LDL-C with soluble fiber. Significant reductions in total and LDL-C can be achieved with a diet high in soluble fiber, especially as part of a blood-cholesterol-lowering diet.

Advantages and Disadvantages. High soluble-fiber intake can be integrated into any of the lipid-lowering diets to enhance cholesterol response. The foods recommended are low in fat and energy and offer other nutrients of value (for example, antioxidants in fruit and vegetables and calcium and iron in beans). The lipid response to the addition of soluble fiber can be determined in a short time (2 to 3 weeks).

Individuals with chewing or swallowing difficulties or digestive and gastrointestinal problems may require more individual attention and guidance to increase fiber intake. Gastrointestinal side effects (flatulence, abdominal bloating, and loose stools) may occur as fiber is increased but tend to subside after prolonged use. See Box 6-3 for guidelines to prevent flatulence.

Dietary fibers may bind with certain minerals and decrease their bioavailability, but the effect of this is considered insignificant in healthy adults. A low-dose multivitamin mineral preparation can be used where indicated as a precautionary measure.

Vegetarian Diets

The population most likely to be nefit from vegetarian diets includes

- individuals who are already vegetarian or semivegetarian but require additional guidance to lower fat intake to meet step I and step II guidelines;
- individuals who are willing to give up meat and also to eat a variety of foods from other food groups (such as fruit, vegetables, legumes, and pasta);
- individuals who are willing and have time to learn about vegetarian eating, plan meals, and experiment with new food selections and recipes; and
- individuals who are at high risk for or have existing CVD and are highly motivated to adopt a vegetarian eating style.

Description. Vegetarian diets encompass various degrees of animal food avoidance ranging from semivegetarian (the diet includes red meat occasionally or avoids red meat but not poultry and fish), to lacto-ovo-vegetarian (a diet that is meat free but includes milk and eggs), to strict vegetarian or vegan (one free of all animal products). Other categories of vegetarianism include macrobiotic, fruitarian, raw foods, and natural hygiene (51). Much variation can exist within the categories because of individual preferences and philosophies, so a thorough diet interview of vegetarian clients is recommended to accurately assess eating style and nutritional needs.

Fat intake should be kept at 30% of energy or less, consistent with step I and step II guidelines. For very restrictive diets, recommendations from the New York Medical College Vegetarian Pyramid specify a minimum of 3 to 5 teaspoons of vegetable oil to achieve an adequate intake of energy and essential fatty acids (New York Medical College, NY). Figure 6-2 is the vegetarian pyramid developed by the Third International Congress on Vegetarian Nutrition. Most very-low-fat diets (<10% of energy from fat) are lacto-ovo-vegetarian or vegan.

All of the guidelines for the step I and step II diets can

be applied to vegetarian eating styles. More than the standard 2 to 4 egg yolks per week may be included in the meal plans of vegetarians who consume eggs as long as total dietary cholesterol goals are met. Dietary patterns for lacto-ovo and vegan diets are shown in Tables 6-12 and 6-13, respectively.

Foods with low nutrient density (concentrated sweets and high-fat foods) should be kept to a minimum and foods with high nutrient density should be emphasized. At least half of the grains consumed, for example, should be whole-grain products (52). Variety in food choices is also important; people who limit themselves to a narrow selection of foods increase their risk of developing nutritional problems.

The nutrients most commonly at risk for being too low in vegetarian diets are iron, zinc, calcium, and vitamins B_{12} and D. In general, vegans require a supplementary source of vitamin B_{12}, such as fortified soy milk, cereals, meat analogs, blackstrap molasses, and other supplemented products (eg, nutritional yeast). People following such diets who live in areas with limited sunshine may need vitamin D, which can be obtained from fortified cereals. All other nutrients can usually be obtained in sufficient amounts from the diet. Any additional vitamin and mineral supplementation should be considered on an individual basis.

Protein needs can be met by consuming a variety of plant foods in amounts sufficient to meet energy needs. Mixtures of proteins from grains, vegetables, legumes, seeds, and nuts complement one another in their amino acid profiles. Contrary to popular belief, it is not necessary that amino acid complementation occur at the same meal as long as a varied diet is consumed (53). Soy protein, a high-quality protein, is an excellent alternative to animal protein. An average of 31 to 47 g/day of soy reduced total cholesterol (9%), LDL-C (13%), and triglycerides (11%) in patients with hypercholesterolemia (54). See Chapter 12 for a discussion of soy protein as a functional food; the quantity of soy protein and other key nutrients in soy products is shown in Table 12-3.

FIGURE 6-2

The proposed vegetarian food guide pyramid

Source: The Third International Congress on Vegetarian Nutrition, Loma Linda, Calif, 1997.

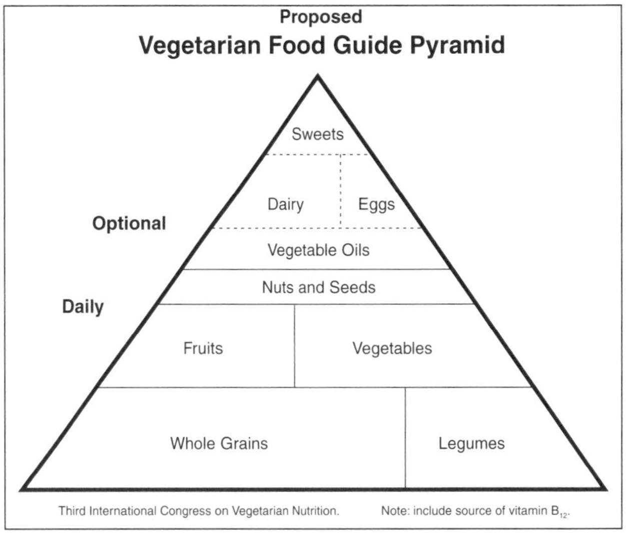

TABLE 6-12

Dietary Patterns for Lacto-ovo-vegetarian Diets at 3 Energy Levels

	1,600 kcal	2,200 kcal	2,800 kcal
	Servings/Day		
Bread, grains, cereals[1]	6	9	11
Legumes, plant proteins	1	2	3
Vegetables	3	4	5
Fruits	2	3	4
Nuts, seeds	1	1	1
Milk, yogurt, cheese	2-3[2]	2-3[2]	2-3[2]
Eggs	½	½	½
Added fats and oils[3]	2	4	6
Added sugar[4]	3	6	9
Approximate composition:			
Protein (g)	70	88	103
Fat (g)	50	62	74
Energy as fat (%)	28	25	24
Saturated fat (g)	16	18	20
Energy as saturated fat (%)	9	7	6

[1] At least half of the servings from whole-grain breads and cereals.

[2] Three servings for women who are pregnant or breast-feeding, for teenagers, and for young adults aged ≤ 24 years.

[3] Fat added to food during food preparation or used as spreads and dressings.

[4] Sugar and other caloric sweeteners (eg, syrup, honey) added to food and bakery items during food preparation and used in drinks, beverages, and desserts.

From: Haddad E (52).

Background. Compared with meat eaters, vegetarians are less obese. They tend to consume less energy; less total fat, saturated fat, and cholesterol; and more unsaturated fat, antioxidants, dietary fiber, and phytochemicals. Vegetarian diets modify blood pressure in both normotensive and hypertensive individuals and appear to blunt the rise in blood pressure that occurs with age. There is also evidence that plant-based vegetarian diets that are low in SFAs and cholesterol have favorable effects on lipids and lipoproteins and can slow or halt the progression of atheromatous plaques as well as contribute to plaque regression (55).

Rationale. There has been increasing interest in vegetarian eating styles for improving cardiovascular health (55-57). Vegetarian diets are usually low in SFAs and cholesterol because of the avoidance of animal products. Plant-based diets also provide significant amounts of complex carbohydrate, fiber, unsaturated fatty acids, and antioxidants. The phytochemicals present in plants may also be protective. In numerous studies, vegetarian diets have been associated with favorable health benefits including those related to CVD (51,55).

Advantages and Disadvantages. Well-designed vegetarian diets can be delicious, heart healthy, and nutritionally adequate. The vegetarian eating style is often also accompanied by other healthful lifestyle characteristics, such as lean body weight, regular physical activity, and abstinence from smoking, alcohol, and illicit drugs. Overall, vegetarian eating styles may not only reduce the risk of CVD but also decrease the risk of gallstones, osteoporosis, kidney disease, and cancer (53). In addition, as noted, vegetarian approaches can be effective for lipid management, weight loss, and blood pressure control. Many individuals may find it easier to take the vegetarian approach of eliminating meat and full-fat animal products altogether (and experience positive results quickly) rather than limit consumption of meat and other animal products (and obtain results more slowly) (19). With some initial dietary guidance from a registered dietitian, the transition to the new eating style can be a positive experience. However, vegetarian eating styles are not for everyone. They require more forethought and planning than nonvegetarian diets and some individuals may consider them to be too extreme. Adherence can also be a challenge at restaurants and social events.

Not all vegetarian diets are low in fat or nutritionally adequate. A lacto-ovo-vegetarian, for example, could have a high intake of SFAs and cholesterol by inclusion of whole milk, eggs, cheese, butter, cream, sweets, desserts, and fried foods. Eating patterns that are too restrictive may lead to nutrient deficiencies, underweight, or other associated health problems. Fruitarian and macrobiotic diets are examples that are often nutritionally inadequate. Careful assessment and planning are necessary to prevent nutrient deficiencies and are especially important in work with infants, children, adolescents, and women who are pregnant, lactating, or trying to conceive (58). Dietary patterns for vegetarian children are shown in Table 6-14.

TABLE 6-13

Dietary Patterns for Vegan Diets at 3 Energy Levels

	1,600 kcal	2,200 kcal	2,800 kcal
	Servings/Day		
Bread, grains, cereals [1]	8	10	12
Legumes, plant proteins	1	2	3
Vegetables	2	3	4
Dark-green leafy vegetables	2	2	2
Fruits	2	4	6
Nuts, seeds	1	1	1
Fortified soy drinks and tofu [2]	2-3[3]	2-3[3]	2-3[3]
Added fats and oils [4]	2	4	6
Added sugar [5]	3	6	9
Approximate composition:			
Protein (g)	60	76	95
Fat (g)	46	58	78
Energy as fat (%)	26	24	25
Saturated fat (g)	8	10	12
Energy as saturated fat (%)	5	4	4

[1] At least half of the servings from whole-grain breads and cereals.

[2] Milk alternatives fortified with calcium, vitamin D, and vitamin B_{12}, and multivitamin and mineral supplements and other supplements.

[3] Three servings for women who are pregnant or breast-feeding, for teenagers, and for young adults aged ≤ 24 years.

[4] Fat added to food during food preparation or used as spreads and dressings.

[5] Sugar and other caloric sweeteners (eg, syrup, honey) added to food and bakery items during food preparation and used in drinks, beverages, and desserts.

From: Haddad E (52).

Sodium-restricted Diets

The population most likely to benefit from a sodium-restricted diet includes patients with hypertension who are salt sensitive and patients with congestive heart failure.

Description. The recommended sodium level in a restricted diet ranges from 2,300 mg/day to 3,000 mg/day depending on the group making the recommendation (1 mEq sodium = 1 mmol sodium = 23 mg sodium). Many Americans (58% of men and 68% of women) are already restricting their salt use at the table (59). To achieve a diet with 2,000 to 3,000 mg of sodium, salt use should be limited and salt should be replaced with herbs and other spices, natural flavorings, and lower-sodium seasonings and condiments. Minimally processed foods should be encouraged because many processed foods (including low-fat choices) can be significant sources of sodium (Box 6-4). Because foods prepared outside of the home often contain added salt, more home preparation of food and care in food selection when dining in restaurants are advised. The easiest approach for monitoring sodium intake is counting milligrams of sodium in foods. Food labels list sodium content, and a book that lists the sodium content of foods is a valuable resource for determining the content of foods that do not have a nutrition label (eg, meat).

Background. In populations with very high sodium intakes (more than 3,450 to 4,600 mg/day), such as Japan, hypertension and stroke are prevalent. In countries characterized by low sodium intakes, the opposite is true. NHBPEP recommends moderate salt restriction (2,300 mg/day) for prevention and treatment of hypertension (8). Consumption of this level of sodium prevented an expected average 9 mm Hg rise in systolic blood pressure seen from age 25 to 55 years (60).

Rationale. The amount of sodium restriction depends on the diagnosis. Patients with hypertension may be salt sensitive, so sodium should be restricted to less than 2,300 mg/day. At present, there is no readily available method for determining salt sensitivity in hypertensive patients or those likely to benefit from sodium restriction. Groups shown to be more salt sensitive are older, overweight, African American, or have low rennin levels (61). Mild congestive heart failure is often treated with a 2,000- to 3,000-mg sodium diet, whereas moderate or severe congestive heart failure often necessitates a 1,000- to 2,000-mg sodium limit (62). The level of sodium and fluid restriction is individualized on the basis of medications and symptom improvement. Very strict sodium restrictions (less than 500 mg) should be avoided if possible because of food palatability concerns. The use of sodium-restricted diets is controversial. Recently, increased myocardial infarctions were observed in the hypertensive patients who had the lowest urinary sodium concentrations (63). The implications of this finding are unknown but warrant further study.

Advantages and Disadvantages. An advantage of a moderate sodium restriction is that in some patients, blood pressure will be normalized by diet changes, eliminating the need for pharmacologic therapy. A disadvantage is that many processed foods must be limited from the diet. Many

TABLE 6-14

Dietary Patterns for Vegetarian Children

	Toddlers Aged 1-2 Yrs (~1,300 kcal)	Preschooler Aged 3-6 Yrs (~1,800 kcal)	Preadolescent Aged 7-10 Yrs (~2,000 kcal)
	Servings/Day		
Bread, grains, cereals	3-4	4-5	5-6
Legumes, plant proteins	½	1	1
Vegetables	1-2	2-3	2-3
Fruits	2-3	2-3	3-4
Nut butters (nuts)	¼	½	1
Milk, yogurt, cheese, or fortified soy milk [1]	2-3	2-3	2-3
Egg	½	½	½
Added margarine and oils [2]	2	3-4	4
Added sugar [3]	3	3-6	6
Approximate composition:			
Protein (g)	54	63	72
Fat (g)	52	52	61
Energy as fat (%)	36	26	27

[1] Whole or full-fat milk and alternatives.

[2] Fat added to food during food preparation or used as spreads and dressings, including margarine fortified with vitamins A and D.

[3] Sugar and other caloric sweeteners (eg, syrup, honey) Added to food and bakery items during food preparation and used in drinks, beverages, and desserts.

From: Haddad E (52).

BOX 6-4 High-Sodium Foods

Each item listed contains approximately 400 mg sodium, and should be used with care.

- **Miscellaneous items**
  ¼ tsp salt
  1 tsp soy sauce
  4 tsp Worcestershire sauce
  2⅓ Tbsp catsup
  2 Tbsp mustard, chili sauce, or barbecue sauce
  4⅔ Tbsp tartar sauce
  4⅔ Tbsp mayonnaise
  4 Tbsp thousand island salad dressing
  3 Tbsp Russian salad dressing
  2 Tbsp French salad dressing
  1⅓ Tbsp Italian salad dressing
  4 medium, 3 extra large, or 2 giant green olives (16 g)
  4 Tbsp sweet pickle relish (60 g)
- **Meat items**
  1 small hot dog
  1 slice lunch meat
  4 slices bacon
  1½ oz cooked pork sausage
  1½ oz ham or corned beef
  1½ oz regular canned tuna
  3 oz regular canned salmon
  1½ oz regular canned crab
  ¾ cup cottage cheese
  2 oz cheese
  ¼ of a 12-inch thin-crust pizza
- **Bread, cereal, dessert items**
  20 pretzels, small
  2 twisted, medium pretzels
  1 Dutch or soft pretzel
- **Vegetable items**
  2 servings (½ cup each) regular canned vegetables
  ⅓ cup canned regular sauerkraut, drained
  ½ large dill pickle (30 g)
  1 oz (approximately 20) potato chips
- **Soup items**
  (All soups listed are canned soups diluted with equal amounts of water)
  ⅔ cup beef broth or vegetarian vegetable
  ½ cup bisque of tomato, clam chowder (Manhattan style), chicken gumbo, cream of asparagus, cream of celery, tomato rice, or tomato
  ⅓ cup cream of mushroom

From: ADA Manual of Clinical Dietetics, 4th edition.

reduced-fat frozen foods, salad dressings, condiments, and soups are high in sodium. Careful reading of food labels is important, especially for patients with lower sodium goals. For some patients these goals are the most difficult to achieve.

Cardiac Diet

The population most likely to benefit from this diet includes individuals hospitalized with some manifestation of CVD and individuals with coronary heart disease.

Description. The cardiac diet is based on the step II diet and provides 2,400 mg of sodium or less. Caffeine is usually restricted. Fluids may be restricted to manage fluid retention or congestive heart failure.

Further modifications should be made as needed to meet individual nutritional needs and deal with potential drug-nutrient interactions. High potassium intake or potassium supplementation (Box 6-5) may be indicated for patients receiving potassium-depleting medications. Salt substitutes can be a significant source of potassium and should be avoided by patients receiving medication that elevates serum potassium levels (potassium-sparing diuretics and angiotensin-converting enzyme inhibitors).

Adjustments in energy level may be needed for weight gain, maintenance, or loss. Although weight reduction for overweight patients is desired, weight maintenance is usually indicated during postsurgical recovery periods. Patients with cardiac cachexia (malnutrition secondary to prolonged myocardial insufficiency) may need additional intervention and nutrition support to promote positive nitrogen balance and anabolism.

The step II diet should be maintained in combination with other dietary modifications. Atherosclerotic disease is progressive and will continue to develop (even after cardiovascular surgery) unless an intervention changes the course of the disease. Dietary intervention can stop disease progression and therefore has a critical role in comprehensive cardiac treatment.

Background. A cardiac diet may be prescribed for patients who have had a myocardial infarction, cardiovascular surgery, or other condition related to CVD. This diet is consistent with overall nutrition recommendations during the acute treatment phase. In the long term this diet can slow progression of CVD; more severe dietary and lifestyle changes may halt or reverse the disease (25).

Rationale. Patients with existing coronary heart disease are in the highest risk category for future disease events. Aggressive cholesterol-lowering therapy is required to reduce LDL-C to the NCEP goal of 100 mg/dL or less. Angiographic studies indicate that reduction of LDL-C to this level retards the rate of progression of atherosclerosis and in some patients can lead to the regression of lesions (2). Sodium restriction is usually advised for cardiac patients because of fluid retention and hypertension. Many lower-fat food products are high in sodium, so guidance in this area is especially helpful.

BOX 6-5 **Potassium Content of Some Common Foods**

Each item listed contains more than 300 mg of potassium.

- **Bread/Cereal**
  Concentrated bran cereal (½ cup)
  Raisin bran (1 cup)

- **Dairy**
  Milk, any fluid (1 cup)
  Yogurt (8 oz)

- **Fruit/Juice**
  Banana (1 medium)
  Cantaloupe (1 cup)
  Figs, dried (3 medium)
  Honeydew (1 cup)
  Orange juice (½ cup)
  Prune juice (½ cup)
  Prunes, dried (5 large)
  Raisins (⅓ cup)
  Tomato juice (½ cup)

- **Meat/Poultry/Fish**
  Flounder (2 oz)

- **Miscellaneous**
  Potato chips (1 oz)
  French fries (1 cup)

- **Vegetables**
  Avocado, raw (⅓ whole)
  Bamboo shoots (½ cup)
  Beans, red (½ cup)
  Beans, lima, cooked (½ cup)
  Celery, raw (1 cup)
  Potato, baked (1 medium)
  Potato, boiled in skin (1 medium)
  Spinach, cooked (½ cup)
  Sweet potato, baked in skin (1 small)
  Tomatoes, canned (½ cup)
  Tomato, raw (1 medium)
  Tomato sauce (½ cup)

From: The Clinical Center Nutrition Department, National Institutes of Health, 1996.

A daily sodium intake of 2,300 mg or less is consistent with the NHBPEP guidelines; lower levels of sodium may be indicated on an individual basis. Caffeine may be restricted because of its stimulating effect on the central nervous system and the risk of cardiac arrhythmias. Small, frequent feedings are suggested for the immediate postsurgical period. Larger meals can increase myocardial oxygen demand, cause abdominal distention, and interfere with breathing by impairing normal diaphragmatic motion. The typical hospital stay for cardiac procedures can be as short as 1 day for angioplasty or 5 days for coronary artery bypass grafting. Thus, time for diet education is limited in the acute care setting. Optimally, patients should be referred to a dietitian who serves outpatients after discharge.

Advantages and Disadvantages. The cardiac diet provides patients with some control over the disease process and can also enhance the efficacy of other concurrent therapies (for example, drug therapy and exercise). Initial adjustment to the new eating style may be difficult, but there are many ways to individualize the diet to suit a patient's eating style and preferences. Successful integration of the diet into a patient's lifestyle takes time and effort on the part of the patient, and often requires social support from family and friends. Frequent follow-up, feedback, and reinforcement from health professionals are essential until the patient successfully adopts the new eating style.

Expected Response to Diet Therapies

Shown in Table 6-15 is the expected response to diet therapy as reported in response to nutrition intervention. Average responses are reported; individuals may have a much greater or lesser response to the diet for the major CVD risk factors. Thus, although diet favorably affects various CVD risk factors, some patients will be able to manage their clinical condition with diet alone, whereas others may have to use diet therapy as an adjunct to drug therapy and other lifestyle modifications.

Summary

Diet intervention is the cornerstone for both prevention and treatment of CVD. The step I diet is the first diet of choice for medical nutrition therapy. If lipid and other physiological goals are not achieved, more aggressive diets are warranted before diet therapy is abandoned. Diet interventions should be consistent with individual lifestyles so that long-term adherence is achieved. Practical applications of the nutritional management of dyslipidemia—three case studies and the lipid profiles for six patients—are presented in the case studies and patient profiles that follow.

Research continues to explore other dietary options for reduction of CVD risk factors. Foods high in n-3 fatty acids, the antioxidant nutrients, and soy protein affect components

TABLE 6-15

Expected Response to Diet Therapy

	Step I	Step II	Very-Low-Fat	High-MUFA
			% Change	
Total cholesterol	↓ 5-15	↓ 5-20	> 20	↓ 5-15
LDL cholesterol	↓ 5-20	↓ 10-25	> 20	↓ 5-20
HDL cholesterol	↓ 0 to -10[1]	↓ 0 to -15[1]	↑ With weight loss ↓ Without weight loss	Slight ↓ or no change [2] or ↑[3]
Triglycerides	+5 to -10[1]	+10 to -10[1]	↓ With weight loss ↑ Without weight loss	No change or slight ↓

[1] Without weight loss or increased exercise. With weight loss, total cholesterol and LDL-C will decrease more; HDL-C will increase and triglycerides will decrease.

[2] Compared with average American diet (high-fat/high-saturated-fat diet).

[3] Compared with low-fat diet.

of the CVD risk profile and may offer additional dietary strategies for the prevention and treatment of CVD. These and other foods with potential significance to CVD are reviewed in Chapter 12.

REFERENCES

1. Chait A, Brunzell JD, Denke MA, Eisenberg D, Ernst ND, Franklin FA Jr, Ginsberg H, Kotchen TA, Kuller L, Mullis RM, Nichaman MZ, Nicolosi RJ, Schaefer EJ, Stone JF, Weidman WH. Rationale of the diet-heart statement of the American Heart Association. Report of the Nutrition Committee. *Circulation*. 1993;88:3008-3029.
2. *Second Report of the Expert Panel on Detection, Evaluation, and Treatment of High Blood Cholesterol in Adults (Adult Treatment Panel II)*. Bethesda, Md: National Institutes of Health; 1993. NIH publication 93-3095.
3. Krummel DA. Cardiovascular disease. In: Krummel DA, Kris-Etherton PM, eds. *Nutrition in Women's Health*. Gaithersburg, Md: Aspen; 1996:383-417.
4. Connor WE, Connor SL. Importance of diet in the treatment of familial hypercholesterolemia. *Am J Cardiol*. 1993;72:42D-53D.
5. Sempos CT, Cleeman JI, Caroll MD, Johnson CL, Bachorik PS, Gordon DJ, Burton VL, Briefel RR, Brown CD, Lippel K, Rifkind BM. Prevalence of high blood cholesterol among US adults. *JAMA*. 1993;269:3009-3014.
6. Van Horn LV, Bujnowski M, Schwaba J, Mathieu-Harris M, Donato K, Cleeman J. Dietitians' contributions to cholesterol education: a decade of progress. *J Am Diet Assoc*. 1995;95:1263-1267.
7. Smith KG, Johnson EQ, eds. *Medical Nutrition Therapy Across the Continuum of Care*. Chicago, Ill: American Dietetic Association, 1996.
8. *The Fifth Report of the Joint National Committee on Detection, Evaluation, and Treatment of High Blood Pressure*. Washington, DC: US Dept of Health and Human Services, National Heart, Lung, and Blood Institute; 1993. NIH publication 93-1088.
9. *Food Guide Pyramid: A Guide to Daily Food Choices*. Washington, DC: US Department of Agriculture, Human Information Service; 1992. Home and Garden Bulletin No. 252.
10. Kris-Etherton PM, Krummel D, Russell ME, Dreon D, Mackey S, Borchers J, Wood PD. The effect of diet on plasma lipids, lipoproteins, and coronary heart disease. *J Am Diet Assoc*. 1988;88:1373-1400.
11. Fredrickson DS. *Dietary Management of Hyperlipoproteinemia: A Handbook for Physicians and Dietitians*. Bethesda, Md: National Heart, Lung, and Blood Institute; 1974. DHEW Publication No. (NIH) 75-110.
12. Ernst N, Cleeman J, Mullis R, Sooter-Bochenek J, Van Horn L. The National Cholesterol Education Program: implications for dietetic practitioners from the Adult Treatment Panel Recommendations. *J Am Diet Assoc*. 1988;88:1401-1411.
13. American Heart Association, Nutrition Committee. Dietary guidelines for healthy American adults. *Circulation*. 1988;77:721A-724A.
14. Watts GF, Jackson P, Mandalia S, Brunt JN, Lewis ES, Coltart DJ, Lewis B. Nutrient intake and progression of coronary artery disease. *Am J Cardiol*. 1994;73:328-333.
15. Watts GF, Jackson P, Burke V, Lewis B. Dietary fatty acids and progression of coronary artery disease in men. *Am J Clin Nutr*. 1996;64:202-209.
16. Connor WE. The decisive influence of diet on the progression and reversibility of coronary heart disease. *Am J Clin Nutr*. 1996;64:253-254.
17. Connor SL, Connor WE. *The New American Diet*. New York, NY: Simon & Schuster; 1986.
18. Pritikin N. *The Pritikin Program for Diet and Exercise*. New York, NY: Grosset & Dunlap; 1982.
19. Ornish D. *Eat More, Weigh Less*. New York, NY: HarperCollins Publishers; 1994.
20. Posner BM, Cobb JL, Belanger AJ, Cupples A, D'Agostino RB, Stokes J. Dietary lipid predictors of coronary heart disease in men. *Arch Intern Med*. 1991;151:1181-1187.
21. McGill HC. *Geographic Pathology of Atherosclerosis*. Baltimore, Md: Williams & Wilkins; 1968.
22. Campbell TC, Junshi C. Diet and chronic degenerative diseases: perspectives from China. *Am J Clin Nutr*. 1994;59(suppl):1153S-1161S.
23. Blankenhorn DH, Johnson RL, Mack WJ, El Zein HA, Vailas LI. The influence of diet on the appearance of new lesions in human coronary arteries. *JAMA*. 1990;263:1646-1652.
24. Schuler G, Hambrecht R, Schlierf G, Niebauer J, Hauer K,

Neumann J, Hoberg E, Drinkmann A, Bacher F, Grunze M, Kubler W. Regular physical exercise and low-fat diet: effects on progression of coronary artery disease. *Circulation.* 1992;86:1-11.
25. Ornish D, Brown SE, Scherwitz LW, Billings JH, Armstrong WT, Ports TA, McLanahan SM, Kirkeeide RL, Brand RJ, Gould KL. Can lifestyle changes reverse coronary heart disease? The Lifestyle Heart Trial. *Lancet*. 1990;336:129-133.
26. Kristal AR, White E, Shattuck AL, Curry S, Anderson GL, Fowler A, Urban N. Long-term maintenance of a low-fat diet: durability of fat-related dietary habits in the Women's Health Trial. *J Am Diet Assoc*. 1992;92:553-559.
27. Connor SL, Gustafson JR, Sexton G, Becker N, Artaud-Wild S, Connor WE. The Diet Habit Survey: a new method of dietary assessment that relates to plasma cholesterol changes. *J Am Diet Assoc*. 1992;92:41-47.
28. Chen YD, Coulston AM, Zhou MY, Hollenbeck CB, Reaven GM. Why do low-fat high-carbohydrate diets accentuate post-prandial lipemia in patients with NIDDM? *Diabetes Care*. 1995;18:10-16.
29. Tinker LF. Dietary fat: is less or more better? *On the Cutting Edge* 1995;16:17-21.
30. Willett WC, Sacks F, Trichopoulou A, Drescher G, Ferro-Luzzi A, Helsing E, Trichopouos D. Mediterranean diet pyramid: a cultural model for healthy eating. *Am J Clin Nutr.* 1995;61:1402S-1406S.
31. Mensink RP. Dietary monounsaturated fatty acids and serum lipoprotein levels in healthy subjects. *Atherosclerosis*. 1994;110:65-68.
32. Nydahl MC, Gustafsson I, Vessby B. Lipid-lowering diets enriched with monounsaturated or polyunsaturated fatty acids but low in saturated fatty acids have similar effects on serum lipid concentrations in hyperlipidemic patients. *Am J Clin Nutr*. 1994;59:115-122.
33. Lichtenstein AH, Ausman LM, Carrasco W, Jenner JL, Gualtieri LJ, Goldin BR, Ordovas JM, Schaefer EJ. Effects of canola, corn, and olive oils on fasting and postprandial plasma lipoproteins in humans and part of a National Cholesterol Education Program Step 2 Diet. *Arterioscler Thromb.* 1993;13:1533-1542.
34. Reaven P, Parthasarathy S, Grasse BJ, Miller E, Almazan F, Mattson FH, Khoo JC, Steinberg D, Witztum JL. Feasibility of using an oleate-rich diet to reduce the susceptibility of low-density lipoprotein to oxidative modification in humans. *Am J Clin Nutr*. 1991;54:701-706.
35. Coulston AM, Hollenbeck CB, Swislocki AL, Chen I, Reaven GM. Persistence of hypertriglyceridemic effects of low-fat, high-carbohydrate diets in NIDDM patients. *JAMA*. 1989;12:94-101.
36. Garg A, Bantle JP, Henry RR, Coulston AM, Griver KA, Raatz SK, Brinkley L, Chen YD, Grundy SM, Haet BA, Reaven GM. Effects of varying carbohydrate content of diet in patients with non-insulin-dependent diabetes mellitus. *JAMA*. 1994;271:1421-1428.
37. Rasmussen OW, Thomsen C, Hansen KW, Vesterlund M, Winther E, Hermansen K. Effects on blood pressure, glucose, and lipid levels of a high-monounsaturated fat diet compared with a high-carbohydrate diet in NIDDM subjects. *Diabetes Care*. 1993;16:1565-1571.
38. Bonanome A, Vison A, Lusiani L, Beltramello G, Confortin L, Biffanti S, Sorgato F, Costa F, Pagnan A. Carbohydrate and lipid metabolism in patients with non-insulin-dependent diabetes mellitus: effects of a low-fat, high-carbohydrate diet vs a diet high in monounsaturated fatty acids. *Am J Clin Nutr*. 1991;54:586-590.
39. Kushi LH, Lenart EB, Willett WC. Health implications of Mediterranean diets in light of contemporary knowledge: 1. Plant foods and dairy products. *Am J Clin Nutr.* 1995;61:1407S-1415S.
40. Anderson JW, Smith BM, Gustafson NJ. Health benefits and practical aspects of high-fiber diets. *Am J Clin Nutr.* 1994;59:1242S-1247S.
41. Anderson JW. *HCF Exchanges: A Sensible Plan for Healthy Eating*. Lexington, Ky: HCF Nutrition Research Foundation, Inc; 1989.
42. Heimendinger J, Van Duyn MA, Chapelsky D, Foerster S, Stables G. The National 5 A Day for Better Health Program: a large-scale nutrition intervention. *J Pub Health Management.* 1996;31:162-170.
43. Diabetes Care and Education Dietetic Practice Group of the American Dietetic Association. *Meal Planning Approaches for Diabetes Management.* Chicago, Ill: American Dietetic Association; 1994.
44. Lanza E, Schatzkin A, Ballard-Barbash R, Clifford DC, Paskett, E, Hayes D, Bote E, Caan B, Shike M, Weissfeld J, Slattery M, Mateski D, Daston C. The Polyp Prevention Trial II: Dietary Intervention Program, participant baseline dietary characteristics. *Cancer Epidemiol Biomarkers Prev.* 996;5:385-392.
45. Khaw KT, Barrett Connor E. Dietary fiber and reduced ischemic heart disease mortality rates in men and women: a 12-year prospective study. *Am J Epidemiol.* 1987;126:1093-1102.
46. Rimm E, Ascherio A, Giovannucci E, Spiegelman D, Stampfer M, Willett W. Vegetable, fruit and cereal intake and risk of coronary heart disease among men. *JAMA*. 1996;275:447-451.
47. Glore SR, Van Treeck D, Knehans AW, Guild M. Soluble fiber and serum lipids: a literature review. *J Am Diet Assoc*. 1994;94:425-436.
48. Ripsin CM, Keenan JM, Jacobs DR, Elmer PJ, Welch RR, Van Horn L, Liu K, Turnbull WH, Thye FW, Kestin M, Hegsted M, Davidson DM, Davidson MH, Dugan LD, Demark Wahnefried W, Beling S. Oat products and lipid lowering: a meta analysis. *JAMA*. 1992;267:3317-3325.
49. Anderson JW, Garrity TF, Wood CL, Whitis SE, Smith BM, Oeltgen PR. Prospective, randomized, controlled comparison of the effects of low fat and low fat plus high fiber diets on serum lipid concentrations. *Am J Clin Nutr*. 1992;56:887-894.
50. Bell LP, Hectorne K, Reynolds H, Balm TK, Hunninghake DB. Cholesterol-lowering effects of psyllium hydrophilic mucilloid. *JAMA*. 1989;261:3419-3423.
51. Messina M, Messina V. *The Dietitian's Guide to Vegetarian Diets.* Gaithersburg, Md: Aspen Publishers, Inc.; 1996.
52. Haddad EH. Development of a vegetarian food guide. *Am J Clin Nutr.* 1995;59:1248S-1254S.
53. Havala S, Dwyer JT. Position of the American Dietetic Association: vegetarian diets. *J Am Diet Assoc*. 1993;93:1317-1319.
54. Anderson JW, Johnstone BM, Cook-Newell M. Meta-analysis of the effects of soy protein intake on serum lipids. *N Engl J Med*. 1995;333:276-282.
55. Whitten C. Vegetarian diets and ischemic heart disease. *Top Clin Nutr*. 1995;10:27-33.
56. Barnard ND, Akhtar A, Nicholson A. Factors that facilitate compliance to lower fat intake. *Arch Fam Med.* 1995;4:153-158.
57. Johnston PK. Vegetarians among us: implications for health

professionals. *Top Clin Nutr*. 1995;10:1-6.

58. Dwyer JT. Vegetarianism for women. In: Krummel DA, Kris-Etherton PM, eds. *Nutrition in Women's Health*. Gaithersburg, Md: Aspen Publishers, 1996:232-262.
59. Federation of American Societies for Experimental Biology, Life Science Research Office. *Third Report on Nutrition Monitoring in the United States: executive summary.* Bethesda, Md: Federation of American Societies for Experimental Biology; 1995.
60. Intersalt Cooperative Research Group. Sodium, potassium, body mass, alcohol, blood pressure: the INTERSALT study. *J Hypertens*. 1988;6:S584-S586.
61. Stern JS. Perspectives on sodium. *Perspect Appl Nutr.* 1995;3:127-129.
62. Krummel DA. Nutritional care in heart failure and transplant. In: Mahan LK, Escott-Stump S, eds. *Food, Nutrition, and Diet Therapy.* Philadelphia: WB Saunders, 1996; 737-750.
63. Alderman MH, Madhavan S, Cohen H, Sealey JE, Laragh JH. Low urinary sodium is associated with greater risk of myocardial infarction among treated hypertensive men. *Hypertension.* 1995;25:1144-1152.

CASE STUDIES: PRACTICAL APPLICATIONS OF THE NUTRITIONAL MANAGEMENT OF DYSLIPIDEMIA

JULIE H. BURNS, MS, RD, AND WAHIDA KARMALLY, MS, RD

Three detailed case studies and six patients' lipid profiles are presented here. The best approach for any patient should be determined by an evaluation of clinical status, a thoughtful assessment of the patient's motivation and barriers to making dietary changes, the patient's responsiveness to diet therapy, his or her ability to understand the basic concepts of nutrition intervention and, most importantly, the support systems available to implement the prescribed eating plan.

Case Study 1: A Middle-aged Man with Type III Dyslipidemia (Carbohydrate-sensitive Inherited Form of Hyperlipoproteinemia)

Mr. X is a single 41-year-old toxicologist with familial dysbetalipoproteinemia (Type III HLP). Although some patients with familial dysbetalipoproteinemia also have diabetes, this patient does not. Before Mr. X relocated to Chicago, he lived in Minnesota and had been treated with 20 mg Mevacor (Merck & Co, Inc, West Point, Pa) and 1,500 mg niacin. His lipid concentrations responded well on this therapy, but his liver function tests were consistently greater than three times the upper limit of normal. As a result, he was switched to 600 mg Lopid bid (Parke-Davis, Morris Plains, NJ). The physical exam was not significant and no xanthomas were observed. Mr. X has a strong family history of premature coronary heart disease (father died at 47 years from a fatal myocardial infarction). When Mr. X was seen by his new Chicago cardiologist for an initial assessment, he was not taking his prescribed medication (Lopid 600 mg bid and aspirin q d) regularly because he was still adjusting to his new job and city. Mr. X exercises aerobically about three times per week (20 to 30 minutes on a treadmill at the health club). The patient was referred by the cardiologist to a registered dietitian; his clinical data are in Table 6-16.

Analysis of Mr. X's baseline diet revealed 39% of total energy was obtained from fat; 12% of his total energy was from saturated fat. Mr. X was also consuming, on average, 380 mg dietary cholesterol and 10 g dietary fiber daily. A liberal step I diet (not energy controlled, medium-fat meats, 2% milk) was prescribed initially to allow Mr. X some time to adjust to a low-fat diet and to improve patient adherence to diet therapy. One to two fish meals per week and the gradual adoption of a high-fiber intake (20 to 35 g) were also encouraged, along with the recommendation to continue his aerobics three times per week for 30 minutes per session and acquire a minimum of 30 minutes of moderate-intensity exercise (such as brisk walking, biking, swimming, yard work, or home repair) on most days of the week. After 6 weeks, Mr. X was moved to a 2,200-kcal step II diet because of his continued elevated lipid concentrations and high risk of premature coronary heart disease.

Because patients with Type III HLP are very sensitive to excess energy intake, Mr. X's energy for the day was distributed among six smaller meals, and alcohol and simple sugar intake were restricted. As noted in Table 6-16, Mr. X experienced an improvement in his lipid profile with aggressive diet therapy and weight loss and a worsening with a higher energy intake and weight gain. His goal weight range is 160-164 lb and his low-density lipoprotein cholesterol (LDL-C) goal is 130 mg/dL or less. The dietitian is optimistic that Mr. X will meet his goals as long as he adheres to his diet (step II hypocaloric diet), takes his lipid-lowering medication, and continues his regular physical activity program. If Mr. X's weight increases or plateaus and his triglycerides (TGs)

TABLE 6-16

Clinical Data for Patient X

Clinical Data[a]	Baseline	After 6 Months	After 8 Months	After 11 Months
TC (mg/dL)	443	279	317	243
TG (mg/dL)	969	146	314	150
HDL (mg/dL)	41	53	51	54
LDL (mg/dL)	N/A[b]	197	203	159
Non-HDL (mg/dL)	402[c]	226	266	189
Weight (lb)	160 (4 years ago) 177 (2 years ago)	172	176	167
Height (in)	69			

[a] TC, total cholesterol; TG, triglycerides; HDL, high-density lipoprotein; LDL, low-density lipoprotein.

[b] LDL cannot be calculated using the Friedewald formula because the triglyceride level exceeds 400 mg/dL.

[c] Non-HDL is calculated by subtracting the high-density lipoprotein (HDL-C) from the total cholesterol (TC).

TABLE 6-17

Clinical Data for Patient Y

Clinical Data	Baseline (on 500 mg Niacin)	After 3 Months on Step II Diet	After Adding Statin, Increasing Niacin to 1,500 mg, and Adhering to a Very-low-fat Diet for 4 Months
TC (mg/dL)	267	211	167
TG (mg/dL)	145	110	79
HDL (mg/dL)	52	46	53
LDL (mg/dL)	186	143	98
Weight (lb)	172	147	141
Height (in)	65		

remain elevated, the dietitian may consider recommending a calorie-controlled diet that is high in monounsaturated fatty acids to reduce production of very-low-density lipoprotein cholesterol (VLDL-C) and TGs.

Note: Although this patient did not tolerate niacin therapy, combining niacin with aggressive dietary therapy is often both efficacious (raises HDL-C levels by as much as 30%) and cost effective. This type of patient would also be a candidate for combined drug therapy using atorvastatin (Lipitor, Parke-Davis, Morris Plains, NJ), a recently approved statin that lowers both LDL-C and TG levels.

Case Study 2: A 61-year-old Man with Angina and Inadequately Treated Hypercholesterolemia

Mr. Y is a married 61-year-old educator in mechanical engineering who has had stable angina for the past 10 years. Mr. Y has a strong family history of coronary artery disease (ie, father died at age 49 from a fatal myocardial infarction and his 79-year-old mother had a coronary artery bypass graft at age 57). Mr. Y's former cardiologist had determined that he needed bypass surgery, which he refused. When first seen by his current cardiologist a year later, Mr. Y told him that he developed chest pain after walking one block. Mr. Y experienced angina after 5 minutes while undergoing a stress test (Bruce protocol). At his initial visit, Mr. Y's medications included 0.125 mg Synthroid (Knoll Pharmaceutical, Mount Olive, NJ), 50 mg Tenormin (Zeneca Pharmaceuticals, Wilmington, Del), aspirin qd, 500 mg niacin, a nitroglycerin patch, 1,000 mg vitamin C, and a multivitamin supplement. Thyroid function tests were normal. Clinical data are given in Table 6-17.

Because of Mr. Y's documented coronary artery disease and strong family history of coronary artery disease, he was instructed on the step II diet initially. Mr. Y had already been close to following a step I diet but needed to reduce his portion sizes of meats to fully comply with the step I guidelines. After meeting with the dietitian, Mr. Y was extremely motivated and, when presented with the option of adopting a very-low-fat diet, felt that this diet was appropriate for him. The dietitian and Mr. Y worked through a few meal plans, devised some sample menus, and determined that a 15% total fat diet was feasible. By making significant changes in his diet and by starting a regular walking program, Mr. Y. lost a significant amount of weight (31 lbs), is within his goal weight range, and has met his LDL goal of 100 mg/dL or less for reversal of heart disease. His angina is stable.

TABLE 6-18

Clinical Data for Patient Z

Clinical Data[a]	Baseline per Patient 3 Years Ago	Before CABG 18 Months Later (on Medications 6 Months)	Post-CABG, on Self-Prescribed VLFD (After 6 Months)	Modified VLFD (After 6 Weeks)
TC (mg/dL)	275	223	208	154
TG (mg/dL)	High 200's	132	359	111
HDL (mg/dL)	N/A	60	48	55
LDL (mg/dL)	N/A	137	89	77
Apo B (mg/dL)[b]	171			
Weight (lb)	172	154	149	143
Height (in)	64.5			

[a] CABG, coronary artery bypass graft; VLFD, very-low-fat diet

[b] Normal range, 62–133 mg/dl.

Case Study 3: A 61-year-old Woman Requiring Multiple-Drug Treatment for Hypercholesterolemia After Coronary Bypass

Mrs. Z is a 61-year-old married clerk with severe coronary artery disease. She has been classified as having a form of familial-combined hyperlipidemia based on her lipid profile and family history. Mrs. Z's father died after his second myocardial infarction at age 58 (first myocardial infarction was at age 45). Her mother died at age 79 of noncardiac causes but had a coronary artery bypass graft at age 61. Mrs. Z has two daughters (ages 34 and 36) without high cholesterol and one son (age 37) with elevated cholesterol who is currently being treated with Mevacor. Mrs. Z had a positive thallium scan on ETT (exercise tolerance test) and subsequently had a PCTA (percutaneous transluminal coronary angioplasty); she had a coronary artery bypass graft 18 months later.

Mrs. Z takes the following medications: 40 mg Zocor (Merck & Co, Inc, West Point, Pa), 500 mg Slo-Niacin tid (Upsher-Smith Laboratories, Inc, Minneapolis, Minn), 2 capsules fish oil qd, 0.625 mg Premarin (Wyeth-Ayerst Laboratories, Philadelphia, Pa), 0.1 mg Synthroid, 20 mg Pepsid (Merck & Co, Inc, West Point, Pa) bid, 1 aspirin qd, 1,000 mg calcium, 400 IU vitamin E, and 30 mg β-carotene. Mrs. Z's thyroid-stimulating hormone level was checked and was within the normal range.

Baseline lipids are not available because the patient had been on drug therapy before going to the cardiologist for treatment. According to the patient, before drug therapy her total cholesterol level was about 275 mg/dL and her triglycerides were in the high 200s (mg/dL); clinical data are given in Table 6-18. Mrs. Z had been taking niacin regularly but had stomach distress, which was improved by the change to a sustained-release formulation. Mrs. Z is sedentary and has struggled with her weight since she was in high school, but has made great progress in her weight loss goals over the last 3 years.

Mrs. Z was instructed to follow a step I diet initially, although with her medical history and her strong family history of coronary artery disease she could have gone directly to a step II diet. Because of her past unsuccessful weight-loss attempts, the dietitian opted for progressive diet therapy to improve long-term dietary compliance.

After her coronary artery bypass graft, Mrs. Z's dietary records were evaluated; her nutrient intake was found to be within the step II diet guidelines. She was provided with additional dietary instructions and received positive reinforcement for her efforts. She also met with an exercise physiologist to fine-tune her walking program.

Mrs. Z was advised to discontinue her β-carotene supplement to reduce the risk of impaired absorption of other potentially beneficial carotenoids. She was allowed to continue her fish-oil capsules because she was also receiving a statin (Zocor), which would help to offset any increase in LDL-C levels that may occur with the fish oil capsules (see Davidson, 1997 in the Case Study and Patient Profile Resources). (Comment: The major advantage for coronary patients taking fish oil may be their effects on reducing sudden death; thus, the dietitian and physician could have opted to recommend the discontinuation of the fish-oil supplements because the long-term effects of this combination therapy are not known. Some practitioners may elect to use this type of combination therapy [statin with fish oils] for those who need treatment for secondary prevention versus primary prevention of CHD.)

After discussing and receiving instruction on the step II diet from the dietitian, Mrs. Z read an article by Dr. Dean Ornish and decided to adopt his very-low-fat diet on her own. Mrs. Z modified Dr. Ornish's plan and consumed excessive carbohydrate (predominantly refined) and too little protein and fat. She reduced her fat intake to 6% of energy, protein to 10%, and carbohydrate to 84%. This disproportionate diet most likely led to an increased hepatic production of VLDL-C, which in turn increased her plasma TG level.

With the typical very-low-fat diet, the percentage of carbohydrate is increased while the fat content is decreased to not greater than 20% of energy; the Ornish plan limits fat intake to approximately 10%. Although Mrs. Z had lost a significant amount of weight over the past three years, at 149 lbs she was still well above her goal weight of 125 to 130 lbs. To reduce her TG level, Mrs. Z was instructed to gradually increase her fat intake (using mostly monounsaturated fat) from her current 8% of total calories to closer to 15% to 20% of energy. A high-fiber diet (20 to 35 g) and one to two fish meals (both low and higher fat) per week were also recommended. The dietitian and Mrs. Z constructed a mildly hypoenergetic meal plan together to meet the revised diet prescription. The dietitian also encouraged Mrs. Z to continue her walking program for a minimum of 30 minutes on most days of the week.

Mrs. Z will return for a follow-up visit in 6 weeks and bring food records with her. At that time the dietitian will assess Mrs. Z's understanding and execution of the very-low-fat diet. The dietitian may consider a diet high in monounsaturated fatty acids (a change in composition of the hypoenergetic diet) with a carbohydrate intake of not greater than 50% of her energy intake if Mrs. Z's TG levels become elevated on the modified very-low-fat diet or if her weight plateaus.

(Note: Because Mrs. Z has always struggled with her weight, long-term maintenance of a weight in her goal range of 125 to 130 lb may be unrealistic. Prevention of weight gain might be a more practical goal.)

Diet Therapy Options for Select Patient Profiles

The following abbreviations are used in the patient profiles: AHA, American Heart Association; CAD, coronary artery disease; CHD, coronary heart disease; HDL, high-density lipoprotein; HRT, hormone replacement therapy; LDL, low-density lipoprotein; MI, myocardial infarction; MUFA, monounsaturated fatty acid; NCEP, National Cholesterol Education Program; PA, physical activity; TC, total cholesterol; VLFD, very-low-fat diet.

PATIENT PROFILE 1: High TC and LDL, Normal TG, Normal Weight

AHA/NCEP Step I Diet. Initiate a step I diet to reduce saturated fat and dietary cholesterol. Encourage a high fiber intake (20 to 35 g/day or 10 to 13 g/1,000 kcal), with an emphasis on obtaining ≥5 g/day of a viscous soluble fiber. Promote PA (ie, at least 30 minutes of moderate-intensity activity on most days).

AHA/NCEP Step II Diet. Proceed from a step I to step II diet if LDL goals are not met to further reduce the saturated fat and cholesterol content of diet. Some motivated patients with established CAD, those who have had a recent myocardial infarction, or patients who are already following a step I diet may choose to go directly to the step II diet. Promote a high fiber intake and PA as described under the step I diet.

VLFD (<20% of total kcal). Consider a VLFD for the patient with a strong family history of premature CHD, multiple risk factors for CHD, or established CHD. Promote PA as described under a step I diet.

High-MUFA Diet (with decreased intake of carbohydrates). May be used in place of a step I or step II diet to enhance diet acceptability and prevent a slight increase in TGs and a slight decrease in HDL. Energy must remain constant to ensure weight maintenance.

PATIENT PROFILE 2: High TC and LDL, Normal TG, Normal Weight

AHA/NCEP Step I Diet. Initiate an energy-controlled step I diet to reduce saturated fat and dietary cholesterol and promote weight loss for TG-lowering and HDL-raising effects. Encourage consumption of one to two fish meals per week (both low- and higher-fat fish) and a high fiber intake (20 to 35 g or 10 to 13 g per 1,000 kcal), with an emphasis on obtaining at least 5 g/day of a viscous soluble fiber. Restrict alcohol and simple sugars. Recommend PA (ie, at least 30 minutes of moderate-intensity activity on most days) and aerobic activity for an HDL-raising effect (requires approximately 1,000 to 2,000 kcal expended per week).

AHA/NCEP Step II Diet. Proceed from a step I to a step II diet if LDL goals are not met to further reduce the saturated fat and cholesterol content of the diet. Promote fish meals, high fiber intake, and PA as described above. Note that some patients' TG levels may increase if weight loss is not achieved. *See* high-MUFA diet.

VLFD (<20% of total kcal). Consider a VLFD for the patient with a strong family history of premature CHD, multiple risk factors for CHD, or established CHD. Promote weight loss, PA, and consumption of one to two fish meals per week if not on a vegan plan as described under step I diet.

High-MUFA Diet (with decreased intake of carbohydrates). Consider an isoenergetic high-MUFA diet for patients resistant to weight loss or unable to lose weight and to enhance dietary adherence to a blood-cholesterol-lowering diet. A high-MUFA diet that maintains weight may help decrease TG levels.

PATIENT PROFILE 3: High TC and LDL, high TG, low HDL, normal weight

AHA/NCEP Step I Diet. Initiate a step I diet to reduce saturated fat and dietary cholesterol. Restrict alcohol and simple sugars. Encourage consumption of one to two fish meals per week (both low- and higher-fat fish) and a high fiber intake (20 to 35 g or 10 to 13 g per 1,000 kcal), with an emphasis on obtaining ≥5 g/day of a viscous soluble fiber. Recommend PA (ie, at least 30 minutes of moderate-intensity activity on most days) and aerobic activity for HDL-raising effect (requires approximately 1,000 to 2,000 kcal expended per week). This type of patient often requires diet therapy plus combination drug therapy to lower LDL and TG effectively.

AHA/NCEP Step II Diet. Proceed from a step I to step II diet if LDL goals are not met to further reduce saturated fat and cholesterol content of diet. Some motivated patients with established CAD, those who have had a recent MI, or patients who are already following a step I diet may choose to go directly to the step II diet. Promote fish meals, a high fiber intake, and PA as described above.

VLFD (<20% of total kcal). Consider a VLFD for the patient with a strong family history of premature CHD, multiple risk factors for CHD, or established CHD. Promote PA and consumption of one to two low-fat fish meals per week if not on a vegan plan as described under the step I diet.

High-MUFA Diet (with decreased intake of carbohydrates). The high-MUFA diet may be considered as an alternative to the step I and step II diets to enhance dietary adherence. Energy must be held constant to maintain weight. Promote PA as described under the step I diet.

PATIENT PROFILE 4: High TG, low HDL, LDL not accurate as a result of high TG, Type 2 diabetes, overweight

AHA/NCEP Step I Diet. Initiate an energy-controlled step I diet to reduce saturated fat and dietary cholesterol and promote weight loss for TG-lowering and HDL-raising effects. Encourage consumption of one to two fish meals per week (both low- and higher-fat fish) and a high fiber intake (20 to 35 g or 10 to 13 g per 1,000 kcal), with an emphasis on obtaining ≥5 g/day of a viscous soluble fiber for better glucose control. Restrict alcohol and simple sugars. Promote PA (ie, at least 30 minutes of moderate-intensity activity on most days) and emphasize the gradual incorporation of aerobic activity into the patient's lifestyle for an HDL-raising effect (requires approximately 1,000 to 2,000 kcal expended per week).

AHA/NCEP Step II Diet. Proceed from a step I to step II diet if LDL goals are not met to further reduce saturated fat and cholesterol content of diet. Promote fish meals, a high fiber intake, and PA as described above. Some patients' TG levels may increase on a step I and step II diet if weight loss is not achieved. *See* high-MUFA diet.

VLFD (<20% of total kcal). Consider a VLFD for the patient with a strong family history of premature CHD, multiple risk factors for CHD, or established CHD. Encourage consumption of one to two fish meals per week if not on a vegan plan, and promote weight loss and PA as described under the step I diet. A VLFD may worsen diabetes control and adversely affect the lipid profile in patients with a high TG level and Type 2 diabetes.

High-MUFA Diet (with decreased intake of carbohydrates). Consider an isoenergetic high-MUFA diet for patients who are resistant to weight loss or unable to lose weight. An isoenergetic high-MUFA diet may help with blood sugar control even when weight loss is not achieved. A moderate carbohydrate intake (50% of energy intake) and a high-MUFA diet may help reduce TG levels.

PATIENT PROFILE 5: High TG, low HDL, overweight

AHA/NCEP Step I Diet. Initiate an energy-controlled step I diet to reduce saturated fat and dietary cholesterol and promote weight loss for TG-lowering and HDL-raising effects. Encourage consumption of one to two fish meals per week (both low- and higher-fat fish) and a high fiber intake (20 to 35 g or 10 to 13 g per 1,000 kcal), with an emphasis on obtaining ≥5 g/day of a viscous soluble fiber. Restrict alcohol and simple sugars. Recommend PA (ie, at least 30 minutes of moderate-intensity activity on most days) and incrementally incorporating aerobic activity into lifestyle for an HDL-raising effect (requires approximately 1,000 to 2,000 kcal expended per week).

AHA/NCEP Step II Diet. Proceed from a step I to step II diet if LDL goals are not met to further reduce saturated fat content of diet. Restrict alcohol and simple sugars. Promote fish meals, a high fiber intake, and PA as described above. Some patients' TG levels may increase on the step I and step II diets if weight is not lost. *See* high-MUFA diet.

VLFD (<20% of total kcal). Consider a VLFD for the patient with a strong family history of premature CHD, multiple risk factors for CHD, or established CHD. Encourage consumption of one to two fish meals per week if not on a vegan plan, and promote weight loss and PA as described under the step I diet.

High-MUFA Diet (with decreased intake of carbohydrates). Consider an isoenergetic high-MUFA diet for patients resistant to weight loss or unable to lose weight. Strict diet adherence combined with drug therapy (niacin or gemfibrozil) is often required in patients with markedly elevated TG of 400 mg/dL or greater.

PATIENT PROFILE 6: Patient with elevated TG after starting on HRT

NCEP Step I Diet. Initiate a step I diet for general risk reduction. Restrict alcohol and simple sugars. Encourage consumption of one to two fish meals per week (both low- and higher-fat fish) and a high fiber intake (20 to 35 g or 10 to 13 g per 1,000 kcal). Recommend low-fat soy products for cardiac, bone, and general health. Promote PA (ie, at least 30 minutes of moderate-intensity activity on most days).

NCEP Step II Diet. Not applicable.

VLFD (<20% of total kcal). Not applicable.

High-MUFA Diet (with decreased intake carbohydrates). A high-MUFA diet may be considered as an alternative to the step I diet to enhance diet acceptability. Energy must be held constant to maintain weight. Consider a high-MUFA diet if TG level continues to be elevated on the step I diet (along with alcohol and simple sugar restriction and an increase in PA). A high-MUFA diet will not further increase TG level when weight remains stable.

Resources for Case Studies and Patient Profiles

American Heart Association, Nutrition Committee. Dietary guidelines for healthy American adults. *Circulation.* 1988;77:721A.

Bakker-Arkema RG, Davidson MH, Goldstein RJ, Davignon J, Isaacsohn JL, Weiss SR, Keilson LM, Brown V, Miller VT, Shurzinske MS, Black DM. Efficacy and safety of a new HMG-CoA reductase inhibitor, atorvastatin, in patients with hypertriglyceridemia. *JAMA.* 1996;275:128-133.

Connor, WE. The decisive influence of diet on the progression and reversibility of coronary heart disease. *Am J Clin Nutr.* 1996; 64: 253-254.

Connor SL, Connor WE. *The New American Diet.* New York, NY: Simon & Schuster; 1986.

Davidson MH, Maki KC, Kalkowski J, Schaefer EJ, Torri SA, Drennan KB. Effects of docosahexaenoic acid on serum lipoproteins in patients with combined hyperlipidemia; a randomized, double-blind, placebo-controlled trial. *J Am Col Nutr.* 1997; 16(3):236-243.

Davidson MH, Macariola-Coad JR, McDonald, AM, Maki, KC, Hall, HA. Separate and joint effects of marine oil and simvastatin in patients with combined hyerlipidemia. *Am J Cardiol.* 1997; 80:797-798.

Franz MJ, Horton ES, Bantle JP, Beebe CA, Brunzell JD, Coulston AM, Henry RR, Hoogwerf BJ, Stacpoole PW. Nutrition principles for the management of diabetes and related complications. *Diabetes Care.* 1994;17(5):490-518.

Garg A, Bonanome A, Grundy SM, Unger RH. Consumption of a high carbohydrate diet with a high monounsaturated fat diet in patients with non-insulin dependent diabetes mellitus. *N Engl J Med.* 1988;319:829-834.

Ornish D. *Eat More, Weigh Less.* New York: HarperCollins Publishers, 1994.

Pearson TA. Alcohol and heart disease. *Circulation.* 1996; 94:3023-3025.

Pritikin N. *The Pritikin Program for Diet and Exercise.* New York, NY: Grosset & Dunlap; 1982.

Rimm EB, Ascherio A, Giovannucci E, Spiegelman D, Stampfer MJ, Willet WC. Vegetable, fruit and cereal fiber intake and risk among men. *JAMA.* 1996;275:447-451.

Ripsin CM, Keenan JM, Jacobs, Jr. DR, Elmer PJ, Welch RR, Van Horn L, Liu K, Turnbull WH, Thye FW, Kestin M, Hegsted M, Davidson DM, Davidson MH, Dugan LD, Demark-Wahnefried W, Beling S. Oat Products and Lipid Lowering—a meta-analysis.

JAMA. 1992; 267:3317-3325.

Second Report of the Expert Panel on Detection, Evaluation, and Treatment of High Blood Cholesterol (Adult Treatment Panel II). National Institutes of Health, National Heart, Lung and Blood Institute, 1993, NIH publication 93-3095.

Stone NJ. Fish consumption, fish oil, lipids, and coronary heart disease. *Circulation*. 1997;94:2337-2340.

Van Horn L. Fiber, lipids, and coronary heart disease: a statement for healthcare professionals from the nutrition committee, American Heart Association. *Circulation*. 1997;95:2701-2704.

CHAPTER 7

Weight Management and Cardiovascular Disease

Brenda Eissenstat, MS, RD; Madeleine Sigman-Grant, PhD, RD; and Karen Reznik Dolins, MS, RD

The achievement and maintenance of a healthy weight contribute significantly to the reduction of risk factors for cardiovascular disease (CVD). However, opinions vary widely on what a healthful weight is, how it is determined, and how it is most effectively achieved. Recommended ideal weights based on population norms (which have been moving upward) are not necessarily relevant to the prevention of chronic diseases and are unattainable for many obese individuals.

Most overweight people are frustrated and disheartened by their lack of long-term success at achieving and maintaining an ideal weight. Strategies aimed at reducing the incidence of obesity and the morbidity and mortality from associated chronic diseases may be more effective if success is redefined to reflect health outcome and quality of life rather than the number of pounds lost.

Overview of Obesity and Overweight

The incidence of obesity and overweight continues to rise despite public education efforts. This chapter provides an overview of the multidimensional nature of obesity and strategies for reducing CVD through weight management. Toward this goal, dietitians are encouraged to identify relevant psychological, social, and physical components of the condition and to address these issues during nutrition therapy. Examples of the inclusion of these components in a comprehensive weight management program are provided, along with practical tools for planning, implementing, monitoring, and assessing such a program. Finally, educational resources and medications to aid weight loss are briefly reviewed.

Defining Obesity

Although the terms *obesity* and *overweight* are used interchangeably, these conditions are different. *Obesity* is defined by the National Institutes of Health consensus panel as an excess of body fat frequently resulting in a significant impairment of health, whereas *overweight* refers to an excess of weight compared with height (1). Because excess body fat, or adipose tissue, is less easily measured than weight, most measures of mortality used in large population studies are based on overweight, not obesity.

Determining Body Fat Percentages

The body fat percentages associated with the lowest morbidity and mortality rates are 12% to 20% for men and 20% to 30% for women. Percent body fat can be determined by several indirect techniques: hydrostatic weighing, caliper measurements, electrical impedance, and infrared interactance (2). These indirect methods are based on assumptions about the chemical and physical properties of fat-free mass or lean body mass. Once fat-free mass is measured, body fat is estimated by subtracting from body weight; percent body fat can then be calculated.

Results obtained with these techniques should be interpreted with caution, however, because measures of lean body mass and fat-free mass can be affected by hydration status, the experience of the personnel performing the tests, and assumptions inherent in the equations developed to calculate percent body fat. For example, lean body mass density often increases with increasing physical fitness and decreases with age (3) and may vary by sex, race, and degree of obesity (2), thus making the equations inaccurate.

Body Mass Index as a Measure of Overweight

Health care teams use body mass index (BMI) to assess relative body weight. BMI is calculated by dividing weight in kilograms by height in meters squared. The body mass index of an individual who is 5'5" tall and weighs 190 pounds is calculated as follows:

$$65 \text{ in} \times 2.54 \text{ cm/in} = 165.1 \text{ cm} = 1.65 \text{ m}$$

$$190 \text{ lb} \div 2.2 \text{ kg/lb} = 86.4 \text{ kg}$$

$$\text{BMI} = \text{kg/m}^2 = 86.4 \div (1.65)^2 = 31.7$$

TABLE 7-1

Body Mass Indexes Frequently Used to Define Desirable and Obese Weights in Adults

Source	Recommended Males	Recommended Females	Overweight/Obese Males	Overweight/Obese Females
Metropolitan Life 1959 (4)	22.0	21.5	26.4	25.8
Metropolitan Life 1983 (5)	22.7	22.4	27.2	26.9
NHANES I (6)	24.5	23.0	—	—
NHANES II (6)	24.3	23.2	27.8	27.3
NHANES III (6)	24.9	24.1	—	—
Guidelines for Americans				
<35 years (7)	19-25	19-25	—	—
≥35 years (7)	21-27	21-27	—	—
Guidelines for all Adult Americans (8)	19-25	19-25	—	—

A consensus panel convened by the American Institute of Nutrition (AIN) to develop preventive weight guidelines for healthy adults concluded that individuals with BMIs of 19 to 25 have the lowest health risk (Table 7-1) (9). Separate guidelines were recommended for the achievement of a more healthful weight in obese individuals.

AIN allowed for an increase of 1 BMI unit or less, or 2 to 5 kg (5 to 10 lb), throughout adulthood; however, health professionals have not reached a consensus on this point (10). Although increases in body weight are customary with age, they may not be inevitable or physiological. Most weight gain in older adults is in the form of adipose tissue, whereas lean body mass decreases. In many non-Western populations, weight loss with increasing age is the norm and lean body mass loss begins in early adulthood. Exercise can promote the retention of lean body mass in older adults. The fourth edition of the *Dietary Guidelines for Americans* emphasizes the importance of maintaining a healthy weight as one ages by including regular activity and balancing energy consumption with energy intake (8).

The most significant limitation of BMI is that it does not account for differences in either leg length or lean body mass. Some individuals with a high BMI may be very fit and, conversely, some individuals with a low BMI may be excessively fat and underweight. Despite these limitations, BMI is highly correlated with body fatness in most populations and is the scientific tool most commonly used to represent relative weight.

Categorizing Excess Weight

The National Center for Health Statistics (NCHS) identified two categories of excess weight: overweight and severe overweight. On the basis of data collected in the second National Health and Nutrition Examination Survey (NHANES II), the cutoff points for overweight and severe overweight were the 85th and 95th percentiles, respectively, of BMI in adults aged 20 to 29 years (27.8 and 31.1 for males; 27.3 and 32.3 for females) (11). These values are comparable with 120% and 140% of the ideal body weight determined from the weight-for-height tables of the Metropolitan Life Insurance Company in 1983 (5). Researchers recognize, however, that values based on population norms at a given time do not necessarily represent healthful weights or weights that minimize disease risk factors today. Mean weights in the adult population exceed the weight standards that are based on the lowest risk for cardiovascular disease (12).

Prevalence of Overweight in the United States

The distribution of weight within the U.S. population appears to be moving away from, rather than toward, a more healthful mean (6). In NCHS surveys the increase in the prevalence of overweight has been dramatic. When values from NHANES III (1988 to 1994) are compared with the BMI cutoff points from NHANES II, 33% of men and 36% of women age 20 and older in the United States were overweight (13). Among adults, the prevalence of overweight increased 3.3 percentage points for men and 3.6 percentage points for women between phase 1 and phase 2 of NHANES III. These findings are consistent with data from the Centers for Disease Control and Prevention's (CDC's) Behavioral Risk Factor Surveillance System, which indicate that from 1987 to 1993 the age-adjusted prevalence of overweight among adults (based on self-reports) increased by 0.9% per year (14).

Obesity is also a major pediatric health problem. A CDC study found that the prevalence of obesity in children (ages 6 to 11 years) was 13.7% and in adolescents (ages 12 to 17 years) was 11.5% (13). In this study *obesity* was defined as a BMI at or above the sex- and age-specific 95th percentile derived from the National Health Examination Surveys cycles 2 and 3, respectively. To account for growth spurts and other physiological changes that occur in children and adolescents, the study used a more conservative definition of overweight than is used for adults.

Paradoxically, as the trend toward overweight continues, more people are dieting than ever before. An estimated $33 billion per year is spent on weight-reduction products (including diet foods, diet soft drinks, artificial sweeteners, and diet books) and services such as fitness clubs and weight-loss programs (15). One study reported that if obesity could be prevented, the United States could have saved about $45.8 billion in 1990—6.8% of health care expenditures that year. Lost employee productivity was estimated at 52.9 million days, at a cost to employers of about $4 billion in 1990 (16).

THEORIES ABOUT THE CAUSES OF OBESITY

It has been well established that genetic factors influence human obesity (17). Recent scientific breakthroughs have identified components of the physiological system that regulate adiposity. The *ob* gene, which is expressed only in fat cells, releases the hormone leptin in response to nutritional status. Studies with laboratory animals have shown that leptin is released from adipocytes and acts centrally to inhibit food intake and increase thermogenesis. The *db* gene is believed to be responsible for encoding the leptin receptor.

Much of the research on these genes has been conducted in mice; however, homologues to these genes are found in the human genome. It appears likely that some form of negative feedback system including the *ob* and *db* genes is responsible for the regulation of fat stores (18). Additional hormonal factors are known to affect satiety and food intake. Biochemical defects at one or more points in the body fat regulatory system are the likely cause of many forms of obesity. Researchers continue to analyze specific chromosomal segments and gene loci that may affect obesity. It is probable that several genes will be discovered that affect human obesity.

A recent model proposed by Meyer and Stunkard (17) suggests that only genetically predisposed persons who are exposed to adverse environmental conditions develop obesity. The difficulty that genetically predisposed individuals have in controlling their weight may be largely of environmental origin. Therapeutic intervention can change adverse environmental conditions such as sedentary lifestyles, overconsumption of food, cultural expectations, and an increase in eating disorders (specifically binge-eating disorder and bulimia nervosa), all of which contribute to the high incidence of obesity.

Improving the energy balance equation by increasing physical exercise can significantly enhance weight management efforts. In addition, exercise can enhance fat oxidation and insulin sensitivity, two major metabolic risk factors for obesity.

The amount of energy expended by physical activity varies widely. Although obese individuals usually expend more energy than do nonobese individuals in a given physical activity (19), this is likely to be offset by a decrease in the duration of the activity. Regular physical activity is essential to long-term success in weight loss and weight management (see Chapter 8) (20,21).

Dietary composition in Westernized nations is thought to contribute to the increase in obesity. These diets are high in fat (especially animal fat), sugar, and alcohol and low in complex carbohydrates. Many developing nations are now experiencing an increasing prevalence of obesity-related diseases as population moves to urban centers impose lifestyle and dietary changes (22).

Another trend that may be contributing to America's increasing obesity is a greater reliance on convenience foods and foods consumed away from home. Easily prepared processed foods often supply more fat, sodium, sugars, and calories and less fiber than do minimally processed foods prepared at home. Fat-free products have recently proliferated in the marketplace. (See Chapter 14 for a discussion of these products.)

Economics and cultural values may be partly responsible for the prevalence of overweight among some ethnic groups. Although obesity has been increasing in all population groups, its incidence is disproportionately higher for African-American and Hispanic women, particularly those with a lower income. NHANES III data reveal that 52% of African-American women and 50% of Mexican-American women are overweight (13).

Fatness is stigmatized in the dominant US culture; an obese individual may be viewed as having failed to exercise self-control. Slimness, especially in women, signifies greater self-control and is associated with affluence. However, many members of ethnic minorities do not hold these beliefs. In many societies, fatness represents success. For example, in Puerto Rican society, weight gain after marriage reflects a husband's success as a provider and a woman's role as wife and mother. Similarly, African-American women often view plumpness as a sign of health, prosperity, and success in the domestic arts. Large body size also promotes respect and allows greater freedom away from home and fewer hassles from young males on the street (23). In other societies, weight loss is associated with serious illness or decreased sexual attractiveness. Individuals who lose weight commonly experience subtle but strong social pressure to regain it.

Although cultural influences may be less important than genetics as a cause of obesity, they are extremely important in prevention and treatment because they are changeable. An understanding of the cultural beliefs and practices of the client or community being served is essential for appropriate and effective treatment of obesity (see Chapter 16).

Eating disorders are another major contributor to the epidemic of obesity in the United States. Although psychological disorders associated with obesity were described by Stunkard (24) in 1959, the American Psychiatric Association did not recognize the diagnosis of binge-eating disorder until 1994 (25). The diagnostic criteria for binge-eating disorder are shown in Box 7-1.

Researchers have suggested that 25% to 50% of the people who seek treatment in weight-loss programs are suf-

BOX 7-1 **Diagnostic Criteria for Binge-Eating Disorder from the *Diagnostic and Statistical Manual*—4th Edition (25)**

A. Recurrent episodes of binge eating. An episode of binge eating is characterized by both of the following:
   1. Eating, in a discrete period of time (ie, within any 2-hour period), an amount of food that is definitely larger than most people would eat in a similar period of time under similar circumstances; and
   2. A sense of lack of control over eating during the episode (ie, a feeling that one cannot stop eating or control what or how much one is eating).
B. The binge eating episodes are associated with at least three of the following:
   1. Eating much more rapidly than normal
   2. Eating until feeling uncomfortably full
   3. Eating large amounts of food when not feeling physically hungry
   4. Eating alone because of being embarrassed by how much one is eating
   5. Feeling disgusted with oneself, depressed, or feeling very guilty after overeating
C. Marked distress regarding binge eating.
D. The binge eating occurs, on average, at least 2 days a week for 6 months.
E. The binge eating is not associated with the regular use of inappropriate compensatory behaviors (ie, purging, fasting, excessive exercise) and does not occur exclusively during the course of anorexia nervosa or bulimia nervosa.

Based on information from the *Diagnostic and Statistical Manual of Mental Disorders,* 4th ed. Copyright 1994 the American Psychiatric Association.

fering from problems associated with binge-eating disorder. The disorder affects both men and women although it is slightly more common in women. Binge-eating disorder has a broader demographic distribution than do anorexia nervosa and bulimia nervosa (26,27).

The most significant difference between people who are and are not classified as binge eaters is the degree of psychological distress experienced. Distorted body images and lifetime histories of depression, anxiety, panic disorder, and personality disorders are common in this population. Binge eaters are reportedly heavier (28) and younger than those who do not binge eat (29). Binge eating often begins in late adolescence or early adulthood, but many binge eaters do not seek treatment until they reach their mid- to late 30s.

Bulimia nervosa also can be present in obese patients. Individuals who have struggled with weight for many years may engage in destructive weight-loss methods such as purging by vomiting, using laxatives or diuretics, or exercising excessively. Box 7-2 provides questions that can be used during a patient's initial assessment to elicit information about disordered eating behaviors.

Awareness of the possibility that obesity may be a physical symptom of a psychological disorder is essential for the treatment of individuals who suffer from eating disorders. For these individuals, food is a coping mechanism that enables the achievement of a degree of normalcy in their lives. Removing food and the rituals surrounding it without providing appropriate new coping skills destines these individuals to failure and may exacerbate their physical and mental health problems.

Recognition of the multifactorial nature of obesity is also essential for effective treatment. Different therapies are required based on the suspected etiology of the disease. Adjunct therapies such as psychotherapy, marital counseling, and other social services are often required. Occasionally, consideration of the client's overall health may mean that these therapies take precedence over dietary

BOX 7-2 **Assessment Questions to Elicit Disordered Eating Behaviors**

- Are there times you feel you cannot stop eating, even though you want to?
- Do you ever eat unusually large amounts of food in a short period of time?
- Do you ever feel extremely guilty or depressed afterwards?
- Do you feel embarrassed by how much you eat and eat alone whenever possible?
- After eating do you ever feel compelled to get rid of the food you have just eaten?
- Do you ever misuse (ie, take more than is recommended or prescribed, or use when it would not normally be needed) diuretics, laxatives, or other medications; induce vomiting; fast; or exercise excessively to prevent weight gain?

treatment. Instructing an obese binge eater to consume a low-fat, low-sodium diet will be ineffective if the overeating is caused by severe depression. An appropriate treatment plan can be implemented only after a thorough assessment. Assessment procedures are discussed later in this chapter.

CARDIOVASCULAR CONSEQUENCES OF OBESITY

Because obesity increases several risk factors for CVD—including hypertension, insulin-resistant glucose intolerance, dyslipidemia, left-ventricular hypertrophy, and thrombogenic factors—it is associated with an increased incidence of morbidity and mortality from CVD (30). Researchers are studying additional mechanisms that may contribute to the development of CVD in the presence of a diet habitually high in fats and cholesterol (see Chapter 1).

As weight increases, the lipid profile becomes more atherogenic. Weight gain increases the levels of blood lipids, including total cholesterol, triglycerides, and low-density lipoprotein cholesterol (LDL-C); weight gain decreases the levels of high-density lipoprotein cholesterol (HDL-C) (31-33).

Data from the Framingham Heart Study show increased total cholesterol, blood pressure, and glucose values for people with a BMI in the higher-BMI quintiles and improvement in these values with a 10% loss of body weight (34). In obese white men ages 20 to 44, total cholesterol concentrations were 23 mg/dL higher and LDL-C levels are 23 mg/dL higher than those in normal-weight men (35). For obese men of all age groups, triglyceride and HDL-C concentrations were 62 to 118 mg/dL higher and 7 to 15 mg/dL lower, respectively, compared with those of normal-weight men (36). In premenopausal white women whose BMI was 27.1 to 30, total cholesterol concentrations were 18 mg/dL higher and LDL-C concentrations were 17 mg/dL higher than they were in similar women whose BMI was 21.1 to 23 (36).

Body fat distribution also influences the plasma lipid profile. Individuals who have a primarily upper-body fat distribution (characterized by an android or apple shape) are more likely to have elevated concentrations of total cholesterol, triglycerides, and apolipoprotein B and lower concentrations of HDL-C than those who have more gluteofemoral fat deposits (gynoid or pear shape).

Estrogen and testosterone influence fat distribution. For example, fat deposits tend to be gynoid in premenopausal women; when estrogen concentrations fall at menopause, however, women are at increased risk of developing android fat deposits. Deep body fat rather than subcutaneous fat is associated with the highest risk.

The metabolic basis for increased risk with abdominal adiposity is believed to be related to the observed increase in insulin resistance (36). Insulin resistance and hyperinsulinemia cause fat cells to be less responsive to the stimulatory effects of insulin on glucose uptakes. Although the mechanisms are not yet clear, it appears that elevated insulin concentrations may lead to increased triglyceride and decreased HDL-C concentrations (37). Finally, insulin resistance may have a role in the development of hypertension by increasing sodium reabsorption and expanding blood volume.

The most common method of measuring abdominal adipose deposits is the waist-to-hip ratio. For men, waist circumference is measured at the navel and hip circumference is measured at the top of the hip bone. For women, waist circumference is measured midway between the bottom of the ribs and the top of the hip bone and hip circumference is measured at the widest point between the hips and the buttocks. A waist-to-hip ratio greater than 0.95 for men and 0.80 for women has been associated with increased CHD risk.

Waist circumference, which is a composite of subcutaneous and deep adipose tissue, is another clinical indicator of CHD. Increased risk was reported with waist circumferences exceeding 102 cm for men and 88 cm for women (38).

Effective weight management strategies, including diet, exercise, and behavior modification, are vital for risk reduction. Weight loss reduces blood lipids, including cholesterol, triglycerides, and LDL-C, and weight loss increases HDL-C, resulting in a more favorable LDL-HDL ratio. A meta-analysis of studies of the effects of weight reduction on blood lipids and lipoproteins found a significant negative correlation (39). A weight loss of 1 kg was associated with a 0.5 mmol/L (approximately 2 mg/dL) decrease in total cholesterol, a 0.02 mmol/L (approximately 0.08 mg/dL) decrease in LDL-C, and a 0.015 mmol/L (approximately 0.06 mg/dL) decrease in triglyceride concentrations. HDL decreased during the active weight-loss phase but increased by 0.009 mmol/L (approximately 0.036 mg/dL) per kilogram when weight loss was maintained (39).

An optimal weight that minimizes cardiovascular risk factors is difficult to determine. The most comprehensive data available (from the American Cancer Society and studies by insurance companies) suggest that the lowest mortality is achieved when weight is slightly less than average (40). A weight that optimizes the cardiovascular risk profile has been determined to correspond with a BMI of 22.6 in men and 21.1 in women. Ideal subscapular thicknesses were less than 12 mm in men and less than 15 mm in women (41).

Ideally, excessive weight gain should be prevented and a weight corresponding to a BMI less than 25 should be maintained, even as one ages. However, recognizing that a large portion of the population is already overweight, a more-healthful-weight goal is needed. Most researchers agree that a sustained weight loss of approximately 10% can significantly reduce an individual's cardiovascular risk profile (42). A loss of as little as 2.3 to 4.5 kg (5 to 10 lb) can help to reduce blood pressure and improve blood lipid levels, insulin resistance, and glucose tolerance while protecting heart muscle mass (36).

The American Health Foundation's Expert Panel on Healthy Weight concluded that for individuals not currently diagnosed with a weight-related disease (ie, hypertension,

CVD, diabetes, or osteoarthritis), a weight loss of 4.5 to 7.3 kg (10 to 16 lb) or the equivalent of 2 BMI units is appropriate. For most healthy individuals, a weight loss of more than 2 BMI units should not be encouraged. However, if it is necessary, the original weight loss should be maintained for at least 6 months before additional weight loss is attempted. The panel encouraged individuals who are at high risk or who have been diagnosed with a chronic disease to consult their physician about setting an appropriate weight goal (42).

THE EMOTIONAL IMPACT OF OBESITY

In addition to bearing the serious medical consequences associated with obesity, obese individuals in the United States are often subjected to prejudice, discrimination, and disrespect. Even among medical professionals, obese individuals may be treated disrespectfully because of their weight (39). The belief that the level of body fat is under voluntary control is both common and mistaken. Individuals struggling with weight loss are often depicted as lacking both the willpower and the desire to lose weight. Alternatively, they may be perceived as having a psychological need to be obese or low self-esteem that prevents appropriate self-care. In reality, the incidence of psychological problems is no higher among obese individuals than in the general population (43).

As previously discussed, genetics, culture, physiological factors, and behavioral factors also affect obesity. Dietitians must confront any personal stereotypes they may harbor about obesity that could be subtly communicated to clients.

Most clients are anxious about beginning a new medical treatment, and in obese patients with a history of weight problems this anxiety can be exaggerated. For some individuals the thought of beginning a new diet recalls previous unsuccessful dieting attempts. Many clients who have experienced previous weight loss and subsequent regain are reluctant to begin a new program and often feel disgusted with or ashamed of themselves.

An understanding of the emotional baggage that is often carried by obese clients can lead to a more supportive and successful relationship. The recognition that obesity is a chronic condition that requires long-term care compels the weight-loss practitioner to focus on an individual's needs and work to improve the individual's self-esteem. Trust and mutual respect facilitate a successful long-term relationship in which clients feel free to return, even after weight regain, without experiencing guilt and shame (44).

Recently, interest in the nondiet approach to weight management has increased. In contrast to the traditional view that fatness is a result of medical or moral negligence, this approach encourages obese individuals to take control and to set their own goals. Accepting that body sizes vary and that each individual's metabolism is unique has helped to reduce the guilt and inadequacy felt by many obese people.

Programs that promote the nondiet approach vary widely, but they all reject the notion that health and happiness can be achieved through slenderness. Rather, they advocate self-acceptance. Some programs emphasize behavior change and weight reduction; however, any weight-loss effort must focus strictly on the relief of health problems (45). Given the relative lack of success of long-term weight loss and the physical and psychological toll inflicted by endless dieting, an approach that emphasizes improving clients' health and happiness may produce the best results.

STRATEGIES FOR IMPROVING CARDIOVASCULAR HEALTH THROUGH WEIGHT MODIFICATION

The following are appropriate guiding principles for a weight modification treatment plan.

- Begin at the client's level of knowledge, motivation, and ability and willingness to change (see Chapter 13).
- Individualize goals and nutrition prescriptions. Work with the client to determine realistic short- and long-term goals.
- Determine energy needs by calculating basal metabolic rate and activity factors.
- Identify the emotional and social support systems available to help the client succeed.
- Identify physical and emotional barriers to success and potential solutions.
- Discuss your assessment and proposed treatment plan with other health professionals who are also working with the client (see Chapter 11).

The improvement of cardiovascular health through weight modification includes assessment, goal setting, nutritional therapy, exercise, program implementation, educational support, medications, and maintenance.

Assessment

The first step in the development of an individualized weight modification program is a thorough assessment that encompasses all of the issues discussed earlier. The assessment combines information obtained from the medical record, the physician, and the client interview. Shape Up America! and the American Obesity Association have prepared a useful manual, *Guidance for Treatment of Adult Obesity*, which reviews assessment and treatment modalities for weight reduction and maintenance (46). The document can be downloaded from the World Wide Web at http://www.shapeup.org/sua or obtained from Shape Up America!, 6707 Democracy Blvd., Suite 107, Bethesda, MD 20817 (send $3 to cover shipping and handling).

The client's medical record or physician can provide medical history (assessment of comorbid conditions such as cardiovascular disease, hypertension, dyslipidemia, Type 2 diabetes, sleep apnea, osteoarthritis, infertility, hyperinsulinemia, cancer, and menopause), medications, diet prescription laboratory data (with dates), and the physician's goals for the client. Information that can be obtained from the patient interview includes weight history, nutrition history, exercise and activity history, social and economic factors, anthropometric values, the existence of any temporary or permanent weight reduction exclusions, and the client's expectations and motivations.

Weight history includes previous weight-loss attempts, methods—including purging behaviors—and outcomes; weight of close biological relatives; and periods of significant weight gain and causes, including binging behaviors. Nutrition history covers knowledge, attitudes, and practices (see Chapter 4). Exercise and activity history covers type, frequency, duration, motivation, and associated illness or injury and other barriers to increasing physical activity. Social and economic factors include living situation, cooking facilities, finances, education, employment, literacy, ethnic or religious considerations, and family interaction.

Anthropometric values include height, weight, BMI, waist-to-hip ratio, and percent body fat. Clients should be active participants in the process of taking measurements; they should be told why the measurements are useful and they should give permission before measurements that require physical contact are initiated. Measurements that may be perceived as intrusive or humiliating should be avoided as should group weighing or measuring. Some measurements, such as skinfold measurements, may be inaccurate in severely obese individuals.

Temporary weight-reduction exclusions include pregnancy, lactation (weight reduction may be attempted if milk production is well established and intervention is not aggressive), unstable mental illness, and unstable medical conditions. Permanent exclusions include anorexia nervosa and terminal illness.

Goal Setting

Clients should be involved in establishing goals. It is important to find out what the client expects to gain from counseling and in what time frame. The client's motivation should also be considered (see Chapter 13 for a discussion of stages of change).

Both real and perceived barriers can impede success. Dietitians can help clients to set realistic short-term goals that reduce perceived barriers and build self-esteem. The setting of flexible long-term goals should be encouraged; these goals may be to prevent further weight gain, stabilize weight, or reduce health risks. As previously noted, a weight loss of 10% or less can achieve a more healthful weight and an associated reduction in CVD risk factors. A weight that reduces health risk can be determined by repeating the baseline measurements after every 5 to 10 lb of weight loss.

Generally, the goal weight should be no lower than the lowest weight that the client has sustained for a year since age 21 (47). Clients often intertwine the goals of weight loss for improved health and weight loss for cosmetic purposes. Society's emphasis on a lean appearance makes separation of these two issues more difficult. Dietitian and client should discuss these issues and together set appropriate goals.

The expected rate of weight loss also must be discussed. Clients often believe that "fast is best"—a belief that is reinforced by the diet industry. Dietitians can help clients to understand the difference between body weight loss and fat loss. Quick weight loss generally indicates loss of lean body tissue and fluids that results in a lowered metabolic rate. A realistic rate of weight loss is generally estimated to be 0.5 to 2 lb per week. Most women can lose 0.5 to 1 lb per week if they exercise and consume a low-fat, high-fiber diet. Larger men may be able to lose up to 2 to 3 lb per week.

It is useful to demonstrate expected weight loss by determining energy requirements. Explain to the client that about 3,500 kcals of energy must be expended to shed 1 lb of fat. Clients who are analytically inclined may find it interesting to review the calculation of energy requirements. Daily energy needs can be calculated on the basis of either the client's initial weight loss goal of 2 BMI units or the client's initial weight (Box 7-3). The calculation should be adjusted periodically as the client loses weight. Establishing a calorie level based on the initial goal weight means that weight loss will be slower but dietary changes will be less dramatic.

Nutritional Therapy

The National Cholesterol Education Program (NCEP) guidelines and the American Heart Association's step I and step II diets should be the basis of the client's food plan. A food plan that provides fewer than 1,500 kcal/day is unrealistic for most men; likewise, women should not consume fewer than 1,200 kcal/day.

Ideally, an energy deficit should result from combining a decrease in energy input (food) with an increase in energy output (exercise). The deficit should be distributed among three meals plus snacks according to the NCEP guidelines, which recommend that 55% or more of calories be obtained from carbohydrate, 30% or less from fat (8% to 10% of calories from saturated fat on the step I diet and less than 7% of calories from saturated fat on the step II diet), and the remainder from protein. Cholesterol intake should be less than 300 mg/day on a step I diet and less than 200 mg/day on a step II diet. See Chapter 6 for a thorough review of the step I and II diets and other therapies designed for specific needs.

Typical nutrition education strategies for weight loss include counting fat grams or calories, weighing and measuring food, using food exchange lists and food pyramids, following a menu, and adhering to mutually agreed-on goals (eg, "For 5 days I will not take second helpings at meals"). The addition of behavioral modification principles to conventional dietary therapy significantly enhances the success of the program (48).

Exercise

Increased activity is critical to the success of any weight-loss program. Exercise is consistently reported to be positively

BOX 7-3 Calculating Daily Energy Requirements

1. BY GOAL WEIGHT

Men: BMR = 66 + (13.7 × wt kg) + (5 × ht cm) – (6.8 × age)

Women: BMR = 665 + (9.6 × wt kg) + (1.7 × ht cm) – (4.7 × age)

Activity levels for typical daily activities, excluding exercise: 20% for sedentary behavior, 30% for light activity, 40% for moderate activity, and 50% for very active. Example: A sedentary 45-year-old male is 5'8" tall and weighs 200 lb. His BMI = 30.5. Energy need at his goal weight (initial weight – 2 BMI units) is calculated as follows:

Goal BMI = 30.5 – 2 = 28.5 (BMI, calculated as kg/m^2)

Height (m) = 68 in × (2.54 in/cm) = 173 cm = 1.73 m

Goal weight (kg) = BMI × (m^2) = 28.5 × (1.73^2) = 85 kg (188 lb)

Daily needs = 66 + (13.7 × 85) + (5 × 173) – (6.8 × 45) = 1,790 + 20% = 2,148 kcal

To lose 1½ lb per week, or 2 BMI units (12 lb) in 9 weeks, energy intake must be reduced by 400 kcal: 2,148 – 400 = 1,748 calories. Increase activity by 250 kcal, for a total deficit of 650 calories daily. Weight loss would be expected to be 1 to 1.5 lb per week. (Clients may choose to increase exercise to achieve a weight loss rate of 1.5 lb per week.)

2. BY INITIAL WEIGHT

Daily need = 66 + (13.7 × 91) + (5 × 173) – (6.8 × 45) = 1,872 + 20% = 2,246 kcal

Reduce caloric intake by 400 kcal: 2,246 – 400 = 1,846 kcal. Increase activity 250 calories for a total deficit of 650 kcal daily.

correlated with weight loss and is considered the best predictor of successful maintenance of reduced body weight (49).

As previously discussed, obesity results from an imbalance between energy intake and energy expenditure, and exercise contributes to weight loss by increasing energy expenditure. Some studies have indicated that exercise may offset the reduction in resting metabolic rate that is seen with energy restriction, presumably by preserving fat-free mass. Hormonal and enzymatic changes that occur with exercise improve the body's ability to mobilize fat stores as an energy source (50). Moderate physical activity has both short-term and sustained effects on psychological well-being that may lead to increased dietary adherence (49).

Knowledge of the multiple benefits of exercise is often not sufficient to motivate obese clients to begin and maintain an effective exercise program. Awareness of and sensitivity to the barriers that prevent obese patients from exercising is essential. Psychological barriers may include previous negative experiences with peers, poor performance, feelings of inadequacy, lack of knowledge or experience, and shame at being observed exercising and wearing exercise clothes. Excess weight itself is a physical barrier to exercise, as is a generally poor fitness level. Walking even a short distance may be tiring and painful (49).

As always, care should be taken to make goals flexible and reasonable. Light to moderate exercise routines should be encouraged. See Chapter 8 for examples of appropriate exercise options. Frequent, positive feedback and reinforcement promotes adherence. Dietitians should stress the importance of both aerobic exercise and resistance training. The latter plays a significant role in weight reduction by sparing or even increasing fat-free mass and thereby preserving resting metabolic rate (51,52). This combined approach is most effective in conjunction with modest, rather than severe, caloric restriction.

Recent studies have raised doubts that exercise without nutrition intervention can significantly promote weight loss in the overweight population (53). Although a lean subject may run 10 miles daily and expend about 1,000 kcal doing so, an obese person is likely to do much less strenuous exercise and therefore expend considerably less energy. Recent work also suggests that in overweight individuals weight loss has a more beneficial effect than aerobic exercise alone on coronary artery disease risk factors (54). The combined benefit of dietary modification and aerobic exercise is clearly greater than the individual benefit of either.

Program Implementation

Figure 7-1 provides a treatment model for reduction of health risk and disease through weight reduction and prevention of weight gain. A weight-loss program may be implemented in a variety of ways, and a combination of approaches may work best. The intuitive practitioner can guide clients to the most effective approach while encouraging them to take responsibility for their treatment. Making a commitment to attend a predetermined number of sessions, agreeing to maintain a food diary, and other assignments encourage clients to take responsibility. A client's willingness to commit to attending additional sessions is a good indicator of readiness to change.

Individuals who are 5% to 20% overweight often are successful with a program that includes exercise, behavior modification, and instruction on healthful food choices. As the degree of obesity increases, additional support and a longer time commitment are usually needed for success. Group settings are most cost-effective and offer additional advantages that are discussed later in this chapter. Conventional food plans of 1,000 to 1,500 kcal or less, which restrict clients to certain approved foods, may produce short-term weight loss but are usually unsustainable and result in rapid weight regain.

Patients with severe obesity (40% to 100% overweight or BMI greater than 30) require extensive individual counseling and are often candidates for very-low-calorie diets, drug therapy, hospital-based programs, or residential treatment. Surgery is reserved for morbidly obese individuals (more than 100% overweight or BMI greater than 40) but may be an option at BMI greater than 35 if severe obesity-related comorbid conditions exist (47). The use of pharmaceuticals for weight loss has become an adjunct to dietary therapy and is discussed briefly later in this chapter.

The nutrition history should illuminate the interventions that are most appropriate for the client. Concrete goals can be developed that target specific behaviors, and the client can develop a sample meal plan that incorporates these goals. For a motivated client who is in the Action stage of change (see Chapter 13), the initial intervention would include development of a food plan and instruction on appropriate low-fat food choices. A review of the energy content of protein, carbohydrates, fat, and alcohol can be included to illustrate the importance of the type of energy consumed. Teaching materials should be geared to clients' educational level, literacy, and ability and willingness to change.

The initial counseling session should conclude with a review of the basic objectives of the new eating pattern, an opportunity to ask questions, a review of the client's goals for the coming weeks, and an appointment for a follow-up visit. Ideally, clients who are attempting weight management and reduction of CVD risk factors attend several educational sessions after their initial evaluation. If, for financial or other reasons, clients cannot attend additional sessions, they should be encouraged to call the dietitian with questions. Follow-up by phone or mail is not ideal but in some circumstances it may be the best or only alternative.

At follow-up sessions the food and exercise plan can be adjusted and problems discussed. Additional nutrition education interventions may include instruction about eating out and ordering from a restaurant menu, recipe modification, low-fat cooking techniques, proper use of food labels, and the addition of fiber to the diet.

Anthropometric measurements (waist, hips, body fat, etc.) can be used to assess progress. Reminding clients of the initial goals that were set reinforces the ultimate goal of improving health (not losing weight for cosmetic reasons). Substantial weight loss and improved laboratory values positively reinforce new behaviors.

Behavioral modification components of a weight-loss program include self-monitoring, problem-solving, controlling stimuli, and slowing the rate of eating. Cognitive therapy may help to reduce self-defeating thoughts (47). Appropriate behaviors that the client has developed to assist weight loss should be reinforced. Efforts to increase clients' self-esteem and self-efficacy help to ensure a positive attitude toward the lifestyle changes to which they are committing.

Diaries are excellent self-monitoring tools. Clients can be encouraged to note not only what they eat but also how they feel (ie, when and where they feel hungry, tired, angry, upset, and so on). Behavior patterns may emerge that the individual is unaware of. Identifying these patterns is instrumental to initiating change.

Because overweight clients tend to underestimate food intake (47), they should be encouraged to weigh and measure all foods for at least several days. Along with the use of food models, this will help to clarify portion sizes. By weighing a bagel or a slice of whole grain bread and measuring the amount of oil or margarine added to food, clients can be more certain that the food intake they are recording in a food diary is accurate.

Problem-solving skills enable clients to deal with and learn from problems they encounter in their program. Developing and reinforcing these skills is important if clients are to succeed on their own (47). A problem can be examined critically in a series of steps: identification and definition (eg, inconsistent exercise routine); generation and evaluation of possible solutions (eg, find an exercise buddy, change exercise routine, time, or place); choice and implementation of a solution (eg, call a friend and set up a time to walk); and evaluation of the outcome (eg, maintained program 4 of 5 days).

Slowing the rate of eating is helpful for many clients. Among the reported benefits are feelings of satiety, increased enjoyment of the flavor and texture of food, and a greater sense of self-control while eating (47). Suggested techniques include putting the fork down between bites, chewing food thoroughly before swallowing, pausing during the meal to notice the taste and texture of the food, and eating in a relaxed setting.

Stimulus control involves removing unnecessary exposure to tempting foods. Practices that reduce impulse eating include using a list to do grocery shopping, storing food out of sight, eating only in a designated location, limiting distractions (eg, turning off the television), planning ahead for

FIGURE 7-1

The treatment model to reduce health risk and disease burden through weight reduction and prevention of weight gain.

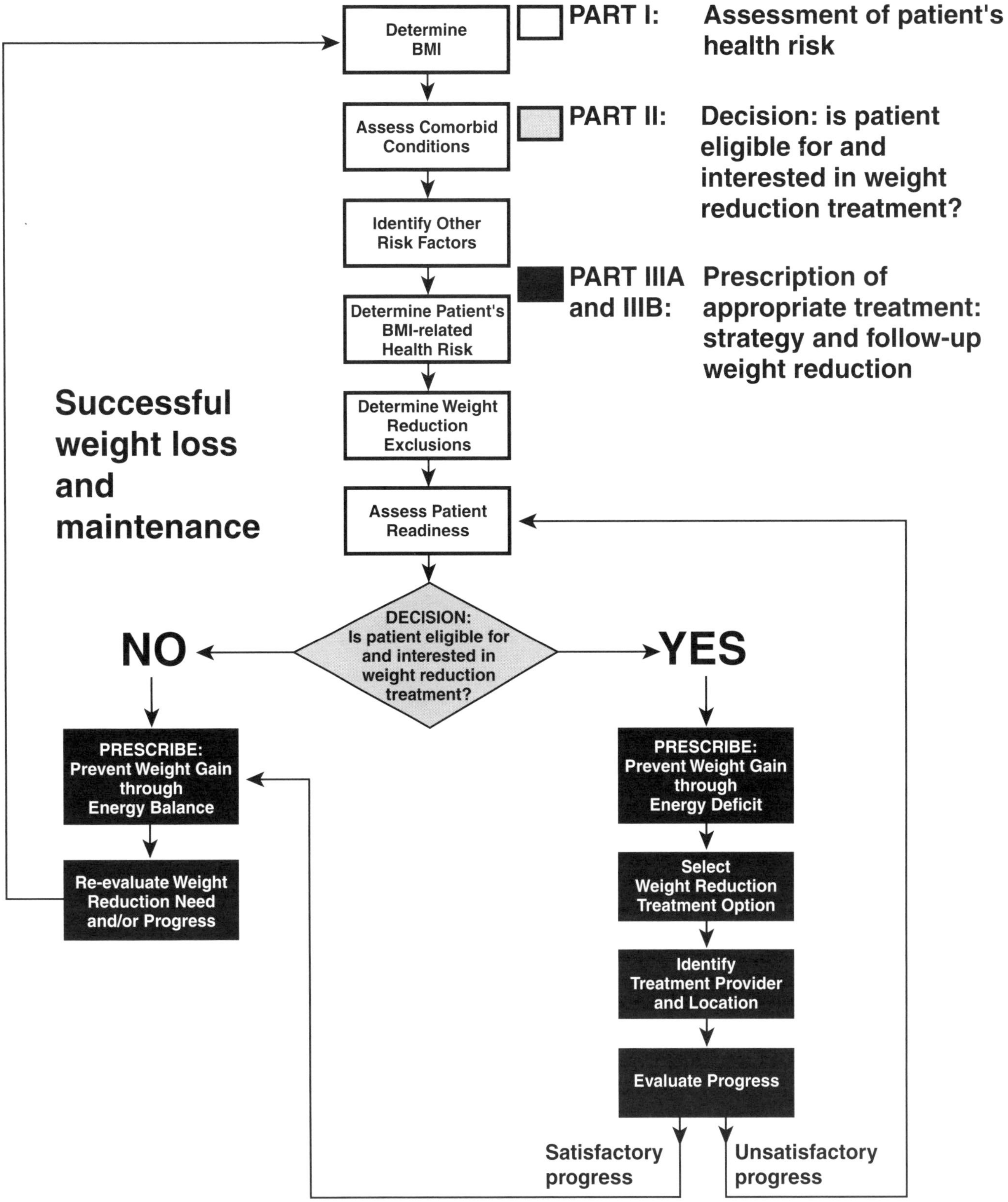

social situations involving food, and resisting the urge to clean your plate (or anyone else's) (55).

Cognitive therapy helps clients to identify and change negative, self-defeating thoughts. Although research is limited on the benefits of cognitive therapy for obese individuals, the technique has been successfully used to treat depression and other mood disorders (56). Burns (57) presents practical applications of cognitive therapy in depression that can easily be adapted for use with weight management clients. A form of cognitive therapy is also found in Brownell's *The LEARN Program for Weight Control* (55).

Educational Support

Group treatment is easily the most cost-effective form of therapy for weight management. Beyond the economic benefits, the support of other group members can be invaluable for individuals who feel alone and ashamed of their weight problem. A good group facilitator can encourage problem-sharing and cooperative development of solutions. Sharing experiences with other group members increases self-awareness, which is empowering and can improve resolve and self-esteem. Group activities such as cooking demonstrations, grocery store tours, and exercise demonstrations are opportunities for hands-on-learning that are not practical in individual counseling.

An effective group requires a leader who is self-assured, enthusiastic, empathetic, kind, and patient. Beyond the necessary professional skills, these personal skills are essential when working with weight-loss clients. Psychosocial issues can be pivotal to the success or failure of a client's program. Addressing these issues requires understanding and identifying with clients' feelings. An atmosphere of empathy, kindness, and optimism helps to assure clients that they are safe discussing personal issues. Skill at putting people at ease and drawing them out during discussions maximizes effective group interaction.

Leaders need to recognize that not all participants will lose weight. Some participants will not choose to use the techniques taught and may try to sabotage the efforts of others. A good leader offers positive reinforcement to those who are trying and shows restraint in admonishing those who are not ready for change. Table 7-2 offers suggestions for dealing with difficult participant behaviors.

Group composition can be an important factor in the success of weight management efforts. Individuals who are extremely obese may quickly drop out of weight-loss classes in which the other participants are only moderately obese. A group whose members have similar needs and goals is usually the most successful. Because most weight management programs have a strong behavioral component in which each lesson builds on previous topics, effectiveness can be diminished when individuals are at different stages of change. However, it is often not possible to control group composition, and extra effort may be required to meet the needs of a diverse group. Chapter 15 addresses some issues to consider in group composition.

Closed groups that meet for a predetermined length of time often have the highest rate of success. In a closed group, all members begin the program together, which helps to build cohesiveness among participants.

Class size is important; large classes (more than 20 participants) often reduce the participation of quieter group members and are less likely to encourage social bonds and interaction among participants. In large classes, it can be difficult to avoid a lecture format in which the advantages of group therapy are lost. By contrast, small classes that stress discussion and sharing can be uncomfortable for some people. Dropouts can threaten the survival of a small group.

A good workable group size is 8 to 12 people. Larger groups are possible, but record keeping and weekly weighing will require more time. Having an assistant perform private weigh-ins and collect and record dietary records and assignments can help to reduce client waiting time in large groups.

Programs can run from 8 to 24 weeks. It takes time to learn and incorporate new behaviors. Brownell (55) reported that a 16-week format was optimal: 10 weeks was too short for participants to make lifestyle changes and more than 16 weeks required a greater time commitment than most people found comfortable. Generally, longer programs result in greater weight loss and provide additional psychological support, but there is a point of diminishing returns as the rate of weight loss slows and costs increase.

Class topics vary based on clients' needs. A comprehensive program addresses the multifactorial nature of obesity and includes discussion of nutrition, exercise, and behavior modification (Table 7-3). Most programs include some sort of weekly homework such as a food and exercise diary, an attitude assessment worksheet, or a behavior-modification monitoring exercise. Skill-building assignments provide a convenient starting place to discuss difficulties faced during the week. Some participants may be uncomfortable filling out forms; alternatives should be available to prevent individuals from dropping out because they have lower literacy skills. (See Chapter 16 for a discussion of techniques appropriate for individuals with lower literacy skills.)

Many professionally designed weight management programs are available, including the LEARN program (55), *The Balancing Act Nutrition and Weight Guide* (58), *My New Weigh of Life* (59), and many others (see Chapter 15). It is rarely cost-effective to develop a new noncommercial program. Topics related to cardiovascular health and group-specific issues can easily be added to commercial programs.

Pharmacotherapy in the Management of Obesity

The treatment of obesity is challenging because success rates are notoriously low when traditional interventions such as diet, exercise, and behavior modification are used. This has prompted recent interest in the use of pharmacotherapy for the management of obesity. The use of weight-loss medications has been shown to result in as

TABLE 7-2

Suggestions for Dealing with Difficult Participants

Participant Behavior	Problem or Possible Motive	Action
Participant statement is definitely wrong	Comes up with a comment that is obviously incorrect	Must be handled delicately. Say: "I can see how you feel" or "That's one way of looking at it" or "I see your point, but let's try looking at it this way."
Searching for your opinion	Trying to put you on the spot Trying to have you support one view May be simply seeking your advice	Generally, you should avoid solving problems. Never take sides. Point out that your view is relatively unimportant. There are times you must and should give a direct answer. Before you determine their reason for asking your view, say, "Fine, let's first get some other opinions." Say: "How do you look upon this point?" (Select someone to reply.)
Won't talk	Bored Indifferent Feels superior Timid	Your action will depend on what is motivating the participant. Arouse participant's interest by asking for their opinion. Draw out the person next to participant. Ask the quiet person for an opinion of what was said. If the participant is seated near you, ask a question so that the person is talking to you, not the group. Ask an easy question. Then say, "Nice answer, thank you."
Griper	Has pet peeve Professional griper Has legitimate complaint	Point out we can't change policy here and that we must operate as best we can under the system. Say you'll discuss problems with person privately later. Ask group, "How do the rest of you feel?"
Side conversations	May be related to the subject May be personal Distracting to the group and you	Don't embarrass participants. Call one participant by name, ask an easy question, or restate last opinion expressed and ask for an opinion. If, during class, you are in the habit of moving around the room, saunter over and stand casually behind or next to the participants who are talking.
Inarticulate	Lacks ability to put thought in order	Say, "Thank you, let me repeat that." Then put it in better language.

Adapted from Burns DD (57).

TABLE 7-3

Topics and Objectives in a 12-Week Weight Management Class

Lesson	Weekly Topics	Weekly Objectives
1	Introduction Self-assessment Goal setting Physical activity	To introduce participants to overall program setup and goals To assist participants in self-assessment To develop realistic goals To teach basic health benefits of weight management To provide basic nutrition information To initiate record keeping as daily routine To introduce concept of need for increased physical activity To determine a personal more healthful weight
2	Energy balance Exchange system	To review activity behavior To determine individual caloric needs To introduce concept of food exchanges/serving sizes
3	Behavior Physical activity	To review exchange system To identify high-risk food situations To determine individual activity plans To raise awareness of physical and emotional components of eating
4	Behavior Fat connection Relapse plans	To continue review of eating behavior patterns To introduce metabolic necessity for lowering fat intake To focus participants on preparing for and managing behavior change To recognize physical and emotional signs of hunger To prepare for lapses and slips
5	Choices Exercise	To develop self-determination and flexibility in thinking and behavior To determine forms of exercise to choose
6	Shopping Food labels	To develop strategies for shopping To determine nutrient content of foods To learn how to read and use food labels To learn the function of fat in foods
7	Recipe modification Scales "lie" Plateaus	To show how to alter favorite recipes to lower-fat versions To identify why "scale weight" is not always accurate To prepare participants for plateaus To develop recipe book for class
8	Eating out Relapse plans	To develop coping mechanisms for dining out To learn to plan for eating out (food selection, amount, etc.)
9	Eating for special events Relapse plans	To form coping strategies for holiday meals, parties, and social occasions To develop strategies for handling sabotage
10	Social support	To institute plans for attaining appropriate social support To learn communication skills
11	Stress/relapse	To prepare for coping with stress and relapse
12	Survival Reassessment Evaluation	To continue preparation for maintenance stage To determine participants' next steps; recalculate BMI To evaluate individual progress To evaluate the program To plan for a reunion

Adapted from Sigman-Grant M (59).

much as a 10% reduction in body weight. Most weight loss occurs during the first 6 months of treatment. When used in conjunction with a calorie-restricted diet and a program of physical activity, pharmacotherapy helps some obese patients lose weight and maintain weight loss. Upon cessation of drug therapy, however, the evidence is clear that patients regain body weight. The criteria for the use of drug therapy for the treatment of obesity include a BMI ≥27, a body fat percentage of 30 or more for women and 25 or more for men, and a weight gain of 13.5 kg or more since 18 years of age (60). In September 1997, two popular diet drugs were withdrawn from the market because of serious adverse side effects, illustrating the importance of close medical supervision for patients on drug therapy for the treatment of obesity.

Presently, there are three classes of drugs used to treat obesity: (1) appetite suppressants that affect the catecholaminergic system (eg, amphetamines, benzphetamine, phendimetrazine, phentermine, mazindol, diethylpropion, and phenlypropanolamine) or the serotonergic system (eg, fenfluramine, dexfenfluramine, fluoxetine, sertraline, and other antidepressant selective serotonin reuptake inhibitors), (2) drugs that reduce nutrient absorption by blocking the action of digestive enzymes or the absorption of nutrients such as fat (these have not yet been approved by the FDA for sale), and (3) drugs that increase energy expenditure by increasing the metabolic rate via changes in sympathetic nervous system tone or uncoupling of oxidative phosphorylation (these have also not yet been approved by the FDA for sale) (60).

It is important to appreciate that more work is needed to demonstrate the long-term safety and efficacy of these drugs. Selective use of these drugs for certain patients may prove to be an effective adjunct to medical nutrition therapy that includes diet, exercise, and behavior modification.

Maintenance

Clients who lose weight are at high risk of regaining most of it, or even of adding additional pounds, unless a relapse prevention program is in place. Research clearly identifies continued self-monitoring of food consumption and exercise habits and frequent client-therapist follow-up contact as prerequisites for weight loss maintenance (61). Follow-up may be by telephone or mail or may take the form of occasional class reunions or a scheduled relapse-prevention group. Intensive maintenance programs that include psychosocial support and nutrition and exercise reinforcement have been shown to be effective but are usually available only through a multidisciplinary weight-loss treatment center. When initial therapy is followed by a maintenance program, a higher level of weight loss is maintained and better adherence to management skills is seen (61).

The primary goal of a maintenance program is to help clients maintain their new healthful weight within the framework of a healthful, enjoyable lifestyle. Some degree of relapse is inevitable. Although relapse is often equated with failure, it can be a valuable learning tool. It can be useful to present this experience as recycling rather than as relapsing. Recycling provides an opportunity to work through a problem again and develop a better solution. Reminding clients that recycling is part of the process of change can help to provide the incentive to reexamine problems and develop effective solutions without eliciting feelings of guilt or failure. Clients need to be reminded of and practice the new lifestyle skills they learned during the treatment program.

Many clients lose weight by severely restricting their food intake. Though this may produce the desired result (ie, quick weight loss), clients lack the skills to maintain the loss once they resume normal eating. Many rigid-restraint eaters are at risk for binge-eating disorder and bulimia (62). These practices may also account for the high frequency of relapse that is typically seen in dieters. Rigid-restraint eaters may require extensive help with the lifestyle skills that promote sustained weight loss.

Weight maintenance programs should focus on the following:

- flexible but intelligent food choices,
- problem-solving,
- changing self-defeating thoughts into positive self-talk,
- stress management,
- self-monitoring,
- maintaining a support system,
- improving social skills and relationships,
- exercise,
- managing anger and loneliness, and
- dealing with depression and anxiety.

Groups such as Overeaters Anonymous are a potential source of lifelong support for individuals who are attempting to sustain weight loss. Overeaters Anonymous is especially helpful for individuals struggling with binge eating or bulimia. It does not offer nutritional therapy or medical care but provides a supportive nonjudgmental atmosphere in which clients can discuss their feelings and share experiences, strength, and hope. Information on local chapters can usually be found in local telephone directories. Additional information can be obtained by contacting the Overeaters Anonymous World Service Office, P.O. Box 44020, Rio Rancho, NM 87174-4020, or by calling (505) 891-2664.

CONCLUSION

Assisting clients to achieve and maintain a more healthful weight that reduces their risk of CVD and other chronic diseases can be the dietitian's greatest challenge and most rewarding experience. The complex nature of obesity and overweight requires dietitians to broaden their traditional role as nutrition educators and to be cognizant of the limitations of their training and expertise. Additional training in counseling skills can be extremely helpful. Working closely with other relevant health professionals is in the best interest of both clients and dietitians.

When the chronic, multifactorial nature of obesity is

addressed, clients can achieve a healthier life and reduce the risk factors associated with the condition. Although no cure exists for obesity, various tools are available for clients to use to achieve a healthier weight and lifestyle.

REFERENCES

1. Burton BT, Foster WR. Health Implications of Obesity: an NIH consensus development conference. *J Am Diet Assoc.* 1985;85:1117.
2. Sjostrom L. Recent methods in the study of body composition. In: Tanner JM, ed. *Perspectives in the Science of Growth and Development.* London: Smith-Gordon; 1989:353-366.
3. Womersley J, Durnin JVGA, Boddy K, Mahaffy M. Influence of muscular development, obesity and age on the fat-free mass of adults. *J Appl Physiol.* 1976;41:223-229.
4. Metropolitan Life Insurance Company. New standards for men and women. *Stat Bull Metropol Life Insur Co.* 1959;40:1-4.
5. Metropolitan Life Insurance Company. 1983 Height and weight tables. *Stat Bull Metropol Insur Co.* 1984;64:2-9.
6. Kuczmarski RJ, Flegal KM, Campbell SM, Johnson CL. Increasing prevalence of overweight among US adults: the National Health and Nutrition Examination Surveys, 1960-1991. *JAMA.* 1994;272:205-211.
7. *Nutrition and Your Health: Dietary Guidelines for Americans.* 3rd ed. Washington, DC: US Depts of Agriculture and Health and Human Services; 1990. Home and Garden Bulletin No. 232.
8. *Nutrition and Your Health: Dietary Guidelines for Americans.* 4th ed. Washington, DC: US Depts of Agriculture and Health and Human Services; 1995. Home and Garden Bulletin No. 232.
9. Blackburn GL, Dwyer JT, Flanders WD. Report of the American Institute of Nutrition Steering Committee on Healthy Weight. *J Nutr.* 1994;124:2240-2243.
10. Must A, Dallal GE, Dietz WH. Reference data for obesity: 85th and 95th percentiles of body mass index (wt/ht^2) and triceps skinfold thickness. *Am J Clin Nutr.* 1991;53:839-846.
11. Garn SM. Fractionating healthy weight. *Am J Clin Nutr.* 1996;63(suppl):412S-414S.
12. Simopoulos AP. Obesity and body weight standards. *Annu Rev Public Health.* 1987;7:481.
13. US Department of Health and Human Services, Centers for Disease Control and Prevention. Update: prevalence of overweight among children, adolescents, and adults—United States, 1988-1994. *Morbid Mortal Weekly Rep.* 1997;46(9):199-202.
14. Galuska DA, Sercula M, Pamuk E, Siegel PZ, Byers T. Trends in overweight among US adults from 1987 to 1993: a multistate telephone survey. *Am J Public Health.* 1996;86:1729-1735.
15. US Congress, House. *Deception and Fraud in the Diet Industry.* Part I. Hearing before the Subcommittee on Regulation, Business Opportunities, and Energy Committee on Small Business. 101st Congress, 2nd Session. Washington, DC: US Government Printing Office; 1990:101-150.
16. Wolf AM, Colditz GA. The costs of obesity: the US perspective. *Pharmacoeconomics.* 1994;5:34-37.
17. Meyer JM, Stunkard AJ. Genetics and human obesity. In: Stunkard AJ, Walden TA, eds. *Obesity Theory and Therapy.* 2nd ed. New York, NY: Raven Press; 1993:137-149.
18. Schwartz MW, Seeley RJ. The new biology of body weight regulation. *J Am Diet Assoc.* 1997;97:54-58.
19. Ferraro R, Boyce VL, Swinburn B, DeGregorio M, Ravussin E. Energy cost of physical activity on a metabolic ward in relationship to obesity. *Am J Clin Nutr.* 1991;53:1368-1371.
20. Wood PD, Stefanick ML, Williams P, Haskell WL. The effects on plasma lipoproteins of a prudent weight-reducing diet, with or without exercise, in overweight men and women. *N Engl J Med.* 1991;325:461-466.
21. King AC, Tribble DL. The role of exercise in weight regulation in nonathletes. *Sports Med.* 1991;11(5):331-349.
22. World Health Organization. *Diet, Nutrition and the Prevention of Chronic Diseases.* Report of a WHO study group, Series 797. Geneva: World Health Organization, 1990.
23. Brown PJ. Cultural perspectives on the etiology and treatment of obesity. In: Stunkard AJ, Walden TA, eds. *Obesity Theory and Therapy.* 2nd ed. New York, NY: Raven Press; 1993:179-193.
24. Stunkard AJ. Eating patterns and obesity. *Psychiatr Q.* 1959;33:284-292.
25. American Psychiatric Association. *Diagnostic and Statistical Manual* (DSM-IV). 4th ed. Washington, DC: American Psychiatric Association; 1994.
26. Marcus MD, Wing RR. Binge eating among the obese. *Ann Behav Med.* 1987;9:23-27.
27. Spitzer RL, Devlin M, Walsh BT, Hasin D, Wing R, Marcus M, Stunkard AJ, Wadden T, Yanovski S, Agras WS, Mitchell J, Nonas C. Binge-eating disorder: a multisite field trial for the diagnostic criteria. *Int J Eat Disord.* 1992;11:191-204.
28. Telch CF, Agras WS, Rossiter EM. Binge eating with increasing adiposity. *Int J Eat Disord.* 1988;7:115-119.
29. Lowe MR, Caputo GC. Binge eating in obesity: toward the specification of predictors. *Int J Eat Disorders.* 1991;10:49-55.
30. Pi-Sunyer FX. Medical hazards of obesity. *Ann Intern Med.* 1993;119:655-660.
31. Glueck CJ, Taylor HL, Jacobs D, Morrison JA, Beaglehole R, Williams D. Plasma high-density lipoprotein cholesterol: association with measurements of body mass. *Circulation.* 1980;62(suppl IV):62-69.
32. Little JA, Graves K, Suchindran CM, Milner J, McGuire V, Beaton G, Feather T, Mattson FH, Christiansen D, Williams OD. Customary diet, anthropometry and dyslipoproteinemia in selected North American populations: the Lipid Research Clinics Program Prevalence Study. *Circulation.* 1986;73(suppl I):1-80.
33. Berchtold P, Berger M, Greiser E, Dohse M, Irmscher K, Gries FA, Zimmerman H. Cardiovascular risk factors in gross obesity. *Int J Obes.* 1977;1:219-229.
34. Ashley FW Jr, Kannel WB. Relation of weight change to changes in atherogenic traits: the Framingham Study. *J Chronic Dis.* 1974;27:103-114.
35. Denke MA, Sempos CT, Grundy SM. Excess body weight: an underrecognized contributor to high blood cholesterol levels in white American men. *Arch Intern Med.* 1993;153:1093-1103.
36. Kannel WB, D'Agostino RB, Cobb JL. Effect of weight on cardiovascular disease. *Am J Clin Nutr.* 1996;63(suppl):419S-422S.
37. Reavens GM. Pathophysiology of insulin resistance in human disease. *Physiol Rev.* 1995;75:473-486.
38. Lean MED, Han TS, Morrison CE. Waist circumference as a measure for indicating need for weight management. *BMJ.* 1995;311:158-161.
39. Dattilo, AM, Kris-Etherton, PM. Effects of weight reduction on blood lipids and lipoproteins: a meta-analysis. *Am J Clin Nutr.* 1992;56:320-328.
40. Lew EA. Mortality and weight: insured lives and the American Cancer Society studies. *Ann Intern Med.* 1985;103:1024-1029.
41. Garrison RJ, Kannel WB. A new approach for estimating healthy body weights. *Int J Obes.* 1993;17:417-423.

42. Meisler JG, St Jeor, S. Summary and recommendations from the American Health Foundations Expert Panel on healthy weight. *Am J Clin Nutr.* 1996;63(suppl):474S-477S.

43. Wadden TA, Stunkard AJ. Psychosocial consequences of obesity and dieting: research and clinical findings. In: Stunkard AJ, Walden TA, eds. *Obesity Theory and Therapy*. 2nd ed. New York, NY: Raven Press; 1993:163-177.

44. Stunkard AJ. Talking with patients. In: Stunkard AJ, Walden TA, eds. *Obesity Theory and Therapy*. 2nd ed. New York, NY: Raven Press; 1993:355-363.

45. Parham ES. Is there a new weight paradigm? *Nutr Today.* 1996;31(4):155-161.

46. *Guidance for Treatment of Adult Obesity*. Bethesda, Md. Shape Up America! and the American Obesity Association; 1996.

47. Wadden TA. The treatment of obesity. In: Stunkard AJ, Walden TA, eds. *Obesity Theory and Therapy*. 2nd ed. New York, NY: Raven Press; 1993:197-217.

48. Brownell KD, Wadden TA. Behavior therapy for obesity: modern approaches and better results. In: Brownell KD, Foreyt JP, eds. *Handbook of Eating Disorders: Physiology, Psychology, and Treatment of Obesity, Anorexia, and Bulimia*. New York, NY: Basic Books, 1986;180-197.

49. Grilo CM, Brownell KD, Stunkard AJ. The metabolic and psychological importance of exercise in weight control. In: Stunkard AJ, Walden TA, eds. *Obesity Theory and Therapy*. 2nd ed. New York, NY: Raven Press; 1993:253-267.

50. Blair SN, Horton E, Leon AS, Lee IM, Drinkwater BL, Dishman RK, Mackey M, Kienholz ML. Physical activity, nutrition and chronic disease. *Med Sci Sports Exerc.* 1996;28:335-349.

51. Ballor DL, Katch VI, Becque MD, Marks CR. Resistance weight training during caloric restriction enhances lean body weight maintenance. *Am J Clin Nutr*. 1988;47:19-25.

52. Donnelly JE, Pronk NP, Jacobsen DJ, Pronk SJ, Jakicic JM. Effects of a very-low-calorie diet and physical-training regimens on body composition and resting metabolic rate in obese females. *Am J Clin Nutr*. 1991;54:56-61.

53. Zalesko, CJ. Exercise for weight loss: what are the facts? *J Am Diet Assoc*. 1995;95:1414-1417.

54. Katzel LI, Bleeker ER, Colman EG, Rogus EM, Sorkin JD, Goldberg AP. Effects of weight loss vs aerobic exercise training on risk factors for coronary disease in healthy, obese, middle-aged and older men. *JAMA*. 1995;274:1915-1921.

55. Brownwell KD. *The LEARN Program for Weight Control.* Dallas, Tex: American Health Publishing Co, 1990.

56. Collins RL, Rothblum ED, Wilson GT. The comparative efficacy of cognitive and behavioral approaches in the treatment of obesity. *Cognitive Ther Res*. 1986;10:299-317.

57. Burns DD. *Feeling Good: The New Mood Therapy*. New York, NY: Avon Books; 1992.

58. Kostas, GG. *The Balancing Act Nutrition and Weight Guide*. Kingsport, Tenn: Quebecor Printing Book Group; 1994.

59. Sigman-Grant M. *My New Weigh of Life*. University Park, Pa: Pennsylvania State University; 1996.

60. National Task Force on the Prevention and Treatment of Obesity. Long-term pharmacotherapy in the management of obesity. *JAMA*. 1996;276:1907-1915.

61. Perri MG, Nezu AM. Preventing relapse following treatment for obesity. In: Stunkard AJ, Walden TA, eds. *Obesity Theory and Therapy.* 2nd ed. New York, NY: Raven Press; 1993:287-299.

62. Pirke KM, Laessle RG. Restrained eating. In: Stunkard AJ, Walden TA, eds. *Obesity Theory and Therapy.* 2nd ed. New York, NY: Raven Press; 1993:151-162.

CHAPTER 8

Promoting a Healthful Lifestyle Through Exercise

Kristine L. Clark, PhD, RD

Increased physical activity is a recognized lifestyle-modification strategy for reducing the incidence of cardiovascular disease (CVD). As discussed in Chapter 1, physical activity beneficially modifies many major CVD risk factors and effectively rehabilitates the cardiovascular system after diagnosis of CVD.

Physical Inactivity — A Modifiable Risk Factor

The relation between physical activity and improved health has become so accepted in the scientific community that *Healthy People 2000* identifies increasing physical activity as one of the top five goals for Americans (1). However, existing data on Americans' exercise habits make bleak reading: Only 22% of all adults appear to participate in physical activity at the levels recommended for obtaining health benefits (30 minutes of moderate-intensity physical activity performed on most days of the week). Another 54% of Americans are insufficiently active and the remaining 24% are entirely sedentary (2). A 1995 report by the President's Council on Physical Fitness stated that Americans were exercising less than they were in 1993 (3).

Motivating individuals to include exercise in their busy and often stress-filled lives can be challenging. The key to helping a person become more physically active is to devise a program that caters to individual needs, desires, and time constraints. This chapter reviews exercise-specific changes that occur in the cardiovascular system and the effect of exercise on the lipid profile and other CVD risk factors. The dietitian's role in developing an exercise program is discussed and activities appropriate for beginning exercisers are provided. Special considerations for exercise in individuals with diabetes are reviewed. Exercise in a cardiac rehabilitation setting is discussed in Chapter 9.

Exercise-specific Changes in the Cardiovascular System

Aerobic activity — any activity in which the heart pumps a continuous supply of oxygen-rich blood to the major muscles — causes enlargement (hypertrophy) of the heart muscle. This enlargement results primarily from an increase in left-ventricular chamber size but also from increases in left-ventricular wall thickness and may be important in promoting improved contractility and increased cardiac work capacity. The capacity of the coronary circulation also appears to increase with aerobic training; the size of the major coronary vessels increases, implying an increased capacity for blood flow to all regions of the heart. Several studies showed that the peak flow rate in the major coronary arteries is increased after an aerobic training program (4). Examples of aerobic activities include walking, jogging, running, swimming, bicycling, stair climbing, dancing, and rowing.

Interest has surged in the use of resistance training — a form of anaerobic exercise — to promote improvement in general health. Resistance training appears to positively affect cardiorespiratory fitness. With resistance training, the heart rate at submaximal rates of exercise is generally reduced, which usually reflects improved cardiorespiratory fitness.

Effect of Physical Activity on the Lipid Profile

People who exercise generally have lower triglyceride levels and higher high-density lipoprotein cholesterol levels (see Chapter 1) than do sedentary individuals. Plasma total cholesterol and low-density lipoprotein cholesterol are less likely to differ. Table 8-1 summarizes the typical lipid profile alterations that result from exercise. The reason for the variation in lipoprotein and plasma lipid responses to exercise is not clear. Exercise alters lipoprotein lipase, hepatic

TABLE 8-1

Differences in Lipoprotein Profile of Exercising vs Sedentary Individuals

	Exercise[a]	Aerobic Exercise	Resistance Training (Anaerobic)	Exercise and Weight Loss
HDL-C[b]	↑	↑	↑	↑↑
LDL-C	–	–	–	↓
VLDL-C	↓	↓↓[c]	↓	↓↓
Triglycerides	↓	↓↓[c]	↓	↓↓
Total-C	–	–	–	↓
Hypertension[d]	↓	↓↓[e]	↓[f]	↓↓

– May or may not change, results variable

↑ = some increase, ↑↑= significant increase, ↓= some decrease, ↓↓= significant decrease.

[a] Exercise defined as moderately hard (60-85% of VO_2 max) 3 to 7 days/week for 10 to 16 weeks (2,4).

[b] HDL_2-C concentrations found to be 5 mg/dL greater relative to inactive individuals, may increase 3-8 mg/dL or more when active adults increase activity beyond their current level (2,4).

[c] Aerobic exercise typically more effective than resistance exercise (2,4).

[d] Mild to moderate hypertension.

[e] Endurance training (90 minutes or more of continuous exercise) reduced systolic and diastolic blood pressure by approximately 10 mmHg (7,8,9,10,11,13).

[f] Wilmore and Costil 1995 (3).

lipase, and lecithin-cholesterol acyltransferase, which are important in triglyceride and cholesterol metabolism (see Chapter 3).

Effect of Physical Activity on Other Cardiovascular Risk Factors

As physical activity becomes part of an individual's lifestyle, there appears to be a concomitant decrease in CVD risk factors such as obesity. Resistance training reduces obesity by decreasing fat mass and increasing fat-free mass (5). Some scientists speculate that increased fat-free mass increases resting metabolic rate and energy expenditure because muscle is more metabolically active than fat. In addition, regular exercise appears to decrease platelet aggregation in men, slowing the development of atherosclerotic plaque and reducing the risk of CVD (6).

Other risk factors, such as smoking, may also be altered with exercise. Currently, few data indicate whether aerobic activity leads to smoking cessation or to a reduction in the number of cigarettes smoked. However, a great deal of anecdotal information suggests that exercise has some effect on the number of cigarettes used.

Effect of Physical Activity on Hypertension

An extensive database supports the effectiveness of exercise in reducing blood pressure in people with mild to moderate hypertension (7-11). In 1994, a task force assembled by the American College of Sports Medicine to investigate the risks of physical activity on hypertension concluded that exercise may normalize blood pressure in some individuals with mildly elevated levels (12,13). Endurance training can reduce both systolic and diastolic blood pressures by approximately 10 mmHg in individuals with moderate essential hypertension (7,8).

A recent meta-analysis of 35 clinical studies involving more than 1,000 adults concluded that aerobic exercise reduces resting systolic and diastolic blood pressure in normotensive adults (14). Across all categories and designs, statistically significant postexercise reductions were found for both systolic (-4.4 ± 6.6 mm Hg) and diastolic (-3.2 ± 3.2 mm Hg) blood pressure. A study conducted through the Honolulu Heart Program found that low-activity subjects had a mean systolic blood pressure 5.9 mm Hg higher than did high-activity subjects (15).

Other Benefits of Exercise

Human immune function undergoes adverse changes with aging, including the development of relative immune deficiency and an immune dysregulated state (16). This immune senescence can lead to an increased risk of infections, autoimmune disorders, and certain cancers in the elderly (16).

The effect of aging has not yet been clearly dissociated from genetic traits and age-related differences in nutritional status, habitual physical activity, and exposure to psychological stressors. Although the role of physical activity in immune function is not completely clear, the belief that appropriate, regular endurance exercise may slow the age-related decline in immune function is growing (16). Because neutrophils, macrophages, and natural killer cells may all play a role in the development of CVD, maintaining optimal immune protection through regular physical activity may be indicated. Further research is needed to clarify the important role of exercise in immune function.

Developing an Exercise Program — The Dietitian's Role

Defining physical activity, explaining its benefits, and discussing the practicality of incorporating physical activity into clients' often busy and stress-filled lives can be among the greatest challenges facing dietitians. Reminding clients of the importance of exercise is unlikely to motivate them to begin exercising. Individuals are more likely to adopt and maintain physical activity if they

- perceive a net benefit from participating in the activity;
- enjoy the chosen activity;
- feel competent and safe while performing the activity;
- can easily fit the activity into their schedule; and
- understand the need to balance the use of convenient, labor-saving devices with activities that require more exertion (ie, the use of a motorized golf cart vs a pull cart).

An activity is more likely to be sustained if it

- is easily accessible on a daily basis;
- does not present an unacceptable financial or social cost to the participant;
- causes few negative effects such as injuries, loss of time, negative peer pressure, and self-identity problems; and
- does not regularly conflict with another time demand.

A dietitian can help clients begin to incorporate physical activity into their daily lives by first assessing their daily activity patterns. For example, ask clients how they spend their mornings, afternoons, and evenings. An entire supplement of *Medicine and Science in Sports and Exercise* is devoted to exercise and activity assessment tools (see the Resources later in this chapter). Use this information to formulate ideas for activities that can be incorporated into each segment of the day.

The American College of Sports Medicine (ACSM), the premier international organization of fitness experts and sports medicine scientists, has devoted years of research to developing guidelines for starting an exercise program. Dietitians who work with individuals with CVD should obtain *The ACSM Fitness Book* (17), an excellent resource that will help dietitians to develop confidence in discussing exercise with clients.

Assessment

The most important question to ask clients before introducing exercise concepts is whether a physician approved participation in an exercise program. Depending on the client's health circumstances, an exercise physiologist may need to prescribe a specific exercise protocol.

Clients who are at high risk for CVD complications during exercise include those who have unstable angina, severe aortic stenosis, uncontrolled cardiac arrhythmia, decompensated congestive heart failure, or other medical conditions that could be aggravated by exercise (eg, acute myocarditis or infectious disease) (7). Clients who are at increased risk who may be able to exercise under direct medical supervision include those with severely depressed left ventricular function, resting complex ventricular arrhythmia, ventricular arrhythmia that appears or increases with exercise, and systolic blood pressure that decreases with exercise, as well as survivors of sudden cardiac arrest, recent myocardial infarction complicated by congestive heart failure, and marked exercise-induced ischemia (see Chapter 9). Planning physical activity for individuals with Type 1 or Type 2 diabetes also presents special challenges and is discussed later in this chapter.

Setting Goals

ACSM recommends use of the term *movement* instead of *physical activity* and recommends accumulating 30 minutes of movement per day. This can be accomplished, for example, by walking for 15 minutes in the morning before work and for an additional 15 minutes later in the day. Individuals can time themselves walking up and down the stairs in their office building for 10 minutes. This kind of exercise break contributes to meeting the goal of 30 minutes of daily movement. Movement of any kind should be encouraged; gardening, mowing the lawn, vacuuming, and dancing around the living room all count toward the goal.

Aerobic Activity

Aerobic exercises use the large muscle groups (eg, the whole leg, arms, back, and gluteals) and promote the greatest cardiovascular benefit when done in a continuous or sustained manner. Although both aerobic and anaerobic activity are important in promoting endurance and strength, aerobic activity appears to provide greater benefits in terms of CVD prevention.

Aerobic activities such as brisk walking, jogging, swimming, stair climbing, and aerobic dance are the best type of exercise to recommend to patients who have hypertension (18). Endurance training reduces both systolic and diastolic blood pressure by about 10 mmHg in individuals with moderate essential hypertension (7-11) but seems to have little effect on those with severe hypertension. The specific mechanisms responsible for the decreases in blood pressure have yet to be determined.

Excellent aerobic exercise equipment is available for indoor or home use. Video exercise programs, aerobic dance programs on cable television, stationary bikes, skiing and rowing machines, stair-climbing equipment, and treadmills make aerobic exercise possible despite difficult schedules or inclement weather. Any one or a combination of these activities can be the foundation of a cardiovascular fitness program.

To obtain the maximum cardiovascular benefit, aerobic activity should be conducted for a minimum of 20 continuous minutes. A common misconception among inactive individuals is that the speed or intensity of aerobic movement must be fast and leave them breathless; aerobic movement can be slow and comfortable.

Clients need to know the level of intensity of movement that is safe for them. A good guide for gauging intensity is the ability to comfortably carry on a conversation with an exercise partner while engaging in the activity. If participants cannot talk comfortably while exercising, they should slow their pace down.

Helping clients to become mentally as well as physically comfortable with movement should be a primary goal. The likelihood of continued physical activity appears to be associated with individuals' perception of their success (19). Additional exercise considerations for overweight and obese individuals are discussed in Chapter 7.

Walking. Walking may be the best introductory exercise for relatively sedentary individuals. Although it is often not regarded as exercise, walking provides excellent cardiovascular and endurance benefits. Clients can expect to expend at least 210 kcal by walking briskly and covering a distance of about 2 miles in 30 minutes. People unaccustomed to walking may not be able to start at this level. However, some clients are motivated by being told how much energy the activity will expend. Sports nutritionists frequently equate a mile of walking or jogging with 100 kcal of energy expenditure. This is approximate because weight and exercise intensity influence energy expenditure, but it gives clients a good idea of the immediate beneficial effect.

Among the advantages of walking for health are that almost anyone can do it, the pace is easily varied, it is free, and it can be done almost anywhere. The only equipment needed is a pair of good walking shoes. Some clients may need information about selecting an appropriate pair of shoes. Shoes should be designed for walking distances that can be covered in 20 to 30 minutes; everyday, comfortable shoes are not appropriate for exercising. Asking clients to bring the shoes they intend to wear for walking to the clinic for evaluation is a good way of ensuring that they have proper shoes. Some clients may find it helpful to receive a list of local stores that stock exercise shoes.

Another important aspect of a walking program is proper posture. The head should be erect and the chin up. Arms should not swing from side to side but rather move in a pumping fashion directly at the sides (but not in a drum-beating motion). Hands should be relaxed, not clenched as if holding a roll of quarters.

Jogging. Jogging is an aerobic activity with benefits equal to those of walking. Because it is a more intense activity, it requires a higher level of motivation and results in greater energy expenditure per minute. According to some exercise scientists, jogging for 30 minutes at a rate of 10 mph expends about 642 kcal (5).

Before beginning a jogging program, clients should participate in a walking program. Many individuals begin a jogging program after participating in a walk-jog program. For example, once individuals can comfortably walk for 60 minutes and feel they could walk more, they may wish to alternate walking a block with jogging a block. Jogging can be done at a slow pace while maintaining a conversation with a partner. Clients should never feel out of breath — although they will feel, appropriately, that they are breathing harder. If any pain is experienced during or after jogging, the participant should stop and a physician should be notified immediately.

Jogging, like walking, only requires a good pair of shoes. Clients should not try to jog in regular walking or tennis shoes. They should be advised to seek professional advice on shoe selection because their gait (supinate or pronate) may influence the type of shoe that should be selected. Other important tips for the beginning jogger include the following:

- Cushioned socks should be worn to protect the foot from excess friction. Very thin socks or socks with holes should not be worn.
- Comfortable shorts or slacks that fit at the ankles, such as sweat pants, should be worn. Bulkiness at the ankles may cause friction between the feet and a general feeling of awkwardness.
- Upper-body clothing should be appropriate for the weather. A tank top or T-shirt can be worn on a warm day. In cooler weather, layered clothing is recommended (eg, a long-sleeved cotton turtleneck shirt and a nylon windbreaker may be appropriate). In cold weather, hats and gloves help to reduce heat loss and nylon or polypropylene fabric helps to wick sweat from the body.
- Large-breasted women may find that a jog bra or a Lycra tank top under a T-shirt reduces discomfort. There are no data to support the need for women to wear a bra when jogging; each woman should be guided by what she finds most comfortable.

Swimming and Water Aerobics. Swimming and water aerobics are excellent options for overweight individuals and others who have difficulty walking or jogging. The main piece of equipment needed for swimming is a swimming suit, a garment that some persons feel uncomfortable wearing. In some swimming facilities, participants may be permitted to wear shorts and a T-shirt. Additional equipment that may be needed includes a bathing cap, a pair of goggles, a towel, and shower shoes.

Swimming is a less convenient form of exercise for most individuals because they must go to a swimming facility and may need to pay a fee. However, swimming is a relaxing activity that puts no stress on joints. Practiced regularly, it decreases body fat and total body weight. The energy expenditure of swimming is approximately 175 kcal for every 30 minutes of continuous movement.

Water aerobics is performed in a swimming pool. Legs and arms circling underwater push against the water, creating resistance that mimics weight training. With life vests or other flotation devices, people can do aerobic exercises in deep water without putting weight on their joints. This form of exercise is ideal for very overweight patients or those with joint problems. Water aerobics classes can provide a social opportunity for participants.

Stair Climbing. Stair climbing gained new popularity with the advent of the stair-climbing machine. Stair climbing is an excellent aerobic activity that primarily uses the major muscles in the lower half of the body (gluteals, quadriceps, hamstrings, and calf muscles). Stair-climbing machines are generally available at health clubs and fitness centers.

Stair-climbing machines operate in a variety of ways; for example, one model has rotating steps whereas another type has two moving steps. A built-in computer enables the user to select the desired duration, level of difficulty, and level of intensity of exercise. Energy expenditure on all types of stair climbers is similar, ranging from approximately 60 to 100 kcal in 10 minutes, depending on the intensity of the movement and the weight of the user. Most stair climbers display the user's pace and energy expended during exercise.

The only other equipment needed for this type of exercise is comfortable shoes; jogging, walking, cross-training, or aerobic dance shoes may be worn. Any comfortable clothing such as a T-shirt and shorts, Lycra tights, or lightweight cotton or nylon sweat pants is appropriate.

Aerobic Dance. Many health clubs feature aerobic dance classes that are designed for individuals of various levels of ability. In addition, aerobic dance programs are often shown on television in the morning and aerobic dance videotapes are available. When purchasing exercise videotapes, clients should read the package description, which should clearly state the fitness level to which the video is geared.

Some clients enjoy the social aspect of aerobic dance classes. A leader encourages attendees and teaches new movements. The presence of others in the class can motivate continued participation.

Aerobic dance may be high or low impact. In low-impact aerobics participants keep one foot on the floor at all times, whereas high-impact aerobics involves jumping or ballistic movements. Both types of aerobic dance promote cardiovascular fitness. These exercises can be adapted to focus on upper-body movement for individuals with limited mobility.

The only equipment needed for aerobic dance is good shoes. Most professionals advise the use of aerobic-dance or cross-training shoes that are designed for back-and-forth and side-to-side movements; most walking and jogging shoes, by contrast, are designed for forward motion. (Clients who are considering several exercise options, such as aerobic dance and walking, should be advised to purchase a cross-training shoe that is designed for multiple activities.)

T-shirts, shorts, Lycra exercise tights, sweat suits, and comfortable cotton slacks and shirts are appropriate apparel for aerobic dance. Clothing should not interfere with movement. Many women are comfortable wearing leotards, but most facilities have no dress code and clothing should be selected on the basis of comfort.

Anaerobic Activity

Unlike aerobic activity, anaerobic activity does not require a continuous supply of oxygen. Activities that are conducted in less than 20 minutes or that require short bursts of energy, such as sprinting, bicycling, and some types of swimming, are considered anaerobic. Other examples include sports characterized by frequent starts and stops, such as tennis, basketball, volleyball, and soccer. These sports are referred to as *high-intensity, intermittent sports*. Weight lifting and resistance training are anaerobic.

Although anaerobic activities are less beneficial than aerobic activities for reducing CVD risk, they are critical for maintaining flexibility, bone health in women, and strength, especially in older people. Resistance training or weight-bearing exercises are part of ACSM's recommendations for a general health and fitness program (19).

Recommendations for Beginning Exercisers

The following guidelines may be useful to dietitians who practice in small facilities where they are the key professionals promoting exercise.

As previously noted, walking is an excellent form of aerobic activity for people who are just beginning to exercise. Most people are able to walk and walking involves all of the major muscle groups. Because it places very little stress on joints, walking is an excellent activity for clients who are out of shape or obese.

If clients have not been walking aerobically for years, ACSM guidelines suggest that the first week of a walking program should consist of a 2-minute warm-up walk (standing in place) followed by a 10-minute walk. The 2-minute warm-up walk should be continued through the sixth week. Walking time may be increased to 15 minutes in weeks 2 and 3 and to 20 minutes in weeks 4, 5, and 6.

Clients should be advised to check their watches after their 2-minute warm-up walk. They should then walk for 5 or 10 minutes in one direction, turn around, and walk directly back to their starting place.

Individuals who are slightly more fit may begin a walking program at level 2 of the ACSM guidelines. This level begins with a daily 2-minute warm-up walk. During weeks 1 and 2, a 20-minute walk is encouraged, increasing to 25 minutes in weeks 3 and 4 and to 30 minutes in weeks 5 and 6.

Level 3 of the ACSM guidelines begins with a daily 2-minute warm-up walk followed by 30 minutes of walking in weeks 1 and 2, 35 minutes in weeks 3 and 4, and 40 minutes in weeks 5 and 6.

The ACSM guidelines include many additional exercises for beginning exercisers that will improve participants' overall fitness level. Exercises such as weight training, which stresses muscular fitness, strength, and flexibility, should be introduced gradually. Clients may become disillusioned with physical activity if they perceive the requirements to be too time intensive.

Beginning a Resistance Training Program. For clients who are interested in starting a resistance training program, dietitians should have available pairs of 1-, 3-, 5-, and 10-pound hand-held dumbbells that can be kept in the office. (Dietitians should be able to tell their clients what hand-held weights cost and where they can be purchased locally.)

Initially, clients can be asked to perform bicep curls with light (1- to 3-pound) dumbbells. A bicep curl involves grasping a weight in each hand (with fingernails facing the body), placing the elbows close to the body at a 90-degree angle, and bringing the forearm toward the shoulder in a slow, smooth movement. The benchmark for progressing to a heavier weight is the ability to perform 8 to 15 repetitions of the movement. When clients can perform an exercise with moderate ease, the number of repetitions should be increased (up to 15) or the next heavier weight should be used. This training technique is referred to as *progressive resistance exercise.*

Other upper-body strengthening exercises that use hand-held weights are the arm extension fly (arms at the sides, raise arms up to shoulder), front arm extension (arms straight in front of body, raise arms slowly up to shoulders), and chest fly (lie on back, bring arms together in front of body, elbows slightly bent).

Performing a series of exercises with a client in the office helps to determine which exercises to perform, how much weight to use, and how many repetitions to do. (See the Resources for two excellent references on assisting clients in the use of hand-held dumbbells.)

Finding Places to Exercise. One of the best exercise resources in the United States is the Young Men's and Women's Christian Association (YMCA and YWCA). Facilities exist in many communities, membership is generally inexpensive, and a wide variety of exercise opportunities are available, ranging from aerobic dance and weight training to jogging and racquet sports.

Free or inexpensive exercise facilities may be available at high schools, community colleges, and universities that have indoor pools and indoor jogging tracks. Some shopping malls allow community members to walk in the mall for exercise early in the morning before the stores open.

EXERCISE CONSIDERATIONS FOR DIABETIC PATIENTS

Exercise and Type 1 Diabetes

Persons with Type 1 (insulin-dependent) diabetes are susceptible to hypoglycemia during and immediately after exercise because the liver fails to release glucose at a rate commensurate with its use. Exercise can thus result in unacceptable swings in plasma glucose levels. Because glycemic control varies widely among individuals with Type 1 dia-

BOX 8-1 Guidelines for Avoiding Hypoglycemia During and After Exercise

- Consume 15 to 30 g carbohydrate for every 30 minutes of moderate-intensity exercise.
  1½ slices of bread = 18 g
  ¾ cup whole-grain flake cereal = 24 g
  4 small ginger snaps = 22 g
  ¼ cup raisins = 33 g
  11 vanilla wafers = 22 g
  10 saltine crackers = 20 g
  1 can (11.5 oz.) of V8 juice = 15 g
  1 medium apple = 21 g
  1 medium banana = 26.7 g
  1 medium orange = 16 g
- Consume a snack of slowly absorbed carbohydrate after prolonged exercise. Slowly absorbed carbohydrates are referred to as low-glycemic foods. Examples include oatmeal, grapes, most dried beans, pasta, ice cream, tomato soup, orange juice, peanuts, barley, apples, carrots, and rye bread.
- Decrease insulin dose. Intermediate-acting insulin: decrease by 30% to 35% on the day of exercise. Short-acting insulin: omit the dose that precedes exercise. Multiple doses of short-acting insulin: reduce the dose that precedes exercise by 30% to 35% and supplement with recommended carbohydrates. Continuous subcutaneous infusion: eliminate the mealtime bolus or the increment that precedes or immediately follows exercise.
- Avoid exercising the muscle underlying the injection site of short-acting insulin for 1 hour after an injection.
- Avoid exercising in the late evening.

Source: Coyle EF, Coyle E (20), and Clark N (21).

betes, careful monitoring of exercise habits, food intake, and timing of food consumption and insulin injection relative to physical activity is necessary to prevent hypoglycemia (20,21) (Box 8-1).

Although exercise does not enhance glycemic control in persons with Type 1 diabetes, it may decrease CVD risk. Persons with Type 1 diabetes are at two to three times the normal risk for developing CVD (20).

Because people with Type 1 diabetes may suffer from nerve damage in the lower extremities that results in loss of sensation in the feet, special attention should be given to the care of the feet. Proper shoes are essential because weight-bearing exercise places additional stress on the feet. Clients with Type 1 diabetes who are considering an exercise program should seek professional advice on shoe selection. A physician who specializes in sports medicine may also be a good resource.

Exercise and Type 2 Diabetes

Most persons with Type 2 (non-insulin-dependent) diabetes suffer from insulin resistance (ie, a lack of target cell response to insulin). As a result, the hormone cannot adequately perform its function of moving glucose across the cell membrane.

Researchers have shown that exercised muscles are more permeable to glucose, possibly because more glucose transporters are associated with the plasma membrane (22,23). Therefore, exercise increases insulin sensitivity and decreases insulin resistance. As a result, it is often possible for persons with diabetes who use insulin to reduce their dose when they begin an exercise program.

Whether these positive benefits are the result of each individual bout of exercise or are the long-term effect of regular exercise is still unclear. However, Neiman (24) found that regular aerobic exercise reduces insulin requirements by 30% to 50% in patients with Type 1 diabetes and by up to 100% when combined with weight reduction in obese patients with Type 2 diabetes. He suggests that the effects are attributable more to the last exercise bout rather than to a general long-term adaptation to exercise. Consequently, to improve diabetes management, all patients with diabetes should be encouraged to adopt a regular, consistent exercise pattern.

RESOURCES

Books

The ACSM Fitness Book can be ordered from Leisure Press, Box 5076, Champaign, Illinois, 61825-5076, phone: 1-800-747-4457 ($11.95 US, $14.95 Canadian). This book contains complete guidelines for assisting patients in designing a fitness program including both anaerobic and aerobic activities. It includes color photographs of clients using hand-held weights.

Free Weights for Women: A Complete Body Sculpting Program, by Bonnie Berger, EdD. 1984, Miller Press, New York. This book has excellent black and white photographs of women using hand-held weights as well as photographs of a variety of strength and conditioning exercises for abdominal, lower-back, leg, torso, and chest muscles. This book is appropriate for showing men and women how to accurately perform a particular exercise.

Assessment Tools

Medicine and Science in Sports and Exercise. 1997;26(6) Suppl:S1-S205. This supplement contains physical activity questionnaires used in health-related research; however, many of the tools can be used in clinical practice. Assessment tools are included for older adults, youth and the general population.

Strong Women Stay Young, by Miriam E. Nelson, PhD (School of Nutrition Science and Policy, Tufts University) and Sarah Wernick. New York, NY: Bantam Books;1997. This book outlines an exercise program based on extensive scientific research, and offers detailed instructions and practical suggestions for beginning and maintaining a strength training exercise program. Written as a popular book, it offers sound advice on nutrition and exercise while motivating women to become active.

Exercise Organizations

International Dance Exercise Association, 6190 Cornerstone Ct. East, Suite 204, San Diego, CA 92121, phone: 619-535-8979.

Institute for Fitness and Health, P.O. Box 98882, Tacoma, WA 98499, phone: 206-584-4481.

International Physical Fitness Association, 415 W. Court Street, Flint, MI 48503, phone: 810-239-2166.

Jazzercise, Inc., 10702 Zion Drive, Fairfax, VA 22032, phone: 703-503-3030

REFERENCES

1. *Healthy People 2000: National Health Promotion and Disease Prevention Objectives.* Washington, DC: US Department of Health and Human Services, 1990. DHHS (PHS) publication 90-50212.
2. American College of Sports Medicine. The recommended quantity and quality of exercise for developing and maintaining cardiorespiratory and muscular fitness in healthy adults. *Med Sci Sports Exerc.* 1990;22:265-274.
3. Wilmore JH, Costil DL. *Physiology of Sport and Exercise.* Champaign, Ill: Human Kinetics; 1994.
4. Stone MH, Fleck SJ, Triplett NT, Kraemer WJ. Health and performance-related potential of resistance training. *Sports Med.* 1991;11:210-231.
5. Haskell WL, Alderman EL, Fair JM, Maron DJ, Mackey SF, Superko HR, Williams PT, Johnstone IM, Champagne ME, Krauss RM, Farquhar JW. Effects of intensive multiple risk factor reduction on coronary atherosclerosis and clinical cardiac events in men and women with coronary artery disease: the Stanford Coronary Risk Intervention Project (SCRIP). *Circulation.* 1994;89:975-990.
6. Hagberg, JM. Exercise, fitness, and hypertension. In:

Bouchard C, Shephard RJ, Stephens T, Sutton JR, McPherson BD eds. Exercise, *Fitness, and Health.* Champaign, Ill: Human Kinetics; 1990:455-466.

7. Hagberg JM, Seals DB. Exercise training and hypertension. *Acta Med Scand Suppl.* 1986;711:131-136.
8. Seals DB, Hagberg JM. The effect of exercise training on human hypertension: a review. *Med Sci Sports Exerc.* 1984;16:207-215.
9. Tipton CM. Exercise, training, and hypertension. *Exerc Sport Sci Rev.* 1984;12:245-306.
10. Tipton CM. Exercise training and hypertension: an update. *Exerc Sport Sci Rev.* 1991;19:447-505.
11. Kaplan NM, Deveraux RB, Miller HS. Systemic hypertension. *Med Sci Sports Exerc.* 1994;26(Suppl);S268-S270.
12. Somers VK, Conway J, Johnston J, Sleight P. Effects of endurance training on baroreflex sensitivity and blood pressure in borderline hypertension. *Lancet.* 1991;337:1363-1368.
13. Kelley G, Tran ZV. Aerobic exercise and normotensive adults: a meta-analysis. *Med Sci Sports Exerc.* 1995;27:1371-1377.
14. Young DR, Sharp DS, Curb JD. Associations among baseline physical activity and subsequent cardiovascular risk factors. *Med Sci Sports Exerc.* 1995;27:1646-1654.
15. Shinkai S, Kohno H, Kimura T, Asai H, Inai R, Oka K, Kurokawa Y, Shepard RJ. Physical activity and immune senescence in men. *Med Sci Sports Exerc.* 1995;27:1516-1526.
16. *The ACSM Fitness Book.* Champaign, Ill: Leisure Press; 1992.
17. McArdle WD, Katch FI, Katch VL. *Exercise Physiology: Energy, Nutrition, and Human Performance.* 3rd ed. Media, Penn: Williams and Wilkins; 1991.
18. Pate R, Pratt M, Blair SN, Haskell WL, Macera CA, Bouchard C, Buchner D, Ettinger W, Heath GW, King AC, Kriska A, Leon AS, Marcus BH, Morris J, Paffenbarger RS, Patrick K, Pollock ML, Rippe JM, Sallis J, Wilmore JH. Physical activity and public health: a recommendation from the Centers for Disease Control and Prevention and the American College of Sports Medicine, a special communication. *JAMA.* 1995;273: 402.
19. Vitug A, Schneider, SH, Ruderman NB. Exercise and Type 1 diabetes mellitus. *Exerc Sport Sci Rev.* 1988;16:285-304.
20. Coyle EF, Coyle E. Carbohydrates that speed recovery from training. *Physician Sportsmed.* 1993;21:111-123.
21. Clark N. Carbohydrates: The complexities of a simple food. *Physician Sportsmed.* 1993;21:49-55.
22. Horton ES. Exercise and diabetes mellitus. *Med Clin North Am.* 1988;72:1301-1321.
23. Ekoe JM. Overview of diabetes mellitus and exercise. *Med Sci Sport Exerc.* 1989;21:353-355.
24. Neiman DC. Physical activity, diabetes, and cancer. In: *Medicine: a Health-Related Approach.* 3rd ed. Palo Alto, CA: Bull Publishing; 1995.

CHAPTER 9

EXERCISE IN A CARDIAC REHABILITATION SETTING

DONNA LOUIE, RN, BSN; AND ROBIN WEDELL, RN, BSN

The US Public Health Service defines cardiac rehabilitation (CR) services as

> comprehensive, long-term programs involving medical evaluation, prescribed exercise, cardiac risk factor modification, [and] education and counseling for individuals with coronary artery disease and congestive heart failure. The programs are designed to limit the physiologic and psychological effects of cardiac illness, reduce the risk for sudden death or reinfarction, control cardiac symptoms, stabilize or reverse the atherosclerotic process, and enhance the psychosocial and vocational status of selected patients. (1)

In a CR program, individuals assume responsibility for their health and wellness through management of their chronic disease. Elements of a comprehensive CR program include the exploration of risk factors, the development of goals that are mutually agreed on by patient and care providers, and the establishment of a mutually acceptable plan to achieve these goals. Participation in a CR program is an opportunity for patients to move beyond cognitive understanding of their risk factors and to change their behavior. It is to be hoped that entry into a CR program marks the beginning of a positive, supportive experience in health maintenance and lifestyle change.

CR uses a multifactorial approach to reduce the risk of heart disease progression, incorporating strategies aimed at achieving the following goals:

- nonsmoker status,
- total cholesterol level less than 200 mg/dL,
- low-density lipoprotein cholesterol (LDL-C) level less than 100 mg/dL (less than 130 mg/dL for individuals without cardiovascular disease [CVD]),
- high-density lipoprotein cholesterol (HDL-C) level greater than 35 mg/dL,
- triglyceride level less than 140 mg/dL,
- blood pressure level below 140/90 mm Hg,
- optimal control of diabetes,
- regular exercise three to five times per week in target heart range,
- maintenance of optimal body weight and body-fat percentage, and
- use of stress-management techniques (2).

This chapter focuses on the exercise component of a CR program. See Chapter 8 for further discussion of the effect of exercise on cardiovascular health and general guidance on promoting a healthful lifestyle through exercise.

ROLE OF EXERCISE IN CARDIAC REHABILITATION

Exercise has traditionally been a cornerstone of CR programs. A sedentary lifestyle is a major risk factor for developing CVD, comparable with other important risk factors such as elevated blood cholesterol, cigarette smoking, and hypertension (3). Fitness level and mortality are inversely related; in general, fitter individuals develop less CVD or develop it later in life (3). Exercise is also helpful in the management of diabetes mellitus, hypertension, dyslipidemias, and obesity.

Proper exercise protects against the development or progression of CVD by improving the coronary risk profile. When combined with other risk factor interventions, exercise improves survival (3). Specific physiological benefits derived from exercise include lower blood pressure, higher HDL-C levels, lower triglyceride levels, enhanced weight reduction and weight maintenance, improved glucose tolerance, decreased platelet aggregation, and improved endothelial function (3). Positive psychosocial effects include reduced depression and anxiety.

Exercise for cardiac patients is not without risk. Physical activity can result in serious cardiovascular complications that might not be apparent at rest. In the interest of safety, specific exercise and risk-reduction guidelines for patients with CVD must be established and explained.

Exercise can be safe and beneficial when these guidelines are followed. Comments such as "Just take it easy" and "You are okay now, you don't have to baby yourself" can be misinterpreted by patients and families and provide no meaningful guidance on safe exercise levels.

The development of an appropriate exercise prescription for a CVD patient includes a thorough assessment of the patient's medical history, health status (including symptoms of angina and arrhythmias), personal beliefs, behavioral characteristics, medications, age, work situation, and response to the exercise stress test (3,4). All participants, especially those who have never valued or understood the importance of exercise in maintaining and promoting health, must be educated about the preventive and physiological benefits of therapeutic physical activity.

PHYSIOLOGICAL BENEFITS OF EXERCISE FOR THE CVD PATIENT

Chronic exercise of appropriate intensity, duration, frequency, and mode increases the maximum amount of oxygen that the body can use. Peripheral changes in the ability of skeletal muscle to extract and use oxygen efficiently contribute significantly to this increase. These changes include increased oxidative enzyme concentrations, capillary density, myoglobin concentration, and muscle fiber adaptations (3). Increased stroke volume and reduction in sympathetic tone are other possible mechanisms by which chronic exercise lowers the risk of sudden cardiac death (3).

The increased efficiency of the cardiovascular system that results from proper exercise training in turn results in a lower heart-rate response to submaximal activities, which allows for longer filling time of the coronary arteries and increased coronary blood flow. Although the potential exists for the development of stimulation of the coronary collateral circulation, this has not been substantiated (3).

Increasing the amount of work that can be maximally performed is not relevant for most individuals with heart disease. However, this increase translates into the ability to do more work at submaximal levels at a lower heart rate and blood pressure level and with less risk of arrhythmia (3). Patients can do more physical activity at a lower cardiovascular cost and can perform more activities of daily life without fatigue or angina.

TYPES OF EXERCISE

Most CR activities include combinations of three types of exercise: isometric, isotonic, and resistive (3). CR professionals can help patients to analyze their leisure and vocational activities and guide them in avoiding, adapting, or integrating activities appropriately according to their exercise tolerance.

Isometric or static exercises are movements that require muscle contraction without movement. The load placed on the cardiovascular system by this type of exercise is thought not to be helpful or protective. Isometric exercise causes vasoconstriction, raising blood pressure (3,4) and creating an abrupt strain on the heart. An example of isometric activity is straining to hold a heavy load, such as a garbage can. Patients with poor exercise tolerance may need to be counseled to avoid carrying such loads and to develop an alternative system such as pulling the load on wheels.

Isotonic exercises (also called dynamic or aerobic exercises) are movements of muscles at a constant weight. Examples are walking, running, swimming, and bicycling, all of which cause the heart to pump at up to five times its resting volume. Done regularly at the appropriate level, dynamic exercises provide the most benefit for cardiovascular patients (3).

Resistive exercises are movements that have both dynamic and static characteristics, combining both muscle contraction and movement. Examples include the use of free weights, plastic bands, and circuit weight-training equipment that challenges muscles yet permits a smooth, full range of motion. For years cardiac patients were advised to avoid resistive exercises because of the risk of arrhythmia and the fear of an exaggerated blood pressure response. However, resistive exercise has been found to be safe and effective for increasing strength in selected cardiac patients and is an important addition to the aerobic component of an exercise program (5).

The cardiovascular response to weight lifting is related to the intensity of the muscle contraction, the size of the muscle group, and the duration of the contraction. Using the leg muscles to the point of fatigue for 1 minute creates a larger blood pressure response than using the arm muscles to the point of fatigue for the same amount of time. Strength training results in thickening of connective tissue and hypertrophy of skeletal muscle fibers. Benefits to the cardiac patient include an increase in muscle strength and a resultant decrease in heart rate and blood pressure response to submaximal work loads, which affect response to activities of daily life. Activities with a resistive component such as gardening, pruning, and vacuuming can be done at a lower cardiovascular cost (3).

To understand the significance of exercise guidelines and precautions, CR patients must first have a basic understanding of the body's response to exercise. A normal response includes an increase in cardiac output, which is caused by increases in both heart rate and stroke volume. During exercise, blood shifts away from the organs to the working muscles. Blood pressure and heart rate rise to meet the body's increased need for oxygen. The heart-rate response is higher for aerobic or dynamic exercise than for static or resistive exercise. Systolic blood pressure normally increases. A drop or no increase in systolic blood pressure with exercise is a significant abnormality that may reflect aortic stenosis, left ventricular dysfunction, myocardial ischemia, or inadequate peripheral resistance. Diastolic blood pressure may decrease, increase, or remain unchanged with exercise. Approximately 6 minutes after cessation of exercise, systolic blood pressure should return to normal or to slightly lower than its preexercise level, and it may remain at that level for several hours (3).

GUIDELINES FOR AN OPTIMALLY EFFECTIVE EXERCISE PROGRAM

The amount of physical activity needed to reduce the risk of disease is much less than is needed to attain a high level of fitness (6). Sedentary individuals can favorably affect their risk profile by increasing their activity by as little as 10 minutes of walking three times daily. However, individuals should be encouraged to strive for an activity level that increases fitness in addition to decreasing the risk of disease.

The key to a good exercise program is the selection of activities that an individual enjoys and will do often enough and at a sufficient duration and intensity to produce a training effect (4). The frequency, intensity, and duration of the exercise program can be modified to meet an individual's goals, needs, and health status. A minimum of 700 kcal/week of physical activity is recommended for improving cardiovascular fitness. For most cardiac patients to obtain the benefits discussed, a goal of 1,000 kcal/week of physical training is suggested. Expending 2,000 kcal/week can promote maximal health benefits and maximal reduction in mortality and morbidity (4), which translates to a goal of an expenditure of 300 kcal/day. Achieving this goal can be especially challenging for working people who have CVD.

To optimize fitness, a comprehensive exercise program incorporates activities that promote aerobic conditioning (the most important component), muscular strength and endurance, and flexibility. Guidelines for an optimally effective exercise program are summarized in Box 9-1. The components of aerobic conditioning — intensity, duration, frequency, mode, progression, and maintenance — are described below (4).

Intensity

The *intensity* of an activity is defined as the amount of energy required to perform the activity relative to the maximum amount of energy that can be provided aerobically. This amount is expressed as a percentage of $V0_2$ max, the maximum amount of oxygen that the body can use. Individuals can monitor their intensity objectively by comparing their heart rate during exercise with their target heart rate and subjectively by perceiving how tired or breathless they are as a result of their exertion (3).

Ideally, exercise intensity for cardiac patients is based on a maximal symptom-limited exercise stress test that is designed to elicit cardiovascular abnormalities. The result of the stress test can be used to calculate a target heart rate by the heart-rate reserve method by using the Karvonen equation (7).

Target heart rate = % of heart-rate reserve × (Max heart rate – Resting heart rate) + Resting heart rate

For most cardiac patients, a moderate level of intensity (60% to 80% of the heart-rate reserve) will provide the benefits of exercise at a low risk of cardiovascular and musculoskeletal complications (4). This level of intensity can be achieved with activities such as walking and bicycling. An

BOX 9-1 **Guidelines for an Optimally Effective Exercise Program**

Frequency: 3-5 times/week
Intensity: Rate of perceived exertion (RPE) should be 13-14 (on Borg scale)
Target heart range (THR) should be 60-80% of maximum heart rate
Time: 5-10 min warm-up
20-40 min in THR
5-10 min cool-down
Type: Use of large muscle groups in a rhythmic, repetitive motion, ie, walking, biking, swimming, jogging, or rowing

PATIENT GOALS:

____

____

____

____

____

____

optimal percentage of heart-rate reserve or exact intensity threshold for improving health and fitness has not yet been established. However, exercise at 35% to 40% of maximal effort can still be beneficial as long as the frequency and duration of the activity are increased (3).

Lower-intensity exercise is often recommended for individuals who are beginning an exercise program at a low fitness level or who have complicating medical conditions. In sedentary people with a low level of fitness, fitness improves with intensities of 50% to 60%. If there are no complications, intensity can gradually be increased to 60% to 80% as an individual's endurance increases. At intensities of 85% to 90%, the anaerobic system provides much of the required energy; resulting fatigue and lactic acid accumulation can reduce exercise duration to less than 15 to 20 minutes. Thus, a 60% to 80% intensity level may be optimal. For individuals not able to achieve this intensity, increased frequency and a gradual increase in duration may be necessary (3,8).

During exercise, participants should achieve a level of exertion that feels challenging. They should feel their heart rate increase and their breathing become deeper but they should not feel unusually short of breath or have symptoms of angina. The Borg scale is widely used as a tool to quantify participants' perception of their rate of exertion (9) (Figure 9-1). This scale ranges from a low of 6 (sitting in a chair) to a high of 20 (maximal effort). A rate of perceived exertion (RPE) of less than 12 is considered light exertion, approximately equivalent to 40% to 60% of maximal capacity. An RPE of 12 to 13 represents moderate exertion, equivalent to about 60% to 75% of maximal capacity. At an RPE of 13, participants should experience slightly labored breathing but still be able to talk comfortably. A range of 12 to 13 RPE is a good general goal for the cardiac patient. An RPE of 14 to 16, which is considered high exertion, is roughly equivalent to 75% to 90% of maximal capacity (3). Once patients perceive the effort that is associated with various exercise intensities, they may have a better understanding of how intensely they should exercise.

FIGURE 9-1

Perceived Exertion Scale (Borg Scale)

6	
7	Extremely light
8	
9	Very light
10	
11	Fairly light
12	
13	Somewhat hard
14	
15	Hard
16	
17	Very Hard
18	
19	Extremely hard
20	

Duration

An optimal exercise program has four phases: warm-up (5 to 10 minutes), aerobic (20 to 60 minutes), resistive (10 to 15 minutes), and cool-down (5 to 10 minutes). The warm-up phase is important for the cardiac patient because it allows the body to increase heart rate and metabolism gradually. Without an adequate warm-up, the patient is at higher risk for cardiac complications such as angina, arrhythmias, fatigue, and sudden cardiac death. Patients must be educated about the importance of performing this critical phase of their exercise session. The cardiovascular warm-up may include range of motion exercises, slow walking, and light-tension bicycling. Circumstances such as cold weather, a recent meal, or low functional capacity dictate a longer warm-up.

The aerobic phase generally follows the warm-up (4). Selecting a variety of aerobic exercises allows for a cross-training effect and may enhance patient compliance.

The resistive training phase can be initiated with individuals who have stable CVD at 4 to 6 weeks after an event. A resistive training program should include 8 to 10 exercises that strengthen the arms, shoulders, chest, abdomen, back, hips, and legs. Box 9-2 lists instructions on resistive training for patients in the CR setting.

The cool-down phase is similar in intensity to the warm-up phase. It usually consists of walking casually and performing standing stretches, followed by floor exercises consisting of stretching and relaxation.

Frequency

To best achieve cardiovascular benefits, aerobic exercise should be performed on a minimum of three nonconsecutive days per week. At intensities of less than 60%, however, exercise should be performed more frequently.

Mode

Activities that rhythmically relax and contract the large muscle groups for prolonged periods of time are best for increasing endurance. Light to moderate activities include walking, cycling, and swimming. Activities characterized by a higher level of exertion include cross-country skiing, jogging, stair-step aerobics, dancing, and rowing. Personal preference, preexisting level of fitness, and orthopedic considerations need to be taken into account in choosing an activity.

The principle of specificity is useful to remember in helping a patient to develop an exercise program. Muscular strength and endurance are achieved in the specific muscles that are trained. If a patient's goal is to achieve a level of fitness and endurance that would make it possible to explore the cities of Europe on foot, a walking, treadmill, or stair-step program would be more relevant than a bicycling and swimming program. Alternatively, a water aerobics program may be more appropriate for a person with back problems and arthritis. Individuals with peripheral vascular disease generally benefit more from weight-bearing exercise. For example, walking helps to improve endurance and reduce the symptoms of peripheral vascular disease.

Progression

Progression depends on baseline functional capacity, health, and motivation. The American College of Sports Medicine's *Guidelines for Exercise Testing and Prescription* breaks progression into three stages: initial conditioning, improvement, and maintenance (4).

To reduce the potential for soreness, discomfort, and injury and to build confidence, the initial conditioning stage should begin at 11 to 12 on the Borg scale, an intensity that is approximately equivalent to 40% to 60% of heart-rate reserve. This level of intensity is maintained as duration is increased to 20 to 30 minutes of continuous activity. This prescription usually lasts for the first 4 to 6 weeks of a new exercise program.

In the improvement stage, intensity increases to 60% to 80% of heart-rate reserve and duration is greater than 20 minutes. Clinically, patients are ready to increase intensity when they are symptom-free, when their RPE is less than 13 on the Borg scale, and when their level of intensity is below their goal of 80% of target heart rate (3).

Maintenance

The maintenance phase usually occurs after about 6 months of rehabilitation. At this point the intensity of physical activity has generally reached a plateau. In the maintenance phase, the emphasis shifts from increasing exercise capacity to maintaining new lifestyle habits. After 3 to 4 months of exercise, patients have learned to self-monitor their activity and appreciate the benefits of CR. Many patients are motivated to maintain lifestyle changes once they observe favorable changes in their risk factor profile, such as an improved blood lipid profile and lower blood pressure, and when they realize that they have more energy and that their clothes fit better.

For some people exercising in a group setting is the only way to stay disciplined, whereas for others an individual exercise program works best. Most importantly, individuals need to feel confident in their self-monitoring skills, exercise prescription, and risk-factor modification regime so that they can take responsibility for their health (4).

INITIAL PATIENT EVALUATION

Most cardiac patients can benefit from participation in a CR program. Box 9-3 summarizes the medical conditions for which CR is appropriate and those that would preclude participation in a CR program. All patients are referred to a CR program by a physician. The initial patient evaluation has three components: reviewing the medical history, identifying learning needs, and establishing risk-factor goals.

Reviewing Medical History

Before participating in an exercise program, all persons with CVD should be carefully evaluated for risk of a future clinical coronary event. Such an evaluation includes assessment of functional capacity, left ventricular function, myocardial blood flow, arrhythmias, pulmonary function, musculoskeletal function, and psychological and social support.

Functional Capacity. Functional capacity is a measure of a patient's ability to perform work. It can be measured with a maximal stress test (on either a bicycle or a treadmill), which starts at a low level and gradually increases to the individual's maximal effort. Functional capacity is measured in METs, the patient's metabolic equivalent (1 MET equals 3.5 ml O_2 consumed per kg of body weight per minute). As functional capacity increases, an individual can achieve more METs before becoming fatigued or experiencing cardiovascular symptoms. Normal functional capacity for adults at their maximal exercise capacity is 7 to 10 METs (8).

BOX 9-2 Instructions for Patients on Resistive Training in the CR Setting

To maximize the safety and effectiveness of an exercise program, participants should be taught to

- hold the weights loosely (gripping can create an exaggerated rise in blood pressure);
- take the contraction through the full range of motion for a slow count of 5 in a smooth, controlled, rhythmic fashion;
- exhale during the contraction and breathe throughout the movement;
- perform 1 set of 10-15 repetitions to moderate fatigue, releasing muscle tension between repetitions to allow for blood flow;
- perform exercises on 2-3 nonconsecutive days per week; and
- increase repetitions when the rate of perceived exertion decreases and the participant feels able to perform more repetitions without unusual fatigue.

BOX 9-3 **Indications and Contraindications for Cardiac Rehabilitation**

Individuals with the following conditions are typically candidates for CR services:

- Myocardial infarction
- Coronary artery bypass surgery
- Angioplasty
- Residual ischemia
- Heart failure
- Arrhythmias
- Dilated cardiomyopathy
- Nonischemic heart disease
- Concomitant pulmonary disease
- Pacemaker or implantable cardioverter defibrillator
- Heart valve repair or replacement
- Aneurysm resection
- Organ transplantation
- Other chronic diseases
- Complex medical problems

The following medical conditions are contraindications to participation in a CR program:

- Unstable angina
- Resting systolic blood pressure greater than 200 mm/Hg or resting diastolic BP greater than 110 mm/Hg
- Significant drop (greater than 20 mm/Hg) in resting systolic blood pressure from patient's average level that is unexplained by medications
- Moderate to severe aortic stenosis
- Acute systemic illness or fever
- Uncontrolled atrial or ventricular arrhythmias
- Uncontrolled tachycardia (greater than 100 bpm)
- Symptoms of congestive heart failure
- Third-degree heart block without pacemaker
- Active pericarditis or myocarditis
- Recent embolism
- Thrombophlebitis
- Resting ST displacement (greater than 3 mm)
- Uncontrolled diabetes
- Orthopedic conditions that prohibit exercise

A patient with a functional capacity of 6 METs or greater 3 weeks or more after a clinical coronary event is considered to be at low risk for recurrence of the clinical event. Such a patient can begin an exercise program at 60% to 70% of maximal functional capacity as measured on the exercise test. A capacity of less than 5 METs is considered to be a moderate level of risk (9).

Patients with a low functional capacity or poor exercise tolerance caused by medical problems or deconditioning should exercise at 40% to 60% of their heart rate reserve. The focus should be on increasing duration gradually to improve endurance. Patients may need to begin with 10-minute walking sessions once or twice daily, progressing to 20 to 40 minutes per session as the patients' tolerance increases. At this point, they can begin to increase their intensity to 60% to 80% (see Intensity, above).

Left Ventricular Function. Left ventricular function is evaluated by the ejection fraction, a measure of the heart's ability to pump blood at rest and during exercise. A normal ejection fraction for a cardiac patient is 58% to 70% (10). After a heart attack, it is not uncommon for the heart to have a decreased ability to effectively pump blood when demand is increased, as occurs with exercise.

An ejection fraction of 50% or greater indicates no significant left ventricular dysfunction. An ejection fraction of 31% to 49% indicates mild to moderately depressed left ventricular function that correlates to moderate risk. An ejection fraction of less than 30% indicates high risk (5). Individuals with a low ejection fraction can benefit from exercise but are at higher risk for cardiovascular complications. It is important to evaluate these patients' performance in a treadmill test. The following factors should be evaluated:

- presence of a normal heart rate and blood pressure response,
- presence of symptoms,
- MET level achieved,
- observation of arrhythmias or ischemic changes,
- level of exertion that produces shortness of breath,
- history of congestive heart failure, and
- medication use.

Patients with a low ejection fraction may be placed on angiotensin-converting enzyme inhibitors, diuretics, digoxin, or vasodilators to enhance cardiovascular performance. Such patients generally demonstrate a low functional capacity. An exercise prescription in which intensity of activity remains low and exercise duration is gradually increased (see Intensity, above) is most appropriate for such patients.

The target heart rate for this high-risk population is usually set at 10 beats per minute below the level at which any abnormality occurred on the treadmill test. Other precautions include instructing patients to take medications 30 minutes to 1 hour before exercising, avoiding large meals before exercising, and drinking adequate fluids to avoid hypotension. Weight is also monitored three to five times a week to assess heart-failure progression. Sudden weight gain, shortness of breath at rest or with minimal exertion, peripheral edema, and increasing fatigue are all symptoms of worsening heart failure. To prevent unnecessary hospitalizations and enhance quality of life, individuals must learn to identify these early warning signs of congestive heart failure (8).

Myocardial Ischemia. *Ischemia* is defined as an imbalance between the supply of and demand for blood flow to the heart muscle. Ischemia can manifest as angina pectoris, ST-T wave abnormalities on electrocardiograms (ECGs), arrhythmias, or left ventricular dysfunction. It can be diagnosed by treadmill testing and characterized by imaging techniques such as Cardiolyte, thallium scans, and echocardiography, which evaluate left ventricular function and coronary artery blood flow to the heart (10).

A patient who has no resting or exercise-induced myocardial ischemia manifested as angina or ST-segment displacement during a treadmill test is considered low risk. A patient who has exercise-induced ST-segment depression of 1-2 mm or abnormalities of blood flow on nuclear stress testing is considered moderate risk. A high-risk patient has severe CVD and marked (greater than 2 mm) exercise-induced ST-segment depression (5).

The patient's anginal pattern (ie, onset, description, frequency, duration, intensity, and triggers), medications, and treatment plan must be reviewed to establish a baseline and ensure a safe exercise prescription. The baseline helps the patient to identify and report to the physician any changes in anginal pattern.

Before patients undergo a treadmill test, the clinician needs to know whether and according to what schedule they take any medications that affect heart rate (eg, digoxin, beta blockers, and calcium channel blockers). Changes in medication can affect the heart rate response to exercise, necessitating a change in the target heart rate.

The patient must be able to exercise within a target heart rate range that is sufficiently challenging but is below the threshold for angina or ischemia. Measures that maximize the safety of exercise and activities of daily life include timing medications, avoiding exercise in extreme temperatures, avoiding large meals, using prophylactic nitroglycerin before exertion, pacing activities, using stress-management techniques, and adopting a blood-cholesterol-lowering diet.

Arrhythmias. Arrhythmias are generally not a significant risk for cardiac patients unless there is a family history of sudden death or a personal history of cardiomyopathy, valvular heart disease, or severe ischemia (3). Exercise can both induce and suppress arrhythmias. Diuretics, digitalis therapy, and recent ingestion of alcohol or caffeine can also induce arrhythmias. Exercise-induced arrhythmias may be generated by enhanced sympathetic tone, increased myocardial oxygen demand, or both. The immediate postexercise period is particularly dangerous because of the high catecholamine levels associated with generalized vasodilation (3). A patient at low risk has no resting or exercise-induced complex arrhythmias, such as three sequential ventricular ectopics in a row, whereas a high-risk patient has complex ventricular arrhythmias at rest or with exercise (5).

The presence and severity of arrhythmias can be determined by patient history, treadmill test, electrophysiologic studies, and ECG testing. It is important to identify the type of arrhythmia, associated symptoms, frequency of occurrence, and the treatment plan. The treatment plan should be confirmed with the patient's physician before an exercise program is started.

Antiarrhythmic agents can effectively suppress or control arrhythmias. However, it is important to differentiate among the possible underlying causes of arrhythmias, which can be related to ischemia, congestive heart failure, or use of stimulants. The treatment depends on the underlying cause of the arrhythmia.

A patient who is at high risk for symptomatic, complex ventricular arrhythmias is an appropriate candidate for continuous telemetry during CR. Telemetry is important for close monitoring in the early phases of CR. Otherwise, patients can be intermittently monitored using Defibrillator LifePak paddles, which allow for a quick and easy evaluation of both symptomatic and asymptomatic patients. ECG rhythm strips are generally obtained before the patient starts exercise to establish a baseline rhythm and are used again during exercise as needed.

Pulmonary Function. A pulmonary history should be taken to evaluate the patient for asthma, bronchitis, emphysema, and other problems. Factors that cause or exacerbate these conditions, such as allergies, bronchospasm, and infection, should be identified and options for the medical management of pulmonary problems should be explored.

TABLE 9-1

Risk Factor Analysis Form

	Normal Values	Your Values
Inhaled Tobacco	0	______________
Blood Pressure	< 140/90 mm Hg	______________
Serum Cholesterol	< 200 mg/dL	______________
HDL-C	> 35 mg/dL	______________
LDL-C	< 100 mg/dL	______________
Triglycerides	< 140 mg/dL	______________
Fasting Blood Sugar	70-120 mg/dL	______________
Level of Fitness (MET level)	______________	______________
Body Composition	Desirable % body fat ________	______________%
	Desirable weight __________	______________
Stress		

Education of patients should emphasize the importance of self-monitoring skills in helping to maximize exercise performance in conjunction with a pulmonary condition.

Factors that contribute to the worsening of a pulmonary problem include cold weather, allergens, stress, infection, medication misuse, exercise, and smoking. Appropriate strategies to minimize the effects of these factors should be discussed with patients. Suggested strategies include:

- consumption of adequate fluids and water to keep the cilia and mucosa in the upper airway moist to reduce coughing and infection;
- proper regular use of inhalers, including prophylactic use to avoid an asthmatic episode;
- avoidance of exercise in cold weather;
- use of precautions to prevent infection such as washing hands, avoiding exposure to illness, and using a peak expiratory flow meter to evaluate breathing capacity;
- use of techniques such as purse-lip breathing and diaphragmatic breathing and relaxation techniques to minimize breathing difficulties, especially in stressful situations; and
- smoking cessation and avoidance of secondhand smoke and other known allergens (8, 11).

Exercise programs for patients with poor pulmonary function should emphasize frequent, short (5 to 10 minutes) periods of low-intensity exercise that slowly increase in duration. These patients will benefit from the use of a pulse oximeter to monitor the oxygen saturation of their blood during exercise (8).

Musculoskeletal Function. Assessing orthopedic limitations can help to prevent the worsening of an existing problem and to maximize the safety of exercise. Orthopedic limitations can affect balance and flexibility as well as ability to perform some aerobic exercises. Activities should be chosen that accommodate any musculoskeletal limitations.

For patients who are recovering from a coronary artery bypass graft, surgical incisions may be a limiting factor. Chest and leg wounds take 6 to 8 weeks to heal. Upper-body exercises that cause sternal tension should be avoided until healing is complete. Following the 6-to-8-week postoperative period, full range-of-motion exercises can be incorporated and resistive exercises using hand weights of 1 to 5 pounds can be added.

Individuals who walk with a cane should use equipment that maintains balance, such as a stationary bicycle, a treadmill with arm rails, or a rowing machine. Some individuals, such as those who find it difficult to get up from and down to the floor, can perform warm-up and cool-down exercises while sitting in a chair. For example, a woman with polio can sit in a chair for the warm-up and cool-down periods and use the stationary bicycle during the aerobic period.

Psychosocial Issues. Patients' perception and understanding of their cardiovascular condition and the level of social support available to them are important factors to assess. Studies show that support from family and friends reduces an individual's morbidity and mortality (1). Fear and depression are common after a heart attack or bypass surgery. Clinicians can validate these feelings and explain that they are generally temporary and will lessen as the patient continues the rehabilitation program. Encouraging patients' family members to attend the initial evaluation often provides emotional support that may strengthen patients' motivation to achieve program goals.

Identifying Learning Needs

Patients participating in a CR program should clearly understand their medical status and the pathophysiology of CVD, know the risk factors that contributed to their CVD, set goals to reduce their risk of future clinical coronary events,

BOX 9-4 **Guidelines for Participation in a Cardiac Rehabilitation Exercise Program**

1. Make a commitment to attend class regularly (schedule other appointments around the time of the class). To improve your endurance, aerobic conditioning must be done at least 3 times a week.
2. Arrive on time for class to get a good warm-up and stay for the cool-down at the end of class. This helps to ensure a safe and optimally effective exercise session.
3. If you have a medical concern, arrive a few minutes early to talk to the nurses about it.
4. Do not eat a meal within 2 hours before class; we do not want your heart to work overtime. (This does not apply to people with diabetes.)
5. Dress in layers according to the weather. Wear loose, comfortable clothing, ie, short-sleeved shirt, tights, thick socks, and supportive athletic shoes.
6. If you have a fever or symptoms of an illness, do not come to class. If you just feel "blah," come to class to be checked out. If you are simply feeling "blue," you should feel better after class.
7. Take your medications at regular times. Taking them late or early can affect your heart's response to exercise.
8. If you feel any unusual symptoms during class (eg, angina, shortness of breath, dizziness, muscle and joint discomfort, loss of balance, or nausea) report them to the nurse and document them on your daily exercise sheet.
9. Tell the nurse if you are unduly tired after class or if you have trouble sleeping at night.
10. Drink plenty of water during the day and bring a water bottle to class.
11. Be patient. It takes time to get into shape and to make lasting changes in your life. Your efforts will be worth it!
12. Count your pulse. There are two primary locations to check your pulse:
    - Your wrist. The radial artery is located at the base of your thumb. It is best felt with two or three fingers of the opposite hand. Do not use your thumb to check your pulse.
    - Your neck. The carotid arteries are large arteries that are located on either side of the windpipe. Use your right hand to check your left carotid pulse and your left hand to check your right carotid pulse. WARNING: Do not press both carotids at the same time! This can cause faintness or irregular heart beat. Also, do not press on the carotid near the jawbone. This can stimulate a sensitive nerve that can cause faintness.

Adapted from and used with the permission of the Cardiac Therapy Foundation of the Mid Peninsula, 655 Arastradero Rd., Palo Alto, CA 94306.

and learn self-monitoring skills that enable them to maintain a safe exercise program.

Important self-monitoring skills include the ability to

- identify angina when it occurs and initiate appropriate treatment;
- use the Borg scale to rate perceived exertion;
- recognize subtle cardiovascular changes such as unusual shortness of breath, increasing fatigue, and decreasing exercise endurance, with and without exercise;
- check weight daily to assess for fluid retention (if a history of congestive heart failure is present);
- understand the meaning and importance of the target heart rate guidelines;
- refrain from exercise when appropriate (ie, during illness or when a change in anginal pattern occurs);
- use available resources to help enhance changes; and
- sustain the motivation to make lifestyle changes.

Appropriate written information can enhance the understanding of both patients and their families. Table 9-1 is a risk-factor analysis form for patients and Box 9-4 is a list of exercise tips for patients in a CR program.

Cardiac rehabilitation has proven to be effective in optimizing patients' emotional, physical, and behavioral responses to the disease process through exercise, risk-factor modification, education, and counseling. Unfortunately, fewer than 30% of candidates use this service. The challenge is to change this pattern and improve the effective delivery of CR services to the individuals who would benefit.

REFERENCES

1. Wenger NK, Froelicher ES, Smith LK, Ades PA, Berra K, Blumenthal JA, Certo CME, Dattilo AM, Davis D, Debusk RF, Drozda JP, Fletcher BJ, Franklin BA, Gaston H, Greenland P, McBride PE, McGregor CGA, Oldridge NB, Piscatella JC, Rogers FJ. *Cardiac Rehabilitation as Secondary Prevention.* Clinical Practice Guideline. Quick Reference Guide for Clinicians, No. 17. Rockville, Md: US Department of Health and Human Services, Public Health Service, Agency for Health Care Policy and Research and National Heart, Lung and Blood Institute; 1995. AHCPR Publication 96-0673.
2. Smith SC, Blair SN, Criqui MH, Fletcher GF, Fuster V, Gersh BJ, Gotto AM. Preventing Heart Attack and Death in Patients with Coronary Disease. *Circulation.* 1995;92:2-4.
3. Scientific Statement, American Heart Association Writing Group: Fletcher GF, Balady G, Froelicher VF, Hartley LH, Haskell WL, Pollock ML. *Exercise Standards: A Statement for Healthcare Professionals From the American Heart Association.* Dallas, Tex: American Heart Association; 1995.
4. American College of Sports Medicine. *ACSM's Guidelines for*

Exercise Testing and Prescription. 5th ed. Baltimore, Md: Williams and Wilkins; 1995.

5. American Association of Cardiovascular and Pulmonary Rehabilitation. *Guidelines for Cardiac Rehabilitation Programs.* 2nd ed. Champaign, Ill: Human Kinetics; 1995.
6. *Healthy People 2000: National Health Promotion and Disease Prevention Objectives.* Washington, DC: US Department of Health and Human Services, 1990. DHHS (PHS) publication 90-50212.
7. Karvonen M, Kental K, Must O. The effects of training on heart rate: a longitudinal study. *Ann Med Exp Biol Fenn.* 1957;35:307-311.
8. Skinner JS. Importance of aging for exercise testing and exercise prescription. In: Skinner JS, ed. *Exercise Testing and Exercise Prescription for Special Cases.* Philadelphia, Penn: Lea and Febiger; 1987:67-74.
9. Borg GA. Psychophysical bases of perceived exertion. *Med Sci Sports Exerc.* 1982;14:377-381.
10. Underhill Motzer SL, Woods SL, Sivarajan Froelicher ES, Halpenny CJ. *Cardiac Nursing.* 3rd ed. Philadelphia, Penn: JB Lippincott Company; 1995.
11. Jones NL, Berman LB, Bartkiewicz PD, Oldridge NB. Chronic obstructive respiratory disorders. In: Skinner JS, ed. *Exercise Testing and Exercise Prescription for Special Cases.* Philadelphia, Penn: Lea and Febiger; 1987:175-186.

CHAPTER 10

Kids and Cholesterol—What Works?

Linda Van Horn, PhD, RD; Niki Gernhofer, MS, RD; and Eileen Peters, MS, RD

In 1992, the National Cholesterol Education Program's (NCEP's) Expert Panel on Blood Cholesterol Levels in Children and Adolescents issued a report that established guidelines for screening, prevention, and treatment of high blood cholesterol in children (1). These guidelines were based on existing evidence from laboratory, clinical, pathological, and epidemiological studies demonstrating that atherosclerosis begins in childhood (2-8). Since then, evidence has accumulated that strengthens the rationale for encouraging a lipid-lowering diet in children to prevent or treat high blood cholesterol levels (9).

The NCEP panel recommended a two-pronged strategy that combines a population approach aimed at optimizing diet and lifestyle behaviors in all children and an individualized approach that targets children and adolescents who are at the greatest risk for developing high blood cholesterol as adults. This chapter summarizes the NCEP guidelines and provides an update on current research on lipids and pediatric diet. Practical advice and suggestions for clinical implementation from both these sources are also provided.

Blood Lipid Levels in American Children

The NCEP report published data from the Lipid Research Clinic Prevalence Study (10). The mean cholesterol and serum triglyceride values by age and sex appear in Tables 10-1 to 10-4. These values influenced the cut points established for determining risk in children (Table 10-5) and continue to guide physicians' decisions regarding treatment. The recommended assessment and treatment schemas are presented in Figures 10-1 to 10-3.

Once it has been established that a child has an elevated total blood cholesterol level (200 mg/dL or higher), a fasting lipoprotein analysis is performed (Figure 10-2). Step I diet therapy is initiated as a preventive measure for all children even if low-density lipoprotein cholesterol (LDL-C) concentrations are below 200 mg/dL. When children are found to be hypercholesterolemic, however, a more deliberate and systematic approach to achieving adherence to the step I diet is taken (Figure 10-2). If the desired lipoprotein response is not achieved after repeated instructions on the step I diet, the step II diet is applied (Figure 10-3). Table 10-6 differentiates the recommended nutrient levels in these two diets; the primary difference between them is that reductions in saturated fat and cholesterol intake are greater in the step II diet.

Population Approach

The population approach is advocated for all American children over the age of 2 years. Specific recommendations include

- achievement of nutritional adequacy by eating a wide variety of foods,
- consumption of energy adequate to support growth and development and reach or maintain desirable body weight, and
- adherence to the step I diet (see Table 10-6).

Children's average daily energy intakes typically range from approximately 1,200 kcal for toddlers to 2,500 kcal for teenagers. This translates to a suggested total fat intake of 40 g/day to 83 g/day (13 g/day to 28 g/day of saturated fat). These values are equivalent to approximately 30% and 10% of energy from total fat and saturated fat, respectively. Table 10-7 summarizes data from the National Health and Nutrition Examination Survey (NHANES III) that illustrate the ranges in energy and relative proportions of fat intake (11). Table 10-8 provides calculated values in grams per day for a full range of energy intakes.

Neither NCEP nor the American Heart Association has yet established specific guidelines for fiber intake in children. The American Health Foundation has recommended the "age plus 5" rule for fiber intake in children ages 2 to 10 (12). This means, for example, a 5-year-old child should eat approximately 5 (age) plus 5 g of fiber every day or 10 g

TABLE 10-1

Serum Total Cholesterol Levels in U.S. Children and Adolescents[a]

Age (years)	n	Overall mean (mg/dL)	Percentiles (mg/dL) 5	10	25	50	75	90	95
Males									
0-4	238	159	117	129	141	156	176	192	209
5-9	1,253	165	125	134	147	164	180	197	209
10-14	2,278	162	123	131	144	160	178	196	208
15-19	1,980	154	116	124	136	150	170	188	203
Females									
0-4	186	161	115	124	143	161	177	195	206
5-9	1,118	169	130	138	150	168	184	201	211
10-14	2,087	164	128	135	148	163	179	196	207
15-19	2,079	162	124	131	144	160	177	197	209

Source: NCEP Report of the Expert Panel on Blood Cholesterol Levels in Children and Adolescents (1).

[a] All values have been converted from plasma to serum. Plasma value x 1.03 = serum value.

TABLE 10-2

Serum LDL-Cholesterol Levels in US Children and Adolescents[a]

Age (years)	n	Overall mean (mg/dL)	Percentiles (mg/dL) 5	10	25	50	75	90	95
White Males									
5-9	131	95	65	71	82	93	106	121	133
10-14	284	99	66	74	83	97	112	126	136
15-19	298	97	64	70	82	96	112	127	134
White Females									
5-9	114	103	70	75	91	101	118	129	144
10-14	244	100	70	75	83	97	113	130	140
15-19	294	99	61	67	80	96	114	133	141

Source: NCEP Report of the Expert Panel on Blood Cholesterol Levels in Children and Adolescents (1).

[a] All values have been converted from plasma to serum. Plasma value x 1.03 = serum value.

Note: The number of children ages 0-4 years who had LDL- and HDL-cholesterol measured was too small to allow calculation of percentiles in this age group. However, the percentiles for total cholesterol (Table 1) for ages 0-4 years and 5-9 years are similar.

TABLE 10-3

Serum HDL-Cholesterol Levels in US Children and Adolescents[a]

Age (years)	n	Overall mean (mg/dL)	Percentiles (mg/dL) 5	10	25	50	75	90	95
White Males									
5-9	142	57	39	43	50	56	65	72	76
10-14	296	57	38	41	47	57	63	73	76
15-19	299	48	31	35	40	47	54	61	65
White Females									
5-9	124	55	37	39	48	54	63	69	75
10-14	247	54	38	41	46	54	60	66	72
15-19	295	54	36	39	44	53	63	70	76

Source: NCEP Report of the Expert Panel on Blood Cholesterol Levels in Children and Adolescents (1).

[a] All values have been converted from plasma to serum. Plasma value x 1.03 = serum value.

Note: The number of children ages 0-4 who had LDL- and HDL-cholesterol measured was too small to allow calculation of percentiles in this age group. However, note that the percentiles for total cholesterol (Table 1) for ages 0-4 and 5-9 are similar.

TABLE 10-4

Serum Triglyceride Levels in US Children and Adolescents [a]

Age (years)	n	Overall mean (mg/dL)	Percentiles (mg/dL) 5	10	25	50	75	90	95
Males									
0-4	238	58	30	34	41	53	69	87	102
5-9	1,253	30	31	34	41	53	67	88	104
10-14	2,278	68	33	38	46	61	80	105	129
15-19	1,980	80	38	44	56	71	94	124	152
Females									
0-4	186	66	35	39	46	61	79	99	115
5-9	1,118	30	33	37	45	57	73	93	108
10-14	2,087	78	38	45	56	72	93	117	135
15-19	2,079	78	40	45	55	70	90	117	136

Source: NCEP Report of the Expert Panel on Blood Cholesterol Levels in Children and Adolescents (1).

[a] All values have been converted from plasma to serum. Plasma value x 1.03 = serum value.

TABLE 10-5

Cut Points of Total and LDL-Cholesterol for Dietary Intervention in Children and Adolescents with a Family History of Hypercholesterolemia or Premature Cardiovascular Disease

Category	Total Cholesterol (mg/dL)	LDL-Cholesterol (mg/dL)	Dietary Intervention
Acceptable	<170	<110	Recommended population eating pattern
Borderline	170-199	110-129	Step I diet prescribed, other risk factor intervention
High	≥ 200	≥130	Step I diet prescribed, then step II diet if necessary

Source: NCEP Report of the Expert Panel on Blood Cholesterol Levels in Children and Adolescents (1).

TABLE 10-6

Characteristics of Step I and Step II Diets for Lowering Blood Cholesterol

Nutrient	Recommended Intake: Step I Diet	Step II Diet
Total fat	Average of no more than 30% of total energy	Same
Saturated fatty acids	Less than 10% of total energy	Less than 7% of total energy
Polyunsaturated fatty acids	Up to 10% of total energy	Same
Monounsaturated fatty acids	Remaining total fat energy	Same
Cholesterol	Less than 300 mg/day	Less than 200 mg/day
Carbohydrates	About 55% of total energy	Same
Protein	About 15%-20% of total energy	Same
Total energy intake	To promote normal growth and development and to reach or maintain desirable body weight	Same

Source: NCEP Report of the Expert Panel on Blood Cholesterol Levels in Children and Adolescents (1).

FIGURE 10-1

Risk assessment

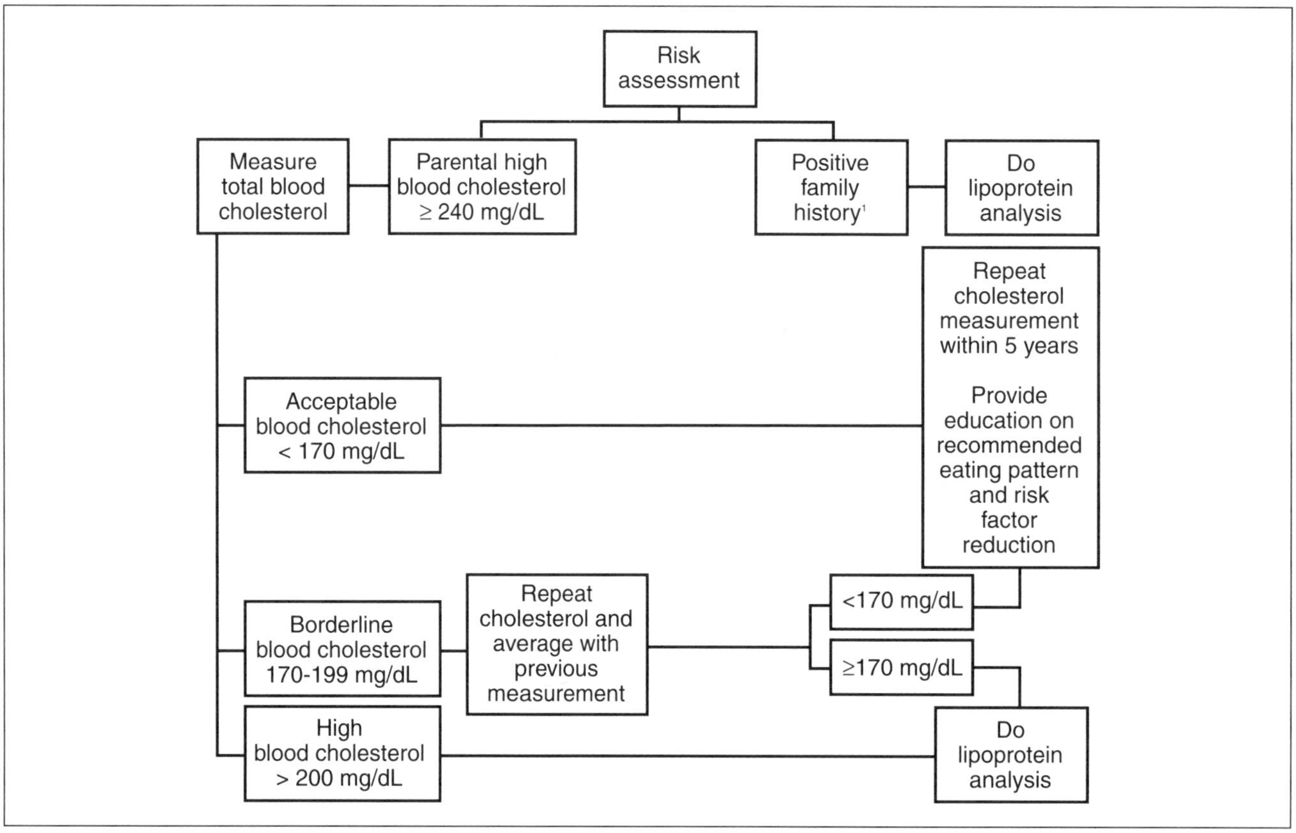

[1] Positive family history is defined as a history of premature (before age 55 years) cardiovascular disease in a parent or grandparent.

Source: National Cholesterol Education Program (NCEP) Report of the Expert Panel on Blood Cholesterol Levels in Children and Adolescents (1).

total. This is easy to accomplish within the recommended step I or step II dietary pattern by emphasizing whole grain cereals, breads, and fruits and vegetables. Once a child's energy intake equals or exceeds that of adults, 25 grams of total dietary fiber should be well tolerated.

Achievement of these population-wide nutrient intake goals requires the support of entities that influence children's eating patterns. These entities include

- schools,
- government agencies,
- the food industry, and
- mass media.

Schools

Because most American schoolchildren consume a significant proportion of their daily food intake at school, schools can serve as a nutrition education laboratory. National school breakfast and lunch programs are now required to provide meals that meet the recommended nutrient levels described earlier. Meal times can introduce students to the nutrient composition, food choices, and preparation techniques that constitute a healthful eating pattern. Dietitians play a vital role in supervising, analyzing, and implementing these nutrition opportunities at the local level. Boxes 10-1 and 10-2 provide examples of appropriate foods for school meal programs.

Since the NCEP report was published in 1992, successful population-based efforts to improve the diets of school children have been reported. The Child and Adolescent Trial on Cardiovascular Health (CATCH) program tested the feasibility of modifying the school lunch program (13-15). CATCH successfully demonstrated reductions in total fat, saturated fat, cholesterol, and sodium consumption by third-grade students. The best results were reported for students who had reinforcement from parents at home as well as nutrition education at school.

CATCH demonstrated that cooperation among school food-service workers, educators, and parents can accomplish adherence to recommended eating patterns. Generalizability of the CATCH results depends on such cooperation. Dietitians can be instrumental in facilitating the coordination of these entities and providing appropriate nutrition education to students and their families.

Another school-based study involved switching children from whole milk to low-fat or skim milk. Whole milk

FIGURE 10-2

Classification, education, and follow-up based on low-density lipoprotein cholesterol

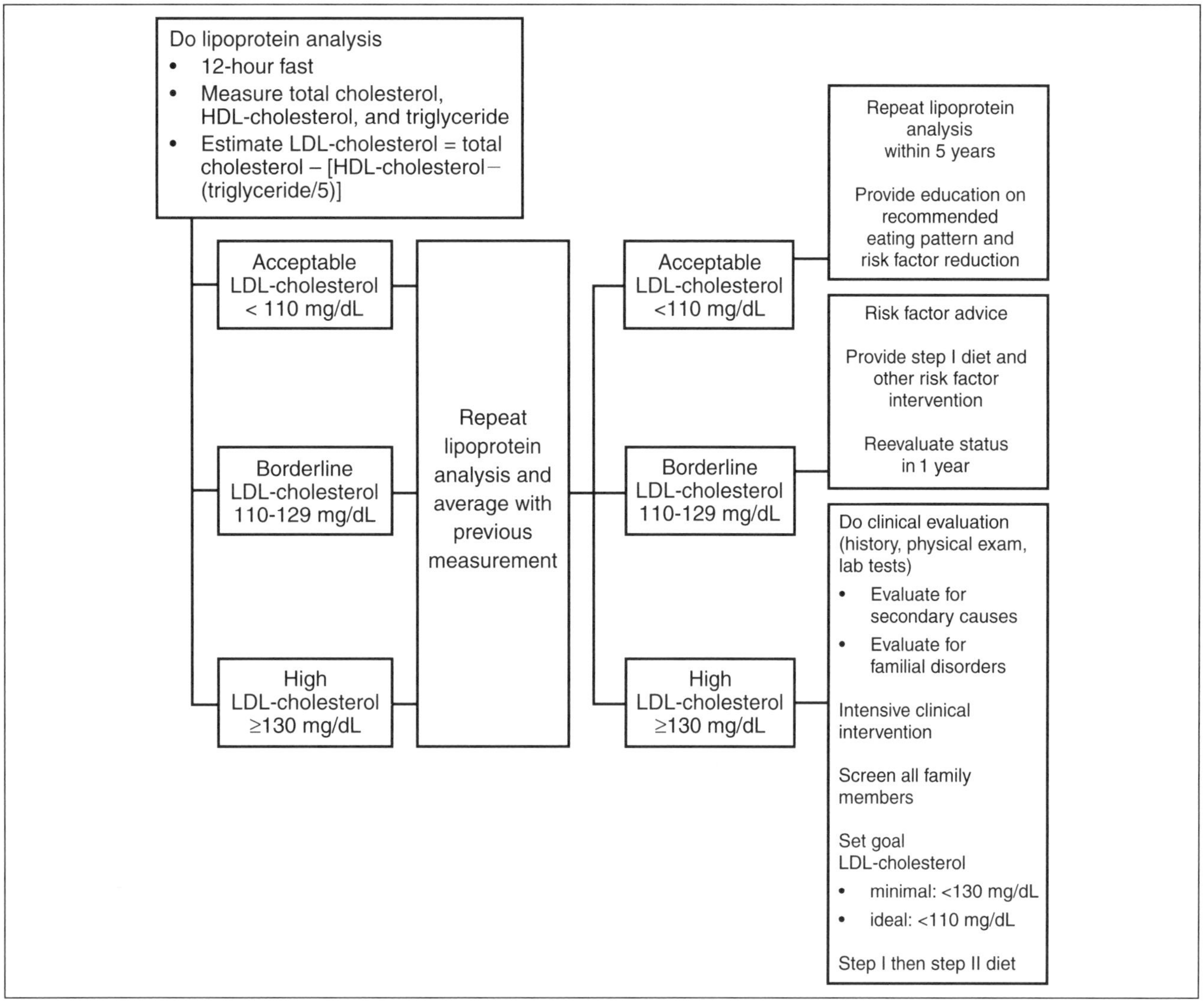

Source: National Cholesterol Education Program (NCEP) Report of the Expert Panel on Blood Cholesterol Levels in Children and Adolescents (1).

is a common source of saturated fat and cholesterol in a child's diet. Such a change requires relatively little nutrition intervention if the concept is marketed in an entertaining way, and it can significantly reduce daily total and saturated fat intake. In one study a live costumed character called Lowfat Lucy the Cow promoted drinking skim milk among schoolchildren (16). Such efforts can have a major impact on the attitudes and behavior of both students and teachers.

Government Agencies

Regulatory policies related to nutrition, nutrition education, and food assistance programs are initiated by government agencies. Perhaps the single most significant contribution of government to improving the country's nutritional status over the past decade was the passage of the Nutrition Labeling and Education Act in 1995. Even among children, standardized, highly specific food labels can facilitate adherence to dietary recommendations concerning consumption of saturated fat. Table 10-8 provides specific fat gram equivalents that correspond to the goal of limiting fat intake to 30% of total energy. This information can help children make food selections that keep fat intake within that range.

Dietitians play an important role in both generating and implementing state and national policies that can affect population-wide nutrition status. As nutrition educators, dietitians can facilitate consumers' ability to make wise decisions at the point of purchase.

Food Industry

The NCEP report encouraged the development of nutritious,

FIGURE 10-3

Diet therapy

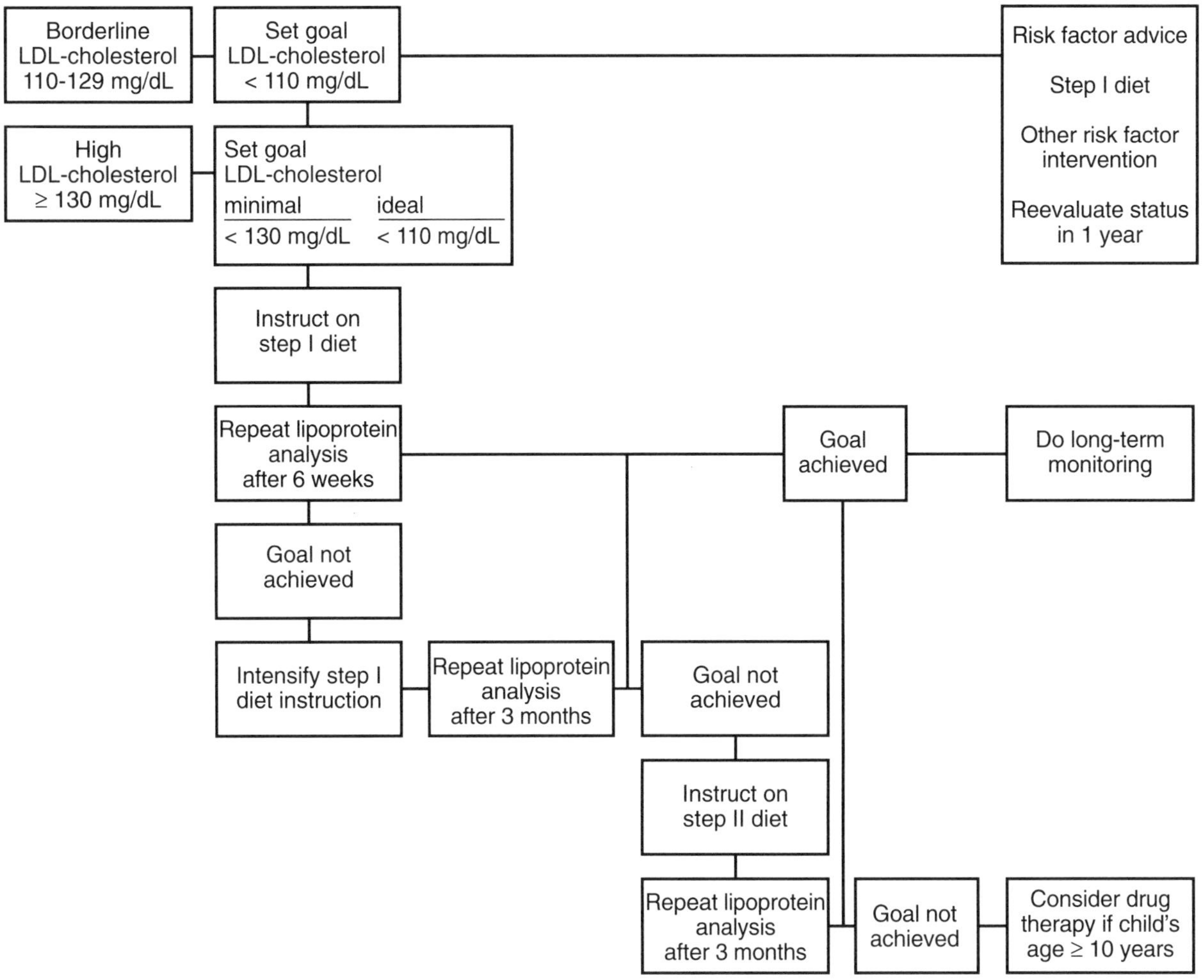

Source: National Cholesterol Education Program (NCEP) Report of the Expert Panel on Blood Cholesterol Levels in Children and Adolescents (1).

TABLE 10-7

Current Mean Energy and Fat Intake by Sex and Age Group: Third National Health and Nutrition Examination Survey (NHANES III)

Age Group	Sample Size		Total Energy (kcal)		Total Fat (% kcal)		Saturated Fat (% kcal)	
	Males	Females	Males	Females	Males	Females	Males	Females
1-2 years	601	630	1339 ± 26.3	1236 ± 26.5	33.5 ± 0.5	34.0 ± 0.5	13.8 ± 0.2	13.9 ± 0.2
3-5 years	744	803	1663 ± 26.5	1516 ± 23.8	32.8 ± 0.4	33.1 ± 0.4	12.6 ± 0.2	12.6 ± 0.2
6-11 years	868	877	2036 ± 44.4	1753 ± 20.4	33.9 ± 0.3	34.2 ± 0.5	12.8 ± 0.2	12.7 ± 0.2
12-15 years	338	373	2578 ± 75.4	1838 ± 48.4	33.1 ± 0.8	33.7 ± 0.7	12.4 ± 0.3	12.0 ± 0.2
16-19 years	368	397	3097 ± 114.4	1958 ± 70.3	34.6 ± 0.7	34.4 ± 0.7	12.6 ± 0.2	12.3 ± 0.4

Source: Morbidity and Mortality Weekly Report 1994;43(7):124-125.

TABLE 10-8

Gram Values to Meet Step I Diet Goals for Different Calorie Levels[a]

	1,200 kcal	1,400 kcal	1,500 kcal	1,800 kcal	2,000 kcal[b]	2,200 kcal	2,500 kcal	2,800 kcal	3,000 kcal
Total fat (g)	40	45	50	60	65	70	80	90	100
Saturated fat (g)	13	15	16	20	20	25	25	30	33
Total carbohydrate (g)	180	210	225	270	300	330	375	420	450
fiber (g)[c]	20-25	20-25	20-25	21-25	25	25	30	30	30
	<300	<300	<300	<300	<300	<300	<300	<300	<300

[a] Numbers may [illegible]nded.

[b] Daily Value on the label for total fat, saturated fat, carbohydrate, dietary fiber, and protein (if listed) is based on a 2,000-kcal reference diet.

[c] American Health Foundation recommends "age plus 5" rule, ie, a 5 year old should eat approximately 5 (age) plus 5 grams or 10 grams of fiber per day.

Reproduced with permission of *Pediatrics* © 1996 (23).

BOX 10-1 **Foods to Provide to Decrease Saturated Fatty Acid and Total Fat Content of School Lunches**

Milk
- Low-fat milk (1%)
- Nonfat milk

Meat and meat alternates
- Lean cuts of meat, such as round steak, round rump roast, round tip roast, and tenderloin roast
- Lean ground beef (85% extra lean) or soy protein added to regular ground beef
- Chicken or turkey without skin, baked, broiled, roasted, or boiled
- Fresh or frozen fish baked, broiled, or poached
- Tuna or salmon
- Cooked dry beans and peas, such as Great Northern, kidney, lima, navy, pinto, red, black, and garbanzo beans, black-eyed peas, lentils, and split peas
- Low-fat and part-nonfat cheeses: farmer, cottage, part-skim ricotta, and mozzarella
- Peanut butter

Bread or bread alternates
- Breads and bread products: bagels, breads, graham crackers, muffins, rolls and pancakes, including whole grain or enriched products
- Noodles, rice, barley, pasta, and bulgur

Fruits and vegetables
- Fresh, frozen, dried, or canned fruits: apricots, cantaloupe, grapefruit, grapes, honeydew melon, peaches, plums, prunes, raisins, tangerines, and strawberries
- Fresh, frozen, or canned fruit juice
- Fresh, frozen, or canned vegetables and salads: broccoli, brussels sprouts, cabbage, carrots, cauliflower, corn, green beans, green peas, green pepper, potatoes, lettuce, okra, spinach, sweet potatoes, tomatoes, winter squash, zucchini

Fats
- Mayonnaise and dressings, including reduced-calorie and modified-fat, light, or low-sodium salad dressings
- Margarine or liquid vegetable oils: canola, corn, cottonseed, olive, peanut, and safflower oils

Other
- Baked goods low in fat: modified cakes and cookies, including angel food cake, fig cookies, ginger snaps, oatmeal cookies, and raisin cookies
- Ice milk, sherbet, low-fat puddings, and low-fat yogurt

Source: NCEP Report of the Expert Panel on Blood Cholesterol Levels in Children and Adolescents (1)

BOX 10-2 **Tips for Reducing Saturated Fatty Acids in Food Preparation and Recipes for School Lunches**

Food preparation

- Prepare beef, pork, chicken, and fish by baking, broiling, roasting, or stewing instead of frying.
- Trim all visible fat from beef and pork before cooking.
- Defat ground meat by cooking meat and then draining off fat.
- Brown meats in pan lightly brushed with oil.
- When preparing stews or soup, start by trimming all visible fat from the meat: when possible, refrigerate the broth and skim off fat with a spoon before reheating and serving.
- Bake or roast meat or meat loaf on a meat rack or on crumpled foil so that the fat can drip off and be discarded.
- Remove skin from chicken before serving.
- Instead of frying fish, try poaching in milk, tomato juice, or water flavored with a little lemon juice, or baking with bread crumb and herb coating.
- When cooking foods such as eggs, French toast, and pancakes, brush the pan with oil just to coat it, or use a nonstick spray made from vegetable oil or a nonstick pan that requires no greasing.

Recipe modifications

- Use low-fat, reduced-fat, or nonfat milk or nonfat dry milk in place of whole milk in recipes.
- In recipes using mayonnaise or sour cream, replace half the mayonnaise or sour cream with nonfat or low-fat plain yogurt.
- Substitute part-nonfat milk cheeses such as mozzarella and farmer cheese for higher fat cheeses such as cheddar, American, and Monterey Jack.
- For desserts and breads, use margarine instead of butter or shortening.
- For fruit cobblers or crisps, reduce the amount of fat by one-fourth.
- Substitute powdered sugar for whipped topping on desserts when appropriate.
- Use margarine instead of butter for white sauces.
- Use defatted ground beef instead of sausage on pizza.
- Use low-fat gravy made with broth or soup base that contains little or no fat.
- Do not add margarine or butter when making sandwiches; do not spread melted butter or margarine on rolls or bread.
- When making toasted or grilled cheese sandwiches, lightly brush only the outside bread with margarine.
- Do not add margarine, butter, or sauces to vegetables; try flavoring vegetables with lemon juice or herbs.

Source: NCEP Report of the Expert Panel on Blood Cholesterol Levels in Children and Adolescents (1)

good-tasting foods low in saturated fat and cholesterol that are appealing to children (1). The food industry has responded by introducing a wide range of fat-modified and fat-free products. However, the sudden influx of these products to the marketplace has generated some new concerns. The incidence of obesity in children is increasing and effective interventions aimed at energy balance are urgently needed. Increased physical activity and a better understanding of nutrient composition are potentially the most effective strategies for weight control.

Children and their parents need to understand that "fat-free" does not mean "calorie-free." Balance, variety, and moderation are still essential principles. In general, intake of fresh fruits, vegetables, and whole grains is woefully inadequate in many children's diets. Increasing consumption of produce often requires more effort and forethought than purchasing a package of cookies, crackers, or chips.

Data from the Bogalusa Heart Study, a long-term pediatric epidemiology study, reported average energy contributions from meals and snacks for 10-year-old children (17-19). Table 10-9, which is adapted from the Bogalusa study, illustrates the importance of snack foods in meeting children's energy needs without increasing total daily fat consumption. Children whose total daily fat intake was less than 30% of energy consumed a greater proportion of energy from snacks than did children whose total daily fat intake was more than 40% of energy (19). Children with the lowest fat intakes also consumed more of their fat energy at breakfast and lunch, whereas children with the highest total fat intakes consumed most of their fat energy at the evening meal. Such data emphasize the need for education about optimal meal patterns as well as the need to encourage the choice of foods lower in fat.

Table 10-10 shows that children with the highest fat intakes consumed most fat energy from meat sources. Children whose fat consumption was 30% or less of total

TABLE 10-9

Energy Contribution by Meal Period for Various Fat Intake Groups (10-Year-Olds)*

	Fat Intake Group			
	1 <30%	2 30%-35%	3 35%-40%	4 >40%
Breakfast	317 (17.7)	355 (18.6)	371 (17.4)	381 (16.2)
Lunch	452 (25.5)	453 (25.0)	492 (24.4)	507 (22.8)
Dinner	530[d] (28.0)[d]	500[c] (26.9)[c]	648[b] (30.5)	871[d] (34.3)[a]
Snacks	638[z] (34.8)	642[y] (33.1)	705 (31.7)	788[x] (31.9)

*Values represent total energy (percentage of energy). Fat intake groups were stratified according to percentage of total energy from fat. Fat intake groups with different superscript letters are statistically different. $a>b$, $P<0.05$; $a>c$, $P<0.05$; $a>d$, $P<0.05$; $b>c$, $P<0.05$; $x>y$, $P<0.05$; $x>z$, $P<0.05$.

Source: Nicklas TA, Webber LS, Srinivasan, SR, Berenson, GS (19). Reproduced with permission of *Pediatrics*, vol 89, p 223, © 1992.

TABLE 10-10

Food Sources of Total Fat by Fat Intake Group (10-Year-Olds)[a]

	Fat Intake Group, g (%)				Pairwise Comparisons[b]	
Food Group	1 <30%	2 30%-35%	3 35%-40%	4 >40%	Amount, g	%
Dairy	12.6 (23.4)	14.2 (21.0)	16.7 (19.7)	18.4 (16.0)	4,3>2,1	1>3,4;2,3>4
Meats[c]	8.1 (15.8)	12.4 (18.3)	20.5 (22.9)	40.5 (30.7)	4>3>2,1	4>3>2,1
Breads/grains	7.1 (13.2)	7.4 (11.1)	7.7 (9.2)	7.7 (6.7)	...	1>2>3>4
Desserts	6.4 (12.4)	8.0 (11.8)	10.8 (11.7)	12.0 (9.4)	4>2,1;3>1	...
Vegetables/soups	5.9 (10.7)	5.4 (8.6)	7.6 (9.0)	11.5 (9.6)	4>3,1,2	...
Fats/oils	4.7 (8.5)	6.2 (9.0)	7.9 (9.3)	13.5 (9.9)	4>3,2,1	4>3,2,1
Snacks	3.0 (5.7)	3.8 (5.7)	3.9 (4.8)	4.9 (4.7)	...	...
Poultry	2.3 (4.3)	4.1 (5.6)	3.6 (4.1)	3.4 (3.4)	...	...
Candy	1.9 (3.6)	2.9 (4.2)	3.8 (4.3)	4.9 (4.4)	4>2,1;3>1	...
Egg	0.7 (1.0)	1.7 (2.2)	2.9 (3.0)	3.8 (3.4)	4>2,1;3>1	4,3>1

Source: Nicklas TA, Webber LS, Srinivasan SR, Berenson GS (19). Reprduced with permission of *Pediatrics*, vol 89, p 221, © 1992.

[a] Fat intake groups were stratified according to percentage of total energy from fat. The total percentage of total fat intake by food group does not equal 100% because of rounding. Not all 21 food groups are represented.

[b] All comparisons indicated are statistically significant, $P<0.05$.

[c] Meats = mixed meat + pork + veal + lamb + beef.

energy derived most of their fat from dairy products. Dietitians can help parents to switch to lower-fat dairy foods and lower-fat cuts of meat without compromising protein or iron intake.

Mass Media

NCEP advocates the promotion of news, educational, and entertainment programming supporting its dietary recommendations. A great need exists for advertising that helps children recognize how processed foods, including fat-modified snacks and desserts, fit within a healthful lifestyle that combines a nutritious diet with regular exercise. Nutrition messages can be entertaining while conveying information about healthful eating behavior.

Computer software that facilitates independent learning and interactive nutrition education is gradually becoming available for both professionals and consumers. Dietitians can be instrumental in providing content for such programs and evaluation tools to document their effectiveness. (See Box 10-3 for references on the dietary assessment of children and adolescents and Appendix 3 for instructional programs that are appropriate for children and adolescents.)

Scientific Rationale for an Individualized Approach

Pediatricians, family practitioners, and other health care team members are advised for both ethical and economic reasons not to conduct universal blood cholesterol screening. NCEP advocates an individualized approach for children who are at greatest risk of developing high blood cholesterol as adults. Included in this at-risk group are children and adolescents whose parents or grandparents

- at age 55 or less underwent diagnostic coronary arteriography and were found to have coronary atherosclerosis or suffered a myocardial infarction or other cardiovascular event, or
- at any age have blood cholesterol levels of 240 mg/dL or higher.

The blood cholesterol levels of these at-risk children

BOX 10-3 Diet Intervention Materials for Children

Special Program in Nutrition (SPIN), Gladstone Institute of Cardiovascular Disease—Good Nutrition for Heart Health for Third and Fourth Grade Students and Their Families
2550 - 23rd Street
P.O. Box 419100
San Francisco, CA 94141-9100
Phone: (415) 826-7500

National Heart, Lung and Blood Institute (NHLBI) Information Center
P.O. Box 30105
Bethesda, MD 20824-0105
Phone: (301) 251-1222
Fax: (301) 251-1223
(For recorded heart health information, call 1-800-575-WELL.)

The Cardiovascular Health Promotion Project (CHPP) (part of NHLBI) offers many products as part of its community outreach, including

- A special edition of *Heart Memo* on CHPP. Issued in 1996, it describes 14 research projects that encourage cardiovascular health behaviors in children and adolescents.
- CATCH curricula: CATCH Physical Education Curriculum (composed of a guidebook, activity box, and videotapes); Heart-Health Classroom Curricula and Family Components for Grades 3, 4, and 5; and Eat Smart-School Cafeteria Program Guide.
- CHPP Resource Guide: offers guidance for working with a variety of age groups in such varied sites as schools, parks, inner cities, and the home.

Child and Adolescent Trial for Cardiovascular Health (CATCH):
Center for Health Promotion Research and Development
University of Texas Health Sciences Center
P.O. Box 20186
Houston, TX 77225
Phone: (713) 792-8547
Fax: (713) 794-1756

Materials developed by CHPP and CATCH are available at cost by requesting an order form from:

NHLBI Information Center
P.O. Box 30105
Bethesda, MD 20824-0105

***Sat Fat Tracking* Book:** Smith K, Ahrens L, Stickney L, Siglin D. *Sat Fat Tracking.* The Lipid Disorders Training Program, University of Iowa College of Medicine, Iowa City, Iowa (based on Sat Fat...Keeping Track). August 1995. (See also Chapters 4 and Appendixes 1 and 3.)

should be tested. In children whose blood cholesterol level is greater than 200 mg/dL, a lipoprotein analysis should also be done (Table 10-5).

Both prevention and treatment begin with diet therapy. Figures 10-1 to 10-3 and Table 10-6 explain the objectives of the dietary intervention process. The overriding goal is to support the child's growth and development while reducing blood cholesterol levels. If careful adherence to the step I diet for at least 3 months does not adequately reduce the child's blood cholesterol level, the step II diet is prescribed. In this diet, saturated fat intake is less than 7% of total energy and cholesterol intake is less than 200 mg/day.

Half of the primary care physicians (including pediatricians) who responded to a national survey said that they felt the prudent step I type diet was healthful for children older than age 2 (Table 10-11) (20). However, only 35% of pediatricians felt prepared to use dietary interventions for their patients and only 13% believed that they had been successful with such interventions. These responses indicate a clear need for dietitians to facilitate such interventions.

TABLE 10-11

Percentage of Physicians Who Strongly Agree with Statements

	FP (%)	GP (%)	PD (%)	All (%)
CHD risk factors predict adult CHD	66	65	57	63
Diet might interfere with growth	7	9	10	8
Prudent diet for > age 2 years is healthy	52	52	53	52
I feel prepared to intervene with diet	46	56	35	45
I am successful with diet intervention	13	18	13	14

FP = family physician; GP = general practitioner; PD = pediatrician; CHD = coronary heart disease.

Source: Adapted from Kimm SY, Payne G, Lakatos E, Darby C, Sparrow A (20).

SAFETY AND EFFICACY OF INDIVIDUALIZED APPROACH

Since the NCEP report was published, further evidence of the usefulness of the individualized approach for at-risk children has been documented. The Dietary Intervention Study in Children (DISC) was a randomized, controlled clinical trial in 663 children with elevated baseline total cholesterol and LDL-C levels. After 3 years on a diet similar to the NCEP step II diet, prepubescent children with elevated LDL cholesterol at baseline decreased their LDL-C levels by 3.3 mg/dL, significantly more than children in the control group, without compromising their growth, cognitive ability, or development (21). Dietitians, behaviorists, and health educators provided intensive dietary intervention to both children and their parents in the intervention group and dietary adherence and adequacy were carefully monitored (22). Concerns about failure to thrive in children on low-fat diets were present as a result of earlier case studies in which lack of effective nutrition education for parents and inadequate nutrient intake by children yielded adverse outcomes. However, such outcomes were not observed in DISC (23).

Some gender-specific differences in response were observed in DISC. Further multivariate regression analyses showed that LDL-C decreased by 0.70 mg/dL for each 10 mg/kcal decrease in dietary cholesterol ($P < 0.05$) for boys; for girls, no single nutrient was significant in the analyses but a treatment effect was evident for the intervention group ($P < 0.05$) (24). Effective input by a dietitian is key to achieving desirable results without jeopardizing the growth and health of these children.

In the Children's Health Project, a clinical study of preadolescent children with elevated baseline LDL-C, participants reduced their LDL-C levels with the use of a parent-child autotutorial intervention that involved nutrition education via a tape recorder and an accompanying workbook (25,26).

THE DIETITIAN'S ROLE IN ENSURING DIETARY ADEQUACY AND ADHERENCE

The clinical trials described earlier have demonstrated the efficacy and safety of step I and step II diets in growing children. Dietary intervention provided by trained, qualified dietitians and health educators was essential to ensuring both adherence and nutrient adequacy.

Because existing consumer-oriented nutrition education is often limited at best and fallacious or misleading at worst, health care teams must take great care to deliver appropriate messages. By overzealously emphasizing fat restriction, well-meaning parents can unintentionally deny their children the energy, protein, and other essential nutrients that the children need for growth. Excessive use of fat-modified or fat-free products without considering serving size, total energy intake, and a proper balance among all the food groups can lead to nutrient deficiencies and obesity.

ESTIMATING CHILDREN'S ENERGY NEEDS

The Recommended Dietary Allowances (RDAs) for energy are based on the resting energy expenditure estimated by height and weight (27). Table 10-12 presents the reference values for children.

Infants from birth to 6 months need approximately 95 kcal/kg; from 6 months to 12 months, the RDA decreases to 84 kcal/kg. In preterm infants or infants born small for gestational age, energy needs are increased to better accommodate catch-up growth; protein and other nutrient requirements are increased accordingly. Table 10-13 gives the RDAs for protein and other nutrients for children.

Until age 10, energy estimates are the same for boys and girls. From age 11 onward, energy estimates are higher for males, reflecting their proportionately greater lean body mass. Beginning at age 11, sex-specific activity factors are applied to the resting energy expenditure to better reflect

TABLE 10-12

Recommended Energy Intake for Children and Adolescents

Category	Age (Yrs)	Weight kg	Weight lb	Height cm	Height in	REE[a] (kcal/day)	Average Energy Allowance (kcal)[b] Multiples of REE[c]	Per kg	Per day[d]
Infants	0.0-0.5	6	13	60	24	320		108	650
	0.5-1.0	9	20	71	28	500		98	850
Children	1-3	13	29	90	35	740		102	1300
	4-6	20	44	112	44	950		90	1800
	7-10	28	62	132	52	1130		70	2000
Males	11-14	45	99	157	62	1440	1.70	55	2500
	15-18	66	145	176	69	1760	1.67	45	3000
Females	11-14	46	101	157	62	1310	1.67	47	2200
	15-18	55	120	163	64	1370	1.60	40	2200

Source: Recommended Dietary Allowances, 10th ed. (27).

[a] REE, Resting energy expenditure. Calculation based on WHO equations, then rounded.

[b] Activity factor multiplied by REE.

[c] In the range of light to moderate activity, the coefficient of variation is ±20%.

[d] Number is rounded.

TABLE 10-13

Recommended Nutrient Intake for Children and Adolescents

Category	Age (Yrs)	Weight[a] kg	Weight[a] lb	Height[b] cm	Height[b] in	Protein[a] (g)	Fat-Soluble Vitamins: Vitamin A (mg RE)[b]	Vitamin D (mg)[c]	Vitamin E (mg a-TE)[d]	Vitamin K (mg)
Children	1-3	13	29	90	35	16	400	10.0	6	15
	4-6	20	44	112	44	24	500	10.0	7	20
	7-10	28	62	132	52	28	700	10.0	7	30
Males	11-14	45	99	157	62	45	1000	10.0	10	45
	15-18	66	145	176	69	59	1000	10.0	10	65
Females	11-14	46	101	157	62	46	800	10.0	8	45
	15-18	55	120	163	64	44	800	10.0	8	55

Category	Water-Soluble Vitamins: Vitamin C (mg)	Thiamin (mg)	Riboflavin (mg)	Niacin (mg NE)[e]	Vitamin B_6 (mg)	Folate (mg)	Vitamin B_{12} (mg)	Minerals: Calcium (mg)	Phosphorus (mg)	Magnesium (mg)	Iron (mg)	Zinc (mg)	Iodine (µg)
Children	40	0.7	0.8	9	1.0	50	0.7	800	800	80	10	10	70
	45	0.9	1.1	12	1.1	75	1.0	800	800	120	10	10	90
	45	1.0	1.2	13	1.4	100	1.4	800	800	170	10	10	120
Males	50	1.3	1.5	17	1.7	150	2.0	1200	1200	270	12	15	150
	60	1.5	1.8	20	2.0	200	2.0	1200	1200	400	12	15	150
Females	50	1.1	1.3	15	1.4	150	2.0	1200	1200	280	15	12	150
	60	1.1	1.3	15	1.5	180	2.0	1200	1200	300	15	12	150

[a]Weights and heights of Reference Adults are actual medians for the U.S. population of the designated age, as reported by NHANES II. The median weights and heights of those under 19 years of age were taken from Hamill et al. (1979). The use of these figures does not imply that the height-to-weight ratios are ideal.

[b]Retinol equivalents. 1 retinol equivalent = 1 µg retinol or 6 µg β-carotene.

[c]As cholecalciferol. 10 mg cholecalciferol = 400 IU of vitamin D.

[d]α-Tocopherol equivalents. 1µg d-α tocopherol = 1 α-TE.

[e]1 NE (niacin equivalent) is equal to 1 mg of niacin or 60 mg of dietary tryptophan.

Source: Adapted from *Recommended Dietary Allowances,* 10th ed. (27).

average energy allowance. The normal variation in these levels is ± 20% of the RDA.

GROWTH: THE ULTIMATE MEASURE OF DIETARY ADEQUACY IN CHILDREN

The National Center for Health Statistics has generated standard growth curves on the basis of height and weight data charted through time for thousands of boys and girls. These data provide useful comparisons for determining the adequacy of a child's growth rate. Regardless of the specific curve a child may be following (ie, 10th percentile or 95th percentile), the key factor in evaluating a child's growth rate over time is whether the child maintains the same position on the curve. Growth standards for girls and boys at different ages are given in Figures 10-4 to 10-7. Monitoring a child's position on the relevant growth curve permits any deviation from the norm to be identified and addressed.

PREVENTION OF OBESITY

The prevalence of obesity among children and adults has increased to epidemic proportions during the past decade despite declines in both total and saturated fat intake (28,29). NHANES III data show a 21% prevalence of overweight in children, where overweight is defined as sex- and age-specific values above the 85th percentile (Table 10-14). Recently, a more conservative definition of overweight was used for children and adolescents, compared with adults, to account for growth spurts and other physiologic changes. A Centers for Disease Control and Prevention study reported when obesity is defined as a BMI at or above the sex- and age-specific 95th percentile the prevalence of obesity in children (ages 6 to 11 years) was 13.7% and in adolescents (ages 12 to 17) was 11.5% (30). Because obese adults are at increased risk for cardiovascular and other diseases, primary prevention in childhood is highly desirable (31,32). Such prevention is efficacious, safe, and feasible even in very young children if skilled dietary intervention and medical monitoring are employed (33).

PRACTICAL RECOMMENDATIONS FOR FACILITATING DIETARY CHANGE

Some of the strategies used and lessons learned in the research studies described earlier can be safely applied in clinical practice. The first step in providing the most effective interventions is to differentiate on the basis of age and level of independence. Adolescents and children are not usually at immediate risk for cardiovascular disease. Motivating factors for establishing a healthful eating pattern are usually related to appearance, fitness, or sports performance rather than to the long-term benefit of reduced cardiovascular risk status in adulthood. When the emphasis is placed on the ways in which a diet rich in fruits, vegetables, and grains can help to control body weight, fight infection, and improve endurance, children and adolescents can recognize the personal benefits of maintaining a healthful diet.

Dietitians can act at multiple levels to help ensure both dietary adherence and nutrient adequacy. They can also reinforce the benefits of physical activity; an active lifestyle is imperative to successful long-term weight control. Clinically, dietitians can work with medical practitioners to perform detailed dietary assessments and initiate sensible but palatable eating behaviors in pediatric patients. School-based feeding programs can be monitored to ensure that meals generally provide less than 30% of total energy from fat, food service personnel are trained to answer questions, students have input on menu selections, and teachers have every opportunity to teach nutrition in traditional and alternative class settings.

Computerized independent-learning tools, which are increasingly popular, may be the most efficient means of standardizing nutrition education messages. For example, a CD-ROM describes the 5-A-Day Program and is geared to children (Dole Food Company, San Mateo, Calif). Point-of-purchase nutrient information will become more prevalent as more consumers use computerized shopping lists and services.

Dietitians can provide expertise in numerous arenas outside traditional office-based practice. Children who are educated about the benefits of a healthy diet and an active lifestyle will consider it natural to choose good-tasting, lower-fat foods and to be physically active. Research is badly needed to identify the most successful approaches to achieving population-wide adherence to the dietary guidelines among children.

Preadolescent children may influence the choice of food at the point of purchase and can opt not to eat food that is served, but in general parents have a key role in determining their children's diets. Because most parents want to help their children maximize their growth and health and prevent obesity, they are usually receptive to dietary intervention efforts targeted to children. Because modeling behavior and supporting the child's efforts are major objectives of this targeted approach, the entire family's nutritional status may benefit.

The pediatric research studies cited earlier emphasized the importance of parental intervention. In DISC, parents attended separate sessions that were held simultaneously with the children's groups to discuss specific food groups and the appropriate choices (21). A "train-the-trainer" approach was emphasized for the parents. Parents were partners with the nutritionists and were told what their children were learning so that they could complement and reinforce these lessons at home. Parents were also encouraged to provide incentives and rewards for dietary adherence and to use self-monitoring exercises and other diet-related behaviors. This was a useful strategy because it simplified the dietary messages given to parents and created a positive relationship between parents and children as they implemented the DISC diet. Even parents with no prior nutrition knowledge learned to shop, cook, and motivate adherence without feeling patronized. These behaviors were reinforced by eating heart-healthy meals together at the 90-minute DISC sessions. Often this meal included foods that had been prepared by the children.

Once children can read, they can be introduced to food

FIGURE 10-4

BOYS: 2 TO 18 YEARS
PHYSICAL GROWTH
NCHS PERCENTILES*

NAME ______________________ RECORD # ____________

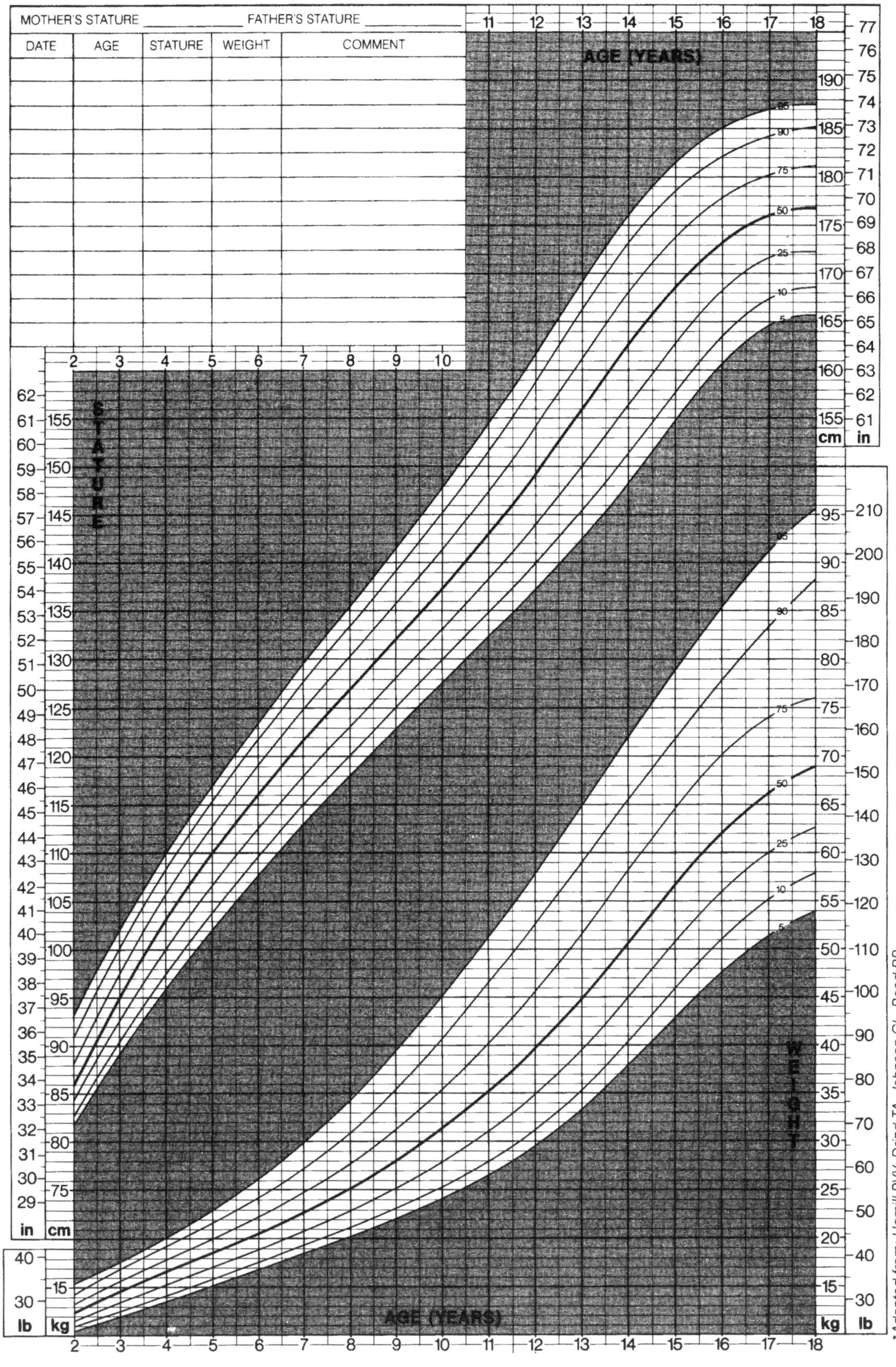

*Adapted from: Hamill PVV, Drizd TA, Johnson CL, Reed RB, Roche AF, Moore WM: Physical growth: National Center for Health Statistics percentiles. AM J CLIN NUTR 32:607-629, 1979. Data from the National Center for Health Statistics (NCHS), Hyattsville, Maryland.

FIGURE 10-5

BOYS: PREPUBESCENT PHYSICAL GROWTH NCHS PERCENTILES*

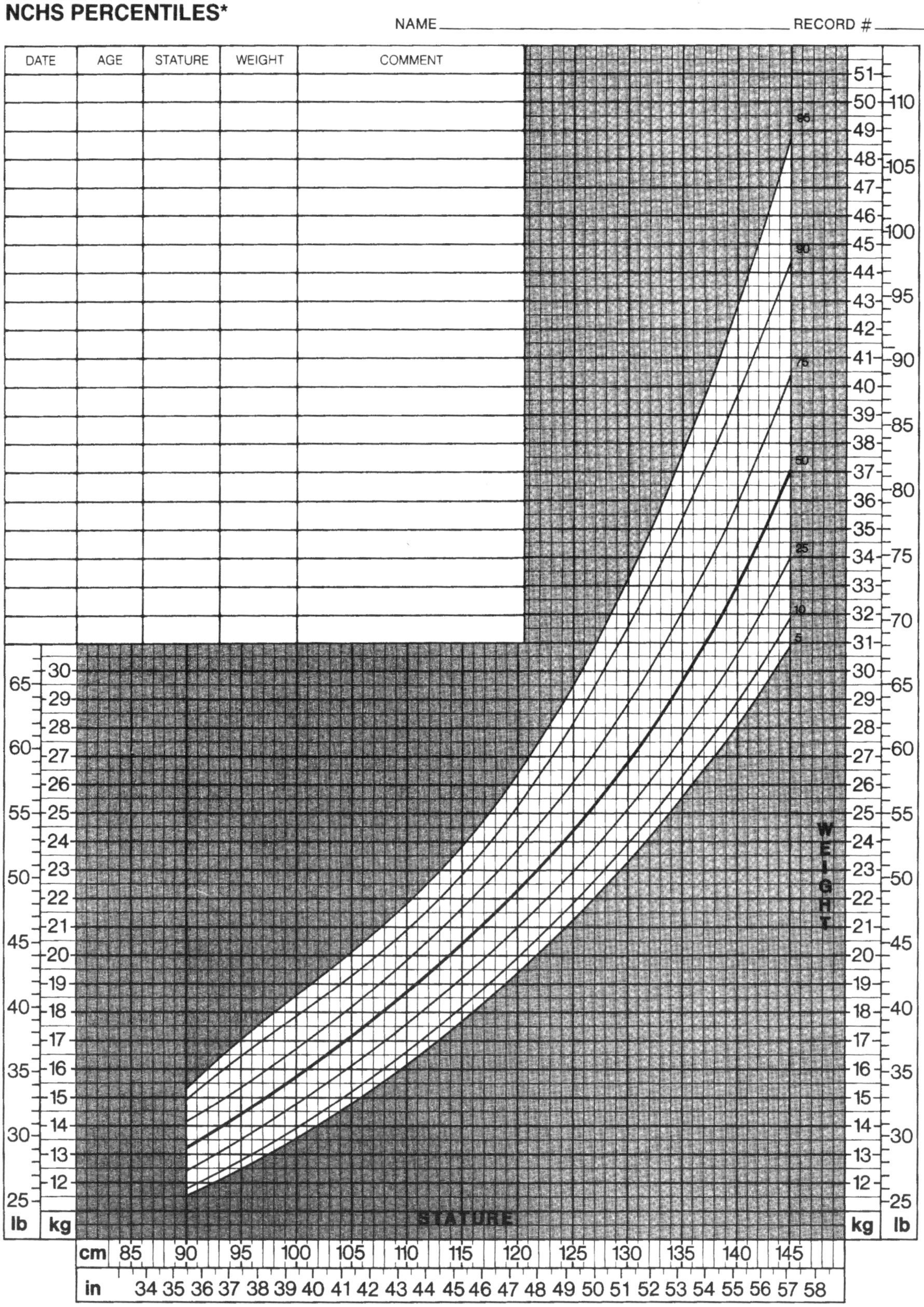

*Adapted from: Hamill PVV, Drizd TA, Johnson CL, Reed RB, Roche AF, Moore WM: Physical growth: National Center for Health Statistics percentiles. AM J CLIN NUTR 32:607-629, 1979. Data from the National Center for Health Statistics (NCHS), Hyattsville,

SIMILAC® WITH IRON
Infant Formula

ISOMIL®
Soy Protein Formula with Iron

Reprinted with permission of Ross Laboratories

FIGURE 10-6

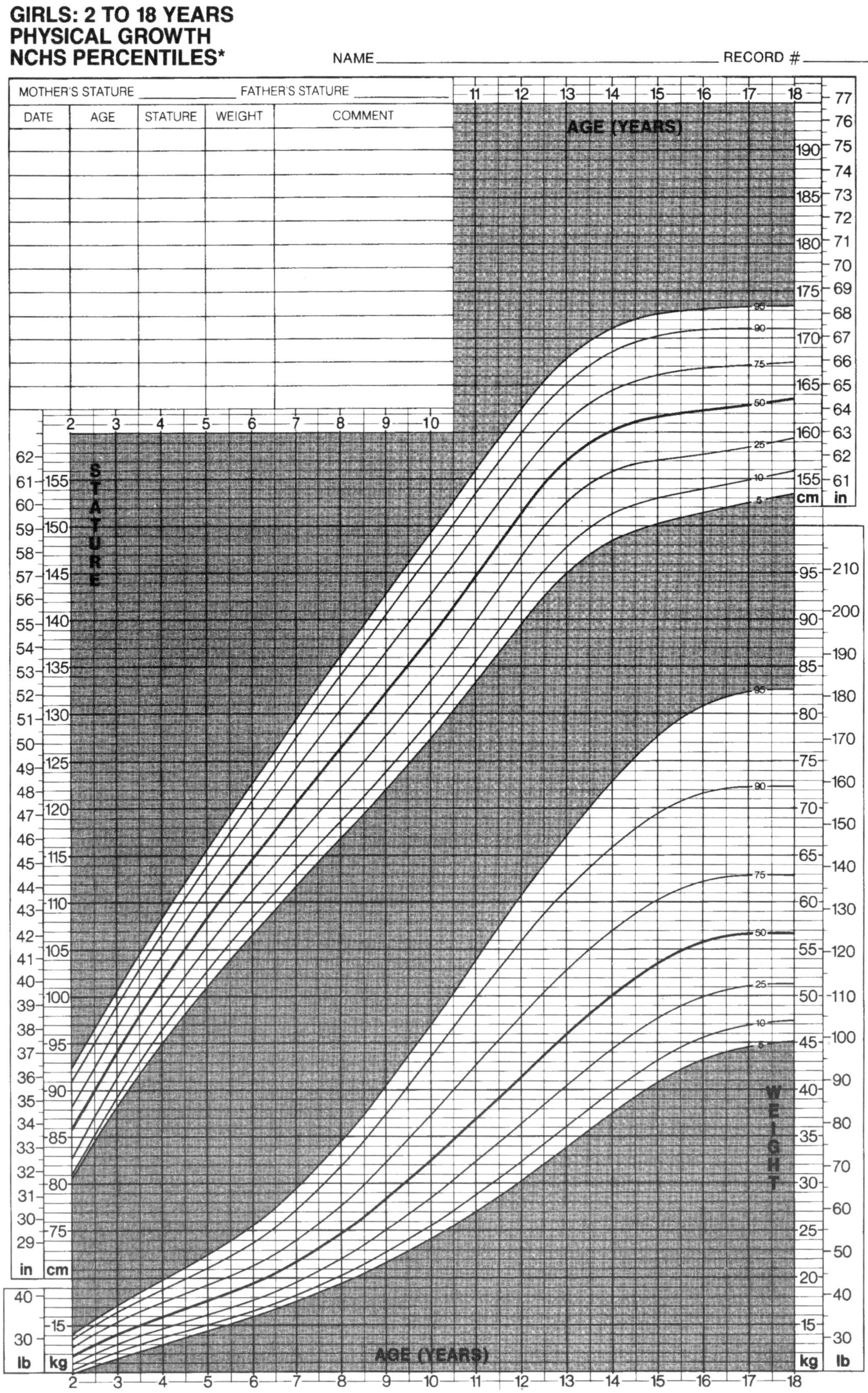

*Adapted from: Hamill PVV, Drizd TA, Johnson CL, Reed RB, Roche AF, Moore WM: Physical growth: National Center for Health Statistics percentiles. AM J CLIN NUTR 32:607-629, 1979. Data from the National Center for Health Statistics (NCHS), Hyattsville, Maryland.

FIGURE 10-7

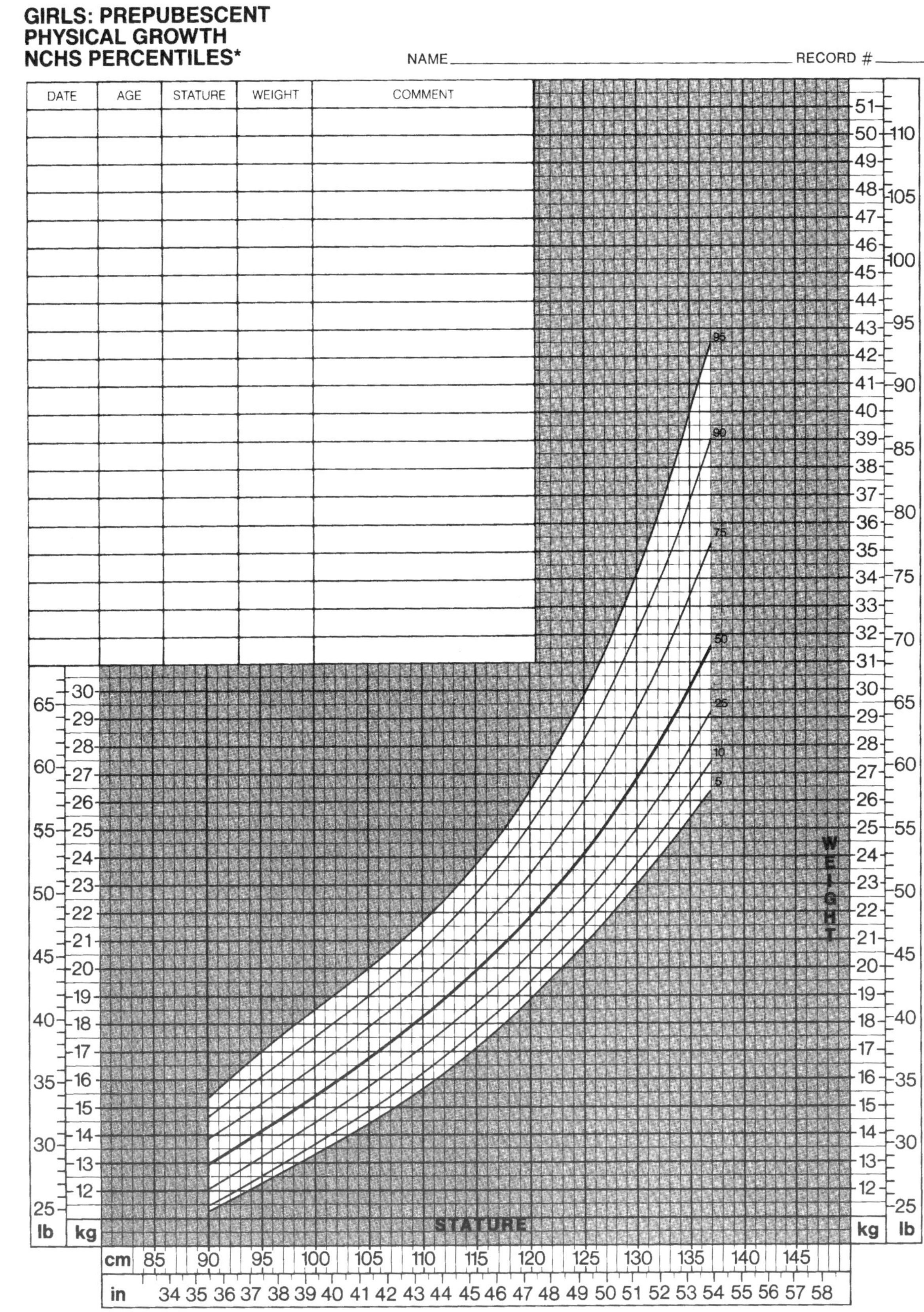

*Adapted from: Hamill PVV, Drizd TA, Johnson CL, Reed RB, Roche AF, Moore WM: Physical growth: National Center for Health Statistics percentiles. AM J CLIN NUTR 32:607-629, 1979. Data from the National Center for Health Statistics (NCHS), Hyattsville, Maryland

Reprinted with permission of Ross Laboratories

TABLE 10-14

Unadjusted Prevalence of Overweight for NHANES III, from Sex- and Age-specific 85th and 95th Percentile Cutoff Points of NHES II and NHES III[a]

Category	No.	85th Percentile	95th Percentile
Sex and Age, y			
Both sexes	2920	22.0±1.1	10.9±0.8
6-11	1817	22.3±1.5	11.0±1.0
12-17	1103	21.7±1.9	10.8±1.3
Boys			
6-8	442	21.3±4.3	11.7±3.6
9-11	467	22.7±2.7	10.9±2.3
12-14	253	23.5±3.3	12.0±2.6
15-17	289	20.7±2.9	13.5±2.8
Girls			
6-8	450	24.2±3.6	13.7±2.7
9-11	458	21.4±4.1	8.2±2.1
12-14	288	21.5±2.8	8.5±2.0
15-17	273	21.4±3.1	9.0±1.4
Sex, Age, y, and Race-Ethnicity			
Boys aged 6-11			
Total[b]	909	21.9±2.4	11.3±1.8
Non-Hispanic white	267	20.5±2.8	10.4±2.4
Non-Hispanic black	257	26.5±2.7	13.4±2.3
Mexican-American	350	33.3±3.0	17.7±2.3
Boys aged 12-17			
Total[b]	542	22.0±2.2	12.8±1.9
Non-Hispanic white	155	23.1±3.1	14.4±2.7
Non-Hispanic black	163	21.1±3.7	9.3±2.4
Mexican-American	203	26.7±4.6	12.8±3.2
Girls aged 6-11			
Total[b]	908	22.7±2.4	10.6±1.3
Non-Hispanic white	270	21.5±3.7	9.8±2.0
Non-Hispanic black	224	31.4±4.0	16.9±2.8
Mexican-American	389	29.0±2.1	14.3±1.7
Girls aged 12-17			
Total[b]	561	21.4±2.7	8.8±1.4
Non-Hispanic white	191	20.3±3.5	8.3±1.6
Non-Hispanic black	147	29.9±4.5	14.4±3.1
Mexican-American	198	23.4±3.0	8.7±2.5

[a] Values are prevalences—SEMs. NHANES indicates National Health and Nutrition Examination Survey; NHES (National Health Examination Survey).

[b] Includes data for race-ethnicity groups not shown separately.

Source: Trocano R, Flegal K, Kuczmarski R, Campbell S, Johnson C (29).

labels and taught how to count fat grams. (See Table 10-15 for guidelines given to DISC participants and parents.) Establishing individual goals for grams of fat and fiber on the basis of energy needs is important for generating self-monitoring objectives.

Even though food labels are now much more informative than they used to be, children of all ages need direction in choosing and balancing appropriate foods. DISC developed the Go Guide (Figure 10-8) to better differentiate preferred foods and to reinforce the importance of eating foods from all food groups daily. The Go Guide accomplished two purposes: It illustrates the components of a complete eating pattern and specifies the recommended number of servings per food group, and it differentiates high-fat (Whoa) foods from preferred (Go) choices without eliminating favorite foods. Table 10-16 provides some examples of Go versus Whoa foods from the grain group.

In addition to label reading, educational tours of the grocery store can be immensely valuable for school-age and older children. The grocery store can be a living nutrition

TABLE 10-15

Shopping Guide to Reading Labels and Choosing Foods Wisely

Food Items	Guidelines for Selection
Cereals	Less than or equal to 2 grams of fat per cup
Cheeses	3 grams or less fat per ounce; part-skim cheeses 4-5 grams fat per ounce
Packaged side dishes (rice, pasta, noodles)	2 grams or less of fat per ½ cup of dry mixture
Packaged foods (with added meat, chicken, or fish)	2 grams of fat or less per serving
Sauces	1 gram of fat or less per serving
Soups	3 grams of fat or less per serving
Cake mixes	5 grams of fat or less per dry serving
Cookies	Low-fat: 3 grams or less per ounce; medium-fat: 5 grams or less per ounce
Crackers	Low-fat: 3 grams or less per ounce; high-fat: 6 grams of fat per ounce
Frozen dairy desserts	3 grams of fat or less per ½ cup
Lunch meats	3 grams of fat or less per ounce
Yogurt	4 grams of fat or less per cup

laboratory for anyone who needs to make dietary changes. If such a tour is not possible, providing a virtual grocery store by means of a collection of food labels to sort through can be equally informative. Role-play about social situations such as parties and sports events can prepare a child to resist temptations to indulge in high-fat foods. "Sat Fat Tracking," a booklet developed at the University of Iowa College of Medicine, is a useful tool for self-monitoring total and saturated fat intake by food group (35) (Boxes 10-3 and 10-4).

Establishing a system of self-monitoring and self-rewards is important to maintaining adherence. In DISC, tokens ("DISC dollars") were awarded for achieving predetermined objectives, record keeping, trying new Go foods, and so on (36). Children could exchange the tokens for balls, books, stickers, and other trinkets. As they grew older, they saved their tokens to buy more significant items such as compact discs, tapes, radios, and cameras. Parents were encouraged to give nonmonetary rewards, such as permission to invite a friend over for dinner, a sleepover, or a camp-out.

Target Foods

Because children should have at least three to four servings of dairy products daily to meet their needs for calcium, protein, and other nutrients, the dairy food group is often a major source of saturated fat and cholesterol in children's diets. This problem can be simply remedied by switching to non-fat, reduced-fat, or low-fat dairy products. Similarly, shifting from hamburger to ground round, ground sirloin, or ground white-meat turkey or chicken also significantly reduces saturated fat intake. Parents can learn to accommodate occasional high-fat meals in an otherwise low-fat diet. Table 10-17 illustrates how to balance higher- and lower-fat meals throughout the day.

Despite progress in modifying national school lunch menus, eating at school (or eating out in a restaurant) can still be challenging. Learning to look for hidden fats in foods can help children to select lower-fat options. Tables 10-18 to 10-21 illustrate different fat sources and suggest lower-fat options. Table 10-21 also provides recipe substitutions for parents who prepare foods at home.

Goal Setting

The concept of setting and achieving goals for dietary behavior may be new to many children and their parents. Parents need guidance to help their children cut back gradually but progressively on foods that are high in fat and cholesterol. The skillful dietitian can encourage families to establish and meet realistic goals. The followng paragraphs explain how goal-setting was explained to parents and children in DISC (unpublished DISC intervention manual).

What Is Goal Setting?

Goal setting is a process of breaking down a large task into small steps that are more easily attainable. Planning and accomplishing a steady series of small successes is an important part of DISC. Achievement of many small successes promotes a feeling of accomplishment and instills confidence in one's future ability to succeed.

How Do I Set a Goal?

First, think of a big, long-term goal that you would like to achieve. Examples of long-term goals might include lowering your blood cholesterol, reducing energy from fat sources, or changing other habits during the next year. To accomplish your long-term goal, set a short-term goal each week.

A good short-term goal meets several important criteria. First, it is specific, concrete, observable, and measurable. This means that it is something that you (or others) can actually do—something you have direct control over—and it has clear results when you accomplish it. Second, it must

FIGURE 10-8

Disc Go! Guide

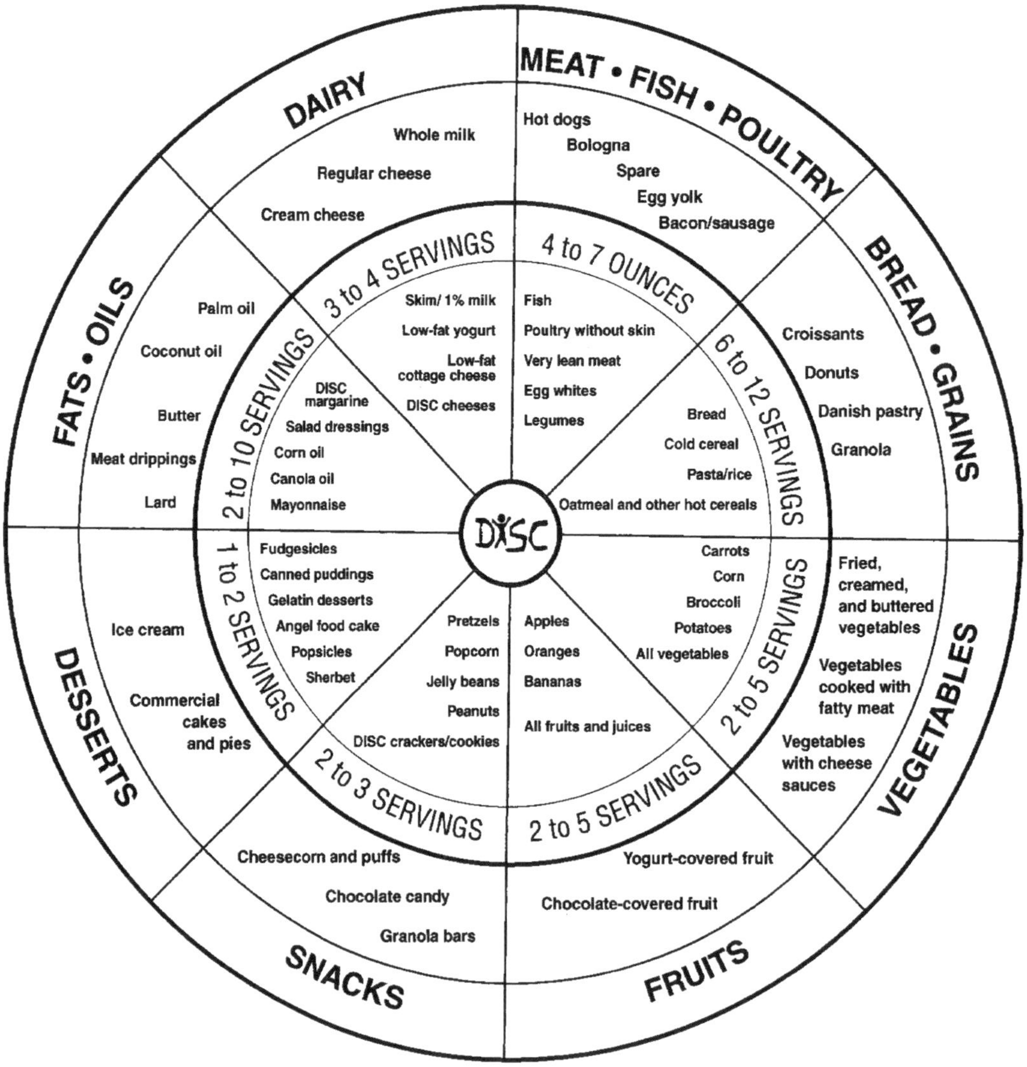

This is your **DISC Go! Guide.** It is designed to help you learn about good nutrition and how to select foods with less saturated fat and cholesterol. These foods are **Go!** foods.

Each day select the recommended variety of **Go!** foods from each food group on the circle. Select **Go!** foods from the center of the circle and **Go!** for them. Use the DISC **Go!** Guide to keep yourself **Go!**-ing and growing Your dietitian will help you determine the number of servings that is best for you.

The foods on the outer edge are **Whoa!** foods. Eat them less often or eat **Go!** foods instead. DISC will teach you how to eat more **Go!** foods and fewer **Whoa!** foods.

Sometimes **Go!** foods become **Whoa!** foods is they are prepared with **Whoa!** ingredients. DISC will teach you how to prepare foods the **Go!** way.

be a positive action rather than the avoidance of doing something. Third, it must have a high probability of success. Ask yourself, "Are my chances of success 85% or more?" If the answer is no, choose a more reasonable goal. We tend to tell ourselves that our achievements are not important unless they take lots of effort or willpower. However, relying on extreme willpower to achieve change is a strategy that is doomed to fail. Changes can become lifelong habits if they are reasonable and enjoyable and if they allow you to experience success in achieving your goals most of the time.

What Is the Next Step?

Once you have selected a good goal, you need to do two more things. First, break down the accomplishment of your goal into

TABLE 10-16

Quick Grain Guide

Go! Foods	Whoa! Foods
Bagels	Cakes (rich)
Dinner rolls	Coffee cake
English muffins	Cookies (high fat)
French bread	Croissant
Pita bread (pocket bread)	Danish pastry
Pumpernickel bread	Doughnuts
Raisin bread	Fritter
Rye bread	Hush puppies
Sourdough bread	Sweet roll
Tortilla	Croutons
Whole wheat bread	Fettucini alfredo
White bread	Noodles Romanoff
Breadsticks	
Graham crackers	
Matzo crackers	
Oyster crackers	
Pasta	
Pretzels	
Popcorn (with GO! fat)	
Rice cakes	
Saltine crackers	
Vanilla wafers	
Dry cereal	
Hot cereal	
Wheat germ	
Corn	
Macaroni	
Rice	
Spaghetti noodles	

Source: Adapted from the *Dietary Intervention Study in Children (DISC) Child Guidebook: Nutrition Guidelines (C), Grains 1-89.* (34)

achievable steps. Second, think of a way to reward yourself for accomplishing the goal. When goals are not accomplished, it is usually because the first step was skipped. The first step should be very specific in time, place, and action.

For example, if a child sets the goal of eating at least one apple every day, the steps to accomplishing that goal might be (1) ask Mom to buy apples, (2) pack two apples for lunch, and (3) eat one apple at lunch and one after school instead of raiding the vending machine. Many people say that the feeling of success is reward enough, but goals are more likely to become regular habits if there is an occasional reward. A reward could be a preferred activity, event, or something that you will do for yourself (eg, an activity with a friend or buying a music disc). It is tempting to use food as a reward for small accomplishments, but this defeats the purpose of changing dietary behavior.

How Do I Recognize a Good Goal?

The following are examples of ineffective and better short-term goals for children:

Ineffective: "I will start thinking about trying to cut down on the amount of fat in my diet."

Better: "I will choose to eat a broiled fish dinner on Tuesday night and a bean dinner on Thursday night this week. This will replace my usual beef dinner to help reduce the fat in my diet."

Ineffective: "I will eat less cholesterol this week."

Better: "I will identify three high cholesterol foods that I usually eat and substitute low-cholesterol alternatives."

Ineffective: "I will relax more and be less anxious so I won't do so much nervous eating."

Better: "I will listen to my relaxation tape every evening after dinner because it helps me to put worrisome thoughts out of my head."

Ineffective: "I will not eat candy bars from the vending machine at my 3:00 p.m. break."

Better: "I will bring an apple to school each day and eat it at my 3:00 p.m. break to replace the candy bar I usually eat."

Ineffective: "The only thing I did last week was substitute low-fat milk for reduced-fat milk, so this week I will eat fish

BOX 10-4 **Sat Fat Tracking**

Sample Day Sat Fat Record

Name:________________ Date:________ Day:________

This sample day shows you how to record foods you have eaten, where to find sat fat grams in this book, and how to total the sat fat grams eaten in a day.

Food	Amount	Look here to find sat fat grams	Sat fat grams
MORNING:			
Corn flakes	1 1/4 cup	Breads, cereals, p. 13	0
Low-fat milk	1 cup	Dairy, p. 12	3
Orange juice	1/2 cup	Fruits, p. 16	0
Toast	1 slice	Breads, p. 13	0
Margarine -tub, soy	1 tsp	Fats, p. 17	1
Jelly	1 Tbs	Zero sat fat, p. 6	0
MIDDAY (Fast Food):			
Grilled chicken breast sandwich	1	Fast food, p.37	1
French fries	medium	Fast food, p. 39	4
Cola	medium	Zero sat fat, p. 6	0
Walnut Brownie™	1	Fast food, p. 40	10
Nonfat milk	1 cup	Dairy, p. 12	0
EVENING:			
Won ton soup	1 cup	Restaurant, p. 42	1
Beef, vegetable stir fry	1 cup	Restaurant, p. 42	5
Rice, plain	1 1/2 cups	Restaurant, p. 42	0
Ice cream (see below)	1/2 cup	Desserts, p. 28	5
Fortune cookie	1	Restaurant, p. 42	0
		Total sat fat	30

Note: 1/2 cup ice cream = 4 1/2 sat fat grams (p. 12, 1 cup ice cream = 9 sat fat gm).
You may count the sat fat grams as 4 1/2 or round up to 5, the nearest whole number.

Source: Smith et al (35).

every evening and not go out for lunch at all."

Better: "I substituted low-fat milk for reduced-fat milk last week, so this week I will continue to drink low-fat milk, and I will also eat fish or chicken twice instead of beef. I will eat fish on Monday and chicken on Thursday. I will help Mom by reminding her to buy fresh fish on the way home from work for Monday's dinner and chicken for Thursday. I will look in our low-fat cookbook to help select the fish and chicken recipes."

INTERVENING IN ADOLESCENCE

Adolescence can be an exciting and highly relevant time to initiate or reinforce dietary change and an active lifestyle. At this age, peers and self-image are crucial concerns. Adolescents are interested in improving their appearance and fitness and in being on the leading edge of knowledge relevant to their peer group. Participation in sports, games, and other vigorous activities provides social as well as physical benefits and is a logical accompaniment to a healthful dietary pattern.

DISC is the only intervention study that has followed children who were counseled on a low-fat diet at age 8 to 10 through puberty and into adolescence (to age 18). Because participants were originally enrolled in the study by their parents, it was important to establish renewed cooperation from the participants themselves when they became teenagers. Because continued adherence to the diet was key to the study outcome measures, it was necessary to identify techniques that sustained adherence for teenagers who had a degree of independence and money to make at least some of their own food choices.

To address this challenge, the DISC interventionists adapted a variety of behavioral models that had been successfully used in treating addictive behaviors unrelated to nutrition. Their methodology, which can be adapted to the clinical setting, combines Prochaska's (39, 40) transtheoretical model of stages of change with techniques developed by Miller and Rollnick (41) for use in motivational interviewing (see Chapter 13 for additional information on the stages of change model in nutrition). S Berg-Smith and col-

TABLE 10-17

Sample Meal Plans That Meet the DISC Diet Criteria[a]

Sample Menu: Balanced Fat in Meals	Sample Menu: High-Fat Lunch, Low-Fat Dinner
Breakfast	**Breakfast**
1½ cups cold cereal (Cheerios)[b]	¾ cup orange juice
1 cup nonfat milk	¾ cup cold cereal (Life)
½ banana, sliced	1 cup nonfat milk
½ English muffin	½ English muffin
1 tsp Go margarine	1 tsp Go margarine
Lunch	**Lunch**
2 slices rye bread	1 hot dog
2 oz dark meat chicken (no skin)	1 hot dog roll
2 tsp mayonnaise	1 large carrot
½ cup carrot sticks	¾ cup potato tots
1 cup nonfat milk	1 cup low-fat milk
1 apple	½ cup canned pears
Snack	**Snack**
3 cups air popped popcorn	2 fig bars
1 tsp melted Go margarine	1 cup nonfat milk
½ cup orange juice	1 apple
Dinner	**Dinner**
3 oz lean roast beef (trimmed)	3 oz broiled haddock
1 cup string beans	½ cup rice
1 cup mashed potatoes	2 tsp Go margarine
1 tsp Go margarine	½ cup broccoli
1 cup lettuce salad	1 cup mixed green salad
2 tsp GO! oil (plus vinegar)	1 Tbsp low-fat dressing
½ cup ice milk	1 cup nonfat milk
Snack	**Snack**
1 cup nonfat milk	3 squares graham crackers
4 Tbsp peanuts	½ cup unsweetened grape juice
2 fig bars	

Source: Dietary Intervention Study in Children (DISC) Adult Guidebook: Nutrition Guidelines (A), Overview/Eggs 2-89 (37).

[a] The examples on this page are not meant to be "the diet" that your child must follow, but they do give you an idea of the types of foods that fit into the DISC diet. Both days provide approximately 2,000 calories with less than 28% of calories from total fat and less than 8% from saturated fat. The second menu shows that even foods high in saturated fat can occasionally be incorporated into the dietary pattern if you plan ahead. Because it was known that a high-fat hot dog would be eaten for lunch, fish was planned for dinner to keep the overall fat intake for the day at goal.

[b] General Mills Foodservice, Minneapolis, Minn.

leagues developed an intervention program for DISC (unpublished DISC Intervention Manual). The essential components are described here.

Although it is important that participants understand the composition of the recommended diet, knowledge alone does not produce behavior change. The next step is to evaluate how well participants follow the diet and why. By asking participants to self-rate adherence, the interventionist can determine how best to proceed.

If the self-assessed adherence rating is high (ie, 8 to 10 on a scale of 1 to 12), the interventionist can encourage maintenance, help fine-tune remaining problems, and offer possible improvements. A thorough dietary assessment is valuable in helping adolescents to identify how well their self-assessment matches objective criteria. For example, deviations from the recommended diet may occur only at sporting events, parties, and other occasions when it is not possible to control the foods that are served. In these cases, eating before the event or bringing an acceptable snack to the event to share can be effective approaches.

A low self-assessment score (2 to 5) may signal indifference, ambivalence, or embarrassment. A sensitive interventionist gently but firmly probes to determine the underlying problem and helps the adolescent to choose a realistic but pro-

TABLE 10-18

Hidden Fats in Foods[a]

Food	Fat Amount (g)
Bagel	2
White bread	1
Biscuit	7
Croissant	12
American cheese (1 oz)	9
Part-nonfat mozzarella (1 oz)	5
Buttermilk (1 cup)	2
Whole milk (1 cup)	8
Reduced-fat milk (1 cup)	5
Low-fat milk (1 cup)	3
Nonfat milk (1 cup)	0.4
Angel food cake	0.1
Cheesecake	29
Layer cake with icing	12
Apple pie	20
Danish pastry	13
Yeast doughnut	14
Chocolate chip cookie (each)	3
Fig bar (each)	0.9

Source: Dietary Intervention Study in Children (DISC) Adult Guidebook: Nutrition Guidelines, Fats 3-89 (1995) (38).

[a] Nutrition Coding Center Database Information.

TABLE 10-19

Added Fats in Foods[a]

Food	Fat Amount (g)
Italian salad dressing (1 Tbsp)	7
Low-cal Italian dressing (1 Tbsp)	1
Mayonnaise (1 Tbsp)	11
Mayonnaise-type salad dressing (1 Tbsp)	7
Low-cal mayonnaise (1 Tbsp)	4
Canola oil (1 Tbsp)	15
Margarine (1 Tbsp)	11

Source: Dietary Intervention Study in Children (DISC) Adult Guidebook: Nutrition Guidelines (A), Fats 3-89 (1995) (38).

[a] Nutrition Coding Center Database Information.

gressive goal aimed at improving adherence, even if only slightly. Sometimes other matters take priority over concern about following the diet. Interventionists who can respect that need and support the participant's struggle often find that the individual later becomes open to making changes. A one-size intervention does not fit all circumstances.

Rating adherence, determining stage of change, and assessing the self-perceived level of confidence (39-41) are useful techniques to help the interventionist and the adolescent mutually develop an individually tailored action plan. More frequent visits (ie, weekly for the first month, then monthly) with the interventionist are useful during the first 6 months after adopting the diet. Once adherence is achieved, less frequent maintenance sessions, quarterly or semiannually, can be adequate.

SUMMARY AND FUTURE DIRECTIONS

The following strategies are useful in helping children and adolescents achieve dietary adherence to a fat-modified diet without compromising growth or health:

- Monitoring growth carefully and continually with the use of growth charts;
- Assessing participants' self-perceived level of adherence and stage of change;
- Mutually establishing realistic but progressive goals;
- Developing a self-monitoring system (ie, fat gram or fiber gram counters);
- Encouraging family support and role modeling;
- Developing appropriate rewards and incentives;
- Reassessing and renewing action plans as needed;

TABLE 10-20

Cholesterol

- Cholesterol in food raises blood cholesterol. Saturated fat also raises blood cholesterol. All animal products contain cholesterol, except egg whites. Organ meats are especially high in cholesterol.
- A major source of cholesterol in the diet is egg yolks. In fact, one egg yolk contains almost twice the amount of cholesterol that we want your child to eat in a day. You'll be getting additional dietary cholesterol in the lean meats and other foods that we suggest you eat.
- You don't need to eat any cholesterol because your body makes all that it needs. So there is no need for egg yolk in the diet at all. Because all of the cholesterol in the egg is in the yolk, you may eat all of the egg whites you wish. They are an inexpensive source of very good protein.
- To keep the cholesterol content of the diet down, keep as many egg yolks out of the diet as possible. Use egg white or egg substitutes in cooking instead.
- Some examples of the cholesterol content of various foods are as follows:

Item	Cholesterol Content (mg)
Chicken breast meat (per oz)	22
Chicken thigh meat (per oz)	25
Beef, 10% fat (per oz)	25
Tuna, water packed (per oz)	18
Flounder (per oz)	17
Shrimp (per oz)	43
Scallops (per oz)	11
Egg yolk (per egg)	230
Egg white (per egg)	0
Milk, nonfat (per cup)	4
Milk, low-fat (per cup)	10
Milk, 2% (per cup)	20
Milk, whole (per cup)	34

Adapted from the *Dietary Intervention Study in Children (DISC) Adult Guidebook: Nutrition Guidelines (A), Overview/Eggs* 2-89 (1995) (37).

TABLE 10-21

Recipe Substitution for Fats

Recipe Calls for:	Substitute:
Whole egg	2 egg whites, or 1 egg white plus 2 tsp nonfat milk powder plus 2 tsp oil, or ¼ cup egg substitute
Whole milk (1 cup)	1 cup nonfat milk, or 1 cup nonfat milk plus 2 tsp oil
Sour cream	Plain nonfat or low-fat yogurt, or 1 cup low-fat cottage cheese blended with 2 tsp lemon juice
Butter or shortening or lard	Equal measure of Go margarine
Cream cheese	1 cup low-fat cottage cheese, rinsed under water and then blended with ¼ cup of Go margarine
Baking chocolate (1 oz)	3 Tbsp unsweetened cocoa powder plus 1 Tbsp Go margarine
Cream in a recipe	Equal measure of canned evaporated nonfat milk, or equal measure of Go nondairy creamer
Bacon	Bacon-like bits (texturized vegetable protein), extra lean turkey bacon

Source: Dietary Intervention Study in Children (DISC) Adult Guidebook: Nutrition Guidelines (A), Fats 3-89 (1995) (38).

- Improving access to desired foods and enhancing proper choices at the point of purchase;
- Targeting problem eating occasions and suggesting alternatives, such as eating dinner before attending an evening party where high-fat foods will be served;
- Encouraging and reinforcing daily physical activity; and
- Praising positive behaviors to enhance self-esteem and build confidence.

Dietitians play a vital role in implementing these strategies in clinical settings. They can also influence and shape policy development aimed at assessing and treating children who are at risk for high blood cholesterol. Evidence for the benefits and safety of a fat-modified diet has never been as compelling as it is now.

The authors wish to acknowledge the outstanding contributions of the investigators, interventionists, and participants in DISC, which was sponsored by the National Heart, Lung, and Blood Institute, who collaborated on the production of many of the materials and strategies presented in this chapter.

REFERENCES

1. National Cholesterol Education Program. Report of the expert panel on blood cholesterol levels in children and adolescents. *Pediatrics*. 1992;89:525-584.
2. National Cholesterol Education Program. *Report of the Expert Panel on Population Strategies for Blood Cholesterol Reduction*. Bethesda, Md: US Department of Health and Human Services, National Institutes of Health; 1990. NIH 90-3046.
3. LaRosa JC, Hunninghake D, Bush D, Criqui MH, Getz GS, Gotto AM Jr, Grundy SM, Rakita L, Robertson RM, Weisfeldt ML, Cleeman JI, Wilson PW, Clarkson TB, Hay JW, Goodman DS. The cholesterol facts: a summary of the evidence relating dietary fats, serum cholesterol, and coronary heart disease. A joint statement by the American Heart Association and the National Heart, Lung, and Blood Institute. *Circulation*. 1990;81:1721-1733.
4. Strong JP. Coronary atherosclerosis in soldiers: a clue to the natural history of atherosclerosis in the young. *JAMA*. 1986; 256:2863-2866.
5. McNamara JJ, Molot MA, Stremple JF, Cutting RT. Coronary artery disease in combat casualties in Vietnam. *JAMA*. 1971;216:1185-1187.
6. Newman WP III, Freedman DS, Voors AW, Guard PD, Srinivasan SR, Cresanta JL, Williamson GD, Webber LS, Berenson GS. Relation of serum lipoprotein levels and systolic blood pressure to early atherosclerosis: The Bogalusa Heart Study. *N Engl J Med*. 1986;314:138-144.
7. Newman WP III, Wattigney W, Berenson GS. Autopsy studies in US children and adolescents: relationship of risk factors to atherosclerotic lesions. *Ann NY Acad Sci*. 1991;623:16-25.
8. PDAY Research Group. Relationship of atherosclerosis in young men to serum lipoprotein cholesterol concentrations and smoking: a preliminary report from the Pathobiological Determinants of Atherosclerosis in Youth (PDAY) Research Group. *JAMA*. 1990;264:3018-3024.
9. Gidding S. The rationale for lowering serum cholesterol levels in American children. *Am J Dis Child*. 1993;147:386-392.
10. National Heart, Lung, and Blood Institute. *The Lipid Research Clinics Population Studies Data Book: Volume I—The Prevalence Study*. Bethesda, Md: US Department of Health and Human Services, National Institutes of Health; 1980. NIH publication 80-1527.
11. McDowell M, Briefel RR, Warren RA, Buzzard IM, Feskanich D, Gardner SN. *The Dietary Data Collection System: An Automated Interview and Coding System for NHANES III*. Proceedings of the 14th National Nutrient Databank Conference. Ithaca, NY: CBORD Group, Inc.; 1990.
12. Williams CL, Bollella M, Wyneler EL. A new recommendation for dietary fiber in childhood. *Pediatrics*. 1995;96:985-988.
13. Perry CL, Stone EJ, Parcel GS, Ellison RC, Nader PR, Webber LS, Luepker RV. School-based cardiovascular health promotion: the Child and Adolescent Trial for Cardiovascular Health (CATCH). *J Sch Health*. 1990;60(8):406-413.
14. Webber LS, Osganian SK, Luepker RV, Feldman HA, Stone EJ, Elder JP, Perry CL, Nader PR, Parcel GS, Broyles SL, McKinlay SM. Cardiovascular risk factors among third grade children in four regions of the United States. *Am J Epidemiol*. 1995;141(5):428-439.
15. Lytle LA, Johnson CC, Bachman K, Wambsgans K, Perry CL, Stone EJ, Budman S. Successful recruitment strategies for school-based health promotion: experiences from CATCH. *J Sch Health*. 1994;64(10):405-409.
16. Wechsler H, Wernick SM. A social marketing campaign to promote low-fat milk consumption in an inner-city Latino community. *Public Health Rep*. 1992;107:202-207.
17. Berenson GS, McMahan CA, Voors AW, Webber LS, Srinivasan SR, Frank GC, Foster TA, Blonde CV. *Cardiovascular Risk Factors in Children: The Early Natural History of Atherosclerosis and Essential Hypertension*. New York, NY: Oxford University Press; 1980.
18. Berenson GS, ed. *Causation of Cardiovascular Risk Factors in Children: Perspectives on Cardiovascular Risk in Early Life*. New York, NY: Raven Press; 1986.
19. Nicklas TA, Webber LS, Srinivasan SR, Berenson GS. Secular trends in dietary intakes and cardiovascular risk factors of 10-year-old children: the Bogalusa Heart Study (1973-1988). *Am J Clin Nutr*. 1993;57:930-937.
20. Kimm SY, Payne G, Lakatos E, Darby C, Sparrow A. Management of cardiovascular disease risk factors in children: a national survey of primary care physicians. *Am J Dis Child*. 1990;144:967-972.
21. The DISC Collaborative Research Group. Cholesterol-lowering diet is effective and safe in children with elevated LDL-cholesterol: three-year results of the dietary intervention study in children (DISC). *Circulation*. 1994;90(4):I-8, 39a. Abstract.
22. Hartmuller V, Snetselaar L, Van Horn L, Steinmuller P, Smith K, Gernhofer N, Evans M, Lasser V, Cecil M, Brown K, Craddick S, Stevens V, von Almen K, Chrostri J, Moag-Stahlberg A. Creative approaches to cholesterol lowering used in the Dietary Intervention Study in Children (DISC). *Topics Clin Nutr*. 1994;10:1.
23. Obarzanek E, Hunsberger SA, Van Horn L, Hartmuller VV, Barton BA, Stevens VJ, Kwiterovich PO, Franklin FA, Kimm SYS, Lasser NL, Simons-Morton DG, Lauer RM. Safety of a fat-reduced diet: the Dietary Intervention Study in Children (DISC). *Pediatrics*. 1997;100:51-59.
24. Kwiterovich PO, Barton BA, McMahon RP, Obarzanek E, Hunsberger S, Simons-Morton D, Kimm SYS, Aaronson Friedman L, Lasser N, Robson A, Lauer R, Stevens V, Van Horn L, Gidding S, Snetselaar L, Hartmuller VV, Franklin F. Effects of diet and sexual maturation on LDL-cholesterol during puberty: the Dietary Intervention Study in Children (DISC). *Circulation*. In press.
25. Shannon BM, Tershakovec AM, Martel JK, Achterberg CL, Cortner JA, Smiciklas-Wright HS. Reduction of elevated LDL-cholesterol levels of 4- to 10-year-old children through home-based dietary education. *Pediatrics*. 1994;94:923-927.
26. Tershakovec AM, Mitchell DC, Smiciklas-Wright H, Hartzel J, Shannon BM. Lower fat intake in children. *Circulation*. 1994;90(4):I-8, 37a. Abstract.
27. National Research Council. *Recommended Dietary Allowances*. 10th ed. Washington, DC: National Academy Press; 1989.

28. National Center for Health Statistics. Plan and operation of the Third National Health and Nutrition Examination Survey. 1988-1994. *Vital Health Stat 1*. 1994;32:1-407.
29. Trocano R, Flegal K, Kuczmarski R, Campbell S, Johnson C. Overweight prevalence and trends for children and adolescents. *Arch Pediatr Adolesc Med.* 1995;149:1085-1091.
30. US Department of Health and Human Services, Centers for Disease Control and Prevention. Update: Prevalence of overweight among children, adolescents, and adults—United States, 1988-1994. *Morbid Mortal Weekly Rep.* 1997;46(9):199-202.
31. Himes JH, Dietz WH. Guidelines for overweight in adolescent preventive services—recommendations from an expert committee: the Expert Committee on Clinical Guidelines for Overweight in Adolescent Preventive Services. *Am J Clin Nutr.* 1994;59:307-316.
32. Rolland-Cachera MF, Deheeger M, Guiloud-Bataille M, Avons P, Patois E, Sempe M. Tracking the development of adiposity from one month of age to adulthood. *Ann Hum Biol.* 1987;14:219-229.
33. Davis K, Christoffel KK. Obesity in preschool and school-age children. Treatment early and often may be best. *Arch Pediatr Adolesc Med.* 1994;148:1257-1261.
34. The DISC Intervention Committee. *Dietary Intervention Study in Children (DISC) Child Guidebook:* Nutrition Guidelines (C), Grains 1-89; Baltimore, Md; 1995.
35. Smith K, Ahrens L, Stickney L, Siglin D. *Sat Fat Tracking*. The Lipid Disorders Training Program, University of Iowa College of Medicine; Iowa City, Iowa. August 1995.
36. Stevens VJ, Obarzanek E, Franklin FA, Steinmuller P, Snetselaar L, Lavigne J, Batey D, von Almen K, Hartmuller V, Reimers T, Lasser VI, Craddick S, Gernhofer N. Dietary Intervention Study in Children (DISC): Intervention design and participation. *J Nutr Educ*. 1995;27:133-139.
37. The DISC Intervention Committee. *Dietary Intervention Study in Children (DISC) Adult Guidebook*: Nutrition Guidelines (A), Overview/Eggs 2-89; Baltimore, Md: 1995.
38. The DISC Intervention Committee. *Dietary Intervention Study in Children (DISC) Adult Guidebook:* Nutrition Guidelines (A), Fats 3-89; Baltimore, Md: 1995.
39. Prochaska JO, DiClemente CC. Transtheoretical therapy: toward a more integrative model of change. *Psychother Theory Res Practice.* 1982;19:276-288.
40. Prochaska JO, Velicer WF, Rossi JS, Goldstein MG, Marcus BH, Rakowski W, Fiore C, Harlow LL, Redding CA, Rosenbloom D, Rossi SR. Stages of change and decisional balance for twelve problem behaviors. *Health Psychol.* 1994;13:1-8.
41. Miller W, Rollnick S. *Motivational Interviewing: Preparing People to Change Addictive Behaviors*. New York, NY: The Guilford Press; 1991.

CHAPTER 11

Management of Cardiovascular Patients in a Hospital Setting

Karen Balnicki, MS, RD; and
Lori Silver-Kolodin, MPH, RD

Management of patients with cardiovascular disease (CVD) can be a challenge. The type-A, overachieving personality of many cardiac patients can be a causative factor for the disease. These patients and their families have usually read the latest magazine and newspaper articles about cardiac disease prevention and treatment. For other patients, a long-term high-fat diet and a sedentary lifestyle have contributed significantly to their disease.

Dietitians' credibility and effectiveness hinge on being aware of pertinent new research, food products, medications, and supplements that relate to cardiovascular health. Dietitians also need to be able and willing to teach basic nutrition principles and simple methods of preparing lower-fat foods that are compatible with a patient's tastes.

The roles and responsibilities of dietitians are evolving as the health care system changes. For example, as the length of hospital stays is reduced, traditional inpatient clinical positions are being moved into expanded outpatient programs, which emphasize the team approach. This chapter discusses the team approach to management of CVD patients and the development of an outpatient cardiac nutrition program, with reference to insurance reimbursement issues that are relevant to dietitians.

The Cardiac Health Care Team

Although cardiology emerged as a specialty in the 1920s, the team approach to patient care did not begin until the 1950s. The Vocational Rehabilitation Act of 1954 was the government's first effort to fund rehabilitation programs in post-World War II America.

The cardiac health care team is a select group of health care professionals who may interact daily and meet at regularly scheduled times to share and compare medical information about their patients. In a team approach, all team members contribute their knowledge, perspectives, and personal styles to the patient's care. When team members communicate a clear, well-reinforced plan to the patient, quality of care can be enhanced beyond what team members could achieve individually.

Being part of a cardiac health care team is a valuable and educational experience. The dietitian, an important member of the cardiac team, has the opportunity to share information with others and, in turn, learn valuable skills from other team members.

Benefits of a Team Approach

The way a health care team functions depends on the health care setting in which it operates. An inpatient setting enables the dietitian and other health care professionals to attend medical rounds together. Rounds provide an excellent opportunity for team members to interact and contribute to better patient care. In an outpatient setting, the physician, nurse, and dietitian may see a patient at consecutive, same-day appointments in the cardiac or lipid clinic. Such grouping of appointments is preferred because it is more convenient for the patient. In addition, it enables the dietitian to communicate any concerns to the physician or nurse immediately, when the other team member has just seen the patient and reviewed the medical chart.

The physician's trust in the working relationship with the dietitian is facilitated when the dietitian consistently demonstrates competence, knowledge of the field, clarity of expression, energy, and commitment. Rapid delivery of more effective, less costly patient care results when the physician makes use of the dietitian's nutrition and dietary assessments. For example, when the physician is familiar with the dietitian's in-depth assessment of the patient's consumption of energy and saturated and total fat, the physician can make a better informed decision to prescribe or adjust lipid-lowering medication.

Team members gain knowledge and appreciation of their colleagues' disciplines, approaches, and personal insights, enabling each member to more easily identify patients who could benefit from other team members' services.

Another important benefit of the team approach is that the responsibilities of team members overlap. For example, a dietitian, nurse, or social worker may conduct the initial interview with a cardiac patient, using a questionnaire that the team has developed for this purpose (Box 11-1). This questionnaire, which may be administered by any team member, asks about medications and supplements; cardiac lab results; exercise, smoking, alcohol, and food habits; and stress and social support. All team members are trained to interview patients, field questions from patients, and provide appropriate general information about the disciplines of other team members.

For the patient, working with a health care team whose members are in regular communication with one another and are aware of the patient's progress strengthens trust and instills positive feelings toward team members. This results in significantly enhanced compliance with dietary recommendations, medications, exercise, and stress management techniques as well as improved lipid status and overall feelings of well-being.

Members of the Health Care Team

Table 11-1 summarizes the roles of the members of the cardiac health care team. The team must include a physician, who may be a preventive medicine specialist; a cardiologist; an endocrinologist specializing in lipid disorders; or a physiatrist (a specialist in physical and rehabilitation medicine). The team must also include at least one nurse who is competent in exercise physiology or wellness. The dietitian is a critical team member because recovery from cardiac disease is strongly influenced by nutrition practices.

An exercise physiologist or physical therapist is valuable in a cardiac rehabilitation setting to evaluate and provide instruction to patients with specific physical limitations. A behavioral medicine professional is also an essential team member. This individual may be a psychiatrist, who can provide prescriptions for depression and stress-related needs; a psychologist, who is trained in behavioral and lifestyle-change counseling; or a social worker, who can address patients' social-support needs.

Managers and support staff are also important team members. In some situations, a nurse or dietitian may function as the program manager or coordinator. The responsibilities and challenges of management provide personal satisfaction and professional rewards to individuals who have an interest in and a talent for administration. In outpatient programs, the dietitian may function as both administrator and nutritionist. Additional responsibilities that may be delegated to the dietitian-administrator include preparing budgets, hiring and scheduling staff, contracting with consultants, developing educational programs, marketing, administering patient surveys, collecting measurements of program results, and generating monthly and annual reports.

Key support staff positions include the administrative assistant, who may schedule appointments and manage information about patients (ie, insurance approvals and reimbursements, medical records, and results of laboratory tests), as well as billing and insurance specialists, medical record transcriptionists, and data entry personnel.

Nontraditional team members may include a consultant chef, who performs cooking demonstrations of heart-healthy food; students, including dietetic interns; and other food professionals in the community. Former patients of an outpatient cardiac program may volunteer to teach a novel nutrition class, which may be inspiring for patients. (See The Team Approach to Group Classes, below; refer also to Chapter 15.)

Team Interactions and Treatment Plans

Communication is the key to successful team interaction. All forms of oral and written communication should be used: meetings, conference calls, e-mails, faxes, documentation in the medical record, or letters and memos.

In meetings or on rounds, the dietitian interacts with the team by reporting on the patient's nutrition assessment and treatment plan (Table 11-2). Usually the nurse or physician presents the patient's case, including risk factors and medical treatment, and other team members provide their comments and propose a plan or course of treatment. The team meeting provides team members with an opportunity to promote the importance of their specialty in advancing patient wellness. An appreciation of each member's specialty evolves as these interactions continue.

Team meetings often include discussion of treatment priorities. Nutrition receives high priority when the patient's risk factors include hyperlipidemia, hypertension, diabetes, or obesity. The dietitian plays an important role in devising the treatment plan for weight loss and managing these disorders.

Nutrition may not be the primary concern in the treatment plan. For example, in the case of a young man of desirable weight who smokes, has high levels of cholesterol, and has had a heart attack, the team may decide to address smoking cessation first and follow up with a plan of action to modify other risk factors. Even when nutrition is not a top priority for a patient, dietary therapy is the mainstay of managing CVD and the dietitian should continually promote good nutrition practices.

Nutrition and Behavioral Medicine

Ideally, a behavioral medicine professional should be directing the emotional health component of the patient's treatment plan. This team member's input is pertinent to all members because much of the effectiveness of the team is through the patient's change of behavior. The following anecdote illustrates the importance of having a behavioral medicine professional as a member of the health care team.

During a nutrition evaluation, a woman reported that her appetite, eating habits, and weight had changed significantly when her husband died. After further inquiry, the patient revealed to the dietitian conducting the initial interview that her husband had become depressed and had shot himself three years previously. She reported that she

BOX 11-1 Sample Patient Questionnaire for Initial Interview

PATIENT QUESTIONNAIRE

Name: ______ Medical Record #: ______
Date of Birth: ______ Age: ______ Sex: ______
Medical Problems/Cardiac Risk Factors: ______

______

______

WEIGHT HISTORY

Highest Adult Weight: ______ Date: ______ Lowest Adult Weight: ______ Date: ______
Height: ______ Today's Weight: ______ Desirable Weight Range: ______ Pts Goal Weight: ______
Pounds Overweight: ______ Short-Term Weight Goal: ______ Long-Term Weight Goal: ______

EXERCISE HISTORY

List all exercise activities done regularly.
Activity/Frequency/Duration: ______
Activity/Frequency/Duration: ______
Activity/Frequency/Duration: ______

MEDICATIONS AND LAB RESULTS

Medications:	Labs:			
HTN: ______	Blood pressure: ______			
______	Systolic BP >150 mm Hg		yes	no
______	Diastolic BP > 90 mm Hg		yes	no
Cholesterol: ______	TC ______	> 200 mg/dL	yes	no
______	HDL ______	< 35 mg/dL	yes	no
______	LDL ______	> 120 mg/dL	yes	no
______	TG ______	> 150 mg/dL	yes	no
	TC/HDL ratio ______	> 4.5	yes	no
Diabetes: ______	FBS ______	> 140 mg/dL	yes	no
______	Hgb A_1C ______	> 8%	yes	no

Aspirin: ______
Hormone replacement therapy (women only):
______

Vitamin/mineral supplements:
______
______

SUBSTANCE HABITS

Cigarette smoking, amount/years: yes no former

Alcohol type/frequency: ______ yes no former

Caffeine type/frequency: ______ yes no

CURRENT EATING HABITS

Estimated daily calories: ______
Low saturated fat/cholesterol: ______ yes no
Low sodium: ______ yes no
Diabetic: ______ yes no

SOCIAL HISTORY

Lives with: ______
Adequate social support? yes no
Stresses: ______ yes no
Occupation: ______

SUMMARY

______
______
______

Interviewed by: ______ Date: ______

TABLE 11-1

Cardiac Health Care Team Members and Their Roles

Team Member	Roles
Physician Cardiologist, Endocrinologist, or Physiatrist	Responsible for patient's overall treatment plan Assesses CVD status and informs patient of findings Prescribes and adjusts medications as necessary Authorizes exercise prescription (for cardiac rehabilitation) Monitors effectiveness of treatment plan Makes appropriate referrals to health care team members Reviews patient issues during cardiac rounds or clinic Communicates status and findings with all members of the team
Registered Nurse Nurse Practitioner Physician Assistant	Responsible for day-to-day overall management and communication with patient and other team members Gathers medical data and assesses patient status Provides education and clarification of the treatment plan Supervises exercise sessions (for cardiac rehabilitation) Educates patient about cardiac health and medications, exercise, smoking cessation, and stress management Reinforces nutrition messages Reviews patient issues during rounds or clinic
Registered Dietitian	Responsible for the patient's medical nutrition therapy Performs in-depth nutrition and dietary assessment Assesses patient's percent body fat and waist-to-hip ratio (in cardiac rehabilitation, may be done by registered nurse) Develops individualized nutrition care plan, educates patients and family, documents intervention Develops and conducts nutrition education classes (usually 1 class for inpatient, 5-10 for outpatient) Reviews patient issues during cardiac rounds or clinic Communicates any change in care plan with other team members
Exercise Professional (Physical Therapist or Exercise Physiologist)	Develops patient's exercise program Assesses patient's physical status Reviews patient's exercise pattern, making treatment recommendations and providing follow-up Supervises exercise sessions with registered nurse or physician Provides education regarding implementing an exercise program Communicates needs and progress of patient's exercise program to the health care team
Behavioral Medicine Professional (Psychiatrist, Psychologist, or Social Worker)	Assesses psychosocial status of patient Assesses and/or identifies patient's functional capacity for behavior change, management of stress, degree of anger, hostility, depression, coping skills, and social support May provide behavioral component of smoking cessation and weight management programs Communicates patient's status with other team members and makes recommendations for appropriate follow-up and/or referrals
Patient (the core of the team)	Responsible for working cooperatively with the entire health care team Provides accurate medical information to all team members Makes best effort to adhere with the treatment plans Complies with the follow-up plan identified Identifies problems with health care team members and communicates needs to team members in a timely fashion Involves family/support members in care plan when appropriate and possible

TABLE 11-2

Dietitian's Oral Report on the Patient's Nutrition Assessment and Treatment Plan

Nutrition Assessment	Dietary Assessment*	Lifestyle Factors†	Treatment Plan‡	Follow-up§
Height	Total calories	Exercise	Eating goals	Weekly nutrition education classes
Weight	Total fat grams	Smoking	Behavioral goals	Midpoint evaluation
% body fat	Saturated fat gm	Alcohol use	Weight loss goals	Phone calls
BMI	Cholesterol	Caffeine use	Exercise goals	
Waist-to-hip ratio	Sodium	Family relationships		
Weight history		Levels of depression		
		Degree of motivation		

*May include soluble fiber, soy, alcohol, vitamin E, beta-carotene, garlic, fish oils.

†May provide information confirming or conflicting with RN/MD report; this information often generates team discussion regarding the patient's treatment plan.

‡Report on nutrition education highlighting messages that others (particularly RN and psychosocial members) can reinforce.

§To support dietary behavior change and monitoring of patient's weight, lipids, and body composition.

dreamed of her husband nightly and was upset and stressed during sleep.

To develop the best treatment plan for a patient, all health care team members must know about circumstances such as this in a patient's history. If a team meeting is imminent, the dietitian may report this information at that time. Alternatively, if the patient is seeing another member of the health care team before a team meeting is scheduled to take place, the dietitian may convey the information to that team member. In the case described above, the woman had not been seeing a behavioral medicine professional and was referred to one.

Interactions Among Dietitians, Nurses, and Physicians

As stated earlier, in outpatient settings patients typically see various members of the health care team at consecutive, same-day appointments. If the physician or nurse sees the patient first, it is important that the dietitian be informed of any concerns about lipid changes or the patient's understanding of or adherence to the prescribed diet. The dietitian should address these concerns at the patient's appointment and communicate the findings of the nutrition assessment to the physician or nurse. If the dietitian sees the patient first, it is the dietitian's responsibility to communicate concerns to the nurse or physician. The medical record, often referred to as the team logbook, is the vehicle for written communication among members of the health care team.

The nurse usually is the team member with whom the dietitian communicates most frequently. In a cardiac rehabilitation setting, the nurse often monitors the patient three times per week at exercise sessions. Patient care will be enhanced if, before making a follow-up visit, the dietitian obtains an update from the nurse on the patient's progress and, after the visit, reports back to the nurse. In addition to reporting on the patient's progress in making dietary changes, the dietitian may share information and seek feedback from the nurse regarding the patient's motivation, attitude, and family situation.

Dietitians and nurses frequently interact in group education classes. The nurse may lead classes on cardiac signs, symptoms, and medications, whereas the dietitian leads classes on nutrition. (See Chapter 15 for suggested nutrition education topics.) Because cardiac health care and nutrition overlap considerably, curricula for group classes should be jointly planned and some classes co-led by a nurse and a dietitian.

The Team Approach to Group Classes

In addition to allowing patients to share ideas and learn from each other, group classes offer many opportunities for members of the health care team to work together. The dietitian and the physical therapist, exercise physiologist, or social worker may co-lead behavioral weight-loss programs that include an exercise component. The nurse, physician, and social worker may conduct smoking cessation programs in which the dietitian participates by discussing strategies to prevent weight gain.

A physical therapist or exercise physiologist can provide education on the health benefits of exercise and demonstrate exercises for safe and effective movement. A social worker or psychologist can discuss the psychological impact of cardiac disease, coping strategies, and techniques for improving communication skills and changing behavior. To reduce stress and promote healing, a psychologist or nurse trained in wellness can offer relaxation techniques, lead meditation sessions, and guide participants in creative visualization.

Guest speakers add variety and interest to group classes. For example, the dietitian may team up with a chef to conduct a cooking demonstration. A seafood buyer may present tips on the purchase and safe preparation of fish. A restaurant owner may be able to help patients to make lower-fat menu selections and discuss alternatives to fat for flavor enhancement. A spe-

BOX 11-2 Sample Program Survey for Evaluation

CARDIAC REHABILITATION PROGRAM EVALUATION

Today's Date: ____________________

1. How long have you been in our program? (circle one)

   (a) < 3 months (b) 3-6 months (c) 6-12 months (d) 1 year or more

2. How helpful have you found the following? Please rate using the numbers 1, 2, 3, or 4.

   1 = very helpful 2 = somewhat helpful 3 = not helpful 4 = did not attend

   ____ (a) Individual session(s) with the doctor
   ____ (b) Individual session(s) with the nurse
   ____ (c) Individual session(s) with the nutritionist
   ____ (d) Individual psychosocial session(s)
   ____ (e) Exercise instruction and sessions
   ____ (f) Nursing education classes
   ____ (g) Nutrition education classes
   ____ (h) Cooking/food demonstrations
   ____ (i) Supermarket tour
   ____ (j) Other ____________________

3. Are you satisfied with our program curriculum? (circle one)

   (a) yes (b) no (c) unsure

4. What would you like to see added to our program?

   ____
   ____
   ____

5. Would you recommend our program to friends and family? (circle one)

   (a) yes (b) no (c) unsure

   Why? ____________________________________
   ____

Thank you for your time and commitment to our program!

cialty food shop owner may be able to demonstrate the use of specialty mustards and vinegars in low-fat cooking.

Former patients who have successfully completed cardiac rehabilitation can provide inspiration by discussing their own case histories, the difficulties that they encountered and conquered, and the positive outcomes that they achieved, such as weight loss and lipid reduction. Such testimonials often provide valuable reinforcement of the health care team's message about the way to achieve a heart-healthy lifestyle.

Confronting Difficulties in Team Relations

Some team members may be unaware of the added benefit that a dietitian can bring to a health care team. A meeting or observational session with the dietitian may help such individuals to better understand the dietitian's role. Another strategy may be to offer the team member an individual nutrition counseling session. Every meeting of team members is an opportunity for individuals on the team to educate one another about the skills and tools each uses to provide quality patient care.

DEVELOPMENT OF AN OUTPATIENT CARDIAC NUTRITION PROGRAM

Most outpatient cardiac nutrition programs incorporate the principles of reducing consumption of fat and calories and increasing physical activity. Effective nutrition education empowers people to eat healthfully. It requires that the dietitian be knowledgeable, engaging, and creative. It is the dietitian's job to translate current scientific nutrition information into everyday language and provide specific, practical guidelines that patients can apply to the daily tasks of selecting, preparing, and enjoying food. Throughout the program, the dietitian should emphasize the importance of regular exercise as well as a low-fat diet in maintaining a heart-healthy lifestyle.

Initial Visit

An in-depth nutrition and dietary assessment by a dietitian is standard practice for all new cardiac patients (see Chapter 4). Anthropometric measurements to determine the patient's percentage of body fat and waist-to-hip ratio are also part of an outpatient nutrition assessment. An individual nutrition plan is designed to incorporate the patient's calorie and fat gram prescription and, if appropriate, carbohydrate or sodium restriction. It may be helpful to use the Food Guide Pyramid or diabetic exchanges to help the patient select appropriate portions of foods from the various food groups. Some patients find that counting grams of total or saturated fat consumed per day is a simple and effective way of monitoring a heart-healthy intake.

American Heart Association nutrition education materials based on National Cholesterol Education Program guidelines and those from other sources (see Appendix 3) provide a wealth of patient education information. After the patient receives nutrition education materials, a follow-up visit is scheduled and the assessment and nutrition care plan are documented in the medical record.

Program Design

Initially, patients in cardiac rehab should be seen for a 1-hour assessment and education session. If the patient is scheduled for cardiac rehabilitation three times per week and anticipates being in the program for at least 3 months, a midpoint nutrition follow-up visit is recommended to assess dietary change and reduction in weight, lipid levels, and body-fat percentage. At this second meeting, the patient may be more open to discussing difficulties with dietary compliance, and the dietitian can provide new and potentially more effective behavioral strategies.

Compliance with weekly nutrition education classes is better if these classes are scheduled before or after patients' exercise classes. For example, if 10 patients are scheduled for exercise sessions at 9:00 a.m. and 11:00 a.m., all 20 patients can be scheduled for nutrition education classes at 10:00 a.m.

Program Completion and Planning for the Future

An exit evaluation is important to document positive outcomes and assist in the preparation of an ongoing diet and exercise plan. Measurements of body-fat percentage and waist-to-hip ratio should be repeated and the results compared with the original and midpoint values. Changes in body weight and blood lipids should be assessed and documented. Blood pressure and blood glucose changes should also be noted if these values are significant for the patient.

Separate weight-loss classes are sometimes available in a hospital outpatient setting. The exit evaluation is a good time to refer patients to such classes if they still have weight to lose and could benefit from continued support. Although these programs are often not covered by health insurance, they are usually not costly.

To obtain feedback and suggestions for program improvements, many programs ask patients to complete a program survey (Box 11-2).

Reimbursement, Follow-up, and Outcomes

Nutrition follow-up is important for achieving positive outcomes such as reduced weight and body fat percentage and improved lipid levels. Unfortunately, the number of follow-up visits scheduled is often determined by the level of reimbursement available. Coverage varies greatly from state to state and among insurance carriers. Most carriers reimburse for cardiac rehabilitation only after a cardiac event such as a heart attack or angioplasty.

Carriers generally require that cardiac rehabilitation sessions include a specific nutrition education component, which justifies paying for dietitian services. However, the carrier does not pay the dietitian directly. Often a hospital agrees to pay for a fixed number of dietitian hours. It is then up to the dietitian to provide individual, group, and follow-up visits; attend weekly rounds; develop new educational materials; and document productivity and positive outcomes within the allotted funds. This arrangement gives the dietitian the flexibility to set priorities relative to the resources available.

To create a successful nutrition component in a cardiac rehabilitation program that enrolls approximately 40 patients four times per year, a minimum of 10 to 12 dietitian hours per week is recommended; 15 to 20 hours per week is ideal. Table 11-3 outlines how one cardiac rehabilitation program allocates dietitian time for nutrition care.

Without an adequate contribution of dietitian time, it will be difficult to achieve significant patient progress. The ultimate cost of the cardiac event is likely to increase far beyond the cost of the dietitian component. Dietitian intervention is a noninvasive, reliable, cost-efficient long-term approach to CVD management. In an effort to reduce overall health care costs, the American Dietetic Association is pursuing third-party reimbursement for dietitian services nationally.

Insurance Coverage for Nutrition Services

Some health insurers will pay for between 2 and 5 nutrition visits per year, regardless of whether a cardiac event occurs, if there is medical justification for the visit. Many carriers, however, will not pay for any dietitian services, even those

TABLE 11-3

Dietitian's Time Allocation for Nutrition Care of Cardiac Rehabilitation Patients (sample)

RD Roles	Time and Frequency	Hours per Week
Initial Assessment and Counseling	1 hour	2
Nutrition and dietary analysis	2 new patients per week	
Lipid and body fat assessment		
Nutrition education		
Dietary goals		
Midpoint Evaluation	½ hour	1
(conducted at week 6)	2 patients per week	
Body weight		
Lipid profile		
Body fat		
Dietary changes		
Dietary goals revised and reinforced		
Exit Evaluation	½ hour	1
(conducted during the last two weeks of the 13 week program)	2 patients per week	
Body weight		
Lipid profile		
Body fat		
Dietary changes		
Dietary goals		
Long-term strategy designed		
Nutrition Education Classes	1 hour classes	2
5-10 nutrition topics	Twice weekly	
Individual Follow-up for High-risk Patients	20 to 30 minutes	1 to 1½
Severe dyslipidemia	2 to 3 patients per week	
Hypertension		
Obesity		
Uncontrolled diabetes		
Patient Rounds/Team Meetings	1-hour meeting per week	1
Communication with Team Members	Varies	1
Patient issues		
Lab results		
Medical record documentation		
Development of Handouts/ Lesson Plans	Varies	1 to 1½
Initial development		
Revision of materials		
Total Hours		10 to 12

that are medically justified. Other insurers pay a lump sum to the physician for the care of a patient; the physician then determines how best to spend the available funds. This system is known as *capitation*. Nutrition services are reimbursable in a capitation system when physicians understand the value of dietitian intervention and actively use the services. It is expected that by 2005, 75% of health insurers will be using a capitation system.

It is in the best interests of patient care, cost containment, and the future of dietetics that dietitians document the beneficial outcomes of nutrition intervention and the potential cost savings to both patients and insurers. This information can be used to promote the value of dietitian services and medical nutrition therapy to physicians, insurers, legislators, and potential clients.

SUMMARY

A well-functioning health care team can greatly enhance the health management of the CVD patient. All team members—and most importantly, the patient—benefit from the team's interactions.

Participating in a cardiac health care team affords dietitians the opportunity to share information with patients and other team members while expanding their counseling, teaching, management, and communication skills. Team participation is challenging, personally rewarding, and fun.

To document results and outcomes, it is essential to perform a thorough assessment at both the beginning and the completion of a cardiac nutrition program. These data will ensure that the program serves its participants and will also provide justification for insurance reimbursement.

CHAPTER 12

Functional Foods and Their Application in the Prevention of Cardiovascular Disease

Jill Upton-Stocki, MS, RD; Valerie Fishell, MS; Kristin Moriarty, MS, RD; and John Milner, PhD

For years people in the United States have been searching for the perfect diet—a diet that promotes well-being and prevents diseases—but only recently has this holistic approach to medicine received scientific endorsement. New clinical and epidemiologic studies are reporting the benefits of specific foods or ingredients for preventing disease as well as new technologies that are making foods more healthful. Foods that have health-promoting properties are now being classified as functional foods.

Functional foods are foods that contain ingredients that aid specific bodily functions in addition to being nutritious (1). A functional food is any food that has a positive effect on a person's health, physical performance, or state of mind (2).

Consumers, health professionals, and the food and health care industries have become increasingly interested in functional foods. As our population ages, consumers are looking for nonpharmacologic ways to prevent diseases and slow the aging process, and health care professionals want to know how to prevent the terrible and costly diseases that affect patients. The food and pharmaceutical industries are interested in functional foods because they see a tremendous opportunity for profit in producing and marketing healthful food products that may prevent diseases.

This chapter reviews six of the more recognized functional foods, their potential health benefits, and their application in a health care professional's practice.

Fish Oil and Fish-oil Supplements

The possible health benefits of fish and fish oils were first suspected when it was discovered that Greenland Eskimos had very low morbidity and mortality from cardiovascular disease (CVD) despite their high fat intake (3-6). Bang and Dyerberg (3-5) studied the Eskimos' diet in the early 1970s and observed that it was low in carbohydrates and high in fat, with most of the fat coming from fish and other marine animals that have a high n-3 (omega-3) fatty acid content. Epidemiologic studies of the Japanese (who also traditionally have high fish intakes) demonstrated that high intakes of n-3 fatty acids correlated with a low incidence of CVD (7). This led the investigators to hypothesize that marine oils, which are high in n-3 fatty acids, have antiatherogenic properties (3,4,7). Since then retrospective, prospective, and clinical studies have examined the role of n-3 fatty acids (from fish consumption and fish-oil supplementation) in the prevention of CVD. A recent American Heart Association Science Advisory, authored by Stone (8) summarizes the studies that have been conducted to date.

The n-3 fatty acid content of fish depends on the species of fish as well as whether it was wild or farm raised. Wild fish generally have higher amounts of n-3 fatty acids than do farm-raised fish. Box 4-8 lists the amounts of n-3 fatty acids in commonly eaten fish as well as the amounts supplied by some commercially available fish-oil supplements.

The fat in fish and fish oils is predominantly the highly unsaturated n-3 fatty acids eicosapentaenoic acid (EPA) and docosahexaenoic acid (DHA). Small amounts of EPA and DHA can be formed in humans from α-linolenic acid (LN) (9,10), but most of the health benefits attributed to n-3 fatty acids are thought to be attributable to the consumption of EPA and DHA and not LN (11-13). However, the Lyon Diet-Heart Study reported remarkable effects of an LN-enriched diet on secondary prevention of coronary events and sudden death (14). In the experimental group, 302 patients who had experienced a myocardial infarct followed a Mediterranean-type diet high in LN for 5 years. The risk of cardiac death was reduced by 76% in the treatment group compared with the control group.

Because LN competes with the other polyunsaturated fatty acid family (the n-6 family) for the enzymes responsible for desaturating and elongating it to form EPA and DHA, increasing the amount of LN relative to the n-6 fatty acid linoleic acid (LA) in the diet increases the concentration of highly unsaturated n-3 fatty acids in the body.

Biological Effects of N-3 Fatty Acids

EPA is a precursor to the metabolically active eicosanoids. Eicosanoids, consisting of prostaglandins, thromboxanes, and leukotrienes, are involved in inflammation and blood clotting, both of which play critical roles in the etiology of CVD. Eicosanoids are formed from either arachidonic acid (a highly unsaturated n-6 fatty acid) or EPA. The type of eicosanoid formed and its subsequent action depend on the fatty acid from which it is formed. Arachidonic acid gives rise to the 2-series of prostaglandins and thromboxanes and to the 4-series of leukotrienes, whereas EPA gives rise to the 3- and 5-series, respectively. Figure 12-1 illustrates the functional consequences of the different eicosanoid series. The actions of EPA-derived eicosanoids on platelets, endothelial cells, and leukocytes are more desirable than those of eicosanoids derived from arachidonic acid. Thus, increasing cell EPA levels by emphasizing n-3 fatty acids in the diet results in a more beneficial eicosanoid profile. One study indicated that consumption of fish oils is 10 times more efficient than consumption of LN for increasing tissue EPA levels (15).

Beneficial Effects

Coronary Heart Disease and Stroke Risk. Epidemiologic and prospective cohort studies reported beneficial effects of n-3 fatty acids on CVD. Kromhout, Bosschieter, and Coulander (16) reported a 50% reduction in coronary mortality in 852 Dutch men who consumed more than 30 g of fish each day compared with those who consumed no fish. These investigators concluded that consumption of as few as one to two fish meals per week may protect against the development of coronary heart disease (CHD). Shekelle, Shryock, Paul, Lepper, Stamler, Liu, and Raynor (17) reported similar results for 1,931 American men followed in the Western Electric Study.

Dolecek (18) examined the relationship between the intake of various polyunsaturated fatty acids (as estimated from four dietary recall interviews at baseline and follow-up years one, two, and three) in the usual care group of the men who participated in the Multiple Risk Factor Intervention Trial (MRFIT). Significant inverse relationships between intake and CHD and CVD mortality were observed for both the parent n-3 fatty acid (LN) and the sum of the fatty acids derived from fish and fish oils (EPA and DHA). This study did not directly assess fish intake and suggested that total n-3 fatty acids are associated with decreased mortality from CVD (no significant associations were observed for the parent n-6 fatty acid, LA).

In a prospective dietary intervention study, the Diet and Reinfarction Trial (DART), 2,033 men who had just recovered from a myocardial infarction were randomly assigned to a treatment or control group (19). The treatment group, who received dietary advice about increasing their fish consumption (ie, to 300 g/week or about three servings), had a 29% reduction in 2-year all-cause mortality and a 33% reduction in ischemic heart disease mortality. Interestingly, early death rates were decreased in men assigned to the fish supplemented diet.

These studies suggest that individuals who consume fish at moderate levels (20 g/day to 30 g/day; the equivalent of one to two fish meals per week) are at lower risk of developing CVD than those who do not eat any fish and are at lower risk of sudden death from coronary disease. Two other major clinical trials, however, failed to report an association between fish consumption (Health Professionals Follow-up Study [20]) and fish-oil intake (Physicians' Health Study [21]) and the incidence of CHD and myocardial infarction. The reasons for these discrepant findings are not apparent. Further studies are needed to clarify the effect of fish and fish-oil consumption on risk and incidence of CHD. In addition, because of the conflicting findings of clinical trials that reported beneficial effects (22) of fish-oil supplementation on the rate of restenosis in patients who had undergone angioplasty and those that reported no significant effect (23), further studies are warranted. Another clinical trial reported no changes in the coronary artery diameter of normocholesterolemic men with CHD who took

FIGURE 12-1

Simplified scheme of eicosanoid formation from arachidonic acid (AA) or eicosapenteanoic acid (EPA) in different cell types

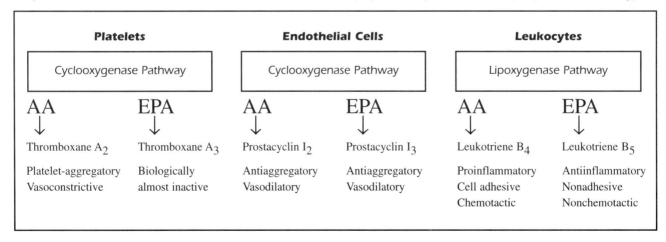

Platelets		Endothelial Cells		Leukocytes	
Cyclooxygenase Pathway		Cyclooxygenase Pathway		Lipoxygenase Pathway	
AA	EPA	AA	EPA	AA	EPA
↓	↓	↓	↓	↓	↓
Thromboxane A_2	Thromboxane A_3	Prostacyclin I_2	Prostacyclin I_3	Leukotriene B_4	Leukotriene B_5
Platelet-aggregatory Vasoconstrictive	Biologically almost inactive	Antiaggregatory Vasodilatory	Antiaggregatory Vasodilatory	Proinflammatory Cell adhesive Chemotactic	Antiinflammatory Nonadhesive Nonchemotactic

6 g of n-3 fatty acids daily for 2 years, which might suggest that the reported beneficial effects of fish and fish oil on CHD may be attributable to mechanisms unrelated to atherosclerosis (24). Thus, the evidence to date indicates that fish consumption is associated with a reduced incidence of CHD in certain population groups. The evidence suggests that fish consumption favorably affects the rate of sudden death from coronary disease. In contrast, it has not been shown consistently to reduce rates of restenosis after angioplasty.

Blood Lipids. The variability in the effect of fish oils on blood lipids is related to the presence of primary hyperlipoproteinemia (25-27). Harris (25,26) summarized the literature evaluating the effects of n-3 fatty acids on serum lipids in subjects with hyperlipoproteinemia and hypertriglyceridemia. Data from normal subjects as well as subjects with Type IIa, IIb, and IV/V lipoproteinemias are presented in Table 12-1.

Regardless of condition, consumption of 5 g to 8 g of n-3 fatty acids (equivalent to one to two fish meals per day or 12 to 20, 1-g fish-oil capsules per day) markedly decreased triglyceride levels (approximately 20% to 52%). The effects of fish oils on other blood lipids are less marked and vary considerably among normal and hyperlipidemic individuals. In normolipidemic individuals n-3 fatty acids had no significant effect on low-density lipoprotein cholesterol (LDL-C) or high-density lipoprotein cholesterol (HDL-C). However, in individuals with Type IV/V hyperlipoproteinemia, LDL-C increased markedly despite a significant decrease in triglycerides. More recently, Harris (26) reported greater triglyceride-lowering effects of n-3 fatty acids in hypertriglyceridemic (-34%) than in normotriglyceridemic (-25%) subjects.

Thrombus Formation. Thrombus (or blood clot) formation, the precipitating event in a myocardial infarction, occurs when a blood clot blocks blood flow in an artery that is occluded by a plaque. Prevention of plaque and thrombus formation reduces the risk of myocardial infarction as well as stroke and peripheral artery disease. Platelet aggregation is a key step in thrombus formation. As discussed previously, EPA is the precursor to the class of eicosanoids that have antiaggregatory, vasodilatory, and nonadhesive effects. This effectively makes the platelets less sticky, which decreases thrombus formation so that the risk of occlusion is less.

Hypertension. A meta-analysis of controlled clinical trials by Morris, Sacks, and Rosner (28) showed that fish-oil supplementation resulted in a small but significant decrease in blood pressure (-0.66/-0.35 mmHg/g n-3 fatty acids). This beneficial effect was observed in patients with preexisting hypertension or heart disease; subjects with normal blood pressure were not affected by fish oil. Whether such a small benefit warrants widespread supplementation of individuals with hypertension remains to be resolved.

Antiarrythmias. Dietary n-3 fatty acids may be protective against lethal cardiac arrhythmias (29). An observational study (30) showed that low levels of fish-oil intake (approximately one fish meal per week) were associated with a 50% reduction in the risk of cardiac arrest. Two small placebo-controlled studies corroborated these findings (31, 32). Animal studies have demonstrated that n-3 fatty acids are antiarrhythmic (29). Because cardiac arrhythmias are thought to precipitate a large proportion of sudden cardiac deaths, consumption of at least one fish meal per week by high-risk populations may confer protective effects.

Adverse Effects

One potential adverse effect of a high fish-oil intake is that bleeding time is prolonged as a result of decreased platelet aggregation (5). Nosebleeds can be a serious problem for the Eskimos, who have an extremely high intake of n-3 fatty acids (14 g/day) (3). However, studies in Westernized populations found an inverse relationship between n-3 fatty acid intake and stroke in African-American men and women and in white women and no association in white men (33), most likely because of a reduction in stroke caused by atherosclerotic lesions in vessels supplying the brain. In addition, abnormal bleeding times were not observed in studies that prescribed large doses of n-3 fatty acids (up to 9 g/day). Thus, consumption of fish oil in the recommended range of 3 g/day to 4 g/day does not increase the likelihood of prolonged bleeding and may actually decrease the risk of stroke. Care should be taken to monitor individuals who are also receiving pharmacological anticoagulative therapy (eg, aspirin or coumadin). Minor side effects of fish-oil capsule consumption are a fishy aftertaste and indigestion, which can be lessened by consuming the capsules with meals. Other potential side effects of fish-oil capsules were described recently by Stone (8) (Box 12-1).

TABLE 12-1

Effect of n-3 Fatty Acids on Blood Lipids in Normal Individuals and Those with Familial Hyperlipidemias

Subject	% Change Total-C	LDL-C	HDL-C	TG	n (# studies)	n-3/day (g)
Normal	–1.8	+0.03	+3.4	–25.2	596(14)	5.3
Type IIa	+1.3	+2.3	+3.8	–20.3	37(3)	4.9
Type IIb	–2.0	+5.6	+7.3	–38.0	194(12)	6.4
Type IV/V	–7.8	+29.9	+9.7	–52.2	101(12)	8.0

Adapted from Harris WS (25).

BOX 12-1 Potential Side Effects of Fish-oil Capsules

General:	Fishy odor, gastrointestinal upset
Coagulation:	Increased bleeding time may result in nosebleeds, easy bruising
Metabolism:	Can increase cholesterol in those with combined hyperlipidemia Can increase calorie intake and hence weight gain Some preparations have added cholesterol Some lack vitamin E (alpha tocopherol); concern for oxidation
Immune response:	Various parameters are decreased (uncertain significance)
Toxicity:	Vitamin A and D toxicity with some preparations Some fish oils (not highly refined) may contain pesticides Concerns regarding effects on immune response
Cost:	Expensive compared with dietary fish intake

Source: Stone NJ (8).

Recommendations

Currently, the American Medical Association and the American Dietetic Association do not promote the use of fish-oil supplements. A recent American Heart Association Science Advisory recommended fish-oil capsules only for the rare patient with severe, treatment-resistant hypertriglyceridemia at increased risk for pancreatitis (8). Increasing fish consumption is an appropriate alternative to supplementation. Fish are a nutrient-dense food, are low in saturated fat, and vary in levels of n-3 fatty acids. Although higher in total fat, fattier fish contain more n-3 fatty acids. Substituting fish for red meat can reduce saturated fat intake. Because fish consumption beneficially affects CVD mortality and the incidence of sudden death from coronary disease, the recommendation to increase fish consumption can benefit many individuals and, in turn, reduce the incidence of CVD morbidity and mortality in certain populations.

Nutritionists have been hesitant to recommend fish-oil supplementation for a variety of reasons. Although fish-oil capsules are available over the counter with vitamin supplements, fish oil taken in large doses is a pharmacological-type therapy. There is no clearly prescribed dosage of fish-oil supplements to guide the practitioner. The Greenland Eskimos consume approximately 14 g of fish oils a day in their diet (3), which is equivalent to approximately 13 to 26 capsules per day—a difficult regime to follow. This translates to divided doses of 6 to 9, 1-g capsules of fish oils taken 2 to 3 times per day. Clinical studies have shown beneficial effects with fish oils at levels of 3 g to 4 g of EPA and DHA per day (25-27), a level that could be managed by most people.

Because of the data linking fish consumption and reduction in CVD mortality, especially a reduction in the rate of sudden death, a prudent recommendation would be to eat fish at least once each week and preferably more often. The emphasis should be on ingesting fish high in n-3 fatty acids, such as salmon, sardines, and mackerel, but lower-fat fish is also recommended. Certain patients with severe hypertriglyceridemia (more than 1,000 mg/dL) may benefit from fish-oil supplementation, especially when attempts to treat secondary causes (through diet, exercise, and gemfibrozil) are unsuccessful, but close follow-up by a lipid specialist familiar with marine oil therapy is advisable.

TRANS FATTY ACIDS

Trans fatty acids are not typical functional foods; *trans* and *cis* fatty acids are two isomeric forms of unsaturated fatty acids found in the diet. The *trans-cis* nomenclature reflects the arrangement of the hydrogen at the site of the double bond. In the *trans* configuration the hydrogen atoms are on opposite sides of the double bond; in the *cis* configuration they are on the same side (Figure 12-2). The public discussion about the relationship between *trans* fatty acids and LDL-C levels has led to questions about the role that margarine and shortening (the major sources of *trans* fatty acids in the diet) should play in a healthful diet. Our current understanding of *trans* fatty acid effects on serum cholesterol levels and, in turn, the incidence of CVD is discussed below.

Trans Fatty Acid Consumption in the United States

Small amounts of *trans* fatty acids occur naturally in meats and dairy products, but the most abundant source of *trans* fatty acids is partially hydrogenated vegetable oils, such as margarine and shortening (34). Hydrogenation converts liquid vegetable oils to fats that are solid at room temperature and is used by the food industry to make fats with valuable functional, sensory, and stability properties.

The consumption of *trans* fatty acids has changed little since the 1970s despite an appreciable increase in the intake of vegetable fat, in the form of shortening and margarine, and a concomitant decrease in intake of animal fat. This is partly because new products tend to contain fewer *trans* fatty acids (eg, tub margarine vs stick margarine) as a result of advances in food technology. Current *trans* fatty acid intake in the US diet is estimated to be between 8.1 g/day and 12.8 g/day, or approximately 5% to 6% of total fat intake and 2% to 4% of energy (35). The most abundant food sources are stick margarines, commercial shortenings, bakery cookies, snack chips, and some fast foods (eg, french fries) (see Box 4-9).

Biological Effects

The health effects of *trans* fatty acids in partially hydrogenated oils in the diet have received considerable scientific and consumer attention during the past few years (36-40). Epidemiologic and metabolic studies suggested that *trans* fatty acids may be like saturated fat and raise plasma total cholesterol and LDL-C levels (36-40). These studies, however, have several limitations (34). In particular, there are questions about the accuracy of the *trans* fatty acid intake data as a result of an incomplete food composition database for *trans* fatty acids and limitations in dietary assessment methodologies. In some of the clinical studies conducted, there were significant design issues because *trans* fatty acids were substituted for unsaturated fatty acids, thus raising questions about whether the plasma effects were due to including *trans* fatty acids in the diet or to decreasing unsaturated fatty acids.

Epidemiologic Studies. Epidemiologic studies have shown a weak correlation between *trans* fatty acid intake and the incidence of CHD or CHD risk factors. Troisi, Willet, and Weiss (37) examined data from the Normative Aging Study and assessed the relations among *trans* fatty acid intake and serum cholesterol, LDL-C, HDL-C, triglycerides, the ratio of total cholesterol to HDL-C, and the ratio of LDL-C to HDL-C. *Trans* fatty acid intake was assessed with a food frequency questionnaire. The results indicated that there was a small, positive, significant correlation ($r = 0.03$ and $r = 0.9$, for unadjusted and partial correlations, respectively) between *trans* fatty acid intake and blood LDL-C levels. The results of the relation between *trans* fat and HDL-C was not significant after confounding variables were controlled for (37).

Another study (40) examined data from the Nurse's Health Study. *Trans* fatty acid intake was again determined with use of a food frequency questionnaire. As *trans* fatty acid intake increased from the lowest quintile of intake to the highest quintile, there was an associated increase in CHD risk. However, the *trans* fatty acid intake and CHD risk relationship was J-shaped, ie, the lowest CHD risk was associated with the middle quintile of *trans* fatty acid consumption (3.9 g/day) whereas higher risk of CHD was associated with both lower (2.4 g/day) and higher (5.7 g/day) intakes of *trans* fatty acids. *Trans* fatty acid intake by participants in the Nurse's Health Study was below the average intake of typical Americans, even for the high-intake quintile, which likely reflects the use of a food frequency questionnaire to collect these data. Thus, additional epidemiologic studies are needed to more firmly establish the association between *trans* fatty acids and risk of CVD.

Controlled Feeding Studies. The results of clinical studies comparing the effects of *trans* fatty acids on LDL-C with those of saturated fatty acids are inconsistent. Of the five controlled clinical studies (36,39,41-43) specifically designed to evaluate *trans* fatty acid effects on plasma lipids and lipoproteins, three (41-43) reported that saturated fatty acids increased LDL-C compared with *trans* fatty acids whereas two (36,39) reported similar effects of saturated and *trans* fatty acids on LDL-C levels. Clinical studies have consistently shown that, compared with unsaturated fatty acids, *trans* fatty acids raise total and LDL cholesterol (36,39,41,42). Thus, the evidence to date suggests that *trans* fatty acids are hypercholesterolemic compared with unsatu-

FIGURE 12-2
Configuration of cis and trans unsaturated double bonds

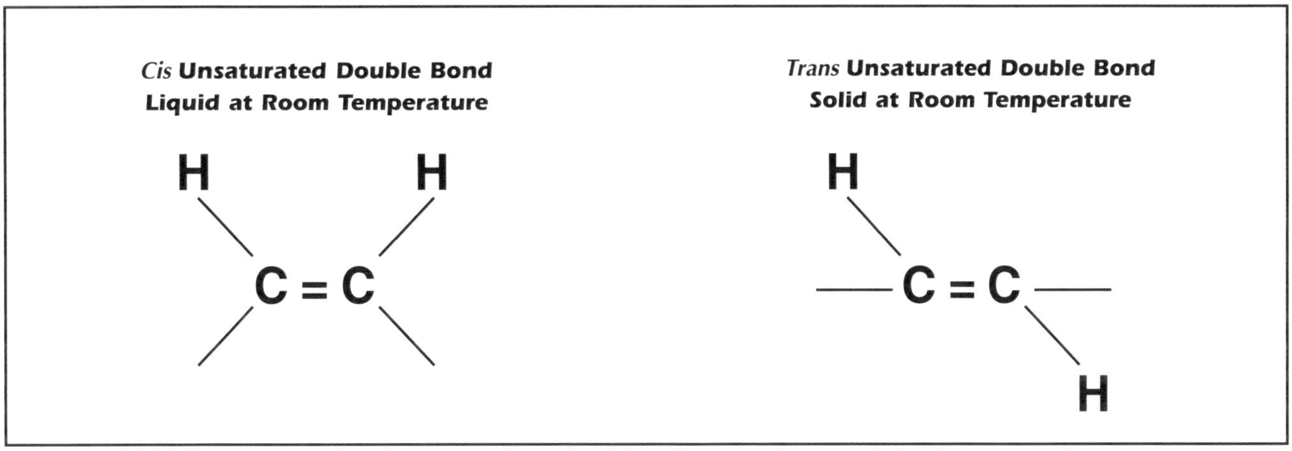

rated fatty acids and either hypocholesterolemic compared with saturated fatty acids or of equal potency to them.

Conflicting data on the effects of *trans* fatty acids on HDL-C were reported. Judd, Clevidance, Muesing, Wittes, Sunkin, and Podczasy (39) found that moderate intakes (4% of energy) of *trans* fatty acids had no effect on HDL-C. High intakes (7% of energy) of *trans* fatty acids, however, resulted in HDL-C levels of 1.38 mmol/L, whereas these values were 1.42 mmol/L for an oleic acid diet and 1.47 mmol/L for a saturated fatty acid diet. Nestel, Noakes, and Belling (41) found that saturated fatty acids increased HDL-C and *trans* fatty acids had no effect, which contrasts with the results of Mensink and Katan (36), who found that saturated fatty acids had no effect on HDL-C and *trans* fatty acids decreased HDL-C. Thus, the evidence to date indicates that compared with both saturated and unsaturated fatty acids, *trans* fatty acids have an unfavorable effect on the ratio of LDL-C to HDL-C.

Effects on Other Coronary Heart Disease Risk Factors

High levels of lipoprotein(a) have been associated with increased CHD risk. Four studies evaluated the effect of *trans* fatty acids on Lp(a) levels (41,43-45). Three studies reported an Lp(a)-raising effect (41, 43, 44) and one showed no effect on Lp(a) (45). Effects have been noted in subjects with high baseline levels of Lp(a); *trans* fatty acids appear not to affect Lp(a) levels in individuals with low baseline levels, which seems to have an underlying genetic basis.

Recommendations

In response to consumer awareness and demand, some fast-food restaurants have switched from using solid vegetable fats (30% *trans* fatty acids) to more liquid oils (approximately 15% *trans* fatty acids) (34). Recent advances in plant technology have produced fats low in *trans* fatty acids; plant breeders are genetically modifying the polyunsaturated fatty acid content of oil seed to reduce the need for hydrogenation (34).

Recently, there has been public discussion about the effects of *trans* fatty acids. Recommending an overall decrease in total fat consumption to no more than 30% of energy will lead to a decrease in both saturated fatty acids and *trans* fatty acids. Because *trans* fatty acids make up a modest proportion of the total fat in the diet it is not appropriate to focus on these acids exclusively and de-emphasize saturated fatty acids. However, it is advisable to counsel patients at high risk for CHD, especially those who are already following a program of intensive dietary therapy to maximally lower total cholesterol and LDL-C levels, about *trans* fatty acids. A recent American Heart Association Science Advisory recommends using naturally occurring unhydrogenated oil when possible and softer margarine instead of harder margarines and cooking fats that are higher in *trans* fatty acids (46) . Unhydrogenated oil and soft margarine are recommended over butter and naturally occurring fats such as palm oil that are solid at room temperature. These recommendations are intended to reduce consumption of saturated fatty acids and *trans* fatty acids, and in turn, reduce the risk of CVD (47).

ANTIOXIDANTS

Antioxidant supplements, including vitamins C and E and beta carotene, are the fastest-growing category of dietary supplements on the market. Their popularity is due to their potential health benefits, including reducing CVD and cancer risk, enhancing immune cell function, improving degenerative disease symptoms, and possibly slowing the aging process.

Oxidation has undesirable side effects such as the generation of peroxides, superoxide anions, and hydroxyl radicals. These byproducts of metabolism are collectively known as *free radicals* and cause cell and tissue damage. Free radicals may directly or indirectly promote atherogenesis by causing oxidation of LDL particles. When free radicals modify fatty acids, a chain reaction is initiated that eventually results in the continued production of peroxides or free radicals. This reaction is terminated only when two free radicals meet and join unpaired electrons (48) or when an antioxidant donates an unpaired electron to stop the reaction.

Although the relationship between LDL and CHD has been known for decades, the role that oxidized LDL plays in CHD progression has been appreciated only more recently (49-51). Oxidized LDL is cytotoxic and damages endothelial cells lining arteries, which facilitates the uptake of circulating monocytes and macrophages by the artery wall. The resident macrophages then take up oxidized LDL, resulting in the formation of foam cells, which eventually leads to the development of plaque. As this process progresses there is a continual narrowing of the artery lumen, eventually leading to the blockage of blood flow through the artery. As LDL levels increase, more LDL is available for oxidation, which in turn increases CVD risk. The fat-soluble antioxidants, vitamin E and beta carotene, are transported in the body in the LDL particle, whereas the water-soluble vitamin, vitamin C, is present in extracellular fluid (52).

Vitamin E

Background. The primary function of vitamin E in the body is to maintain the integrity of cell membranes by preventing the oxidation of polyunsaturated fatty acids. *Vitamin E* is a generic term for all tocol and tocotrienol derivatives that exhibit the biological activity of α-tocopherol, one of the naturally occurring tocopherols. The other naturally occurring tocopherols are beta-, gamma-, and delta-tocopherols. All of the naturally occurring tocopherols have the same molecular configuration around the chiral centers in the phytyl tail and are referred to as R-R-R-tocopherol, d-tocopherol, or (+)-tocopherol. Commercially synthesized tocopherols are a mixture of the eight possible R-L isomers and are referred to as all-rac-tocopherol or [dl]-tocopherol. The distinction among the tocopherol stereoisomers is of biological importance because their potencies vary in vivo (alpha > beta > gamma > delta). One milligram of the acetic ester of an all-rac mixture of alpha-tocopherol has the vitamin E activity of 1 International Unit (IU) and is used as the standard with which to measure all other tocopherols and tocotrienols. On this basis, 1 mg of R-R-R-α-tocopherol acetate (which is more stable than the free form) has a vitamin E activity of 1.36 IU and 1 mg of all-rac-α-tocopherol (a mixture of eight possible isomers) has a vitamin E activity of 1.1 IU.

The tocotrienols have only one chiral center, so they have only *d* and *l* sterioisomers. However, there are two double bonds present in the phytyl tail, which allows for the existence of four *cis*/*trans* isomers. In contrast to the tocopherols, there is little information on the antioxidant effects of tocotrienols.

Exciting evidence is emerging that vitamin E has a beneficial effect on risk of coronary disease (53-56). Observational studies reported a protective effect of vitamin E on CVD risk (53,54) and intervention studies corroborated these findings (55,56). The Cambridge Heart Antioxidant Study reported that patients with severe heart disease who received either 400 or 500 IU of vitamin E per day had a 47% reduction in major cardiovascular events and a 77% decrease in risk of nonfatal myocardial infarction (56). Ongoing intervention studies will clarify the extent of both beneficial and potentially beneficial effects of vitamin E on CVD risk. Besides reducing LDL oxidation as a result of its potent antioxidant properties, vitamin E reduces platelet aggregation and thrombus formation (57).

Dietary Sources and Recommendations. Food sources of vitamin E include vegetable oils, dark green leafy vegetables, nuts, avocados, whole grain cereals, fortified cereals, and eggs (Box 12-2). The current US intake of vitamin E is 7-11 mg/day, but this varies widely depending on fat intake (59). The current Recommended Dietary Allowance (RDA) for vitamin E is 8 mg/day to 10 mg/day (59). Levels of vitamin E below 100 mg/day do not appear to reduce CVD risk (51). Clinical trials have shown that 400–800 IU/day of vitamin E reduces CHD by ~40% (51).

Carotenoids and Beta Carotene

Background. Beta carotene, a member of the carotenoid family, is synthesized by plants and converted into vitamin A by the body in the intestinal mucosa. Of the more than 500 carotenoids found naturally, only about 50 have provitamin A activity. Beta carotene is the most abundant and biologically active carotenoid. Beta carotene functions as an antioxidant (60,61) and of the carotenoids makes the most important quantitative contribution to human nutrition. The bioavailability of beta carotene in food is not as great as that of retinol (another form of vitamin A) or of pure carotenoid substances but is increased with cooking (62).

The biological effectiveness of beta carotene and retinol is such that 6 μg of dietary beta carotene is equivalent to 1 μg of retinol. The vitamin A activity in foods is currently expressed as retinol equivalents (REs): 1 RE is equal to 1 μg of all-*trans*-retinol, 6 μg of all-*trans*-beta carotene, or 12 mg of other vitamin A carotenoids. Ingestion of high doses of preformed vitamin A, either acutely or chronically, is toxic. Signs of toxicity usually appear with sustained daily intakes of 50,000 IU. Carotenoids are not known to be toxic even when large amounts are ingested for weeks to years. This lack of toxicity is mainly attributable to a reduced efficiency of absorption at high doses and a limited conversion to vitamin A in the intestine, liver, and other organs. However, carotenoids taken in large doses over several weeks are absorbed well enough to color adipose tissue stores and cause a yellow discoloration of the skin.

Beta carotene is a fat-soluble antioxidant that quenches singlet oxygen and reacts directly with free radicals generated during lipid peroxidation (63). Although beta carotene is less reactive toward free radicals than is α-tocopherol, both may exert a cooperative effect by residing in and scavenging free radicals at different positions in the lipophilic compartment: α-tocopherol at the membrane surface and beta carotene in the interior of membranes (63).

A multicenter, case-control study that compared the beta carotene concentration in adipose tissue of subjects who had experienced an acute myocardial infarction and in control subjects was conducted in Europe (64). Investigators found that beta carotene was higher in adipose tissue of control subjects and concluded that a higher beta carotene intake reduced the risk of myocardial infarction. Because this was an epidemiologic study, cause and effect cannot be inferred because adipose tissue beta carotene levels may be indicative of a particular lifestyle (ie, consumption of foods such as carrots and leafy green vegetables that contain beta carotene and other compounds) that may affect risk of myocardial infarction. In contrast, two subsequent controlled, clinical studies found that beta carotene did not reduce mortality from CVD (65) or decrease incidence of angina (66).

The results of studies evaluating beta carotene have not been encouraging with respect to cancer. The Beta-carotene and Retinol Efficacy Trial (CARET) was prematurely terminated after preliminary data showed that the beta carotene intervention provided no benefit and could actually be harmful (67). Because of these negative results, the Women's Health Study being conducted at Harvard involving 20,000 female health professionals is removing beta carotene from the study's intervention group (68).

Although the CARET results showed no benefits of beta carotene, these results must be interpreted with caution because the subjects were smokers, and therefore at increased risk for cancer. It is known that at high partial pressures of oxygen, as occurs in the lungs, beta carotene acts as a pro-oxidant and may induce cancer and therefore may put smokers at increased risk.

Dietary Sources and Recommendations. Rich sources of beta carotene are leafy green and yellow vegeta-

BOX 12-2 Food Sources of Vitamin E as Alpha-Tocopherol (mg)

Eggs, chicken	**Serving**	**mg/serving**
fresh/frozen	1 large	0.88
yolk		0.87
Vegetable oils		
almond oil	1 T (14g)	5.30
corn oil (brand A)	1 T (14g)	1.90
corn oil (brand B)	1 T (14g)	3.00
cottonseed oil	1 T (14g)	4.80
olive oil	1 T (14g)	1.60
palm oil	1 T (14g)	2.60
safflower oil	1 T (14g)	4.60
sunflower oil	1 T (14g)	6.10
wheat-germ oil	1 T (14g)	20.30
Fruits		
apple, raw with skin	1 med (138g)	0.81
apricots, cnd in heavy syrup	4 halves	0.80
banana	1 med	0.31
mango, raw	1 med (207g)	2.32
Grain products		
pasta	1 cup	1.03
Nuts		
almonds, dried	1 oz (24 nuts)	6.72
almonds, oil roasted	1 oz (22 nuts)	1.55
cashews, dry roasted	1 oz	0.16
filberts (hazelnuts), dried	1 oz	6.70
peanut butter	1 T (16g)	3.00
pistachio, dried	1 oz	1.46
Vegetables		
asparagus, raw	4 spears (58g)	1.15
avocado, raw	1 med (173g)	2.32
beet greens, raw	1 cup (38g)	0.57
carrots, raw	1 med (72g)	0.32
mustard greens, raw	½ cup (28g)	0.56
sweet potato, raw	1 med (130g)	5.93

Source: Pennington JAT (58).

bles. The average daily consumption of beta carotene in the United States is approximately 1.5 mg, yet the US National Cancer Institute and the US Department of Agriculture references suggest that the average diet should provide 6 mg/day (69). The RDA for vitamin A is 800 RE to 1,000 RE or approximately 4.8 mg to 6.0 mg beta carotene daily, the equivalent of two medium carrots or 2 cups of cooked broccoli.

Most epidemiologic studies suggest that beta carotene may protect against CVD. Long-term clinical trials presently underway are designed to test the effectiveness of beta carotene supplements in reducing CVD risk. Currently five or more servings of fruits and vegetables are recommended daily to reduce the risk of chronic disease. On average, five servings of fruits and vegetables would provide 0 mg to 3 mg of beta carotene daily. The extent to which this nutrient reduces CVD risk remains to be resolved. At this time, patients should be advised to get their beta carotene via the diet, consume at least the recommended amount of fruits and vegetables per day, and focus on eating at least three to four servings of foods high in beta carotene every week.

Vitamin C

Background. Vitamin C (ascorbic acid), a water-soluble antioxidant found in the blood and cytosol of cells, reduces the damage caused by free radicals during the oxidation process (60). Vitamin C, beta carotene, and vitamin E may work synergistically in preventing cellular oxidation. Vitamin C has been shown to regenerate tocopherol from the tocopheroxy radical, whereas beta carotene and vitamin C probably do not interact (63).

Several epidemiologic studies showed a significant inverse correlation between plasma vitamin C levels and

TABLE 12-2

Vitamin C Content of Selected Foods

Food	Serving	Mg/Serving
Broccoli, raw	½ cup	41
Grapefruit, pink	1 medium	94
Lemon	1 medium	31
Orange	1 medium	80
Potato, with skin	1 medium	26
Strawberries	1 cup	85
Tomato, raw	1 medium	24

Source: Pennington JAT (58).

CVD mortality. The Basel Prospective Study found that men with low plasma vitamin C concentrations (22.7 μmol/L) had an increased risk of death from ischemic heart disease (70). Other epidemiologic studies reported an apparent decreased risk of CVD with an increased consumption of vitamin C (71-74) but still others found no such relation (53,75,76). Additional studies are needed to determine whether vitamin C is effective in decreasing the risk of CVD.

Dietary Sources and Recommendations. Many fruits and vegetables are good sources of vitamin C. The best sources include citrus fruits, strawberries, broccoli, green peppers, tomatoes, and potatoes (Table 12-2). Vitamin C is heat sensitive; losses during food preparation can be minimized by steaming or by cooking in a minimal amount of water for the shortest time possible.

The RDA for vitamin C is 60 mg/day for nonsmokers and 100 mg/day for smokers. However, therapeutic doses are much greater, ranging from 200 mg/day to 18,000 mg/day. Optimal vitamin C intake is difficult to assess and may be within the range of 180 mg/day to 750 mg/day (76), although an intake of 140 mg/day appears necessary to saturate the total body vitamin C pool (77). Current US daily intake is estimated to be 77 mg/day to 109 mg/day (59). Although vitamin C is not toxic, abdominal bloating and diarrhea have been reported when doses of 2 g or more are consumed (78). Individuals consuming large doses of vitamin C also are susceptible to rebound scurvy or clinical vitamin C deficiency if they abruptly discontinue their intake.

Other Antioxidants

Selenium. Selenium is an essential trace mineral necessary for the production of glutathione peroxidase, the enzyme that catalyzes the breakdown of hyperoxides. In this reaction selenium functions as an antioxidant. Selenium and vitamin E also work synergistically as antioxidants. Vitamin E protects against oxidative stress, providing an environment that enhances the action of selenium (79).

Selenium intakes as high as 900 μg/day were reportedly consumed without side effects (80). However, selenium can be toxic when taken in excess of 1000 mg/day. This toxicity can be offset if vitamin E and selenium are taken together. The RDA for selenium is 55 μg/day to 75 μg/day (59); however, the average US intake of selenium is approximately 110 μg/day. Seafood, kidney, and liver are consistently good sources of selenium. The selenium content of grains and seeds varies with the selenium content of the soil in which they are grown. Generally, fruits and vegetables are poor sources of selenium.

Co-Enzyme Q10. Co-enzyme Q10 (or ubiquinone) is lipid soluble and structurally similar to vitamin E. Like vitamin E, it may protect membrane phospholipids and LDL from oxidation (81). In addition, co-enzyme Q10 may protect and regenerate vitamin E (82). Co-enzyme Q10 is not considered a vitamin because it is synthesized in the body from the precursors of cholesterol synthesis. The synthesis of co-enzyme Q10 increases with age. Good sources of co-enzyme Q10 include fresh, unprocessed foods such as meats, fish, nuts, and seed oils (83).

Recommendations

Although clinical trials have been inconclusive, accumulating evidence suggests that antioxidants, particularly vitamin E, play a role in the prevention and progression of CVD. Ongoing clinical trials will provide information about the potential benefits of the antioxidant vitamins. It is appropriate to recommend foods high in antioxidants (ie, carrots, broccoli, nuts, oranges, and many other fruits and vegetables) that may confer additional cardiovascular benefits via their antioxidant potential as an important part of a healthful diet.

CARDIOVASCULAR BENEFITS OF ALCOHOL CONSUMPTION

Background

The 1995 *Dietary Guidelines for Americans* recommended moderation for those who drink alcohol (84). The previous edition of the guidelines stated that alcohol has "no net benefit" and "is not recommended." However, the Expert Scientific Committee revised the guidelines to acknowledge the large body of evidence demonstrating that "moderate drinking...is associated with a lower risk for heart disease..."

...ompared with alcohol consumption.
FIGURE ...rve shows that moderate drinkers appear
Total m... than either heavy drinkers or abstainers.
The Jm Klatsky, 1981, *Ann Intern Med* (88). Adapted with
t...on from *Annals of Internal Medicine* © 1981.

FIGURE 12-3

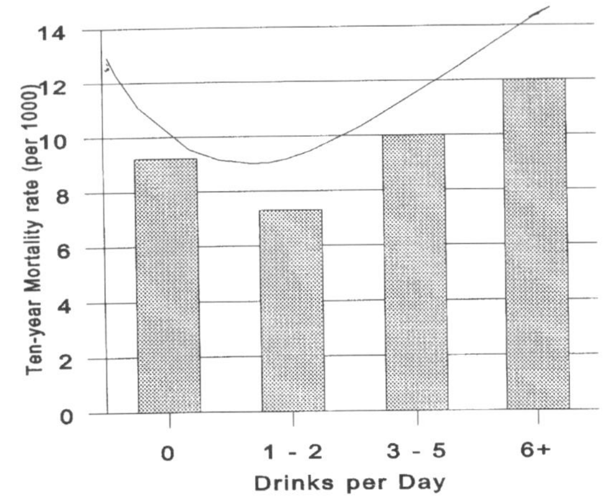

(85). The current dietary guidelines state that "moderate alcohol intake may enhance enjoyment of meals and offer some protection from coronary heart disease." However, the committee does not recommend that nondrinkers begin drinking alcohol and emphasizes that alcohol consumption is inappropriate for children and adolescents. Pregnant women are strongly cautioned against alcohol consumption because of the potential adverse effects on fetal development and growth. Similar recommendations have been made by the American Heart Association (86).

Numerous epidemiologic and prospective studies support the J-shaped relationship of alcohol consumption and cardiovascular disease (85,86,87). Nondrinkers and heavy drinkers have higher rates of CVD mortality than do moderate drinkers (Figure 12-3). Diseases related to alcoholism and excessive alcohol intake include stroke, alcoholic cardiomyopathy, certain cancers, cirrhosis, and pancreatitis (86). Many of the epidemiologic studies focus on the phenomenon referred to as the French paradox, which is based on the observation that despite the consumption of a high-fat diet, France has one of the lowest rates of CHD and CHD-related mortalities of the industrialized nations (89). This paradox may, in part, be explained by the large amounts of red wine consumed by the French compared with people living in other countries (Figure 12-4) (90). In France, where daily alcohol intake averages 1.5 to 2 glasses of primarily red wine (20 g/day to 30 g/day), the incidence of CHD is 40% less than it is in other Western societies (89).

Biological Effects

Alcoholic beverages have various bioactive ingredients that may be cardioprotective. Resveratrol, a natural antifungal ingredient in grape skins, elevates HDL-C levels, decreases platelet aggregation, and inhibits LDL oxidation (91,92). Some studies suggest that red wine has a greater cardiovascular protective effect relative to other alcoholic beverages because it is processed longer with the grape skins that contain resveratrol (93). Red wine also contains tannins, phenolic compounds, anthocyanin, and bioflavonoids that serve as powerful antioxidants and free radical scavengers (94). The bioflavonoid quercetin found in some beers and wines is an even more potent antioxidant than vitamin E (94).

Beneficial Effects

Blood Lipids and Lipoproteins. Alcohol consumption has consistently been shown to increase HDL-C (92,95) and many epidemiologists suggest this HDL-C raising effect may explain up to 50% of the CHD risk reduction associated with alcohol consumption (95). A 15-day study (92) compared the effects of alcohol, red wine, and white wine using volunteers. The researchers found that both red and white wine increased HDL-C similarly.

Alcoholic beverages and their constituents inhibit LDL oxidation (93). Wine contains natural flavonoids that exhibit antioxidant properties such as donating hydrogen to superoxide anions, hydroxyl radicals, and lipid peroxyl radicals, thereby decreasing lipid oxidation in vivo (93). It is believed that regular consumption of wine, which contains these flavonoids, collectively reduces the oxidation of LDL-C and other lipoproteins.

Thrombus Formation and Hemostasis. Platelet aggregation is associated with the development of CHD because platelets that interact or adhere to the damaged arterial walls increase the rate of atherosclerosis development. Acute damage to the plaque can lead to platelet-mediated

FIGURE 12-4

Heart disease rates in 18 Western countries

Reproduced with permission from AS St Leger et al, *Lancet* 1979; 1(8124):1017-1020 (90).

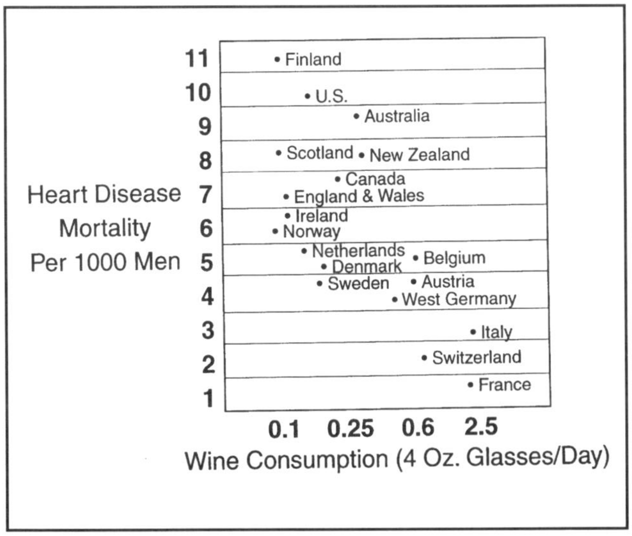

thrombosis, which can produce unstable angina, silent ischemia, and fatal or nonfatal myocardial infarction (96). Alcohol favorably reduces platelet aggregability and thus reduces the incidence of these cardiovascular events (92,96-98). In the Caerphilly Prospective Heart Disease Study, platelet aggregation was measured in 1,600 men and a much lower risk of platelet aggregation was observed in men who consumed alcohol than in those who did not (97).

Hypertension. Heavy alcohol consumption is a risk factor for hypertension. The alcohol in two drinks will raise blood pressure in many individuals (99) and also increase risk of all-cause mortality (100). The mechanisms by which this occurs are not clear. Interestingly, mortality is lower for light drinkers than for nondrinkers for reasons that appear to be unrelated to the effects of alcohol on blood pressure.

Recommendations

As a result of the extensive literature showing the cardioprotective effects of moderate alcohol consumption (two 12-oz beers, two 4-oz glasses of wine, or 1½ oz distilled spirits), alcohol in moderation can be included as a part of a heart-healthy meal plan. Because of the compelling research on alcohol and its CHD benefits, the Mediterranean Diet Pyramid (see Figure 6-1) includes moderate alcohol consumption. However, because of the serious social and medical consequences of excessive and abusive alcohol consumption, health professionals must be cautious when making recommendations about alcohol intake. Experts agree that it is inappropriate to recommend moderate alcohol consumption to a nondrinker in order to reduce the risk of CVD (85).

SOY PROTEIN

Background

Different dietary proteins exert different effects on plasma cholesterol concentrations. Substituting soy protein for mixed protein reduces the plasma total cholesterol concentration in hypercholesterolemic subjects but causes only a small, insignificant change in subjects with normal plasma cholesterol concentrations (101). The mechanism responsible for the effects of different proteins on plasma cholesterol concentrations has not been elucidated but several hypotheses have been proposed. Some suggest that soy protein impairs cholesterol absorption or bile acid reabsorption (102,103); this was observed in rabbits and rats (104) but not consistently in humans (105,106). Others suggest that changes in endocrine status, such as alterations in the ratio of insulin to glucagon (107) and thyroid hormone concentrations (108) are responsible for the hypocholesterolemic effects of soy protein.

Another hypothesis proposes that the different amino acids from animal and soy protein are responsible for changes in cholesterol metabolism (109); further research in this area led researchers to propose that it is the nonprotein components, that is, saponons (110), fiber (111), phytic acid (112), and phytoestrogens (113) that are responsible for soy protein's cardioprotective effects.

Phytoestrogens are naturally occurring plant substances that are structurally or functionally similar to estradiol, the active form of estrogen. Because of this, they can bind to estrogen receptors and produce effects similar to estrogen, though weaker. Estrogens are beneficial in reducing the risk of cardiovascular disease (114). The protective effects of estrogen may be manifested through lipid changes—specifically, a decrease in LDL-C and an increase in HDL-C—and vascular effects—namely changes in vasomotor tone and vessel wall function.

Phytoestrogens comprise a number of classes of compounds, including lignans and isoflavones. The isoflavones genistein and daidzein occur in high concentrations in soybeans. Plasma concentrations of genistein and daidzein are increased by diets rich in soy proteins (115,116). Genistein has several properties that suggest its potential as a cardioprotective compound. In vitro genistein blocks the action of platelet-derived growth factor (PDGF) and other growth factors (117), thereby inhibiting the proliferation and migration of arterial smooth muscle cells and halting the transition of fatty streaks to advanced lesions. Genistein may also reduce overall thrombosis associated with atherosclerosis by interfering with the activation of platelets (118,119) as well as the platelet-activation (120), platelet-aggregation (121), and growth-factor (122) functions of thrombin. If genistein has similar actions in vivo, it may effectively slow the development or progression of atherosclerosis. Daidzein is a potent antioxidant and may also slow the development or progression of atherosclerosis (123).

Soy Protein Sources

Soy protein sources include soy milk, tofu, soy sauce, isolated and textured soy protein supplements, and meat analogues (Table 12-3). These products can be incorporated into a diet by substituting soy milk for regular milk, using tofu in stir-fry recipes, and barbecuing tempeh (a fermented soy bean cake) or meat analogues. (See Chapter 6.)

The *US Soyfoods Directory,* published by the Indiana Soybean Development Council, offers a comprehensive list of soy foods available in the US, including descriptions of soy foods, the nutritional content of specific soy foods, and recipes. A free copy of the directory can be obtained by writing Stevens & Associates, Inc, 4816 North Pennsylvania Street, Indianapolis, IN 46205; by phone at 1-800-301-3153 or 317-926-6272, or by e-mail at info@soyfoods.com. A searchable version is available on the Internet at http://www.soyfoods.com.

Recommendations

In conclusion, evidence appears to be mounting on the reduction of cholesterol and other cardiovascular benefits of soy protein consumption. Although no large multicenter, long-term (longer than 6 months) clinical studies have been conducted on soy protein's safety and effectiveness, it

TABLE 12-3

Nutrient Composition of Soy Foods

Product	Carbohydrate (g)	Protein (g)	Fat (g)
Soybeans, ½ c boiled	8.5	14.3	7.7
Soy protein concentrate, 1 oz	8.7	16.3	0.13
Soy milk, ½ c	2.2	3.3	2.3
Tempeh, ½ c	14.1	15.7	6.4
Tofu, ¼ raw block	3.5	12.8	7.1
Soy protein isolate 1 oz	2.1	22.6	0.95

appears that low-fat soy foods are an appropriate addition to cardiac patients' diets, especially if the patients have high blood cholesterol levels. Phytoestrogens present in soy foods appear to reduce the arthogenicity of low-density lipoprotein. Genestein and daidzein may protect the arterial wall by reducing platelet aggregation, cellular adhesion, and thrombus formation.

GARLIC AND CARDIOVASCULAR DISEASE

Investigations during the past decade have heightened interest in scientists and consumers about the potential benefits of garlic as a modifier of cardiovascular disease. These studies have largely concentrated on the effect of garlic on serum cholesterol, low-density lipoprotein (LDL), high-density lipoprotein (HDL), and triglyceride concentrations. Although considerable variability exists across these studies, most provide evidence that increased garlic consumption is accompanied by a decrease in circulating cholesterol and triglyceride concentrations. Part of the variability among these studies arises from the lack of consistency in the preparations examined, variation in the total quantity consumed, and differences in the duration of treatment (124,125,126). The variability also reflects a host of environmental and genetic factors influencing cholesterol and triglyceride homeostasis. Nevertheless, garlic consumption in some individuals for extended periods of time is followed by a modest reduction in cholesterol, LDL-cholesterol, and triglyceride concentrations. Most evidence indicates that a more pronounced response occurs in people with moderate to severe hypercholesterolemia. Greater attention to factors contributing to individual responses should shed light on the circumstances where enhanced garlic consumption produces maximum benefits.

Intake Amount

Although the consumption of garlic varies widely among individuals, intakes as high as 20g/day occur without apparently ill consequences (127). However, substantially lower intakes may be sufficient to produce a response in hypercholesterolemic individuals. Some evidence suggested that as little as one-half to one clove of garlic per day is sufficient to reduce cholesterol levels, possibly by about 10% (128,129). Interestingly, the size of this effect is comparable with that observed with other cholesterol-lowering dietary manipulations. Thus, increased garlic consumption may hypercholesterolemia in some individuals.

Response to Various Preparations

In a double-blind study with 42 adult men and women, Jain, Vargas, Gotzkowsky, and McMahon (124) found that providing a garlic powder tablet (300 mg three times daily) significantly depressed circulating cholesterol, LDL-cholesterol, and fatty acids compared with a placebo. To date, more than 40 studies have examined the ability of garlic to modify plasma cholesterol and triglycerides. The response has varied from no significant response in a few investigations to an approximate 30% reduction in both cholesterol and triglycerides in others. In most cases, the consumption of fresh uncooked garlic, garlic powder tablets, spray-dried garlic, or a garlic extract lowered cholesterol and triglyceride concentrations. Steiner, Khan, Holbert, and Lin (130), using a double-blind crossover study with 41 moderately hypercholesterolemic men, found that providing 7.2g of a deodorized preparation (aged garlic extract) reduced total serum cholesterol by 7% compared with the baseline period. A modest reduction in LDL cholesterol was also observed in subjects consuming the garlic extract. This study, as well as others, points to the need for prolonged garlic consumption to produce a response in blood cholesterol and triglyceride concentrations. Likewise, a sustained intake appears necessary to maintain this reduction.

Simons (131) found that consumption of 300-mg garlic powder tablets three times daily was not accompanied by a change in plasma cholesterol, LDL cholesterol, HDL cholesterol, or plasma triglycerides in mildly hypercholesterolemic subjects. The degree of hypercholesterolemia may significantly influence the degree and timing of the response to supplemental garlic. Additional studies are needed to determine the conditions of various garlic preparations that are most likely to be beneficial. Although the type of garlic preparation consumed is likely a significant factor in the overall response, it appears that odor is not an absolute prerequisite (130).

Several compounds in garlic may contribute to its ability to depress cholesterol and fatty acid biosynthesis (132). Garlic extracts may block cholesterol biosynthesis at several different locations (133). Sulfur compounds within garlic such as allicin, diallyl disulfide, and allyl mercaptan were all effective in blocking cholesterol biosynthesis, although the magnitude depended on the specific compound examined (134). Allyl sulfur compounds found in garlic can alter cellular thiols (135). More than one mechanism may be occurring because nicotinic acid and adenosine, other compounds found in garlic, are also recognized to depress HMG-CoA reductase activity (133).

Garlic protein contains a high proportion of cysteine residues. Recent studies by Mathew, Daniel, and Augusti (136) showed that garlic protein reduces cholesterol concentrations in rats. Whether this response relates to the protein per se or to the presence of a compound bound to protein remains to be determined (137). Collectively, several agents in garlic likely account for its ability to reduce cholesterol and fatty acids biosynthesis.

Antithrombotic Properties

Garlic extracts and several of its constituents possess significant antithrombotic properties (126). In vitro studies show that sulfur compounds, including allicin and ajoene, likely contribute greatly to these antiplatelet effects, although other compounds, including adenosine, may also contribute. Whether these parent compounds or their metabolites actually account for the antithrombotic activity is not known. Ali and Thomson (138) examined the effect of the consumption of a fresh clove of garlic on platelet thromboxane production in a group of male volunteers aged 40 to 50 years. Consuming one clove (approximately 3 g) of fresh garlic daily for 16 weeks resulted in a reduction of serum cholesterol by approximately 20% and reduction of serum thromboxane by approximately 80%. Changes in the phosphorylation of proteins may account for the alterations in thromboxane concentrations. Villar and Alvarino (139) found ajoene treatment produced nonselective hyperphosphorylation of numerous proteins in platelet lysates.

Blood Pressure

A meta-analysis of seven studies revealed that increased garlic intake modestly influences blood pressure (140). Depending on the study, the effect was principally on systolic or diastolic blood pressure. Collectively, these data suggest that various garlic preparations may be of some value in individuals with mild hypertension. Unfortunately, insufficient information precludes the identification of what circumstances or conditions might derive the greatest benefits. Again, garlic odor does not appear to be a prerequisite because a deodorized garlic preparation was found to cause a 5.5% decrease in systolic blood pressure and a slight decrease in diastolic blood pressure (130).

Recommendations

In conclusion, most evidence points to the probability that increased garlic consumption reduces the risk of cardiovascular disease. Although the evidence of garlic's benefits is more than speculation, severe limitations preclude identifying which individuals and conditions would benefit most. Until this is known, it remains prudent to eat a variety of foods and not to restrict garlic intake.

Summary

A number of foods and nutrients play a role not only in the development of but also in protection from CVD. Through manipulation of food sources and supplements, it is possible to develop an efficacious diet for CVD risk reduction. These strategies, in conjunction with standard diets that lower blood cholesterol (diets that are low in total fat, saturated fat, and cholesterol), offer the potential to markedly reduce CVD risk beyond that currently achievable. Further studies are needed to provide the scientific rationale required for making appropriate dietary recommendations.

References

1. Hassler C. *Functional Foods*. Presented at the NutraCon Functional Foods Conference; 1994; New Orleans, La.
2. Goldberg I. *Functional Foods, Designer Foods, PharmaFoods, Nutraceuticals*. New York, NY: Chapman & Hall; 1994:xv-xvi.
3. Bang HO, Dyerberg J, Hjorne N. The composition of food consumed by Greenlandic Eskimos. *Acta Med Scand*. 1973;200:69-73.
4. Dyerberg J, Bang HO, Hjorne N. Fatty acid composition of plasma lipids in Greenland Eskimos. *Am J Clin Nutr*. 1975;28:958-966.
5. Dyerberg J, Bang HO. Hemostatic function and platelet polyunsaturated acids in Eskimos. *Lancet*. 1979;2:433-435.
6. Kroman N, Green A. Epidemiological studies in the Upernavik district Greenland. *Acta Med Scand*. 1980;208:401-406.
7. Hirai A, Hamazaki T, Terano T, Nishikawa T, Tamura Y, Kumagai A, Sajiki J. Eicosapentaenoic acid and platelet function in Japanese. *Lancet*. 1980;2:1132-1133.
8. Stone NJ. Fish consumption, fish oil, lipids, and coronary heart disease. *Circulation*. 1996;94:2337-2340.
9. Sprecher H, James AT. Biosynthesis of long chain fatty acids in mammalian systems. *In: Geometrical and Positional Fatty Acid Isomers*. Champaign, Ill: American Oil Chemists' Society; 1979:56-90.
10. Emken EA, Adlof RO, Gulley RM. Dietary linoleic acid influences desaturation and acylation of deuterium-labeled linoleic and linolenic acids in young adult males. *Biochimica Biophys Acta*. 1994;1213:277-288.
11. Sanders TAB, Roshani F. The influence of different types of ω-3 polyunsaturated fatty acids on blood lipids and platelet function in healthy volunteers. *Clin Sci*. 1983;64:91-99.
12. Budowski P, Trostler N, Lupo N, Vaisman N, Eldor A. Effect of linseed oil ingestion on plasma lipid fatty acid composition and platelet aggregability in healthy volunteers. *Nutr Res*. 1984;4:343-346.
13. Singer P, Berger I, Wirth M, Godicke W, Jaeger W, Voigt S. Slow desaturation and elongation of linoleic and α-linoleic acids as a rationale of eicosapentanoic acid-rich diet to lower blood pressure and serum lipids in normal, hypertensive and hyperlipidemic subjects. *Prostaglandins Leukot Med*. 1986;24:173-193.
14. de Lorgeril M, Renaud S, Mamelle N, Salen P, Martin J-L,

Monjaud I, Guidollet J, Touboul P, Delaye J. Mediterranean alpha-linolenic acid-rich diet in secondary prevention of coronary heart disease. *Lancet.* 1994;343:1454-1459.

15. Mest HJ, Beitz J, Heinroth I, Block HU, Forster W. The influence of linseed oil diet on fatty acid patterns in phospholipids and thromboxane formation platelets in man. *Klin Wochenschr.* 1983;61:187-191.
16. Kromhout D, Bosschieter EB, Coulander CL. The inverse relationship between fish consumption and 20-year mortality from coronary heart disease. *N Engl J Med.* 1985;312:1205-1209.
17. Shekelle RB, Shryock AM, Paul O, Lepper M, Stamler J, Liu S, Raynor WJ. Diet, serum cholesterol, and death from coronary heart disease: the Western Electric Study. *N Engl J Med.* 1981;304:65-70.
18. Dolecek TA. Epidemiological evidence of relationship between dietary polyunsaturated fatty acids and mortality in the Multiple Risk Factor Intervention Trial. *Proc Soc Exp Biol Med.* 1992;200:177-182.
19. Burr ML, Holiday RM, Fehily AM, Whitehead PJ. Haematological prognostic indices after myocardial infarction: evidence from the Diet and Reinfarction Trial (DART). *Eur Heart J.* 1992:13(2);166-170.
20. Ascherio A, Rimm EB, Stampfer MJ, Giovannucci EL, Willett WC. Dietary intake of marine n-3 fatty acids, fish intake, and the risk of coronary disease among men. *N Engl J Med.* 1995;332:977-982.
21. Gualler E, Hennekens CH, Sacks FM, Willett WC, Stampfer MJ. A prospective study of plasma fish oil levels and incidence of myocardial infarction in US male physicians. *J Am Coll Cardiol.* 1995;25:387-394.
22. Bolibar I, Thompson SG, von Eckardsterin A, Sandkamp M, Assmann G. Dose-response relationships of serum lipid measurements with the extent of coronary stenosis: strong, independent, and comprehensive. *Thomb Vasc Biol.* 1995;15:1035-1042.
23. Leaf A, Jorgensen MB, Jacobs AK, Gote G, Schoenfeld DA, Scheer J, Weiner BH, Slack JD, Kellett MA, Raizner AE, Weber PC, Mahrer PR, Rossouw JE. Do fish oils prevent restenosis after coronary angioplasty? *Circulation.* 1994;90:2248-2257.
24. Sacks FM, Stone PH, Gibson CM, Silverman DI, Rosner B, Pasternak RC. Controlled trial of fish oil for regression of human coronary atherosclerosis: HARP Research Group. *J Am Coll Cardiol.* 1995;25:1492-1498.
25. Harris WS. Fish oils and plasma lipid and lipoprotein metabolism in humans: a critical review. *J Lipid Res.* 1989;30:785-807.
26. Harris WS. n-3 Fatty acids and serum lipoproteins: human studies. *Am J Clin Nutr.* 1997;65(suppl):1645S-1654S.
27. Sanders TAB. Influence of ω-3 fatty acids on blood lipids. *World Rev Nutr Diet.* 1991;66:358-366.
28. Morris SC, Sacks F, Rosner B. Does fish oil lower blood pressure? A meta-analysis of controlled trials. *Circulation.* 1993;88:523-533.
29. Leaf A, Kang JX. Dietary n-3 fatty acids in the prevention of lethal cardiac arrhythmias. *Curr Opin Lipidol.* 1997;8:4-6.
30. Siscovick DS, Raghunathan TE, King I, Weinmann S, Wicklund KG, Albright J, Bovbjerg V, Arbogast P, Smith H, Kushi LH, Cobb LA, Copass MK, Psaty BM, Lemaitre R, Retzlaff B, Childs M, Knopp RH. Dietary intake and all membrane levels of long-chain n-3 polyunsaturated fatty acids and the risk of primary cardiac arrest. *JAMA.* 1995;274:1363-1367.
31. Christensen JH, Gustenhoff P, Kosup E, Aaroe J, Toft E, Moller J, Rasmussen D, Dyerberg J, Schmidt EB. Effect of fish oil on heart rate variability in survivors of myocardial infarction: a double blind randomized controlled trial. BMJ. 1996;312:677-678.
32. Sellmayer A, Witzgall H, Lorenz R, Weber PC. Effects of dietary fish oil on ventricular premature complexes. *Am J Cardiol.* 1995;76:974-977.
33. Gillum RF, Mussolino ME, Madans JH. The relationship between fish consumption and stroke incidence: the NHANES I epidemiologic follow-up study. *Arch Intern Med.* 1996;156:537-542.
34. Expert Panel. Kris-Etherton PM, ed. *Trans* fatty acids and coronary heart disease risk. *Am J Clin Nutr.* 1995;62(suppl):655S-707S.
35. Hunter JE, Applewhite TH. Reassessment of *trans* fatty acid availability in the US diet. Am J Clin Nutr. 1991;54:363-369.
36. Mensink RP, Katan MB. Effect of dietary *trans* fatty acids on high-density and low-density lipoprotein cholesterol levels in healthy subjects. *N Engl J Med.* 1990;323:439-445.
37. Troisi R, Willett WC, Weiss ST. *Trans*-fatty acid intake in relation to serum lipid concentrations in adult men. *Am J Clin Nutr.* 1992;56:1019-1024.
38. Ascherio A, Hennekens CH, Buring JRE, Master C, Stampfer MJ, Willet WC. *Trans*-fatty acid intake and risk of myocardial infarction. *Circulation.* 1994;89:94-101.
39. Judd JT, Clevidance BA, Muesing RA, Wittes J, Sunkin ME, Podczasy JJ. Dietary *trans* fatty acids: effects on plasma lipids and lipoproteins of healthy men and women. *Am J Clin Nutr.* 1994;59:861-868.
40. Willett WC, Stampfer JM, Manson JE, Colditz GA, Speizer FE, Rosner BA, Sampson LA, Hennekens CH. Intakes of *trans* fatty acids and risk of coronary heart disease among women. *Lancet.* 1993;341:581-586.
41. Nestel PJ, Noakes M, Belling B. Plasma lipoprotein lipid and Lp[a] changes with substitution of elaidic acid for oleic acid in the diet. *J Lipid Res.* 1992;33:1029-1036.
42. Zock PL, Katan MB. Hydrogenation alternatives: effects of *trans* fatty acids and stearic acid versus linoleic acid on serum lipids and lipoproteins in humans. *J Lipid Res.* 1992;33:399-410.
43. Aro A, Jauhiainen M, Partanen R, Salminen I, Mutanen M. Stearic acid, *trans* fatty acids, and dairy fat: effects on serum and lipoprotein lipids, apolipoproteins, lipoprotein(a), and lipid transfer proteins in healthy subjects. *Am J Clin Nutr.* 1997;65:1419-1426.
44. Mensink RP, Zock PL, Katan MB, Hornstra G. Effect of dietary *cis* and *trans* fatty acids on serum lipoprotein(a) levels in humans. *J Lipid Res.* 1992;33:1493-1501.
45. Lichtenstein AH, Ausman LM, Carrasco W, Jenner JL, Ordovas JM, Schafer EJ. Hydrogenation impairs the hypolipidemic effect of corn oil in humans. *Arterioscler Thromb.* 1993;13:154-161.
46. Lichtenstein AH. *Trans* fatty acids, plasma lipid levels, and risk of developing cardiovascular disease. *Circulation.* 1997;95:2588-2590.
47. Zock PL, Katan MB. Butter, margarine, and serum lipoprotein. *Atherosclerosis.* 1997;13:7-16.
48. Stocker R. Lipoprotein oxidation: mechanistic aspects, methodological approaches, and clinical relevance. *Curr Opin Lipidol.* 1994;5:422-433.

49. Steinberg D, Parthasarathy S, Carew TE, Khoo JC, Witztum JL. Beyond cholesterol: modifications of low-density lipoprotein that increase its atherogenicity. *N Engl J Med.* 1989;320:915-924.
50. Steinberg D. Antioxidants in the prevention of human atherosclerosis: summary of the proceedings of a National Heart, Lung, and Blood Institute workshop, Sept 5-6, 1991, Bethesda, Md. *Circulation.* 1992;85:2337-2344.
51. Rimm EB, Stampfer MJ. The role of antioxidants in preventive cardiology. *Curr Opin Cardiol.* 1997;12:188-194.
52. Duthie GG, Brown KM. Reducing the risk of cardiovascular disease. In: Goldberg I, ed. *Functional Foods, Designer Foods, PharmaFoods, Nutraceuticals.* New York, NY: Chapman & Hall; 1994:19-38.
53. Rimm EB, Stampfer MJ, Ascherio A, Giovannucci E, Colditz GA, Willett WC. Vitamin E consumption and the risk of coronary disease in women. *N Engl J Med.* 1993;328:1444-1449.
54. Stampfer MJ, Rimm EB. Epidemiological evidence for vitamin E in prevention of cardiovascular disease. *Am J Clin Nutr.* 1995;62(suppl):1365S-1369S.
55. Jialal I, Grundy SM. Effect of dietary supplementation with alpha-tocopherol on the oxidative modification of low-density lipoprotein. *J Lipid Res.* 1992;33:899-906.
56. Stephans NG, Parsons A, Schofield PM, Kelly F, Cheeseman K, Mitchinson MJ. Randomised controlled trial of vitamin E in patients with coronary disease: Cambridge Heart Antioxidant Study (CHAOS). *Lancet.* 1996;347:781-786.
57. Steiner M. Influence of vitamin E on platelet function in humans. *J Am Coll Nutr.* 1991;20:466-473.
58. Pennington JAT. *Food Values of Portions Commonly Used.* Bowes and Church 16th ed. Philadelphia, Penn: Lippincott; 1994.
59. Food and Nutrition Board. *Recommended Dietary Allowances.* 10th ed. Washington, DC: National Academy Press; 1989.
60. Padh H. Vitamins for optimal health. In: Goldberg I, ed. *Functional Foods, Designer Foods, PharmaFoods, Nutraceuticals.* New York, NY: Chapman & Hall; 1994:261-293.
61. Lin RIS. Phytochemicals and antioxidants. In: Goldberg I, ed. *Functional Foods, Designer Foods, PharmaFoods, Nutraceuticals.* New York, NY: Chapman & Hall; 1994:393-449.
62. Erdman Jr JW, Bierer TL, Gugger ET. Absorption and transport of carotenoids. *Ann NY Acad Sci.* 1993;691:76-85.
63. Niki E, Noguchi N, Tsuchihashi H, Gotoh N. Interaction among vitamin C and vitamin E, and β-carotene. *Am J Clin Nutr.* 1995;62(suppl):1322S-1365S.
64. Kardinal AFM, Kok FM, Ringstad J, Aracena G, Mazaev VP, Kohlmeier L, Martin BC, Aro A, Kark J. Antioxidants, adipose tissue, and risk of myocardial infarction: the EURAM study. *Lancet.* 1993;342:1379-1384.
65. Greenburg ER, Baron JA, Kragas MR, Stukel TA, Nierenberg DW, Stevens MM, Mandel JS, Haile RW. Mortality associated with low plasma concentration of beta carotene and the effect of oral supplementation. *JAMA.* 1996;275:699-703.
66. Rapola JM, Virtamo J, Hakka JK, Heinonen OP, Albanes D, Taylor PR, Huttunen JK. Effect of vitamin E and beta carotene on the incidence of angina pectoris. *JAMA.* 1996;275:693-698.
67. Omenn GS, Goodman GE, Thornquist MD, Balmes J, Cullen MR, Glass A, Keogh JP, Meyskens FL, Valanis B, Williams JH Jr, Barnhart S, Hammar S. Effects of a combination of beta carotene and vitamin A on lung cancer and cardiovascular disease. *N Engl J Med.* 1996;334:1150-1155.
68. Anon. *Clinical Investigator News.* 1996;4(2):1.
69. Lachance P. Dietary intake of carotenes and the carotene gap. *Clin Nutr.* 1988;7:118-122.
70. Gey KF, Stahelin HB, Eichholzer M. Poor plasma status of carotene and vitamin C is associated with higher mortality from ischemic heart disease and stroke: Basel Prospective Study. *Clin Invest.* 1993;71:3-6.
71. Frei B. Ascorbic acid protects lipids in human plasma and low-density lipoprotein against oxidative damage. *Am J Clin Nutr.* 1991;54:1113S-1118S.
72. Itoh R, Yamada K, Oka J, Echizen H, Suyama Y, Murakami K. Serum ascorbic acid and HDL cholesterol in a healthy elderly Japanese population. *Int J Vitam Nutr Res.* 1990;60:360-365.
73. Jacques PF, Hartz SC, McGandy RB, Jacob RA, Russell RM. Ascorbic acid, HDL, and total plasma cholesterol in the elderly. *J Am Coll Nutr.* 1987;6:169-174.
74. Riemersma RA, Oliver M, Elton PA, Alfthan G, Vartiainen E, Salo M, Rubba P, Mancini M, Georgi H, Vuilleumier JP, Gey KF. Plasma antioxidants and coronary heart disease: vitamins C and E, and selenium. *Eur J Clin Nutr.* 1990;44:143-150.
75. Aro A, Kyllastinen M, Kostiainen E, Gref CG, Elfving S, Uusitalo U. No effect on serum lipids by moderate and high doses of vitamin C in elderly subjects with low plasma ascorbic acid levels. *Ann Nutr Metab.* 1988;32:133-137.
76. Levine M, Dhariwal KR, Welch RW, Wang Y, Park JB. Determination of optimal vitamin C requirements in humans. *Am J Clin Nutr.* 1995;62(suppl):1347S-1356S.
77. Jacob RA, Skala JH, Omaye ST, Turnlund JR. Effect of varying ascorbic acid intakes on copper absorption and ceruloplasmin levels of young men. *J Nutr.* 1987;117:2109-2115.
78. Milner JA. Reducing the risk of cancer. In: Goldberg I, ed. *Functional Foods, Designer Foods, PharmaFoods, Nutraceuticals.* New York, NY: Chapman & Hall; 1994:39-70.
79. Zhu LZ, He YP, Piao JH. Difference of antioxidative effect between vitamin E and selenium. In: Ong ASH, Packer L. eds. Lipid-soluble antioxidants: biochemistry and clinical applications. Basel: Birkhauser Verlag, 1992:92-104.
80. Goldstrich JD. *The Cardiologist's Painless Prescription for a Healthy Heart and a Longer Life.* Dallas, Tex: 9-Heart; 1994.
81. Stocker R, Bowry VW, Frei B. Ubiquinol-10 protects human low density lipoprotein more efficiently against lipid peroxidation than does α-tocopherol. *Proc Natl Acad Sci USA.* 1991;88:1646-1650.
82. Alleva R, Tomasetti M, Battino M, Curatola G, Littarru GP, Folkers K. The roles of coenzyme Q_{10} and vitamin E on the peroxidation of human low-density lipoprotein subfractions. *Proc Natl Acad Sci USA.* 1995;92:9388-9391.
83. Kamei M, Fujita T, Kanbe T, Sasaki K, Oshibi K, Tani S, Matsui-Yuasi I, Morisawa S. The distribution and content of ubiquinone in foods. *Int J Vitam Nutr Res.* 1986;56:57-63.
84. US Dietary Guideline Committee, US Department of Agriculture, US Department of Health and Human Services. Nutrition and Your Health: Dietary Guidelines for Americans. 4th ed. 1995. Home & Garden Bulletin 232.
85. Moore RD, Pearson TA. Moderate alcohol consumption and coronary artery disease: a review. *Medicine (Baltimore).* 1986;65:242-267.

86. Pearson, TA. Alcohol and heart disease. *Circulation.* 1996;94:3023-3025.
87. Rimm EB, Klatsky A, Grobbee D, Stampfer MJ. Review of moderate alcohol consumption and reduced risk of coronary heart disease: is the effect due to beer, wine, or spirits? *BMJ.* 1996;312:731-736.
88. Klatsky AL, Friedman GD, Siegelaub AB. Alcohol and mortality. A ten-year Kaiser-Permanente experience. *Ann Intern Med.* 1981;95:139-145.
89. Renaud S, DeLogeril M. Wine, alcohol, platelets, and the French paradox for coronary heart disease. *Lancet.* 1992;339:1523-1526.
90. St Leger AS, Cochrane AL, Moore F. Factors associated with cardiac mortality in developed countries with particular reference to the consumption of wine. *Lancet.* 1979;1:1017-1020.
91. Kimura Y, Okuda H, Arichi S. Effect of stilbene derivatives on leukocyte arachadonic acid metabolism. *Waka Lyaku Gakkaishi.* 1985;2:516-517.
92. Seigneur M, Bonnet J, Dorian D, Benchimol F, Drouillet G, Gouverneur J, Larrue R, Crockett M, Boisseau P, Ribereau-Gayon, Bricaud H. Effect of the consumption of alcohol, white wine, and red wine on platelet function and serum lipids. *J Appl Cardiol.* 1990;5:215-222.
93. Frankel EN, Kanner J, German JB, Parks E, Kinsella JE. Inhibition of human low-density lipoprotein by phenol substances in red wine. *Lancet.* 1993;341:454-457.
94. Frankel EN, Waterhouse AL, Kinsella JE. Inhibition of human LDL oxidation by resveratrol. *Lancet.* 1993;341:1103-1104.
95. Gaziano JM, Buring JE, Breslow JL, Goldhaber SZ, Rosner B, VanDenburgh M, Willett W, Hennekens CH. Moderate alcohol intake, increased levels of high-density lipoprotein and its subfractions, and decreased risk of myocardial infarction. *N Engl J Med.* 1993:329:1829-1834.
96. Folts JD, Demrow HS, Slane PR. Moderate alcohol consumption, CAD, and myocardial ischemia. *J Myocard Ischemia.* 1994;6(8):33-40.
97. Renaud SC, Beswick AD, Fehily AM, Sharp DS, Elwood PC. Alcohol and platelet aggregation: the Caerphilly Prospective Heart Disease study. *Am J Clin Nutr.* 1992;55:1012-1017.
98. Marmot MG. Alcohol and coronary heart disease. *Int J Epidemiol.* 1984;13:160-167.
99. Criqui MH, Wallace RB, Mishkel M, Barrett-Connor E, Heiss G. Alcohol consumption and blood pressure: the Lipid Research Clinics Prevalence study. *Hypertension.* 1981;1:342-348.
100. Boffaetta P, Garfinkel L. Alcohol drinking and mortality among men enrolled in an American Cancer Society prospective study. *Epidemiology.* 1990;1:342-348.
101. Carroll KK, Kurowska EM. Soy consumption and cholesterol reduction: a review of animal and human studies. *J Nutr.* 1995;125:5945-5947.
102. Beynen AC. Comparison of the mechanism proposed to explain the hypocholesterolemic effect of soybean protein versus casein in experimental animals. *J Nutr Sci Vitaminol (Tokyo).* 1990;36:587-593.
103. van der Meer R, Beynen AC. Species-dependent responsiveness of serum cholesterol to dietary proteins. *J Am Oil Chem Soc.* 1987;64:1172-1177.
104. van der Meer R, de Vries HT, van Tintelen G. The phosphorylation state of casein and the species-dependency of its hypercholesterolemic effect. *Br J Nutr.* 1988;59:467-473.
105. Fumagalli R, Soleri L, Farini R, Musanti R, Mantero O, Noseda G, Gatti E, Sirtori CR. Fecal cholesterol excretion studies in type II hypercholesterolemic patients treated with soybean protein diet. *Atherosclerosis.* 1982;43:341-353.
106. Roda E, Mazzella G, Cornia GL, Villanova N, Pironi L, Barbara L. Effects of soybean protein-rich diet on biliary lipid composition. In: Barbara L, Miglioli M, Phillips SF, eds. *New Trends in Pathophysiology and Therapy of the Large Bowel.* Amsterdam, The Netherlands: Elsevier/North Holland Biochemical Press; 1983;309-312.
107. Ham JO, Chapman KM, Essex-Sorlie D, Bakhit RM, Prabhudesai M, Winter L, Erdman JW Jr, Potter SM. Endocrinological response to soy protein and fiber in mildly hypercholesterolemic men. *Nutr Res.* 1993;13:873-884.
108. Forsythe WA III. Soy protein, thyroid regulation, and cholesterol metabolism. *J Nutr.* 1995;125:619S-623S.
109. Huff MW, Hamilton RMG, Carroll KK. Plasma cholesterol levels in rabbits fed low-fat, cholesterol-free, semi-purified diets: effects of dietary proteins, protein hydrolysates, and amino acid mixtures. *Atherosclerosis.* 1977;28:187-195.
110. Potter SM, Jimenez-Flores R, Pollack J, Lone TA, Berber-Jimenez MD. Protein-saponin interaction and its influence on blood lipids. *J Agric Food Chem.* 1993;41:1287-1291.
111. Lo GS. Physiological effects and physio-chemical properties of soy cotyledon fiber. In: Furda I, Brine CJ, eds. *New Developments in Dietary Fiber.* New York, NY: Plenum Press; 1990:49-66.
112. Jariwalla RJ, Sabin R, Lawson S, Herman ZS. Lowering of serum cholesterol and triglycerides and modulation of divalent cations by dietary phytate. *J Appl Nutr.* 1990;42:18-28.
113. Lovati MR, Manzoni C, Agostinelle P, Ciappellano S, Mannucci L, Sirtori CR. Studies on the mechanism of the cholesterol lowering activity of soy proteins. *Nutr Metab CVD.* 1991;1:18-24.
114. Stampfer MJ, Colditz GA. Estrogen replacement therapy and coronary heart disease: a quantitative assessment of the epidemiological evidence. *Prev Med.* 1991;20:47-63.
115. Setchell KDR, Adlercreutz H. Mammalian ligans and phytoestrogens: recent studies on their formation, metabolism, and biological role in health and disease. In: Rowland IR, ed. *Role of the gut flora in toxicity and cancer.* New York, N.Y.: Academic Press; 1988:315-345.
116. Adlercreutz H, Markkanen H, Watanabe S. Plasma concentrations of phytoestrogens in Japanese men. *Lancet.* 1993;342:1209-1210.
117. Aklyama T, Ishida J, Nakagawa S, Ogawara H, Watanabe S, Itoh N, Shibuya M, Fukami Y. Genistein, a specific inhibitor of tyrosine-specific protein kinases. *J Biol Chem.* 1987;262:5592-5595.
118. Nakashima S, Koike T, Nozawa Y. Genistein, a protein tyrozin kinase inhibitor, inhibits thromboxane A2-mediated human platelet responses. *Mol Pharmacol.* 1991;39:475-480.
119. Sargeant P, Farndale RW, Sage SO. ADP-and thapsigargin-evoked Ca^{2+} entry and protein-tyrosine kinase inhibitors genisten and methyl-2,5-dihydroxycinnamate in fura-2-loaded human platelets. *J Biol Chem.* 1993;268:18151-18156.
120. Ozaki Y, Yatomi Y, Jinnai Y, Kume S. Effects of genistein, a tyrosine kinase inhibitor, on platelet functions. Genistein attenuates thrombin-induced Ca_{2+} mobilization in human platelets by affecting polyphosphoinositide turnover. *Biochem Pharmacol.* 1993;46:395-403.

121. Asahi M, Yanagi S, Ohta S, Inazu T, Sakai K, Takeuchi F, Taniguchi T, Yamamura H. Thrombin-induced human platelet aggregation is inhibited by protein-tyrosine kinase inhibitors, ST 638 and genistein. *FEBS Lett.* 1992;309:10-14.
122. Linassier C, Pierre M, LePecq JB, Pierre J. Mechanisms of action in NIH-3T3 cells of genistein; an inhibitor of EGF receptor tyrosine kinase activity. *Biochem Pharmacol.* 1990;39:187-193.
123. Wei H, Bowen R, Cai Q, Barnes S, Wang Y. Antioxidant and antipromotional effects of the soybean isoflavone genistein *Proc Soc Exp Biol Med.*
124. Jain AK, Vargas R, Gotzkowsky S, McMahon FG. Can garlic reduce levels of serum lipids? A controlled clinical study. *Amer J Med.* 1993;94:632-635.
125. Silagy C, Neil A. Garlic as a lipid lowering agent—a meta-analysis. *J Royal Coll Phys London.* 1994;8:39-45.
126. Agarwal KC. Therapeutic actions of garlic constituents. *Med Res Rev.* 1996;16:111-124.
127. Mei X, Wang ML, Xu HX, Pan XY, Gao CY, Han N, Fu MY. Garlic and gastric cancer: the influence of garlic on the level of nitrate and nitrite in gastric juice. *Acta Nutrimenta Sinica,* 1982;4:53-56.
128. Gore JM, Dalen JE. Cardiovascular disease. *JAMA.* 1994;271:1660-1661.
129. Warshafsky S, Kamer RS, Sivak SL. Effect of garlic on total serum cholesterol. A meta-analysis. *Ann Intern Med.* 1993;119:599-605.
130. Steiner M, Khan AH, Holbert D, Lin RI. A double-blind crossover study in moderately hypercholesterolemic men that compared the effect of aged garlic extract and placebo administration on blood lipids. *Amer J Clin Nutr.* 1996;64:866-870.
131. Simons LA, Balasubramaniam S, von Konigsmark M, Parfitt A, Simons J, Peters W. On the effect of garlic on plasma lipids and lipoproteins in mild hypercholesterolaemia. *Atherosclerosis.* 1995;113:219-225.
132. Yeh YY, Yeh SM. Garlic reduces plasma lipids by inhibiting hepatic cholesterol and triacylglycerol synthesis. *Lipids.* 1994;29:189-193.
133. Gebhardt R. Multiple inhibitory effects of garlic extracts on cholesterol biosynthesis in hepatocytes. *Lipids.* 1993;28:613-619.
134. Gebhardt R, Beck H. Differential inhibitory effects of garlic-derived organosulfur compounds on cholesterol biosynthesis in primary rat hepatocyte cultures. *Lipids.* 1996;31:1269-1276.
135. Sundaram SG, Milner JA. Diallyl Disulfide Induces Apoptosis of Human Colon Tumor Cells. *Carcinogenesis.* 1996;17:669-673.
136. Mathew BC, Daniel RS, Augusti KT. Hypolipidemic effect of garlic protein substituted for casein in diet of rats compared to those of garlic oil. *Indian J Exper Biol.* 1996;34:337-340.
137. Larner AJ. How does garlic exert its hypocholesterolaemic action? The tellurium hypothesis. *Med Hypo.* 1995;44:295-297.
138. Ali M, Thomson M. Consumption of a garlic clove a day could be beneficial in preventing thrombosis. *Prost Leuko & EFA.* 1995;53:211-212.
139. Villar R, Alvarino MT, Flores R. Inhibition by ajoene of protein tyrosine phosphatase activity in human platelets. *Biochim Biophys Acta.* 1997;1337:233-240.
140. Silagy CA, Neil HA. A meta-analysis of the effect of garlic on blood pressure. *J Hypertension.* 1994;12:463-468.

PART 4

IMPLEMENTATION STRATEGIES

CHAPTER 13

Promoting Dietary Adherence

Michelle Berry, MS, RD; and Debra Krummel, PhD, RD

Maintaining dietary adherence is often difficult as an individual begins the change to a new eating style. Eating habits can be extremely resistant to change because they are often formed early in life and are intricately woven into lifestyle, culture, and environment. Interventions that support behavior change and facilitate long-term adherence are needed to realize the health benefits of medical nutrition therapy.

In a retrospective study, time spent with a dietitian was positively correlated with the degree of cholesterol lowering experienced by patients who had a primary diagnosis of hypercholesterolemia (1). In a lipid clinic, a single counseling session led to significant reductions in plasma low-density lipoprotein cholesterol (LDL-C), but the patients' reduction was not enough to attain lipid goals (2). The authors suggest that longer and more controlled dietary interventions are necessary to achieve lipid goals. Attendance at three feedback sessions based on food frequency data enabled 88% of postmyocardial infarction patients to achieve a step II diet at 90 days after admission (3). However, this study reported neither the amount of dietitian contact time nor the content and format of the nutrition intervention.

Any contact that patients with non-insulin-dependent diabetes mellitus had with a dietitian produced better medical outcomes than no contact (4). Practice guidelines for patients with diabetes included at least three counseling sessions with a dietitian; the number of visits was determined by the patient's success in attaining goals and objectives (5). Four to five sessions have been suggested as necessary for cardiac patients to achieve desired outcomes (6,7). However, a number of factors may prevent patients from receiving diet counseling, including cost (70%), lack of interest (66%), lack of time (56%), lack of support from a significant other (38%), and lack of understanding of the benefits of counseling (36%) (7).

Counseling sessions that are based solely on strict education are less likely to produce adherence (8). A cognitive-behavioral approach that includes goal-setting, self-monitoring, reinforcement, feedback, and individualization was effective in a weight control program (9) and for patients with renal disease (10, 11). Although traditional instruction practices (individualizing diet, assessing previous knowledge, engaging social support, and providing information) remain popular, (7) behavioral strategies (goal-setting, contracting, assessing barriers, and self-monitoring) may facilitate adherence in all patients, including those with hyperlipidemia (12, 13). Many of the behavioral principles for weight management can be applied in counseling patients to decrease cardiovascular disease (CVD) risk regardless of weight status (Box 13-1). For example, stimulus control can be used to reduce the number of high-fat snacks kept in the home.

This chapter presents guidelines to aid the practitioner in supporting and promoting dietary adherence. From the initial client contact through follow-up and long-term monitoring, promoting adherence is an ongoing process that is intended to lead clients to better health and to higher levels of motivation and self-sufficiency.

The Foundations of the Client-Dietitian Relationship

The foundations of the client-dietitian relationship can be divided into the following categories for evaluation: the environment, educational principles, rapport, and nutrition history.

The Environment

Cardiovascular nutrition counseling may occur in a variety of settings, such as a clinic, hospital, health club, worksite, private practice, or home-based office. The availability of sufficient time, space, resources, and support in facilitating client adherence will influence the choice of setting. Clients' adherence is highly related to perceptions of quality of care (15), and initial impressions of quality of care are influenced by the environment in which intervention begins.

The meeting place should be attractive, quiet, comfortable, and conducive to confidentiality. Arrangements should

BOX 13-1 Behavioral Principles for Heart-Healthy Diets

STIMULUS CONTROL

- Instead of snacking, go for a walk.
- Store foods that don't fit your meal plan out of sight.
- Grocery shop when not hungry, using a list of foods appropriate for your meal plan.
- Purchase fat-modified products instead of favorite high-fat equivalents (eg, frozen yogurt instead of ice cream).

REWARD

- Enlist the help of family and friends.
- Use self-monitoring records as the basis for rewards (choose only nonfood rewards).
- Plan specific rewards for certain behaviors.

SELF-MONITORING

- Keep a record of foods consumed or a tally of targeted nutrients (eg, fat grams).
- Use self-monitoring for reinforcement.

RELAPSE PREVENTION

- Use a self-monitoring tool to identify barriers to change.
- Make small changes that you are likely to continue.

NUTRITION EDUCATION

- Learn about fat, saturated fatty acids, fiber, and sodium content of the foods you consume.
- Use the nutrition label.

COGNITIVE RESTRUCTURING

- Set realistic goals.
- Think about the successes, not the failures.
- Avoid use of the words "always" and "never."
- Counter negative thoughts with rational restatements.

Adapted from Stunkard AJ, Berthold HC (14). Used with permission of the American Society for Clinical Nutrition. © 1985 *Am J Clin Nutr.*

be made to ensure that counseling sessions are not interrupted by phone calls or other health care professionals (16). Good lighting and acoustics (especially for elderly clients) are desirable. If the setting is a patient's hospital room, uninterrupted time should be scheduled for nutrition counseling if possible and a screen or curtain should be used for privacy if necessary (17).

Interventions are most successful when they are consistently supported by all members of the health care team. Maintaining good communication with physicians, nurses and nurse practitioners, physician assistants, office staff, pharmacists, physical therapists, occupational therapists, and social workers can help to ensure that these professionals reinforce the importance of nutrition therapy. Clients frequently question each health care provider about the need for therapy—essentially testing the system to ensure that what they are being asked to do is important (16). Delivery of a consistent message by all team members can be a strong reinforcer (see Chapter 11).

It is helpful to let other team members know how they can reinforce adherence. Dietary change is a complex behavioral task. Changes usually must be implemented over time and assimilated into the client's lifestyle—a slow process that involves the gradual replacement of old habits with new ones. Repetition of principles, positive reinforcement, and problem solving are usually most helpful. Negative comments, disapproval, and scare tactics are not helpful and can lead to avoidance and canceled appointments. Care providers should be advised not to focus on dietary mistakes. Rather, they should focus on clients' strengths and accomplishments. Any positive change such as weight loss, improvement in cholesterol values, or effort to improve eating behavior should be acknowledged and praised.

The terms *compliance* and *noncompliance* have been criticized for connoting professional dominance (ie, the physician or nutritionist decides what is best and the client complies). The term *adherence* may be more accurate and less judgmental in tone and may also imply greater participation by the individual. Likewise, the term *patient* may be appropriate in medical settings, but in other settings terms such as *client, participant,* or *member* (for individuals enrolled in a program, group, or club) may imply a more collaborative, active role for the individual. Because for many individuals the word *diet* leads to avoidance, many practitioners prefer terms like *nutrition, healthful eating, eating style,* or *meal plan.*

Appointments for nutrition counseling should be scheduled in advance and should allow adequate time to discuss any questions that arise. A scheduled appointment conveys to the client that this time is important. It is helpful to prepare for appointments by reviewing background information about the client's medical or socioeconomic circumstances and gathering needed materials and resources. Meetings with the client should occur promptly at the scheduled time. Long waiting times are associated with lower adherence and with failure to keep follow-up appointments.

Educational Principles

Successful nutrition intervention involves much more than the provision of nutrition facts. Clients frequently must also learn to change behaviors, habits, personal environments, and lifestyles (17). Following are some teaching principles to keep in mind.

- The teaching style should be appropriate to the learner. The client's literacy level, knowledge, skills, attitudes, and circumstances will influence what, how, and how much is taught.
- Technical language should be avoided. Use terms like *high blood pressure* (instead of *hypertension*) and *high cholesterol* (instead of *hypercholesterolemia*). Learning is diminished when the client does not understand the terms being used.
- Simplicity is the best approach. Complex regimens are associated with lower levels of adherence (15). Keep all instructions and materials concise and easy to understand.
- Appropriate amounts of information should be provided.
- Examples, analogies, and anecdotes can be used to clarify main points. Information that is personalized is much more likely to be remembered.
- Active learning strategies such as role-playing exercises should be used. Clients' reactions can be sought and clients can be asked to describe the relevance of dietary information to their lifestyle.
- Strengths should be identified and built on. Positive attributes in clients' lifestyles can be pointed out. Clients can be taught to apply strengths and skills that they already have to achieve their health goals.
- Enthusiasm, creativity, and a variety of approaches are important in demonstrating that healthful eating can be enjoyable.
- Clients must be encouraged to learn new skills. Information alone seldom results in behavior change. Clients also need to develop and practice new skills such as cooking vegetables, interpreting nutrition labels, and selecting appropriate foods from restaurant menus. Skills can be practiced both during nutrition education sessions (ie, modifying recipes or creating menus for a week) and between sessions (ie, practicing assertiveness with co-workers who offer high-fat snacks).
- Clients should be encouraged to ask questions.
- Important points should be repeated often. It may be necessary to explain the same concept frequently or in several different ways.
- Written materials should be carefully selected. Written materials can aid in client education, but they should not be overused. Do not shower clients with papers, brochures, recipes, and coupons. The chosen materials should meet clients' immediate learning needs.
- Provision of frequent feedback is important. Clients should be informed of their weight, blood pressure reading, laboratory values, dietary assessment results, etc. This information can be used to reinforce concepts, observe progress, and relate behaviors to outcomes.

Rapport

The establishment of rapport is the first step in building a positive, collaborative relationship. Rapport-building helps clients to feel welcome, comfortable, respected, and safe. Nutrition counselors should project warmth, acceptance, sincerity, and empathy so that clients feel free to openly discuss their concerns.

Rapport is an ongoing process of maintaining two-way communication, trust, and mutual cooperation. Counseling skills that promote rapport include listening attentively to clients, being alert not only to what is said but also to body language; summarizing what clients say to demonstrate interest and to clarify meaning; and identifying and acknowledging clients' feelings (Table 13-1). Practitioners should avoid doing most of the talking themselves; the objective is to encourage the client to talk. Open-ended questions (ie, "What…," "How…," or "Tell me…") help clients to better define their thoughts and feelings and enable therapists to better understand clients' views.

Rapport can convey either an authority-centered or a client-centered approach. In an authority-centered approach, the professional is an authority figure who advises a course of action that the client is expected to carry out (eg, by following a 1,500-kcal meal plan that is provided). In a client-centered approach, the client actively participates in clarifying needs and exploring potential solutions (eg, by identifying meals at fast-food restaurants as a contributor to weight and cholesterol concerns and brainstorming ideas for alternative quick meals).

Grommet (18) provides the following example of how

TABLE 13-1

Counseling Skills That Enhance Rapport

Skill	Examples
Nonverbal behavior	Good eye contact Leaning toward the patient Appropriate nodding Facial expressions that match the mood of the client
Attentive listening	Listening without interrupting Concentrating on understanding the client's views and perspective
Nonjudgmental reflection of content	"You've tried to change your eating before (content responses; paraphrasing), but after a couple of weeks it didn't seem to be worth the effort."
Empathic reflection of feelings (affective responses)	"You were really disappointed when you found out that your cholesterol had increased again."
Use of open-ended questions	"What has been most effective when you've tried to lose weight before?"

commonly used behavior modification techniques can differ by approach. Using the authority-centered approach, after reviewing the client's food records the professional advises a behavioral solution such as, "You will need to keep all food in the kitchen cabinets to eliminate visual cues." Using the client-centered approach, after reviewing food records the professional invites the client to identify cues to eating and to explore ways to reduce cues and develop nonfood responses to them. In the client-centered approach, the client's active involvement facilitates learning, aids in problem identification, and can enhance motivation and commitment.

The Nutrition History

Every client contact is an opportunity to gain a greater understanding of the multiple factors that influence the individual's nutrition and cardiovascular health. Initial sources of information may include medical records, other health professionals, a phone call to the individual, and a questionnaire that is completed by the client before the first meeting. Additional information is obtained by using good listening skills and asking open-ended questions. Food records and other dietary instruments provide quantitative information. All of this information contributes to a complete and accurate assessment.

A thorough nutrition history includes assessments of usual dietary intake, weight history, activity levels, psychosocial and economic factors that affect dietary choices (eg, home environment, income, educational level, and ethnic and religious background), nutrition knowledge, and readiness to learn and change (19). An objective measure of nutrient intake should be used for baseline and long-term assessment of adherence (see Chapter 4).

The nutrition history helps the dietitian to understand the client's food preferences, eating environment, and other circumstances that may affect nutrition intervention. More than one session may be required to obtain a complete nutrition history.

STRATEGIES TO PROMOTE ADHERENCE

Individualization of Therapy

Medical nutrition therapy is individualized on the basis of the client's lipid values and goals, medication, and other medical and lifestyle considerations that are identified in the assessment. The dietary assessment may identify specific food groups in which changes would significantly benefit the client; meat, dairy products, baked goods, and desserts are usually the largest contributors of dietary fat, although this varies with the individual. Food records may indicate specific behaviors (eg, eating large portion sizes) or behaviors linked to times of day (eg, eating in the evening) that need to be addressed.

Clients' motivation for seeking nutrition counseling is critical to the success of a nutrition intervention. The Stages of Change model (20) provides a useful framework for individualizing nutrition interventions on the basis of clients' readiness and willingness to change. According to this model, individuals progress through a series of stages before achieving maintenance of desired behaviors (Table 13-2). Theoretically, the use of stage-specific interventions can help clients to progress from one stage to the next (21, 23, 24). Examples of nutrition interventions based on the Stages of Change model are shown in Table 13-3.

The degree to which a client likes a regimen (25) and the degree to which the regimen is tailored to the client's needs (15) strongly influence subsequent adherence. Some clients may be well-suited to making comprehensive changes. For example, a cardiac client who is highly motivated to reduce angina may choose a very-low-fat, near-vegetarian diet to achieve symptomatic relief (26). Other clients may need to begin by making small dietary changes and developing confidence in their ability to adhere. Clients must be very involved in this process because only they know their limitations (16). A client-centered approach enhances the dietitian's ability to effectively individualize therapy.

TABLE 13-2

Stages of Change

Stage	Description	Examples
Precontemplation	There has been no change and there is no intent to change in the foreseeable future (next 6 months). The individual is unaware or underaware of the problem. May be resistant to change or defensive; may deny risk or possibility of complications.	The patient is not aware of cholesterol level and is not interested or concerned. Avoids reading, thinking, or talking about changing eating habits.
Contemplation	The individual is aware that a problem exists, is seriously thinking about working on it, but currently is not prepared to take action. Considering change (within next 6 months). May remain in this stage for an extended period of time until ready to act.	The patient is aware that cholesterol has shown an increase at each annual physical exam and wants to know what this means and what to do about it. Receptive to reading material.
Preparation	The individual commits to taking action within the next month. Willing to set behavioral goals and to begin making some small behavioral changes as a prelude to the next stage. This is a good time to refer the patient to an action-oriented program.	The patient is considering different plans of action to take and is evaluating pros and cons. Switched to a lower-fat milk, is reading, and is comparing food labels.
Action	This is the period of overtly and progressively modifying behavior, experiences, or environment to resolve the problem. The individual actively participates in dietary interventions, exercise interventions, or both. After 6 months of continuous successful action, the individual enters the maintenance stage.	The patient acts on goals that were set with the dietitian. May be counting fat grams and trying to stay below a target level. May pack low-fat lunches daily to take to work.
Maintenance	The individual works to continue the new behaviors, integrate them into lifestyle, and prevent relapse. It is an active (not passive) stage in which the individual continues to modify the environment to maintain the new behaviors.	The patient is pleased with the progress made and is committed to continuing positive eating behaviors. Follow-up sessions with dietitian are reduced to twice a year. It is recognized that eating at social events and during travel pose a challenge, so the patient focuses on learning strategies and skills to handle those situations more effectively and consistently.
Relapse	The individual backslides to former behavior. Recovering from a relapse involves reentering a previous stage.	When spouse became ill, low-fat eating and other lifestyle changes could not be continued. The patient ate frequently in fast-food restaurants, had no time to exercise, and regained some weight.

From Grommet JK (18); Prochaska JO, DiClemente CC (20); Sandoval WM, Heller KE, Wiese WH, Childs DA (21); Clark MM, Pera V, Goldstein MG, Thebarge RW, Guise BJ (22).

TABLE 13-3

Using the Stages of Change Model for Nutrition Interventions

Stage	Goal	Strategies
Precontemplation	Personalize risk for the client.	1. Create a supportive climate for change. 2. Discuss the diet and cardiovascular disease relationship—relate eating behavior to risk factors. 3. Assess nutrition knowledge and attitudes. 4. Build on prior nutrition knowledge.
Contemplation	Increase self-efficacy.	1. Identify problematic behaviors. 2. Prioritize behaviors to change. 3. Discuss coping strategies. 4. Discuss motivations. 5. Identify barriers to change. 6. Identify solutions to barriers. 7. Gain support from family and friends.
Preparation	Initiate change.	1. Set small, attainable goals. 2. Discuss earlier attempts to change. 3. Discuss ways to succeed at change.
Action	Commit to change.	1. Reinforce decision to change. 2. Encourage self-rewarding behavior. 3. Increase coping skills. 4. Discuss relapse prevention techniques.
Maintenance	Continue commitment.	1. Plan follow-up to support changes. 2. Reinforce self-rewarding behaviors. 3. Increase coping skills. 4. Discuss relapse and techniques.
Relapse	Reinforce commitment	1. Reassess motivation and barriers. 2. Discuss importance of maintaining change. 3. Explore new coping strategies.

Adapted with permission from Sandoval WM, Heller KE, Wiese WH, Childs DA, *Top Clin Nutr* 9(3):64-69 (21). © 1994 Aspen Publishers, Inc.

Teaching materials and approaches should be geared to clients' educational and literacy level, lifestyle, and readiness and willingness to change. Approaches to lipid-lowering diets include the use of food lists, individualized menus, exchange lists, and food pyramids and other guides, as well as quantitative approaches such as counting calories or fat grams. An approach should be selected that is appropriate for the client. For some individuals, developing a handwritten, specific plan with the dietitian's assistance may be the most effective strategy (27).

Sensitivity to cultural and ethnic influences is important. When necessary, efforts should be made to locate foreign-language materials and well-illustrated materials that require minimal interpretation. An excellent resource for cultural food practices is the American Dietetic Association/American Diabetes Association series of professional manuals, *Ethnic and Regional Food Practices* (28), which include typical and modified meal patterns, menus, and exchange lists for a variety of ethnic groups including soul/southern, Filipino, Alaskan, Chinese, Jewish, Navajo, Mexican, and others. (See Chapter 16 for a discussion of intervention strategies for special groups.)

Involving Clients in Problem Solving

Clients should be encouraged to be actively involved in developing behavior-change strategies. Dietitians may suggest possibilities, but clients are most committed to a plan of action if they have chosen and planned it themselves. For example, a client prone to eating high-fat restaurant foods during lunch break can be encouraged to identify strategies for changing this behavior and then to select a strategy and develop a plan for implementing it. When clients learn how to solve adherence problems, they gain confidence, skill, and the ability to handle issues that arise in the future (29).

Challenges to the adoption of a low-fat, heart-healthy diet have been identified in long-term intervention studies

BOX 13-2 **Scenario of a Nutrition Counselor Converting General Intentions into Specific Behaviors and Stating the Behavioral Goals in Positive Terms**

Client:	I really just want to lose weight.
Counselor:	Losing weight is important to you for a number of reasons.
Client:	Yes, for my cholesterol, my heart, my appearance. I'll feel better; I will have less arthritis pain in my knees. It's what I really need to do.
Counselor:	You are very determined about succeeding.
Client:	I have to do this! From now on I will watch what I eat—after all, I know what I should eat. I'll watch what I eat and I'll come to these appointments regularly. I know that I will stay on track if I report to someone.
Counselor:	You're motivated and feel ready to start now. But tell me—what do you mean when you say you'll watch what you eat?
Client:	Well, you know what I mean. I'll watch the fat and the sugar. I won't have second helpings.
Counselor:	You will have one serving instead of two.
Client:	That's right. At dinner, I usually eat second and even third helpings. I know I will lose weight if I just take one moderate-size portion of each food.
Counselor:	Great idea! Let's write that down as one of your goals for the next couple of weeks. (The counselor gives the client a pen and paper. The client writes: "At dinner, I will have one moderate size portion of each food.") Now tell me — how do you plan to watch the fat?
Client:	Well, *you* know what I mean. I don't need to put butter on my vegetables, my potatoes, and my bread. I could get lite cream cheese for my morning bagel. I could skip the whipped cream on the jello.
Counselor:	You certainly have a lot of ideas that would reduce your total fat intake. Let's write all of those down. And instead of focusing on what you won't eat, let's describe what you will eat. You plan to enjoy your vegetables, potatoes, bread, and jello plain and you intend to buy lite cream cheese for your morning bagel.

(30, 31) as well as observed in practice. These challenges include a preference for high-fat foods (ie, regular cheese, mayonnaise and salad dressings, and whole milk); an inability to decrease meat portion sizes; difficulty replacing meat meals with vegetarian meals; and increasing consumption of low-fat grains, mixed dishes, and fruits and vegetables without added fat.

Clients can actively confront these challenges by identifying problems, giving them a level of priority, identifying solutions, and setting specific goals. Individuals are more likely to be committed to (32) and take responsibility for goals that they generate (33). The nutrition counselor's role is to ensure that the client's strategy is specific, that it will have an impact on the problem, and that the client is likely to successfully implement the strategy (34).

Positive Reinforcement

Negative words (eg, *no*, *not*, *don't*, *stop*, *avoid*, and *eliminate*) should be avoided. It is preferable to emphasize the foods that can be eaten (eg, breads, cereals, grains, legumes, vegetables, and fruits) rather than those that should be avoided. Dietitians can help clients to choose strong, positive goals ("I would like to eat fruit and popcorn for snacks") instead of weak, negative ones ("I would like to cut out the high-fat chips").

Positive reinforcement is one of the best strategies for shaping behavior. Acknowledging, praising, and encouraging clients who make positive changes, no matter how minor, help to ensure that the behavior is repeated and that other positive changes follow.

Focusing on Behaviors

Behaviors are within clients' control. Outcomes (eg, weight loss, lower cholesterol, and triglyceride control) result from sustained behaviors. For example, a client who has failed in previous attempts to lose weight may say that he wants to lose 30 lb and maintain the loss for a year. This is an outcome, not a behavior. Asking "What actions can you take to achieve that outcome?" helps clients to focus on behaviors rather than on results (29). Box 13-2 contains a scenario in which the nutrition counselor converts general intentions into specific behaviors and states the behavioral goals in positive terms.

An appropriate number of goals may have to be negotiated if the client seems to be taking on too many at once. Establishing satisfactory goals clarifies for both client and counselor the behaviors that will be attempted and reassures the counselor that the client's efforts will indeed decrease total fat and calories. At the next meeting, the counselor can ask about the client's progress in implementing these behaviors. Barriers to the implementation of specific behaviors are more easily resolved than generalized attitudinal barriers such as "I blew it. I didn't lose any weight. I have no discipline."

Activities such as planning menus, modifying recipes, comparing food labels, and role-playing can be incorporated into nutrition counseling sessions to help clients practice new behaviors. Food modeling (providing samples of appropriate low-fat foods to taste) can be an effective way for clients to experience target behaviors (16). Many individuals do not actively seek out new food experiences but are willing to try a new food if it is offered to them. If the experience is positive, they are often willing to eat the food again in their own environment. (See Chapter 15 for a more detailed discussion of food sampling, cooking demonstrations, and cooking classes.)

Teaching Self-monitoring

Self-monitoring is considered one of the most effective behavioral strategies for achieving adherence (35). Whenever a client establishes a new behavioral goal, the dietitian should ask "How will you track that?" Clients can be encouraged to keep records, using food diaries, calendars, checklists, and other self-monitoring tools. Record keeping maintains day-to-day awareness of behavior and helps to alter habits and increase behavioral consistency. It also provides a record of both successes and problems that can be addressed at subsequent counseling sessions.

A variety of self-monitoring techniques may be appropriate, depending on the individual and the behaviors being targeted. Someone who is trying to modify grocery shopping habits might save supermarket register tapes as a record of shopping behavior. Someone who is trying to reduce doughnut-eating at work might pocket a quarter for every piece of fruit eaten instead of a doughnut and count the change at the end of the day or week. Another easy and effective approach is noting on a calendar the amount of time spent exercising or the number of meatless meals eaten in a week.

When clients put time and effort into keeping records, it is important to spend time reviewing the records during counseling sessions. Counselors should avoid expressing judgment or disapproval at the quality or content of clients' records. It is difficult to keep accurate records; some foods (or behaviors) may be omitted, and errors in portion size are common. Records are best used to identify trends, point out strengths, and teach concepts.

At the end of each session, it is helpful to ask clients to explain in their own words what their goals are. It is important to establish that a client understands at least one behavior that can be taken to improve the targeted risk factor.

Follow-up

Adherence after only one session is unlikely. Time is needed to try dietary adjustments through trial and error, to make lifestyle adjustments, and to achieve short-term behavioral goals that eventually lead to long-term adherence. At follow-up sessions the practitioner can answer questions and provide reinforcement. Three sessions at 1-month intervals have been recommended for medical nutrition therapy (19). (See Chapter 15.)

A common problem in nutrition intervention is failure to take follow-up lipid measurements at 6- and 12-month intervals (36). To maintain adherence to therapy, clients need to receive feedback about the progress they are making. Witnessing an improvement in cholesterol level can strongly reinforce behavior change. However, if cholesterol is not measured until 6 months to 1 year after behavior change has occurred, recidivism is likely. Lipid panels (total, low-density lipoprotein, and high-density lipoprotein cholesterol and triglyceride concentrations) are usually much more useful than total cholesterol alone for assessing the effectiveness of an intervention and providing feedback to clients. Nutritionists should communicate with physicians and clients (and in many cases insurance providers) about the value of follow-up measurements.

The second report of the National Cholesterol Education Program recommends that cholesterol measurements be taken at 4 to 6 weeks and 3 months after initiation of nutrition therapy (37). If the response is unsatisfactory, a second trial of dietary therapy is recommended, with measurements taken at 3 to 6 weeks and 3 months. At least 6 months of intensive dietary therapy is indicated before lipid-lowering drug therapy is considered; some clients may require a year or more of instruction and counseling.

Long-term contact, structure, and reinforcement are extremely useful (38); peer support is also effective (39). Group programs can provide a source of ongoing peer and professional support. Clients should be encouraged to become involved in appropriate follow-up programs such as support groups, cardiac rehabilitation programs, and heart-health classes and to meet with nutrition professionals who provide long-term follow-up services. The American Heart Association, local hospitals, medical centers, colleges and universities, the American Dietetic Association National Nutrition Network referral hotline (1-800-366-1655), and Mended Hearts (a national network of cardiac patient support groups based in Dallas, Texas [214-706-1442]) are sources of information about ongoing support. (Also see Chapter 15.)

Monitoring Progress and Outcomes

Indicators of progress are important for the counselor (to evaluate the effectiveness of the intervention), the client (to obtain feedback), and the physician (to make treatment decisions). Indicators of adherence fall into three categories: physiological measures, dietary data, and subjective assessments by counselor and client. No single measure is reliable on its own; eating behavior and physiological response are so dynamic that a combination of measures is always recommended.

Physiological Measures. Objective measures include lipid values, blood pressure, blood glucose concentration, weight, body composition, and other physical and biochemical measurements. Alone, they may not accurately indicate adherence because they are influenced by nondietary factors such as hormonal changes, medications, fluid retention, physical activity, and stress. Because it may take some time for behavior changes to be reflected in changes in physiological measures, overdependence on such measures may underestimate adherence and frustrate clients. For example, weight fluctuates widely depending on hydration and is known to plateau at times during a weight-loss program. Over time, physiological measures generally will corroborate behavior changes. However, care must be taken not to accuse clients of failing to adhere when they simply are nonresponders. Multiple physiological measures should be obtained so that patterns and trends can be observed and evaluated over time.

Changes in Dietary Data. Data on actual eating behavior are a useful indicator of change when compared with baseline data over time. Self-reported food intake data are subject to error unless closely monitored, as may occur in a research setting. Underreporting, omissions, and errors in portion sizes are common problems and should be taken into consideration. In combination with other adherence indicators, however, dietary data are a valuable source of information. (See Chapter 4 for specific recommendations on dietary assessment.)

Subjective Assessments. Client-reported changes are the most immediate indicator of progress. For self-reports to be a reliable part of the clinician's assessment, good rapport and a trusting, collaborative relationship must have been established with the client. Clients' desire to comply may result in overreporting of success (16), but subjective assessments can be useful, especially in documenting progress that is not yet apparent in objective measures (29). Sandoval, Heller, Wiese, and Childs (21) suggest that progress can be expressed as movement from one stage of change to the next: "The client did not lose a significant amount of weight. However, she moved from contemplation to action and made significant changes in diet."

BARRIERS TO CHANGE

Identifying Barriers

Barriers to dietary change take many forms—absence of family support, a life change that disrupts normal eating, a birth, an illness, a new job, travel, beliefs and attitudes, or any other obstacle that interferes with a client's intention to adhere. Barriers must be clearly identified and cognitive and affective issues that the client associates with the problem must be clarified. This is best accomplished by using the counseling skills described earlier. Clarifying the problem often helps the client to more effectively identify possible solutions to the problem.

Once a barrier has been identified, it is important that the client refocus attention on the desired positive outcomes. Frequently clients and counselors dwell on problems rather than on the positive outcomes that they seek (29). A problem orientation might be expressed as, "No matter how I try, I have not been able to do anything positive for my own health since the divorce." Counselors can guide clients to adopt a goal orientation that views the skills, information, resources, and abilities necessary for change as goals that lead to personal development. The problem may be restated as "It is important to do something positive for my own health now—and these are the specific things I want to do," and specific behaviors and time frames can be listed.

Barriers may or may not be related to nutrition. In the previous example, exercise, smoking cessation, and a long-overdue visit to the dentist may make the list, but more healthful eating practices may not yet fit into the client's overall plan. However, the client is better focused and able to chip away at the barrier that is blocking dietary change. Therapists cannot solve problems or overcome barriers for their clients, but they can help to empower clients to take the next step for themselves. It is useful to maintain a list of other professionals (social workers, psychologists, physical therapists, exercise physiologists, etc.) to whom clients can be referred when referral is indicated.

Laquatra and Danish (29) classify barriers, or roadblocks, into four general categories: lack of knowledge, lack of skills, lack of social support, and fear of taking risks. Table 13-4 gives examples of nutrition-related roadblocks. It can be helpful to first classify the type of roadblock that a barrier represents. Too often, practitioners try to give information when the client already knows what to do. Repetition of dietary information is not helpful when the roadblock is a lack of skill, social support, or ability to take risks. Frequently individuals know what to do but not how to do it (a skill roadblock). Alternatively, they may perceive that the costs of change outweigh the benefits (a risk-taking roadblock). Change occurs with the realization that the elimination of roadblocks is under the individual's control (29).

Whether nutrition counseling is short term or long term, counselors who help clients to identify interim goals that chip away at barriers are taking the most effective approach. In long-term counseling, practitioners with more advanced counseling skills can teach skill development, risk-taking, and social support strategies.

Promoting Self-sufficiency

A Chinese proverb says, "Give a man a fish and you feed him for a day. Teach a man to fish and you feed him for a lifetime." The primary objective of nutrition counseling is to equip clients with the skills necessary to sustain a heart-healthy diet and a healthful lifestyle for the rest of their lives. Three levels of motivation have been described that are relevant to nutrition (29, 40).

- Compliance, the lowest level of motivation, occurs when individuals conform to certain behaviors to gain rewards or avoid punishment. Compliance is usually short term and rarely results in maintenance. ("They told me at the hospital that I have to follow this diet.")

TABLE 13-4

Overcoming Roadblocks to Adherence

Example of Barrier	Roadblock	Possible Strategies
The patient consistently underestimates the amount of total fat, saturated fat, and cholesterol consumed.	Lack of knowledge	The patient keeps a record of food intake and uses a counter to self-monitor the targeted nutrients to increase knowledge of food composition and alternative ways to meet nutrient goals.
The patient's active social life and travel schedule result in frequent access to high-fat foods.	Lack of skill	The patient learns how to select the lowest-fat foods at parties and special events, be assertive in social situations and restaurants, and make special requests. Role-playing and practice are used to improve skill level.
The patient's family is not supportive of lower-fat eating. Family members complain when lower-fat foods are served.	Lack of social support	The patient identifies the type of support needed from family and practices requesting the support in a way that increases the likelihood of receiving it. The patient may need to seek other sources of support if family members remain unwilling.
The patient is reluctant to refuse high-fat pastries baked by his mother for fear of hurting her feelings or appearing ungrateful.	Lack of risk taking	After discussing and exploring the risks vs benefits, the patient generates ideas on how to decrease the risks involved. Action is initiated in small steps and outcome is assessed at each step.
The patient's life is in transition because of a recent move to a new community and the patient is depending on convenience and fast foods right now.	Combination of lack of knowledge, skill, social support, and risk taking	After the least amount of change the patient is willing to make is determined, the patient begins with setting a small, achievable behavioral goal and follows up with progressively more challenging goals after each success.

- Identification is a higher level of motivation. Individuals adopt behaviors because they like or respect the counselor or identify with the program. ("I couldn't possibly let the other group members [or my dietitian] down!")
- Internalization is the highest level of motivation. Strategies for change are developed and adopted because they are consistent with the individual's value system. ("I believe in eating the healthiest and freshest foods possible. After all, it is an investment in me.")

Dietitians interact with individuals at all three levels. The skills clients learn—problem solving, setting goals, using feedback, and altering habits—are intended to increase self-sufficiency and self-motivation. These life skills can be used in many different settings.

SUMMARY

Many theory-based tools are available to dietitians to enhance adherence: individualization, client-centered problem-solving, positive reinforcement, goal-setting, self-monitoring, follow-up, social support, and monitoring of progress and outcomes. Use of these tools helps to foster empowered clients who are successful at making dietary changes for life.

CASE STUDY

A recently retired high school teacher was referred for cholesterol reduction. He was motivated to focus time and attention on his health. He felt that multiple stressors and demands on his time during his final years of teaching had led him to neglect his health. As a result, he had gained too much weight. Although he loved sports (including coaching), over the years his level of physical activity had declined almost to zero.

The client began nutrition counseling in January. He reported skipping meals, severely reducing meat consumption, and severely restricting calorie consumption to lose

BOX 13-3 Profile of Client

Age: 63 years
Height: 6'3"
Sex: male

Date	Weight
1/29	284½ lb
2/19	285¼
3/8	283
3/22	285
5/14	Refused to be weighed.
6/1	276¼
7/9	272¾
9/9	261¼ lb

Date	Lipid values:[a]			
	Chol (mg/dL)	LDL (mg/dL)	HDL (mg/dL)	TG (mg/dL)
1/5	243	180	37	130
3/22	248	186	36	128
6/1	242	180	37	125
9/9	214	144	43	137
10/9	212	144	44	122

Date	Food Log Daily Average Food Score:[b]
1/12	7
5/9	16
6/27	9
8/10	7
9/1	4

[a]Chol, cholesterol; LDL, low-density lipoprotein cholesterol; HDL, high-density lipoprotein cholesterol; and TG, triglycerides.
[b]A food score of 10 or below is equivalent to the step I diet. A score of 5 or below is equivalent to the step II diet (Cholesterol Lowering Intervention Program, University of Pittsburgh).

weight quickly. However, he also reported uncontrollable periods of eating in which he regained lost weight. His initial food log score was 7, but at that time he was inexperienced at self-monitoring and it is likely that some underreporting occurred (Box 13-3).

Nutrition counseling was aimed at helping the client to identify goals, monitor his behavior, observe patterns and trends, and use problem solving to achieve his goals. The counselor presented the principles of low-fat eating and healthy weight loss. Increased activity was promoted to aid in weight loss; meal-skipping was discouraged. Although past experience had convinced the client that eliminating meat was the fastest way to lose weight, that type of eating pattern proved to be too restrictive to sustain over the long term. He eventually settled on a pattern of vegetarian eating on most days, with an occasional serving of lean meat.

In April, the client decided to join a supervised exercise program offered at a hospital near his home; the program combined aerobic activity, weight training, and stretching. His attendance was erratic at first, but after making some schedule adjustments and getting acquainted with the program staff, he began working out regularly three times a week. The combination of regular exercise and low-fat eating resulted in significant weight loss as well as a significant increase in his enthusiasm and self-confidence. Low-fat eating and exercise became an integral part of his lifestyle.

During this period, a major life event occurred. The client's son was drafted by a major-league baseball team. The client and his wife traveled frequently to visit their son out-of-state and to attend games. Frequent travel challenged maintenance of his exercise routine and frequent meals away from home challenged maintenance of his low-fat diet. Strategies for maintaining a healthful lifestyle during travel became the main topic of discussion at intervention sessions.

The client currently is continuing all of his efforts. His weight has decreased by 23¼ lb, high-density lipoprotein cholesterol concentration has increased from 37 to 44 mg/dL, and low-density lipoprotein cholesterol concentration has decreased from 180 to 144 mg/dL (a 20% reduction) (Box 13-3). The client continues to return for follow-up nutrition counseling and cholesterol measurements as he attempts to reduce low-density lipoprotein cholesterol to below 130 mg/dL.

REFERENCES

1. McGhee MM, Johnson EQ, Rasmussen HM, Sahyoun N, Lynch MM, Carey M. Benefits and costs of medical nutrition therapy by registered dietitians for patients with hypercholesterolemia. *J Am Diet Assoc.* 1995;95:1041-1043.
2. Dallongeville J, Leboeuf N, Blais C, Touchette J, Gervais N, Davignon J. Short-term response to dietary counseling of hyperlipidemic outpatients of a lipid clinic. *J Am Diet Assoc.* 1994;94:616-621.
3. DeBusk RF, Miller NH, Superko HR, Dennis CA, Thomas RJ, Lew HT, Berger WE, Heller RS, Rompf J, Gee D, Kraemer HC, Bandura A, Ghandour G, Clark M, Shah RV, Fisher L, Taylor CB. A case-management system for coronary risk factor modification after acute myocardial infarction. *Ann Intern Med.* 1994;120:721-729.
4. Franz MJ, Splett PL, Monk A, Barry B, McClain K, Weaver T, Upham P, Bergenstal R, Mazze RS. Cost-effectiveness of medical nutrition therapy provided by dietitians for persons with non-insulin-dependent diabetes mellitus. *J Am Diet Assoc.* 1995;95:1018-1024.
5. Monk A, Barry B, McClain K, Weaver T, Cooper N, Franz MJ. Practice guidelines for medical nutrition therapy provided by dietitians for persons with non-insulin-dependent diabetes mellitus. *J Am Diet Assoc.* 1995;95:999-1006.
6. Plous S, Chesne RB, McDowell AV. Nutrition knowledge and attitudes of cardiac patients. *J Am Diet Assoc.* 1995;95:442-446.
7. Hyman DJ, Clark M, Houston-Miller N, Johannsson M, Ghandour G, Shah R, Debusk RF. Cholesterol-related counseling by registered dietitians in northern California. *Prev Med.* 1992;21:746-753.
8. Neil HAW, Roe L, Godlee RJP, Moore JW, Clark GMG, Brown J, Thorogood M, Stratton IM, Lancaster T, Mant D, Fowler GH. Randomised trial of lipid lowering dietary advice in general practice: the effect on serum lipids, lipoproteins, and antioxidants. *BMJ.* 1995;310:569-573.
9. Skender ML, Goodrick GK, Del Junco DJ, Reeves RS, Darnell L, Gotto AM, Foreyt JP. Comparison of 2-year weight loss trends in behavioral treatments of obesity: diet, exercise, and combination interventions. *J Am Diet Assoc.* 1996;96:342-346.
10. Milas NC, Nowalk MP, Akpele L, Castaldo L, Coyne T, Doroshenko L, Kigawa L, Korzec-Ramirez D, Scherch L, Snetselaar L. Factors associated with adherence to the dietary protein intervention in the modification of diet in renal disease study. *J Am Diet Assoc.* 1995;95:1295-1300.
11. Gillis BP, Caggiula AW, Chiavacci AT, Coyne T, Doroshenko L, Milas C, Nowalk MP, Scherch LK. Nutrition intervention program of the Modification of Diet in Renal Disease study: a self-management approach. *J Am Diet Assoc.* 1995;95:1288-1294.
12. McCann BS, Retzlaff BM, Dowdy AA, Walden CE, Knopp RH. Promoting adherence to low-fat, low-cholesterol diets: review and recommendations. *J Am Diet Assoc.* 1990;90:1408-1417.
13. Baldwin TT, Falciglia GA. Application of cognitive-behavioral theories to dietary change in clients. *J Am Diet Assoc.* 1995;95:1315-1317.
14. Stunkard AJ, Berthold HC. What is behavior therapy: a very short description of behavioral weight control. *Am J Clin Nutr.* 1985;41:821-823.
15. Caggiula AW, Watson JE. Characteristics associated with compliance to cholesterol lowering eating patterns. *Patient Educ Couns.* 1992;19:33-41.
16. Caggiula AW, Milas NC. Approaches to successful nutritional intervention in renal disease. In: Mitch WE, Klahr S, eds. *Nutrition and the Kidney.* 2nd ed. Boston, Mass: Little, Brown; 1993:365-387.
17. Raab C, Tillotson JL, eds. *Heart to Heart: A Manual on Nutrition Counseling for the Reduction of Cardiovascular Disease Risk Factors.* Bethesda, Md: National Institutes of Health; 1983. NIH Publication No. 83-1528.
18. Grommet JK. Weight management: framework for changing behavior. In: Dalton S, ed. *Overweight and Weight Management: The Health Professional's Guide to Understanding and Practice.* Gaithersburg, Md: Aspen Publishers; 1997.
19. Smith KG, Johnson EQ, eds. *Medical Nutrition Therapy Across the Continuum of Care.* Chicago: American Dietetic Association, 1996.
20. Prochaska JO, DiClemente CC. Transtheoretical therapy: toward a more integrative model of change. *Psychother Theory Res Pract.* 1982;19:276-288.
21. Sandoval WM, Heller KE, Wiese WH, Childs DA. Stages of change: a model for nutrition counseling. *Top Clin Nutr.* 1994;9:64-69.
22. Clark MM, Pera V, Goldstein MG, Thebarge RW, Guise BJ. Counseling strategies for obese patients. *Am J Prev Med.* 1996;12:266-270.
23. Thompson B, Shannon J, Beresford SA, Jacobson PE, Ewings JA. Implementation aspects of the Seattle "5 a Day" intervention project: strategies to help employees make dietary changes. *Top Clin Nutr.* 1995;11:58-75.
24. Glanz K, Kristal AR, Sorensen G, Palombo R, Heimendinger J, Probart C. Development and validation of measures of psychosocial factors influencing fat- and fiber-related dietary behavior. *Prev Med.* 1993;22:373-378.
25. Coyne T, Olson M, Bradham K, Garcon M, Gregory P, Scherch L. Dietary satisfaction correlated with adherence in the Modification of Diet in Renal Disease study. *J Am Diet Assoc.* 1995;95:1301-1306.
26. Barnard ND, Akhtar A, Nicholson A. Factors that facilitate compliance to lower fat intake. *Arch Fam Med.* 1995;4:153-158.
27. Diabetes Care and Education Dietetic Practice Group, The American Dietetic Association. *Meal Planning Approaches for Diabetes Management.* 2nd ed. Chicago, Ill: American Dietetic Association; 1994.
28. Diabetes Care and Education Dietetic Practice Group, American Dietetic Association. *Ethnic and Regional Food Practices: A Series.* Chicago, Ill: American Dietetic Association; 1989–present.
29. Laquatra I, Danish SJ. Nutrition counseling in weight management. In: Dalton S, ed. *Overweight and Weight Management: The Health Professional's Guide to Understanding and Practice.* Gaithersburg, Md: Aspen Publishers; 1997.
30. Barnes MS, Terry RD. Adherence to the cardiac diet: attitudes of patients after myocardial infarction. *J Am Diet Assoc.* 1991;91:1435-1439.
31. Kristal AR, White E, Shattuck AL, Curry S, Anderson G,

Fowler A, Urban N. Long-term maintenance of a low-fat diet: durability of fat-related dietary habits in the Women's Health Trial. *J Am Diet Assoc*. 1992;92:553-559.
32. Berry MW, Danish SJ, Rinke WJ, Smiciklas-Wright H. Worksite health promotion: the effects of a goal-setting program on nutrition-related behaviors. *J Am Diet Assoc*. 1989;89:914-923.
33. Lauer L. Enhancing skills for the emerging nutrition therapist. *Ventures* (ADA Nutrition Entrepreneurs DPG newsletter). 1996;12:17-18.
34. Caggiula AW, Milas NC. Nutrition counseling for success. *Top Clin Nutr*. 1986;1:7-13.
35. Baker RC, Kirschenbaum DS. Self-monitoring may be necessary for successful weight control. *Behav Ther*. 1993;24:377-394.
36. Caggiula AW, Watson JE, Kuller LH, Olson MB, Milas NC, Berry M, Germanowski J. Cholesterol Lowering Intervention Program: effect of the step I diet in community office practices. *Arch Intern Med*. 1996;156:1205-1213.
37. National Cholesterol Education Program. *Second Report of the Expert Panel on Detection, Evaluation, and Treatment of High Blood Cholesterol in Adults (Adult Treatment Panel II)*. Bethesda, Md: National Institutes of Health; 1993. NIH Publication No. 93-3095.
38. Wing RR. Behavioral treatment of obesity: its application to Type II diabetes. *Diabetes Care*. 1993;16:193-199.
39. Lefavi R, Kratina K. "Connection" in the therapeutic relationship. *SCAN's Pulse*. 1996;15:16-17.
40. Kelman HC. Compliance, identification, and internalization: three processes of attitude change. In: Hinto BL, Reitz HJ, eds. *Groups and Organizations: Integrated Readings in the Analysis of Social Behavior*. Belmont, Calif: Wadsworth; 1971.

CHAPTER 14

Making Healthful Food Choices to Achieve a Step I Diet

Lynn D. Dugan, MS, RD; Catherine Champagne, PhD, RD; Brenda Eissenstat, MS, RD; and Karen Reznik Dolins, MS, RD

Translating nutrition knowledge into a message that clients will remember and use is a challenging task for dietitians. An effective way to begin is to identify nutrition concepts that clients are familiar with and link new concepts to this existing framework. Focusing on a few target behaviors (usually one to three desired changes) is often adequate to make significant progress toward improved health. Clients who successfully adopt a few fat-reduction strategies are more likely to maintain them and be open to additional changes in the future.

A recent study (1) of individuals who had successfully lowered their fat intake from a mean of 45% to 25% of energy from fat identified the following six significant fat-reduction strategies (listed in descending order of significance):

- decreasing the use of fat as flavoring (eg, in salad dressings, spreads, and gravy);
- decreasing consumption of recreational foods (eg, snacks, hot dogs, cookies, and pizza);
- decreasing the use of added cooking fat;
- decreasing consumption of beef, pork, and cheese and increasing that of rice, beans, and fruit;
- changing breakfast choices to decrease consumption of meats and eggs; and
- using fat-modified foods.

Nutrition recommendations are often presented in terms of percentage (ie, limiting calories from saturated fat to 10% of energy). However, teaching clients to prepare meals and providing suggestions for specific meals and foods are usually more effective strategies for achieving sustained reductions in dietary fat intake.

This chapter provides information relevant to these strategies and other important topics, including using the new food label in diet planning, expanding food choices at the grocery store, preparing food and cooking, and making appropriate restaurant and fast-food choices. Presenting these concepts in a manner that emphasizes clients' individual needs facilitates an enjoyable transition to a more healthful diet.

Using the New Food Label for Diet Planning

Nutrition labeling has been a source of consumer information since the 1970s. However, before 1990, nutrition labels did not provide information about key nutrients that are needed to plan special diets for clients with cardiovascular disease. Furthermore, nutrition labels were not consistently useful because they were not included on all packaged food products. To use the new food label for diet planning, nutritionists and consumers must be familiar with

- the nutrition facts label,
- nutrient content claims and descriptors, and
- health claims.

The Nutrition Facts Label

The Nutrition Labeling and Education Act of 1990 (NLEA) dramatically changed nutrition labeling by requiring the US Food and Drug Administration (FDA) and the US Department of Agriculture (USDA) to significantly revise food labels. These revisions went into effect in mid-1994. (Resources on food labeling are listed in Box 14-1.) Today, approximately 90% of processed foods display the Nutrition Facts Label, which provides information that is useful for planning special diets.

The new food label, illustrated in Figure 14-1, ensures that the same nutrition information is displayed on all products. Whereas the old label highlighted nutrients for the purpose of overcoming dietary deficiencies, the new label provides information about key nutrients that are of public health concern for the purpose of disease prevention—total fat, saturated fat, cholesterol, sodium, and dietary fiber. Serving size and the number of servings per container are

BOX 14-1 Additional Resources on Food Labeling

- Boyd Browne M. *Label Facts for Healthful Eating: Educators' Resource Guide.* Dayton, Ohio: The Mazer Corporation; 1993.
- Food labeling: health claims; oats and coronary heart disease. *Fed Regist.* 1996;61:296-337.
- Food labeling: rules and regulations. *Fed Regist.* 1993;58:667, 17087-17090.
- Guthrie JF, Fox JJ, Cleveland LE, Welsh S. Who uses nutrition labeling, and what effects does label use have on diet quality? *J Nutr Educ.* 1995;27:163-172.
- Kris-Etherton PM, Wozniak-Wowk C, Scott LW, Jaax S. Implementation of blood cholesterol-lowering diets using nutrition labels. *Top Clin Nutr.* 1994;10:14-26.
- *The New Food Label: There's Something in It for Everybody.* Washington, DC: International Food and Information Council, US Department of Health and Human Services, US Food and Drug Administration; 1994.

FIGURE 14-1

Nutrition facts label for chili beans

Nutrition Facts	
Serving Size ½ cup (130 g)	
Servings Per Container about 3	
Amount per Serving	
Calories 110	Calories from Fat 10
	% Daily Value*
Total Fat 1 g	**1%**
Saturated Fat 0 g	**0%**
Cholesterol 0 mg	**0%**
Sodium 460 mg	**19%**
Total Carbohydrate 21 g	**7%**
Dietary Fiber 6 g	**23%**
Sugars 3 g	
Protein 6 g	
Vitamin A 10% •	Vitamin C 0%
Calcium 4% •	Iron 10%
*Percent Daily Values are based on a 2,000 calorie diet.	

listed at the top of the label. Serving sizes are standardized across product categories, making nutrition information more readily comparable for similar foods. Next, total calories and calories from fat are listed. The product's content in grams of carbohydrate, sugars, fat, and protein is listed, as well as the percent daily value (DV) for these nutrients.

The percent DV is a new tool that is designed to quantify how the nutrients of one food serving fit into the 2,000-kcal reference diet. The DV is based on the current nutrition recommendations of the USDA Food Guide Pyramid and the US Dietary Guidelines for Americans (2, 3). For example, the label illustrated in Figure 14-1 indicates that consumers requiring a 2,000-kcal diet would get approximately 1% of their recommended total daily fat intake (65 g of fat or no more than 30% of calories from fat) by consuming one serving of this food. Table 14-1 gives the daily values used to calculate the percent DV for nutrients on the food label.

A recent survey found that only half of the adults questioned understood what percent DV was (4). Consequently, basic nutrition education should include a review of the food label and how to use it. The American Dietetic Association and other professional organizations provide many educational tools that explain the most effective use of the food label (see Appendix 3).

Food labels must also list four micronutrients—vitamin A, vitamin C, calcium, and iron—that were singled out for their impact on disease prevention. The US Recommended Dietary Allowances for these micronutrients were listed on the old food label. On the new label, they are listed as a percentage of DV only.

Also included on the label are the number of kilocalories that the food provides per gram for fat, carbohydrates, and protein. If space permits, some labels may include a footnote with information about nutrient intakes with a 2,000- or 2,500-kcal reference diet.

Dietitians can teach their clients at least two ways of using the information on the nutrition label to plan and implement a low-fat, cholesterol-lowering diet: counting fat grams and using the percent DV. The new labels make it easy for consumers to count grams of total fat and, if appropriate, saturated fat. Polyunsaturated and monounsaturated fat may also be listed on the label if a nutrient content claim is made relating to fatty acids or cholesterol. Clients following the step I or II diet can also use the kilocalorie, cholesterol, sodium, and fiber content information on the label.

The percent DV can be used to compare similar food products or to guide daily food choices. Mathematically inclined clients can add the percent DV of a nutrient in all foods eaten in a day to get a general idea of how their intake fits in with their nutrition goals. For this application of percent DV to be valuable, however, clients must understand

TABLE 14-1

Daily Values Used to Calculate % DV on the Nutrition Label

Food Component	Daily Value[a]
Total fat (g)[b]	65[c]
Saturated fat (g)[b]	20[c]
Cholesterol (mg)[b]	300
Sodium (mg)[b]	2,400
Potassium (mg)	3,500
Total carbohydrate (g)[b]	300[c]
Dietary fiber (g)[b]	25[d]
Protein (g)[b]	50[c]
Vitamin A (IU)[b]	5,000
Vitamin C (mg)[b]	60
Calcium (g)[b]	1
Iron (mg)[b]	18
Vitamin D (IU)	400
Vitamin E (IU)	30
Thiamin (mg)	1.5
Riboflavin (mg)	1.7
Niacin (mg)	20
Vitamin B-6 (mg)	2.0
Folate (mg)	0.4
Vitamin B-12 (μg)	6.0
Biotin (mg)	0.3
Pantothenic acid (mg)	10
Phosphorus (g)	1
Iodine (μg)	150
Magnesium (mg)	400
Zinc (mg)	15

[a]Daily value for adults and children aged 4 or older.

[b]Mandatory component of the nutrition label.

[c]Daily value based on a 2,000-kcal reference diet.

[d]Daily value based on 11.5 g per 1,000 kcal.

their individual nutrition goals.

Remember that the DV on the label relates to the 2,000-kcal reference diet. Therefore, clients must know whether their target consumption level is more or less than 2,000 kcal. For example, clients adopting a 1,600-kcal diet should consume no more than 80% of DV for the nutrients specifically indicated in a cholesterol-lowering diet (ie, fat, saturated fat, cholesterol, and sodium). A client on a 2,500-kcal diet could consume 125% of DV for these same nutrients.

However, many clients do not understand and rarely use percentages. They prefer to know how many grams of key nutrients a food provides. For example, to maintain a goal of 20% to 30% of energy from fat on a 1,600-kcal diet, total fat consumption should be between 35 g and 53 g. For nutrients such as dietary fiber, vitamin C, calcium, and iron, exceeding the recommended DV may be acceptable and even desirable for some clients.

For clients who are following diets that are more restrictive than those outlined by the Dietary Guidelines and the Food Guide Pyramid (eg, step II and very-low-fat diets), DV goals must be adjusted and calculated on an individual basis. Clients with known cardiovascular disease may need to adjust fat, saturated fat, cholesterol, and sodium intakes.

For example, clients following a step II diet would need to reduce their daily saturated fat intake to 70% of DV (ie, 7% of energy from saturated fat instead of 10%). A client whose goal is to consume 20% of energy from fat should not exceed 66% of DV for fat (ie, 20% of total calories from fat instead of 30%). The target consumption level can also be described as a number of fat grams for a given energy level. A client on a diet restricted to 1,500 mg of sodium should not exceed 62% of DV for sodium (ie, 1,500 mg instead of 2,400 mg).

Diets will always include foods that do not carry the nutrition label, such as fresh meat, fish, poultry, and produce as well as ready-to-eat foods such as deli and bakery items, restaurant foods, bulk foods, and foods sold by small businesses. The absence of a label on these products should not discourage the practitioner or the client from using the nutrition label for overall diet planning. Information on the ingredient list of foods missing nutrition labels can be used to assess fat and sodium contents. Clients should understand how to decrease total fat, saturated fat, and cholesterol intake in all foods by

- substituting lower-fat foods for high-fat foods (eg, skim milk for whole milk and lean meats and lower-

TABLE 14-2

Target Levels for Total Fat, Saturated Fat, Cholesterol, and Sodium on Labels with Health Claims

To make a health claim, a product must have no more than:

	Individual Food Product[a]	Main Dish Product[b]	Meal Product[b]
Total fat (g)	13	19.5	26
Saturated fat (g)	4	6	8
Cholesterol (mg)	60	90	120
Sodium (mg)	480	720	960

[a]Per reference amount, per label serving, and for foods for which reference amount is ≤30 g or ≤2 tsp per 50 g.
[b]Per labeled serving.

fat cheeses for their higher-fat counterparts),
- decreasing consumption of high-fat foods,
- using cooking methods that add little or no fat (eg, baking instead of frying), and
- monitoring portion sizes.

The USDA's Food Guide Pyramid can be used to guide serving sizes and proportions of foods in the diet (2). The range of serving sizes given in the Food Guide Pyramid for each food category permits flexibility in planning meals for different calorie levels.

In addition to the Nutrition Facts Label and the listing of ingredients, the NLEA provides two new, strictly defined tools—nutrient content claims and health claims—that can be useful in helping individuals make food choices that promote adherence to a special diet.

Nutrient Content Claims

Nutrient content claims or descriptors are claims used on food packages to describe the amount of a nutrient per serving of the food. Because they have the same meaning for every product on which they appear, consumers can use them as a quick reference when evaluating food choices. However, because nutrient content claims are voluntary, products that carry no claims may be nutritionally similar to those that do carry a content claim—and equally appropriate for a special diet.

Box 14-2 gives the NLEA's definitions of all nutrient content claims. The following are the most important claims for clients following a cholesterol-lowering diet:

- *Lean* and *extra lean* describe the total fat content of meat, poultry, seafood, and game meats. *Lean:* less than 10 g total fat, less than 4 g saturated fat, and less than 95 mg cholesterol per 100 g of meat *or,* for a main dish or meal-type product, 100 g and per labeled serving. *Extra lean:* less than 5 g total fat, less than 2 g saturated fat, and less than 95 mg cholesterol per 100 g of meat *or* 100 g and per labeled serving of a main dish or meal-type product.
- *Free* as in fat free: less than 0.5 g per serving; saturated fat free: less than 0.5 g saturated fat per serving and *trans* fatty acids 1% or less of total fat.
- *Low* as in low fat: 3 g or less per serving; low saturated fat: 1 g or less per serving and 1% or less of calories from saturated fat; low sodium: 140 mg or less per serving; and low cholesterol: 20 mg or less and 2 g or less of saturated fat per serving.
- *Reduced* or *less:* at least 25% less of a nutrient relative to the regular version of the same product.
- *Light:* 50% less of a nutrient relative to the regular version of the same product.

Health Claims

The NLEA authorizes health claims for the following nine nutrient-disease relationships that are supported by research:

1. fiber-containing grain products, fruits, and vegetables *and* cancer;
2. fruits and vegetables *and* cancer;
3. fat *and* cancer;
4. fiber-containing grain products, fruits, and vegetables *and* coronary artery disease;
5. saturated fat and cholesterol *and* coronary artery disease;
6. oat bran and rolled oats *and* coronary artery disease;
7. sodium *and* hypertension;
8. folate *and* neural tube defects; and
9. calcium *and* osteoporosis.

To be eligible to carry a health claim, a food must meet the following three criteria: it must not exceed specific amounts of total fat, saturated fat, cholesterol, and sodium (Table 14-2); it must contain at least 10% of DV (before supplementation) of protein, dietary fiber, vitamin A, vitamin C, calcium, and iron; and it must meet nutrient levels that are specific for each approved health claim.

Health claims provide another tool that clients who are following a cholesterol-lowering diet can use to identify appropriate foods. Products that carry claims related to coronary artery disease are low in total fat, saturated fat, and cholesterol. In Table 14-3, the health claims relevant to cardiovascular disease risk are those numbered 4, 6, and 9.

The American Heart Association (AHA) has developed a point-of-purchase tool to assist consumers in choosing

BOX 14-2 Federal Definitions for Nutrient Content Claims

	Free	Low	Reduced	Other
Calorie	Fewer than 5 calories per Reference Amount. Also labeled **free of calories, no calories, zero calories, without calories, trivial source of calories, dietarily insignificant source of calories.**	40 calories or less per Reference Amount when Reference Amount is more than 30 g *or* more than 2 Tbsp. 40 calories or less per Reference Amount *and* per 50 g when Reference Amount is 30 g or less *or* 2 Tbsp or less. *Exception:* "Low-calorie" sugar substitutes containing 40 calories or less per serving and *not* per 50 g product. Main-dish products and meal products containing 120 calories or less per 100 g. Also labeled **few calories, contains a small amount of calories, low source of calories, low in calories.**	At least 25% fewer calories per Reference Amount. Meal products and main-dish products containing at least 25% fewer calories per 100 g. Also labeled **reduced in calories, calorie reduced, fewer calories, lower calorie.** *Claim Example:* "Reduced calorie cupcakes—33% fewer calories than regular cupcakes. Calorie content has been reduced from 150 to 100 calories per serving."	**Light** or **lite** product has ⅓ fewer calories *or* 50% less fat per Reference Amount; if more than half the calories are from fat, fat content must be reduced by 50% or more. *Claim Example:* "Lite cheese cake—200 calories, 4 g fat. Regular cheese cake—300 calories, 8 g fat per serving." Main-dish products or meal products must meet requirements for **low calorie** *or* **low fat** and must identify nature of the claim. *Claim Example:* "Light Delite Baked Flounder Dinner with Rice and Mixed Vegetables, a low-fat meal." A product for which the reference food contains 40 calories or less and 3 g fat or less per serving may use the term **light** or **lite** without further qualification if it is reduced by 50% or more in sodium content compared to the reference food. Certain nonnutrient claim uses of **light** or **lite** are permitted but must be accompanied by qualifying information. *Other uses:* **light in color, light in texture, light brown sugar, light molasses.** *See* Sodium definitions for **lightly salted** and **light in sodium.**
Fat	Less than 0.5 g fat per Reference Amount and no added ingredient that is a fat or generally understood by consumers to contain fat unless marked by an asterisk referring to the statement "adds a trivial amount of fat," "adds a negligible amount of fat," or "adds a dietarily insignificant amount of fat." Main-dish products and meal products containing less than 0.5 g fat per labeled serving. Also labeled **free of fat, no fat, zero fat, without fat, nonfat, trivial source of fat, negligible source of fat, dietarily insignificant source of fat.**	3 g or less fat per Reference Amount when Reference Amount is more than 30 g or more than 2 Tbsp. 3 g or less fat per serving *and* per 50 g when Reference Amount is 30 g or less or 2 Tbsp or less. Main-dish products and meal products containing 3 g or less total fat per 100 g and not more than 30% calories from fat. Also labeled **low in fat, contains a small amount of fat, low source of fat, little fat.**	At least 25% less fat per Reference Amount. Main-dish products and meal products containing at least 25% less fat per 100 g. Also labeled reduced in fat, fat reduced, less fat, lower fat, lower in fat. *Claim Example:* "Reduced fat - 50% less fat than our regular brownies. Fat content has been reduced from 8 g to 4 g per serving."	**—Percent fat free** permitted if product meets requirements for "low fat." **—Percent lean** permitted for meat and poultry products and main-dish and meal products if products meet requirements for "low fat." **100 percent fat free** meets requirements for "fat free" if product contains less than 0.5 g fat per 100 g and contains no added fat. **Light** or **lite** product has ⅓ fewer calories *or* 50% less fat per Reference Amount. *Claim Example:* "Light mayonnaise, 50% less fat than regular mayonnaise."

(cont)

	Free	Low	Reduced	Other
Saturated Fat	Less than 0.5 g saturated fat per Reference Amount and the level of trans fatty acids does not exceed 1% of the total fat; containing no ingredient that is saturated fat or is generally understood by consumers to contain saturated fat unless marked by an asterisk referring to the statement "adds a trivial amount of saturated fat," "adds a negligible amount of saturated fat," or "adds a dietarily insignificant amount of saturated fat." Main-dish products and meal products containing less than 0.5 g saturated fat per labeled serving and the level of trans fatty acids does not exceed 1% of the total fat. Also labeled **free of saturated fat, no saturated fat, zero saturated fat, without saturated fat, trivial source of saturated fat, negligible source of saturated fat, dietarily insignificant source of saturated fat.**	1 g or less saturated fat per Reference Amount and no more than 15% of calories from saturated fat. Main-dish products and meal products containing 1 g or less saturated fat per 100 g and less than 10% of calories from saturated fat. Also labeled **low in saturated fat, contains a small amount of saturated fat, low source of saturated fat, a little saturated fat.**	At least 25% less saturated fat per Reference Amount. Main-dish products and meal products containing at least 25% less saturated fat per 100 g. Also labeled **reduced in saturated fat, saturated fat reduced, less saturated fat, lower saturated fat, lower in saturated fat.** *Claim Example:* "Reduced saturated fat. Contains 50% less saturated fat than the national average for nondairy creamers. Saturated fat reduced from 3 to 1.5 g per serving."	
Cholesterol	Less than 2 mg cholesterol per Reference Amount and 2 g or less saturated fat per Reference Amount; containing no ingredient generally understood by consumers to contain cholesterol unless marked by an asterisk referring to the statement "adds a trivial amount of cholesterol," "adds a negligible amount of cholesterol," or "adds a dietarily insignificant amount of cholesterol." Main-dish product containing 19.5 g or less total fat per labeled serving, less than 2 mg cholesterol per labeled serving, and less than 2 g saturated fat per labeled serving. Meal product containing 26 g or less total fat per serving, less than 2 mg cholesterol per labeled serving, and less than 2 g saturated fat per labeled serving. When fat exceeds 13 g per Reference Amount, per labeled serving, or per 50 g if Reference Amount is 30 g or less or 2 Tbsp or less, the product must declare the amount of total fat next to claim; also, for main-dish products with	20 mg or less cholesterol per Reference Amount and 2 g or less saturated fat per Reference Amount when Reference Amount is more than 30 g or more than 2 Tbsp; contains 13 g or less total fat per Reference Amount. 20 mg or less cholesterol per Reference Amount *and* per 50 g; and 2 g or less saturated fat per Reference Amount when Reference Amount is 30 g or less or 2 Tbsp or less; contains 13 g or less total fat per Reference Amount. When fat exceeds 13 g per Reference Amount (or per 50 g if Reference Amount is 30 g or less *or* 2 Tbsp or less), the product must declare the total amount of fat in the serving next to claim. Main-dish products containing 19.5 g or less total fat per labeled serving, 20 mg or less cholesterol per 100 g, and 2 g or less saturated fat per 100 g. Meal products containing 26 g or less total fat per labeled serving, 20 mg or less cholesterol per 100 g, and 2 g or less saturated fat per 100 g.	At least 25% less cholesterol and 2 g or less saturated fat per Reference Amount per 50 g if Reference Amount is 30 g or less to 2 Tbsp or less. When fat exceeds 13 g per Reference Amount, per labeled serving, or per 50 g if Reference Amount is 30 g or less or 2 Tbsp or less, the product must declare the total amount of fat in a serving next to claim. For main-dish products, at least 25% less cholesterol per 100 g, and 2 g or less saturated fat per 100 g (product must declare the total amount of fat in a serving if product contains more than 19.5 g fat). For meal products at least 25% less cholesterol per 100 g, and 2 g or less saturated fat per 100 g (product must declare the total amount of fat in a serving if product contains more than 26 g fat). Also labeled **reduced in cholesterol, cholesterol reduced, less cholesterol, lower cholesterol, lower in cholesterol.** *"Reduced Cholesterol" Claim Example (product)*	Cholesterol claims only allowed when food contains 2 g or less saturated fat per Reference Amount.

(cont)

	Free	Low	Reduced	Other
Cholesterol (cont'd)	more than 19.5 g fat and meal products with more than 26 g fat per labeled serving. Also labeled **free of cholesterol, zero cholesterol, without cholesterol, no cholesterol, trivial source of cholesterol, negligible source of cholesterol, dietarily insignificant source of cholesterol.**	Also labeled **low in cholesterol, contains a small amount of cholesterol, low source of cholesterol, little cholesterol.**	*has more than 13 g fat):* "This pound cake contains 30% less cholesterol than our regular pound cake. Cholesterol lowered from 45 mg to 30 mg per serving. Contains 15 g fat per serving."	
Sodium	Less than 5 mg sodium per Reference Amount and containing no ingredient that is sodium chloride (table salt) or is generally understood by consumers to contain sodium unless marked by an asterisk referring to the statement "adds a trivial amount of sodium," "adds a negligible amount of sodium," or "adds a dietarily insignificant amount of sodium." Main-dish products and meal products containing less than 5 mg sodium per labeled serving. Also labeled **free of sodium, no sodium, zero sodium, without sodium, trivial source of sodium, negligible source of sodium, dietarily insignificant source of sodium.**	140 mg or less sodium per Reference Amount when Reference Amount is more than 30 g or more than 2 Tbsp. 140 mg or less sodium per Reference Amount *and* per 50 g when Reference Amount is 30 g or less or 2 Tbsp or less. Main-dish products and meal products containing 140 mg or less sodium per 100 g. Also labeled **low in sodium, little sodium, contains a small amount of sodium, low source of sodium.** **Very Low:** 35 mg or less sodium per Reference Amount when Reference Amount is more than 30 g or more than 2 Tbsp. **Very Low:** 35 mg or less sodium per Reference Amount *and* per 50 g when Reference Amount is 30 g or less or 2 Tbsp or less. **Very Low:** Main-dish products and meal products containing 35 mg or less sodium per 100 g. Also labeled **very low in sodium.**	At least 25% less sodium per Reference Amount. Main-dish products and meal products containing at least 25% less sodium per 100 g. Also labeled **reduced in sodium, sodium reduced, less sodium, lower sodium, lower in sodium.** *Claim Example:* "Reduced sodium spaghetti sauce—50% less sodium than regular spaghetti sauce. Sodium content has been reduced from 300 to 150 mg per serving."	**Light in sodium** or **Lite in sodium** product has 50% less sodium per Reference Amount. For main-dish products and meal products, **Light/Lite in Sodium** means the food is **Low Sodium.** Salt is not synonymous with sodium. Salt refers to sodium chloride, which is 40% sodium. **Salt free** meets requirements for **sodium free.** **Unsalted, Without added salt,** or **No salt added** are permitted if (1) no salt is added during processing, and (2) the product it resembles and substitutes for is normally processed with salt, and (3) the label bears the statement "not a sodium free food" or "not for control of sodium in the diet" if the food is not sodium free. **Lightly salted** has added 50% less sodium than is normally added to the food; label must declare "not a low sodium food" if product is not "low in sodium."
Sugar	Less than 0.5 g sugar per Reference Amount and containing no ingredient that is a sugar or that is generally understood by consumers to contain sugar unless marked by an asterisk referring to the statement "adds a trivial amount of sugar," "adds a negligible amount of sugar," or "adds a dietarily insignificant amount of sugar." Main-dish products and meal products containing less than 0.5 g sugars per labeled serving. Label must also declare	May not be used as a claim.	At least 25% less sugar per Reference Amount. Main-dish products and meal products containing at least 25% less sugar per 100 g. Also labeled **reduced in sugar, sugar reduced, less sugar, lower sugar, lower in sugar.** *Claim Example:* "These corn flakes contain 25% less sugar than our sugar coated corn flakes. Sugar content has been lowered from 12 to 9 g per serving."	**No added sugar, Without added sugar,** or **No sugar added** are permitted if 1) no amount of sugars, or any other ingredient that contains sugars that functionally substitute for added sugars, is added during processing or packaging; 2) the product contains no ingredients that contain added sugars, such as jam, jelly, or concentrated fruit juice; 3) the product it resembles and substitutes for normally contains added sugars; and 4) the label declares that the food is not "low calorie" or "calorie reduced" as appropriate.

(cont)

	Free	Low	Reduced	Other
Sugar (cont'd)	that the product is "not a reduced calorie food," "not a low calorie food," or "not for weight control" unless the food meets the requirements for a low calorie or reduced calorie food. Also labeled **free of sugar, no sugar, zero sugar, without sugar, sugarless, trivial source of sugar, negligible source of sugar, dietarily insignificant source of sugar.**			

Other Terms

Good source, Contains, Provides	Contains 10 to 19% of the Daily Value per Reference Amount. May not be used as a claim for total carbohydrate. Meal products and main-dish products must clearly identify the claim subject (food component). *Claim Example:* "The serving of sweet potatoes in this product is a good source of dietary fiber."
High, Rich in, Excellent source of	Contains 20% or more of the Daily Value per Reference Amount. May not be used as a claim for total carbohydrate. Meal products and main-dish products must clearly identify the claim subject (food component). *Claim Example:* "The serving of broccoli in this product is high in vitamin C."
More, Fortified, Enriched, Added	Contains at least 10% more of the Daily Value for protein, vitamins, minerals, dietary fiber, or potassium per Reference Amount compared to the reference food. Main-dish products and meal products containing at least 10% more of the Daily Value for protein, vitamins, minerals, dietary fiber, or potassium per 100 g. "Fortified" and "enriched" may not be used as a claim on meat or poultry products. *Claim Example:* "Contains 10% more of the daily value for fiber than white bread. Fiber content of white bread is 1 g per serving; (this product) 3.5 g per serving."
Fiber	Product making any fiber claim must qualify for a "good source" or "high" claim; must declare the level of total fat per Reference Amount if food is not "low fat."
Lean	Meat, poultry, seafood, and game meat with less than 10 g total fat, less than 4 g saturated fat, and less than 95 mg cholesterol per Reference Amount and 100 g. Main-dish, meal, and meal-type products with less than 10 g total fat, less than 4 g saturated fat, and less than 95 mg cholesterol per 100 g and per labeled serving.
Extra Lean	Meat, poultry, seafood, and game meat with less than 5 g total fat, less than 2 g saturated fat, and less than 95 mg cholesterol per Reference Amount and 100 g. Main-dish, meal, and meal-type products with less than 5 g total fat, less than 2 g saturated fat, and less than 95 mg cholesterol per 100 g and per labeled serving.

Source: Boyd Browne MG. *Label Facts for Healthful Eating: Educator's Resource Guide.* National Food Processors Association. Dayton, Ohio: The Mazer Corporation, 1993.

TABLE 14-3

Disease-specific Health Claims

Subject of Health Claim	Specific Nutrient Requirements
1. Fiber-containing grain products, fruits, and vegetables *and* cancer	Food must be or must contain a grain product, fruit, or vegetable Food is "low fat" Food is (without fortification) a "good source of dietary fiber"
2. Fruits and vegetables *and* cancer	Food must be or must contain a fruit or vegetable Food is "low fat" Food is a "good source" of at least one of the following: vitamin A, vitamin C, or dietary fiber
3. Fat *and* cancer	Food is low fat or fish and game meats are "extra lean"
4. Fruits, vegetables, and grain products that contain fiber *and* coronary artery disease	Food must be or must contain a fruit, vegetable, or grain product Food is "low saturated fat," "low cholesterol," and "low fat" Food contains (without fortification) at least 0.6 g soluble fiber per reference amount: Soluble fiber must be listed on nutrition information panel
5. Saturated fat and cholesterol *and* coronary artery disease	Food is "low saturated fat," "low cholesterol," and "low-fat" or fish and game meats are "extra lean"
6. Oat bran and rolled oats *and* coronary artery disease	Food must contain 13 g oat bran/serving or 20 g rolled oats/serving and this serving must provide 1 g of beta-glucan soluble fiber; the food must also be low in fat, saturated fat, and cholesterol
7. Sodium *and* hypertension	Food is "low sodium"
8. Folate *and* neural tube defects	Food is a "good source" of folate
9. Calcium *and* osteoporosis	Food is "high calcium" Calcium content is easily absorbed Food contains no more phosphorus than calcium per reference amount

healthful foods. The Heart-Check Program, developed in 1994, helps consumers identify foods that, when used as part of a healthful diet, meet the AHA's dietary guidelines for fat and cholesterol consumption for healthy people over age 2. All food manufacturers except those associated with tobacco companies may participate in the program. Foods that meet the AHA's criteria clearly display the heart-check mark on product packaging. This program provides another practical, visual cue to consumers who are attempting to purchase healthful foods.

The AHA criteria are based on a review of current scientific evidence and are comparable with the dietary guidelines of other major national health organizations. They emphasize dietary moderation and flexibility. Companies that wish to further support the Heart-Check Program and the AHA's research and education efforts can also participate in the Promotional Partners Program, which allows greater use of the heart-check mark in promotional activities.

EXPANDING FOOD CHOICES IN THE GROCERY STORE

One of the first steps in implementing a healthful diet is choosing appropriate foods to bring into the home. Because it contains nutrient information and verifiable health claims, the new food label is a useful tool in sorting through the many choices available in the modern grocery store. In addition to traditional food choices, the consumer now has the option of purchasing foods that have been modified in one or more ways. These include foods with modified fat, cholesterol, or sodium contents and reduced-fat and fat-free foods.

Modified Foods

The earliest modified foods were reduced-sugar jellies and diet foods that lacked taste appeal. During the past three decades, however, many lower-fat, fat-free, low-cholesterol, and lower-sodium products have become available, offering greater choice and variety to individuals who wish to maintain a heart-healthy diet.

Foods and beverages labeled "low sodium" contain 140 mg or less of sodium per serving. Products labeled "no salt added" are usually low in sodium but not sodium free because they contain naturally occurring sodium. In some products, potassium chloride may be substituted for sodium chloride. Although potassium chloride is similar to table salt, many individuals feel it is not a satisfactory substitute. Some people find the taste bitter, and the potassium content may be incompatible with some medications.

Some foods that carry a "low-cholesterol" nutrient content claim are not modified at all. Assuming that no animal products (ie, meat, eggs, or dairy products) have been added to the food in processing, all foods of plant origin are cholesterol free. Products that have been modified to reduce their cholesterol content usually contain less animal fat than the original food or are made with egg whites instead of whole eggs. In addition, to be eligible to carry a low-cholesterol claim, a food must contain 2 g or less of saturated fat per serving.

Many "reduced," "low," and "free" products are appropriate for a cholesterol-lowering diet but there are exceptions, and checking the food label remains important. Some sugar-free foods (eg, dietetic chocolates) are higher in fat and calories than the unmodified food, and reduced-fat products often contain more sodium than the original food.

Instead of being relegated to the diet section, modified foods are now found throughout the grocery store. Appendix 2 lists examples of the types of modified foods likely to be found in a typical grocery store in the United States. In many cases, the foods contain specific descriptors that conform to the federal nutrition-labeling standards.

Reduced-fat and Fat-free Foods

The medical community and public health agencies have conveyed the message that a low-fat diet is a more healthful diet and in so doing have spawned a huge market for fat-free products. However, although data from the third National Health and Nutrition Examination Survey reveal that both fat and cholesterol consumption (as a percentage of energy consumed) and blood lipid levels have declined (5,6), the public has continued to grow fatter. Research has yet to determine whether these new products are an asset or a liability.

Reduced-fat products are not always lower in calories than their unmodified counterparts. Fat-free cakes and cookies often trade added carbohydrates for fat. Persons with diabetes must learn to look past the fat-free label for the food's total carbohydrate content. People on weight-reduction diets should be advised to use reduced-fat and fat-free products cautiously and to account for all the calories they contain.

Fat imparts flavor to foods, as well as a creamy mouth-feel and a sensation of satiety. Food manufacturers seeking to reduce the fat in their products use a variety of fat replacers, which may be carbohydrate based (eg, cellulose, maltodextrins, gums, starches, fiber, and polydextrose), protein based (eg, Simplesse [NutraSweet Company, Deerfield, IL 60015]), or fat based (eg, Olestra [Procter & Gamble, Cincinnati, Ohio]) (7).

Simplesse, developed by the NutraSweet Company, is a protein-based fat substitute that supplies 1-2 kcal/g. Produced by a process called microparticulation, the protein simulates the texture of fat. It has been used in cheese products and ice creams. It can be used in baking but not in frying because it is not a good heat conductor.

Olestra, developed by Procter and Gamble, is a fat-based product made from sucrose and 6 to 8 long-chain fatty acids (8). Although it has many of the properties of fat, it is not absorbed by the human body and is therefore calorie free. Olestra was approved by the FDA for use in snack foods such as potato chips, corn chips, cheese puffs, and crackers.

The American Dietetic Association issued the following position statement on fat replacements (9): "The American Dietetic Association recognizes the innovative development and use of traditional food ingredients and processing methods to reduce or replace fat in foods. Such foods should be used within the context of a diet consistent with the Dietary Guidelines for Americans."

An important question for researchers is whether fat-free products can be formulated that contribute to satiety in a way that reduces total calorie consumption. Certainly, the person who replaces 1 oz of potato chips cooked in oil with 1 oz of potato chips cooked in Olestra, or who eats a low-fat cheese made with Simplesse instead of the high-fat variety, will consume fewer calories. However, one study conducted on normal-weight males found that although consumption of Olestra significantly reduced fat intake, increased carbohydrate consumption resulted in stable total energy intake (10). Further studies are needed to assess the effect of these products on individuals seeking to reduce dietary fat and the risks associated with cardiovascular disease.

Food Preparation and Cooking Tips

Clients frequently have the misconception that a heart-healthy diet is devoid of all their favorite foods and consists of broiled chicken breasts and dry baked potatoes. The wide selection of nutritionally altered foods now available means that lack of dietary variety need not be an issue. Likewise, many of a client's favorite foods can continue to be enjoyed when they are prepared in a healthful manner. For most people, the dietary changes necessary to improve health are appropriate for all family members over age 2. Given that heart disease has a genetic component, the adoption of a heart-healthy diet by the entire family may help to prevent future disease.

One of the easiest ways to reduce intake of both total and saturated fat is to make substitutions. Most high-saturated-fat ingredients have lower-fat counterparts. Substitutions often have little or no effect on the quality (taste and texture) of the final product. Box 14-3 shows effective substitutions for higher-fat traditional ingredients and condiments. Additional

BOX 14-3 Lower-Saturated-Fat Substitutes for High-Fat Ingredients

Traditional Ingredient	Lower Saturated Fat Substitute
Whole milk	Nonfat, low-fat or reduced-fat depending on the extent of reduction needed
Heavy cream	Evaporated nonfat milk Equal amounts of low-fat yogurt and low-fat cottage cheese, blended until smooth
Light cream	Evaporated nonfat milk; 3 Tbsp oil and nonfat milk to equal 1 cup
Sour cream	Low-fat or fat-free plain yogurt Part-nonfat ricotta cheese thinned with yogurt or cultured nonfat buttermilk 1 cup low-fat cottage cheese whipped in a blender to a smooth consistency, add ~ 1 Tbsp lemon juice Fat-free sour cream
Cream cheese	Fat-free or light cream cheese Add 4 Tbsp diet margarine to 1 cup cottage cheese, blend until smooth, add nonfat milk as needed
Cheese	Reduced-fat cheese (<5 grams fat/oz) Use low-cholesterol, low-fat processed cheese Use smaller amount of "stronger" cheese, eg, sharp vs mild cheddar
Whole egg	Egg substitute, commercial 2 egg whites = 1 whole egg 1 egg white + 1 tsp vegetable oil Homemade egg substitute: 6 egg whites + 1 Tbsp vegetable oil + ¼ cup nonfat milk (¼ cup = 1 egg)
Butter	Polyunsaturated margarine in recipes Diet margarine as spread Butter substitute for flavoring (eg, Butter Buds,[a] Molly McButter[b]) In baked goods, use part applesauce and reduce liquids, ½ c applesauce ~ 4 Tbsp fat
Solid vegetable shortening or lard	Polyunsaturated margarine Vegetable oil
Bacon, sausage, salt pork, pork hock, or other high-fat seasoning	Use low-fat smoked sausage, reduce portion size Use meatless bacon bits Use margarine or vegetable oil to sauté Use low-fat meat or vegetable broth with soups, stews, and vegetables
Ground beef	Extra lean ground beef, reduce portion size Ground turkey, lean or extra lean
Beef steak or roast	Top round, eye of round, tip, full cut round, brisket (point section), sirloin, top loin, tenderloin, bottom round, chuck arm; trim all visible fat, reduce portion size
Pork	Tenderloin, Canadian bacon, lean boneless ham, center loin roast or chop; trim all visible fat, reduce portion size
Chocolate	1 oz = 3 Tbsp cocoa or carob powder + 1 Tbsp polyunsaturated vegetable oil or margarine (Note: carob powder is sweeter than cocoa; reduce sugar in recipe by ¼)
Salad dressing	Balsamic vinegar or flavored herb vinegar Fat-free salad dressings
Oil	Use nonstick pans Use nonstick vegetable oil sprays In baked goods, use applesauce for ½ of oil
Coffee creamer	Low-fat or nonfat milk Evaporated nonfat milk Fat-free coffee creamers
Mayonnaise	Plain nonfat yogurt Reduced or fat-free mayonnaise Mustard
Cream soup	Use meat or vegetable stock or wine or a combination thickened with cornstarch, arrowroot, or flour; add nonfat dry milk for creamier consistency Homemade white sauce made with 1 cup nonfat milk, 1 Tbsp margarine, 2 Tbsp flour, with flavors as follows Celery soup: add ¼ cup celery to soup Chicken soup: add bouillon powder or cube Mushroom soup: add canned or sautéed mushrooms 99% fat-free cream soups
Whipped cream	Whip cold evaporated nonfat milk, flavor with honey and vanilla Fat-free frozen whipped topping Reduced-fat or fat-free whipped cream

[a]Butter Buds, Cumberland Packing Corp, Brooklyn, NY 11205.

[b]Molly McButter, Alberto-Culver USA Inc., Melrose Park, IL 60160.

BOX 14-4 **Heart-Healthy Cooking Techniques**

To reduce fat:
- Avoid deep-fat-frying, sautéing, and pan frying.
- Use baking, stir-frying, steaming, broiling, and grilling.
- Avoid the need for added fat by using nonstick pans and nonstick cooking sprays.
- In soups and stews, cool the dish after cooking, remove hardened fat from the surface. Reheat the dish and serve.
- For a low-fat gravy; separate drippings from fat that has risen to the top using a gravy separator. Or add ice cubes to the meat drippings; fat will congeal and adhere to the ice cubes. The fat can be removed with a large slotted spoon or strained through cheese cloth.
- Prepare gravies and sauces from bouillon, or wine and herbs.
- Remove the skin from chicken, keep moist by basting with low-fat sauces, wrapping in foil or cooking with vegetables like tomatoes, green peppers, and mushrooms.
- Reduce by half the fat suggested in traditional recipes.

To reduce sodium:
- Substitute low-sodium soy sauce.
- Use herbs and spices for seasoning instead of salt; try fresh herbs.
- Use salt substitute or reduced sodium salt (in moderation).
- Use no-added-salt soups and canned foods.
- Avoid foods and seasonings containing MSG (monosodium glutamate).
- Reduce by half the salt suggested in traditional recipes.
- Reduce by half the "spice packet" found in commercial boxed grain products.

strategies to reduce fat consumption include

- reducing the portion size of higher-fat foods (eg, using beef as a condiment);
- choosing lean cuts of meat;
- increasing consumption of high-carbohydrate, low-fat foods (eg, whole grains, dried beans, peas, lentils, and rice); and
- reducing the use of fat in cooking.

By changing a few ingredients and using low-fat cooking techniques (Box 14-4), traditional menus can be altered to reduce fat and calorie content. Box 14-5 offers some creative menus that comply with the step I guidelines. Recipes for selected entrees included in these menus are given in Box 14-6.

TIPS FOR DINING OUT

Today, nearly 50% of every food dollar is spent on food eaten away from home. For this reason, clients need to learn how to eat healthy foods in restaurants. As always, balance is a guiding principle. Clients should understand that the total diet is what counts; occasional splurges can be worked into a step I diet. Many choices are available on restaurant menus that allow people to meet their dietary needs.

A recent study showed that, with proper education, clients can fit historically restricted fast foods into a step I cholesterol-lowering diet without compromising the diet's therapeutic effect (11). Hypercholesterolemic subjects could eat at fast-food restaurants five times per week and balance their traditional favorite foods with lower-fat menu choices. Study participants achieved significant decreases in serum lipid levels and dietary fat intake, consistent with the goals of a step I diet. This study supports the concept that all foods can fit into a balanced diet, including a cholesterol-lowering diet.

It may be helpful to give clients a list of recommended local restaurants and copies of Boxes 14-7 (which illustrates how making choices at fast-food restaurants can fit into a step I diet), 14-8 (which lists some preferred choices at sit-down restaurants), 14-9 (which outlines dining-out guidelines), and 14-10 (which provides a sample day's menu that adheres to the step I diet).

Appropriate choices may be found either on a regular menu or on a "healthy" or "lite" menu. Clients should be encouraged to ask for foods they desire when appropriate choices are not on the menu. The more restaurant patrons voice their food preferences, the more likely a restaurant will be to honor those requests or to adapt its menu to reflect those preferences. Clients should also be encouraged to ask questions about how food is prepared and served.

In addition, clients should be counseled about the pitfalls of dining out. These include

- skipping meals before dining out, which can lead to excessive hunger and poor menu choices;
- succumbing to the finish-your-plate syndrome—because restaurant portion sizes are generally larger than is recommended for a step I or II diet, clients

BOX 14-5 Sample 1,600-kcal Menus Complying with Step I Guidelines

Day 1

Breakfast

½ grapefruit, unsweetened	(1 fruit)	Total fat	10 g
1 slice toasted cracked wheat bread	(1 starch)	Saturated fat	2 g
1 cup oatmeal, prepared with water, no salt added	(2 starch)	Protein	15 g
2 tsp margarine[a]	(2 fat)	Carbohydrates	68 g
1 cup nonfat milk	(1 nonfat milk)	Cholesterol	4 mg
		Dietary fiber	7 g
		Energy	428 kcal

Lunch

2 oz turkey breast, roasted	(2 very lean meat)	Total fat	19 g
2 oz Swiss cheese[a]	(2 high fat meat)	Saturated fat	11 g
1 large leaf of lettuce	(free)	Protein	41 g
1 medium tomato slice	(free)	Carbohydrates	46 g
2 slices oat bran bread	(2 starch)	Cholesterol	100 mg
2 tsp fat-free mayonnaise	(free)	Dietary fiber	5 g
½ cup California Waldorf salad[b]	(1 fruit, ¼ nonfat milk)	Energy	520 kcal

Dinner

3 oz beef, top sirloin	(3 lean meat)	Total fat	20 g
1 large baked potato	(2 starch)	Saturated fat	5 g
½ cup green peas	(1 starch)	Protein	36 g
1 small salad (lettuce, tomatoes, carrots)	(free)	Carbohydrates	63 g
1 Tbsp Thousand Island salad dressing[a]	(1 fat)	Cholesterol	80 mg
1 tsp margarine[a]	(1 fat)	Dietary fiber	10 g
1 slice whole-grain bread	(1 starch)	Energy	569 kcal

Snack

1 medium raw apple	(1 fruit)	Total fat	0.5 g
		Carbohydrates	21 g
		Dietary fiber	4 g
		Energy	81 kcal

Daily Totals

		Total fat	49 g
		Saturated fat	18 g
		Protein	93 g
		Carbohydrates	199 g
		Cholesterol	185 mg
		Dietary fiber	26 g
		Energy	1,597 kcal

Day 2

Vegetarian Breakfast

1 blueberry bran muffin (medium)	(1½ starch, 1 fat)	Total fat	7 g
1 cup nonfat milk	(1 nonfat milk)	Saturated fat	1 g
1 cup mixed fruit: honeydew melon, blueberries, orange	(1 fruit)	Protein	13 g
		Carbohydrates	51 g
		Cholesterol	26 mg
		Dietary fiber	6 g
		Energy	308 kcal

Lunch

¼ sliced avocado	(2 fat)	Total fat	22 g
¼ cup mung bean sprouts	(free)	Saturated fat	7 g
1 oz Swiss cheese[a]	(1 high-fat meat)	Protein	18 g
2 slices red and green pepper	(free)	Carbohydrate	64 g
2 slices tomato	(free)	Cholesterol	28 mg
2 tsp mayonnaise-type salad dressing, regular[a]	(1 fat)	Dietary fiber	9 g
mustard 1½ tsp	(free)	Energy	520 kcal
2 slices rye bread	(2 bread)		
1 oz hard pretzels, salted	(1¼ starch)		

Dinner

1 cup Mediterranean pasta[b]	(2 starch, 1 vegetable, 1 fat)	Total fat	20 g
1 cup broccoli, steamed	(1 vegetable)	Saturated fat	4 g
½ cup garbanzo bean salad[b]	(2 starch, 1 fat)	Protein	24 g
1 whole-wheat dinner roll	(1 starch)	Carbohydrate	86 g
2 tsp margarine[a]	(1 fat)	Cholesterol	5 mg
		Dietary fiber	6 g
		Energy	605 kcal

BOX 14-5 Sample 1,600-kcal Menus Complying with Step I Guidelines

Snack			
1 cup grapes, fresh	(1 fruit)	Total fat	3 g
2 fig bar cookies	(1½ carbohydrate)	Saturated fat	1 g
		Protein	2 g
		Carbohydrate	41 g
		Dietary fiber	3 g
		Energy	183 kcal
Daily Totals			
		Total fat	52 g
		Saturated fat	13 g
		Protein	57 g
		Carbohydrate	242 g
		Cholesterol	59 mg
		Dietary fiber	24 g
		Energy	1,615 kcal
Day 3			
Breakfast			
1 medium cinnamon-raisin bagel (56 g)	(2 starch)	Total fat	12 g
1 oz cream cheese, regular[a]	(2 fat)	Saturated fat	7 g
1 cup nonfat milk	(1 nonfat milk)	Protein	17 g
½ banana	(1 fruit)	Carbohydrate	61 g
		Cholesterol	35 mg
		Dietary fiber	4 g
		Energy	405 kcal
Lunch			
1 cup apple-celery-chicken salad[b] for pita sandwich	(5 very lean meat, ½ fruit)	Total fat	7 g
2 slices tomato	(free)	Saturated fat	2 g
1 lettuce leaf	(free)	Protein	39 g
1 small or ½ large whole wheat pita	(1 starch)	Carbohydrate	59 g
½ cup nonfat milk	(½ nonfat milk)	Cholesterol	82 mg
1 medium pear, fresh	(1½ fruit)	Dietary fiber	8 g
		Energy	641 kcal
Dinner			
Fish Canton,[b] 1 fillet plus sauce and garnish	(4 lean meat)	Total fat	28 g
⅓ cup brown rice	(1 starch)	Saturated fat	6 g
½ cup cooked asparagus	(1 vegetable)	Protein	38 g
1 tsp margarine[a]	(1 fat)	Carbohydrate	61 g
1 small french roll	(1¼ starch)	Cholesterol	63 mg
2- 2" oatmeal raisin cookies, prepared from recipe with margarine	(1½ carbohydrate, 1 fat)	Dietary fiber	7 g
		Energy	641 kcal
Snack			
¾ cup or 6 oz low-fat yogurt	(1 nonfat milk)	Total fat	2 g
1 cup strawberries	(1 fruit)	Saturated fat	1 g
		Protein	7 g
		Carbohydrate	48 g
		Cholesterol	188 mg
		Dietary fiber	3 g
		Energy	169 kcal
Daily Totals			
		Total fat	48 g
		Saturated fat	16 g
		Protein	102 g
		Carbohydrate	213 g
		Cholesterol	188 mg
		Dietary fiber	22 g
		Energy	1,655 kcal

Source: Menus courtesy of Pennington Biomedical Research Center.

[a] To further reduce fat and saturated fat, lower-fat alternatives of these foods can be selected, when available.

[b] Recipe for this item can be found in Box 14-6.

BOX 14-6 Recipes for Selected Entrees Listed in Box 14-5

Mediterranean Pasta

16 oz pkg	Penne pasta
2 oz	Sun-dried tomatoes
1 cup	Water, hot
3 cups	Marinated artichoke hearts
1 cup	Scallions, chopped
1/3 cup	Celery, chopped
1/4 cup	Greek black olives, sliced
1 cup	Colored sweet bell peppers, seeded & chopped
1 Tbsp	Oregano, dried
3 Tbsp	Olive oil, extra virgin
4 Tbsp	Balsamic vinegar
2 oz	Feta cheese
1 Tbsp	Parmesan cheese
1/2 tsp	Salt *
1/4 tsp	Cracked black pepper

Boil pasta, submerge in cold ice water. Drain and reserve in separate bowl. Reconstitute the sun-dried tomatoes in hot water for 15-20 minutes; reserve juices. In a large pasta bowl fold artichoke hearts, scallions, celery, olives, peppers, and oregano together. Add olive oil, balsamic vinegar, tomatoes, and juices; stir. Toss with pasta and cheese. Add salt and pepper.
Serves 8.

Source: Recipe courtesy of Kelly Patrick, Chef at Pennington Biomedical Research Center.

* If sodium content is a concern, may omit salt.

1 serving contains: 224 kcal, 7.5 g protein, 36.6 g carbohydrate, 5.8 g total fat, 1.4 g saturated fat, 4.5 mg cholesterol, 2.5 g dietary fiber.
Diabetic exchanges: 1 fat, 2 starch, 1 vegetable.

Garbanzo Bean Salad

5 cups	Garbanzo beans, rinsed and well drained
3 medium	Tomatoes, chopped
1/4 cup	Parsley, chopped
1/4 cup	Green onion, chopped
1/2 cup	Nonfat cottage cheese
1 Tbsp	Peanut oil
3 Tbsp	Vinegar
1 clove	Garlic, minced
1/4 tsp	Salt*
1/2 tsp	Black pepper

Rinse the beans under running water, then drain well. Place in a medium bowl. Add the tomatoes, parsley, and green onion; set aside. In a small bowl, whisk together the cottage cheese, oil, vinegar, garlic, salt, and pepper. Pour over the salad ingredients and toss to combine. Chill before serving, tossing occasionally. Taste and season with additional pepper and vinegar, if necessary.
Serves 8.

Source: Pennington Biomedical Research Center.

* If sodium content is a concern, omit salt.

1 serving contains: 206 kcal, 11.4 g protein, 31.5 g carbohydrate, 4.7 g total fat, 0.68 g saturated fat, 0.62 mg cholesterol, 0.7 g dietary fiber.
Diabetic exchanges: 2 starch, 1 fat.

should be encouraged to split an entree, order an appetizer- or half-size portion, or take leftover food home;

- ignoring nutrition goals when away from home—remind clients that they should always exercise the principles of balance and freedom of choice (most people feel good about eating a meal that meets their dietary needs); and
- not enjoying a restaurant experience or avoiding dining out. Having the tools to make the best restaurant and menu selections leads to an enjoyable culinary experience.

BOX 14-6 Recipes for Selected Entrees Listed in Box 14-5, continued

California Waldorf Salad

½ cup	Low-fat ricotta cheese
½ cup	Plain nonfat yogurt
3 Tbsp	Honey
2 Tbsp	Lemon juice
5	Red-skinned apples, cut into ½" cubes
2 cups	Pineapple chunks, canned in own juice or water
1½ cups	Seedless green grapes
1 cup	Celery, sliced in ¼" pieces

Puree ricotta cheese, yogurt, honey, and juice in blender or food processor. Combine apples, pineapples, grapes, and celery with dressing. Serve on lettuce with mint sprig, if desired.
Serves 8 (1 cup portion); serves 16 (½ cup portion).

Source: Pennington Biomedical Research Center.

1 serving contains: 78 kcal, 1.6 g protein, 17.6 g carbohydrate, 0.85 g total fat, 0.4 g saturated fat, 2.5 mg cholesterol, 1.6 g dietary fiber.

Diabetic exchanges: 1 fruit, ½ nonfat milk.

Apple-Celery Chicken Salad Sandwich

3 cups	Diced, cooked, skinless chicken breast meat
½ cup	Finely chopped fresh spinach (or 3 Tbsp finely chopped frozen spinach, thawed and drained)
⅔ cup	Nonfat yogurt
1 Tbsp	Lemon juice
1 tsp	Dry mustard
¼ cup	Chopped green onions
1 Tbsp	Dried dill
½ cup	Chopped celery
1	Apple, cored and diced
4	Pita breads, halved

In a large bowl combine the spinach, yogurt, lemon juice, mustard, green onion, dill, and celery. Stir to combine. Add the chicken and apple; blend well. Season to taste with salt and pepper if you wish. Spoon approximately ½ cup salad into each pita half, tuck in a lettuce leaf, and serve.
Serves 8.

Source: Pennington Biomedical Research Center.

1 serving contains: 210 kcal, 31.5 g protein, 9.3 g carbohydrate, 4.8 g total fat, 1.2 g saturated fat, 79 g cholesterol, 1.4 g dietary fiber.

Diabetic exchanges: 5 very lean meat, ½ fruit.

Fish Canton

¼ cup	Soy sauce*
2 oz	Sherry
¼ cup	Peanut oil
⅓ cup	Parsley, fresh
1½ Tbsp	Ginger
6 cloves	Garlic, minced
12 filets	Swordfish (3-4 oz filets)
½ cup	Almonds, chopped or slivered
¾ cup	Green onion, sliced

In a bowl stir together soy sauce, sherry, oil, parsley, ginger, and garlic until well combined. Arrange fish fillets on grill; brush liberally with sauce. Grill fish until it flakes easily, turning once and brushing frequently with sauce. During last minute of grilling, sprinkle almonds and green onion over fish. Serve at once, garnish with parsley and lemon or lime slices.
Serves 12.
*If sodium content is a concern substitute low sodium soy sauce.

Source: Pennington Biomedical Research Center.

1 serving provides: 254 kcal, 28.5 g protein, 3.6 g carbohydrate, 13.0 g total fat, 2.6 g saturated fat, 53 g cholesterol, 1.1 g dietary fiber.

Diabetic exchanges: 4 lean meat.

BOX 14-7 **Sample Restaurant Meals That Comply with Step I Guidelines**

Quick Service Restaurants

Chinese meal:		
Chicken chow mein (1 cup)	Total fat	7.5 g
Steamed rice (½ cup)	Saturated fat	1.3 g
Pineapple chunks (½ cup)	Polyunsaturated fatty acids	2.3 g
Fortune cookie (2)	Monounsaturated fatty acids	3.4 g
Tea (1 cup)	Carbohydrates	57 g
	Protein	9.5 g
	Cholesterol	100 mg
	Total calories	326 kcal
Deli meal:		
Roast beef sandwich with	Total fat	12 g
Low-cal mayonnaise (1 Tbsp)	Saturated fat	3 g
Pretzels (1 oz ~ 6 large twists)	Polyunsaturated fatty acids	.5 g
Apple (1)	Monounsaturated fatty acids	4 g
Soft drink (12 fl oz)	Carbohydrates	131 g
	Protein	38 g
	Cholesterol	87 mg
	Total calories	784 kcal
Mexican meal:		
Taco salad (1 serving, 198 g includes tortilla shell)	Total fat	23 g
Spanish rice (1 cup)	Saturated fat	7.8 g
Salsa (1 oz)	Polyunsaturated fatty acids	2.4 g
Melon or other fresh fruit (1 cup)	Monounsaturated fatty acids	5.3 g
Coffee (1 cup)	Carbohydrates	103 g
	Protein	21 g
	Cholesterol	48 mg
	Total calories	676 kcal
Cafeteria or diner meal: breakfast		
Raisin bran (1 cup)	Total fat	11 g
Reduced-fat milk (1 cup)	Saturated fat	3.8 g
English muffin (1)	Polyunsaturated fatty acids	1.2 g
Margarine (1 tsp)	Monounsaturated fatty acids	3.7 g
Preserves (1 tsp)	Carbohydrates	144 g
Banana (1)	Protein	20 g
Orange juice (1 cup)	Cholesterol	18 mg
	Total calories	713 kcal
Cafeteria or diner meal: lunch		
Grilled chicken breast (3 oz)	Total fat	10.7 g
Baked potato (1)	Saturated fat	2.6 g
Broccoli, cooked (½ cup)	Polyunsaturated fatty acids	3.0 g
Fresh fruit salad (1 cup)	Monounsaturated fatty acids	4.1 g
Margarine (1 tsp)	Carbohydrates	104 g
Soft drink, cola (12 oz)	Protein	33.0 g
	Cholesterol	70.9 mg
	Total calories	633 kcal
Burger meal:		
Small hamburger (1)	Total fat	11 g
Tossed green salad with	Saturated fat	3.5 g
low-cal French dressing (2 Tbsp)	Polyunsaturated fatty acids	1.5 g
Low-fat vanilla shake (16 oz)	Monounsaturated fatty acids	6 g
	Carbohydrates	105 g
	Protein	25 g
	Cholesterol	41 mg
	Total calories	614 kcal

Source: Erin Sharp, RD.

BOX 14-8 Ethnic Options for Dining Out

Choose more often...	Choose less often...
American	
Salad bar (lettuce, fresh vegetables, light dressing on the side) Baked potatoes, toppings on the side Steamed vegetables Grilled chicken Small hamburger (avoid high fat toppings, ie, cheese, bacon, mayonnaise) Sorbet Frozen yogurt	Croutons, cheese, mayonnaise-based salads (tuna, macaroni, and egg) Potato chips Fried mozzarella sticks Barbeque ribs Reuben sandwich with corned beef, cheese, and thousand island dressing Hot fudge sundae Cheesecake
Mexican	
Mexican salad with chicken or beef and salsa (hold the shell, cheese, and sour cream) Mexican rice and beans (if not made with lard) Gazpacho soup Chicken soft tacos Pescado de Veracruz (fish with tomato sauce) Chicken fajitas Tropical fruits (mangos, kiwi, bananas, pineapples, and guavas)	Nachos topped with guacamole, cheese, and sour cream Refried beans Chili con queso (chili with cheese) Chimichangas (fried, with beef or chicken and cheese) Carne asada (grilled sirloin steak in an enchilada sauce with guacamole) Cheese quesadillas Sopaipillas (deep-fried dough, tossed in sugar)
Far East (Asian)	
Hot-and-sour soup Steamed Peking ravioli Teriyaki beef Pan-fried noodles with shrimp Steamed white rice Stir-fried chicken with vegetables Beef chow mein Pineapple chunks	Fried jumbo shrimp Egg rolls Crispy fried won tons Pork lo mein Beef fried rice Sweet-and-sour chicken Cashew beef Fried bananas
Mediterranean (Greek)	
Tzatziki (yogurt, mint, and cucumber spread) Dolmades (grape leaves stuffed with rice, onions, and tomatoes) Marinated grilled octopus Tomato and cucumber salad Kibbeh (cracked wheat, meat, onions, and spices) Roast chicken Fresh fruit	Tyrosalata (whipped feta cheese spread) Taramosalata (caviar with olive oil and lemon juice) Fried calamari Greek salad (feta cheese, olive oil) Mousaka (eggplant and tomato casserole with white sauce) Broiled lamb chops Pasticchio (baked macaroni with ground beef, eggs, and cream sauce) Kataif (pastry made with dough, nuts, and sugar)
Southern	
Rolls Boiled potatoes Greens Beef-vegetable stew Baked catfish Chicken creole with vegetables Fresh fruit	Biscuits, cornbread Ham hocks and gravy Sweet potato pie Stuffed cabbage rolls Barbeque ribs Fried catfish Fried chicken Fruit cobbler

Choose more often...	Choose less often...
Middle Eastern	
Couscous	Feta cheese
Tabouli (cracked wheat salad with tomatoes and onions)	Falafel (deep-fried patties of chickpeas and fava beans)
Hummus and pita bread	Kalamata (olives)
Shish kebab (chicken skewered) with tomatoes, onions, and peppers	Spanikopita (spinach and cheese pie with phyllo dough)
Gyros	Omelet (three eggs and feta cheese)
Fresh fruit	Kefta kabob (ground lamb with beef patties, onions, and peppers)
	Baklava
Italian	
Minestrone soup	Lentil and sausage soup
Steamed clams	Fried calamari
Marinated mushrooms	Antipasto (cheese and meats)
Insalata (crunchy greens, vegetables)	Caesar salad
Pasta with red tomato sauces	Pasta with cream sauces (fettucini alfredo)
Pasta primavera	Lasagna
Linguini with white wine clam sauce	Chicken parmigiana (chicken with mozzarella cheese and tomato sauce)
Italian ice	Cannoli
French	
Jellied consomme (clear, light broth)	French onion soup (with cheese)
Shrimp cocktail	Escargot
Grilled asparagus	Stuffed mushrooms
Baby field greens salad (light dressing on the side)	Nicoise (salad with olives, anchovies, tuna, eggs, and olive oil)
Petite filet mignon	Beef Wellington
Poached salmon	Shrimp scampi (made with butter)
Fresh berries	Prime rib
	Chocolate raspberry cake

Source: Erin Sharp, RD.

BOX 14-9 The Dining Out Experience

Eating healthfully while dining out can be easy if you have the right mind-set, know what to look for, and are prepared with the right questions. Use the following guidelines to help ask questions and make requests.

- Ask about ingredients (restaurants usually don't list extras like butter and mayonnaise).
- Request certain items be served on the side, such as salad dressing, sauces, and gravies.
- Bring your own condiments, such as fat-free dressing or seasoning, when possible.
- If available, choose menu items served as small portion sizes, which may be listed as regular, petite, kiddie, or appetizer size.
- Inquire about food preparation and clarify menu descriptors you are unsure of: watch fried, breaded, and creamed descriptors.
- Request that a food be prepared differently (eg, broiled instead of fried).
- Order items from the soups, salads, and appetizer listings: have a salad as an appetizer and ask the waiter to serve your appetizer as the main dish.
- Ask for a doggie bag with your meal and immediately set aside a portion to take home.
- Don't be afraid to ask questions; most restaurants are more than willing to meet special requests.

BOX 14-10 **Sample One-Day Menu That Meets the Step I Diet Guidelines[a]**

A Step I Diet Day

		% kcal of meal
Breakfast	**Meets Step I Guidelines**	**% kcal of meal**
Bagel (plain, 1 medium)	Total fat	20%
Low-fat cream cheese (1 oz)	Saturated fat	9%
Cereal, corn flakes (1 cup)	Polyunsaturated fat	2%
Banana (1 small)	Monounsaturated fat	5%
Low-fat milk (1 cup)	Carbohydrates	68%
Orange juice (1 cup)	Cholesterol	40 mg
	Protein	12%
	Total calories	662 kcal
Lunch	**Does Not Meet Step I Guidelines**	
Pepperoni pizza (1 slice)	Total fat	45%
Garden salad (3 oz)	Saturated fat	9%
Italian dressing (2 Tbsp)	Polyunsaturated fat	20%
Apple (1 medium)	Monounsaturated fat	14%
Diet soft drink (12 oz)	Carbohydrates	44%
	Protein	11%
	Cholesterol	14 mg
	Total calories	416 kcal
Dinner	**Meets Step I Guidelines**	
Baked fish (3 oz)	Total fat	18%
Baked potato (1 medium)	Saturated fat	8%
Nonfat sour cream (1 oz)	Polyunsaturated fat	3%
Peas and carrots (1 cup)	Monounsaturated fat	5%
Dinner roll (1 medium)	Carbohydrates	59%
Margarine (1 tsp)	Protein	23%
Low-fat milk (1 cup)	Cholesterol	68 mg
	Total calories	754 kcal
Daily Totals	**Meets Step I Daily Guidelines**	
	Total fat	25%
	Saturated fat	9%
	Polyunsaturated fat	6%
	Monounsaturated fat	7%
	Carbohydrates	59%
	Protein	16%
	Cholesterol	123 mg
	Total calories	1,835 kcal

[a]Guidelines are as follows: <30% of calories from fat, <10% of calories from saturated fat, and <300 mg of cholesterol.

Source: Erin Sharp, RD.

REFERENCES

1. Keenan DP, Achterberg C, Kris-Etherton PM, Abusabha R, Von Eye A. Use of qualitative and quantitative methods to define behavioral fat-reduction strategies and their relationship to dietary fat reduction in the Patterns of Dietary Change Study. *J Am Diet Assoc.* 1996;96:1245-1251.
2. *Food Guide Pyramid: A Guide to Daily Food Choices.* Washington, DC: US Department of Agriculture, Human Information Service; 1992. Home and Garden Bulletin No. 252.
3. *Nutrition and Your Health: Dietary Guidelines for Americans.* 3rd ed. Washington, DC: US Departments of Agriculture and Health and Human Services; 1990. Home and Garden Bulletin No. 232.
4. Parkwood Research Associates. The PREVENTION Magazine/CNN Poll, August, 1994; The New "Nutrition Facts" Food Label: Is It Making a Difference?
5. Centers for Disease Control and Prevention. Daily dietary fat and total food-energy intakes—NHANES III, Phase 1, 1988-91. *JAMA.* 1994;721:1309.
6. Johnson CL, Rifkind BM, Sempos CT, Carroll MD, Bachorik PS, Briefel RR, Gordon DJ, Burt VL, Brown CD, Lippel K, Cleeman JL. Declining serum total cholesterol levels among US adults: the National Health and Nutrition Examination Surveys. *JAMA.* 1993;269:3002-3008.
7. Miller DL, Rolls BJ. Implications of fat reduction in the diet. In: *Handbook of Fat Replacers.* Roller S, Jones SA, eds. Boca Raton, Fla: CRC Press; 1996:27-44.

8. *Introducing the Breakthrough New Fat Replacer: Olean.* Cincinnati, Ohio: Procter and Gamble; 1996.
9. Hudnall MJ, Connor SL, Connor WE. Position of the American Dietetic Association: fat replacements. *J Am Diet Assoc.* 1991;91:1285-1288.
10. Rolls BJ, Pirraglia PA, Jones MD, Peters JC. Effects of Olestra, a noncaloric fat substitute, on daily energy and fat intakes in lean men. *Am J Clin Nutr.* 1992;56:84-92.
11. Davidson MH, Kong JC, Drennan KB, Story K, Anderson GH. Efficacy of the National Cholesterol Education Program Step 1 Diet. *Arch Intern Med.* 1996;156:305-312.

CHAPTER 15

Spreading the Word — Teaching Classes About the Nutrition-Heart Health Link

Kathryn M. Kolasa, PhD, RD

Nutrition education, counseling, and behavioral intervention efforts can help individuals to reduce fat intake and alter blood lipid levels (1). Dietary education can be successful in both one-on-one and group settings. Dietitians, nutritionists, health educators, cooperative extension service agents, and others provide food and nutrition information to a wide variety of audiences in classes and workshops.

Hospitals, cardiac rehabilitation facilities, physicians' offices, and outpatient facilities present many opportunities for classes for patients with known disease. Worksite and wellness programs, community and cooperative extension service centers, churches, schools, and meetings of civic and service organizations provide opportunities for public education.

Some programs are designed to create awareness of the link between nutrition and heart health; others, to teach participants food skills associated with a healthful lifestyle. Some programs also can help patients lose weight.

To make dietary changes, people must have individualized goals that are usually best defined in one-on-one counseling. Classes cannot replace one-on-one dietary counseling, although they may be both an entry point and an adjunct to it.

Classes can be an efficient way for health care providers to deliver information to clients who are seeking practical day-to-day food-behavior strategies for meeting their personal goals. Successful classes meet the shared information needs of most participants, leaving specific issues to individual counseling sessions. Group classes also provide opportunities for individuals to become aware of a dietary issue, find solutions to dietary problems, practice those solutions, and evaluate them with group support.

Group meetings and workshop settings accommodate teaching techniques such as cooking demonstrations (2), food sampling, game playing, and testimony sharing that are impractical to provide on a one-on-one basis. For some people, the group process is a stronger motivator for adopting nutritional recommendations than is individual counseling.

There are no simple answers to questions about optimal class size, frequency, length, composition, and fees. No definitive research has identified the topics, activities, handouts, and materials that result in behavior change. This chapter provides insights into these issues based on the experience of nutrition educators and the limited published nutrition education research in this area.

A 1- to 2-hour session appears to be appropriate for an introduction to cardiovascular health. At least six sessions are needed to cover all topics related to cardiovascular nutrition and to achieve lifestyle change.

Course Logistics

Audience

Individuals' knowledge of nutrition and motivation for behavior change vary greatly. Expert teaching skills are required to engage a heterogeneous audience. When possible, it is best to target a class to individuals who have similar information and service needs and who are in a similar stage of change (3). (See Chapter 13 for a discussion of the stages-of-change theory.)

Important issues to consider include the current cardiovascular health status of the intended audience. Do participants have known risk or disease? Do they have complications such as a cardiac event, angioplasty, bypass, or transplant? Are they at high risk but without known disease?

The needs of participants who want to reduce their fat intake or follow the step I diet differ from those of participants who want to follow a strict regimen such as that of Dean Ornish (4). An individual who only wants to "cut back" is likely to lose interest in a class that focuses on following a vegetarian diet that provides 10% of energy from fat.

Consider other characteristics of your intended audience members, including their communication and learning styles, gender, education or occupation, living arrange-

TABLE 15-1

Examples of Class Topics and Course Lengths

Program and Length			Topics													
References	Weeks	Time (min)	Orientation Risk Factors	Diet Guidelines	Fat	Substitution	Eating Out/ Holiday Eating	Sodium	Store Tour	Exercise	Lifestyle Change	Food Prep	Food Demo	Meal Plan/ Food Labels	Weight	Other
5	4	90		✘	✘	✘	✘	✘	✘						✘	
6	5	—			✘	✘	✘									Cookoff; follow up monthly
7	6	120	✘	✘						✘	✘			✘		Follow up session @ 12, 24 weeks
8	6	120		✘		✘						✘	✘	✘		
9	1	120	✘		✘			✘	✘		✘		✘			
10	1	180		✘	✘	✘	✘				✘					
11	1	60	✘	✘	✘									✘	✘	

ments, income, and cultural background. Although some researchers theorize that diversity within an audience contributes to problem solving, experienced nutrition educators have observed that men drop out of classes when most of the participants are women, minorities tend to stay away from classes when there are few minority participants, professionals tend to avoid attending classes with laborers, physicians avoid attending classes with other medical personnel, and overweight individuals drop out of classes in which most participants are thin. If it is feasible, it is best to target your classes to specific groups.

Use strategies to reach individuals with like interests. For example, classes for men can be promoted through men's groups and health clubs, whereas classes for patients with heart disease can be promoted through cardiac rehabilitation programs, physicians' offices, and hospital discharge planning services.

Duration

The number of sessions will most likely hinge on issues such as budget, available resources, acceptability of the class method to your intended audience, and expectations (those of the instructors as well as the participants). It is unrealistic to expect significant dietary change to result from participation in one class, but a single class can be an efficient way to deliver information to an interested group. A single 15-minute session, delivered during an employee work break, may increase awareness of the link between diet and heart disease and may motivate some members of the audience to seek additional information.

Table 15-1 lists the number of sessions and topics covered in a sampling of programs. Packaged programs for "heart-smart" nutrition vary from one to eight sessions, with individual sessions lasting from 30 minutes to 2 hours (5-11). Effective weight management programs are usually longer (approximately 16 weeks) and multifaceted (12, 13). Research on the effectiveness of cardiovascular education programs is complicated by participants' diverse needs, which influence the choice of topics and the number of sessions required.

Another major factor to consider in determining course duration is class attrition. Even the most energetic, dynamic nutrition educators experience participant dropout. Attrition rates for nutrition education classes vary greatly; in multiple-session courses, attrition may reach 50%. Studies show that attrition is affected by many factors, including the effectiveness of the program leader, program structure and length, convenience, participant characteristics, costs, and incentives (14). Attrition is discouraging to both the group leader and the remaining participants.

The course duration will affect attendance and learning. It is usually unrealistic to expect participants with complex lifestyles to attend a course that lasts many weeks. Local health care professionals can be good sources of information about experiences with different audiences and may have recommendations regarding course duration. Many cardiac rehabilitation dietitians have found their patients will attend 20-minute nutrition sessions weekly while they are enrolled in a 6- to 12-week phase 2 program when the nutrition sessions are coupled with exercise sessions. Successful healthy-heart evening programs have consisted of six to eight sessions, and individuals in a heart-disease reversal program may participate in weekly sessions for up to a year.

Group Size

The size of informational classes is limited only by the size of the facility and the instructor's ability to engage the crowd. Skill-building classes may need to be restricted to 10 to 15 participants. Budgetary considerations may dictate the size of the group; for example, 25 participants may be needed to generate sufficient revenue for a cooking class. A course that includes a store tour may need to be limited to 6 participants.

Preparation

Nutrition Education in Small Groups: Developing a Learning Community provides clear examples of how to involve adults in their own nutrition education (15). This workbook and companion videotape demonstrate effective group discussion, role playing, case studies, and other ways to actively involve audiences. Balch (16) provides a useful review of research findings that describe effective interventions to achieve dietary change.

The Course

Topics frequently taught in heart-healthy nutrition classes include

- the role of cholesterol in the body,
- the link between blood cholesterol levels and diet,
- dietary self-assessment,
- fat budgeting,
- nutrient label reading,
- portion sizing,
- ingredient substitutions,
- menu planning,
- eating out,
- weight management,
- dietary fiber,
- forming new habits, and
- snacking.

Topics such as increasing consumption of fish and meatless meals, reducing sodium, seasoning, dietary supplementation, and the value and safety of fat substitutes are taught less frequently. Food sampling, recipe modifications, and grocery store tours are highly rated activities that are included when feasible.

Creative variations on the typical topic list can make handouts and promotional materials more interesting. Cookbook titles and the headlines in the food sections of magazines and newspapers can sometimes provide inspiration for topic titles, for example, Choosing a Healthy Eating Style, Making Better Breakfasts, Wellness in Your Kitchen, Making the Most of Fish and Fowl, The Versatile Vegetarian, The Garden Basket — Salads and Vegetables, Cooking for Your Waistline, Eating Light with Red Meat, Cooking Minus the Salt Shaker, New Ideas for Poultry, Guilt-free Snacks and Desserts, Satisfying Your Sweet Tooth — Sanely, Potpourri, Kids Corner, Enjoying Holiday and Restaurant Meals, Fast Foods for Busy Times, and Beware of the Headlines.

Providing the minimum amount of information needed to encourage dietary change is usually more effective than teaching everything relevant to diet and heart disease. For example, if members of an audience are consuming 45% of energy from fat, a discussion that is limited to reducing total fat intake may be more appropriate than a detailed discussion of reducing saturated fat intake.

It is better to focus on the group's information needs and goals rather than on an individual participant's questions. Individuals with specific questions or more advanced information needs should be encouraged to discuss them after class or during a personal counseling session.

Only One Class?

The objective of a one-time class or lecture to a civic or special interest group should be defined clearly. Leading a group through a 30-minute dietary self-assessment often helps participants to realize that their food habits are not consistent with a heart-healthy diet. A short quiz on diet and cholesterol can be an effective tool to help attendees become aware of the extent of their knowledge about diet and heart disease. After participants have completed the quiz, each statement can be reviewed and common misperceptions discussed. The audience can take the quiz home and consider its application in daily life (17).

A nutrition trivia game can be a good way to engage people who are in the precontemplation and contemplation stages of behavior change. At the end of the session, promotional materials for other classes and counseling sessions can be handed out and individuals who are interested in additional classes can be contacted later.

Teaching Tools and Resources

Class participants almost always ask for recommendations of books, cookbooks, videos, and computer programs, and a suggested reading list can be a part of the class outline. Many educational materials focus on nutrition and heart disease (see Resources in this chapter). Additional resources can be found on the World Wide Web site of the Food and Nutrition Information Center of the National Agricultural Library (18).

Individualizing Classes

Individualization of dietary goals is best done in one-on-one counseling sessions, but dietary self-assessment tools can help to personalize a class for participants. A variety of self-scoring dietary assessment tools and simple computerized food frequency tools can be used (19, 20). Questions found in the USDA's *Dietary Guidelines and Your Diet* series of bulletins can be used to assess food habits (21). *The Weight Loss Readiness Quiz* from the National Center for Nutrition and Dietetics is appropriate for a class that emphasizes weight loss (Box 15-1) (22).

BOX 15-1 The Weight-loss Readiness Quiz

Are you ready to lose weight? Your attitude about weight loss affects your ability to succeed. Take this readiness quiz to learn whether you need to make any attitude adjustments before you begin. Mark each item true or false. Be honest! It's important that these answers reflect the way you really are, not how you would like to be. A method for interpreting your readiness for weight loss follows.

1. I have thought a lot about my eating habits and physical activities to pinpoint what I need to change.
2. I have accepted the idea that I need to make permanent, not temporary, changes in my eating and activities to be successful.
3. I will only feel successful if I lose a lot of weight.
4. I accept the idea that it's best if I lose weight slowly.
5. I'm thinking of losing weight now because I really want to, not because someone else thinks I should.
6. I think losing weight will solve other problems in my life.
7. I am willing and able to increase my regular physical activity.
8. I can lose weight successfully if I have no "slip-ups."
9. I am ready to commit some time and effort each week to organizing and planning my food and activity programs.
10. Once I lose some initial weight, I usually lose the motivation to keep going until I reach my goal.
11. I want to start a weight loss program, even though my life is unusually stressful right now.

Scoring the weight-loss readiness quiz

To score the quiz, look at your answers to items 1, 2, 4, 5, 7, 9. Score "1" if you answered "true" and "0" if you answered "false."
For items 3, 6, 8, 10, 11, score "0" for each true answer and "1" for each false answer. To get your total score, add the scores for all questions.
No one score indicates for sure whether you are ready to start losing weight. However, the higher your total score, the more characteristics you have that contribute to success. As a rough guide, consider the following recommendations:

- If you scored 8 or higher, you probably have good reasons for wanting to lose weight now and a good understanding of the steps needed to succeed.
- If you scored 5 to 7, you may need to reevaluate your reasons for losing weight and the methods you would use to do so.
- If you scored 4 or less, now may not be the right time for you to lose weight. Although you might be successful in losing weight initially, your answers suggest that you are unlikely to sustain sufficient effort to lose all the weight you want or to keep off the weight that you do lose.

Adapted from Weight Loss Quiz, Nutrition Fact Sheet, National Center for Nutrition and Dietetics of The American Dietetic Association.

(See Chapter 4 for additional suggestions on assessment tools.)

Some dietitians offer weekly computerized nutrient assessments, but these can be time consuming unless resources are available to assist with data entry and interpretation. If a multimedia computer is available, participants can be invited to evaluate their own diet with the help of a user-friendly food frequency program such as Nutrition DISCovery (20). Many cardiac rehabilitation programs offer nutrient analysis on admission to and at completion of the program.

Getting Started

Programs appropriate for use in group settings are available commercially (23-30). Sample programs are listed in the Resource section of this chapter. Most programs are available in kit form and include an implementation or process guide, manuals for both instructor and participants, and other support materials. The implementation or process guide describes how to make contacts, schedule programs, and recruit participants; it also provides a checklist and schedule for the completion of these tasks. Implementation guides for programs that use volunteer presenters include a train-the-trainer curriculum.

An instructor's manual or facilitator's guide that outlines the curriculum and provides teaching tips is a critical component of the kit. It should include program objectives; a detailed outline; a list of materials needed; a complete description of activities and demonstrations; master copies of overheads, slides, and handouts; posters; incentives; and an evaluation scheme.

Some programs have a participant manual or self-study guide that makes most handouts unnecessary. Participant manuals may also include exercise and diet diaries. These manuals may seem costly, but when the cost of the labor and supplies to duplicate materials is considered, they may be a bargain. In addition, participants place considerable value on receiving a comprehensive reference booklet.

Packaged programs vary greatly in cost. Before a packaged program is selected, a standardized review method should be used to evaluate its educational material, including the material's source, reading level, content, design, quality and technical criteria, manner of presentation, and instructional guides. Tools are available to guide the review of both written and audiovisual nutrition education materials (31).

A packaged program saves preparation time; provides the creativity of others in its quizzes, games, and group activities; and provides professional-quality materials such as graphics, slides, videotapes, and computer programs. Most packages have been developed with input from education specialists and instructional designers, who may also provide suggestions on adapting the program to specific audiences. Some programs have been reviewed or endorsed by organizations such as the American Academy of Family Physicians and the American Heart Association.

Use of a packaged program still requires planning. Although most programs give the impression that they require little preparation, time is required for reviewing the program and handouts; selecting slides and video clips; and ordering and receiving booklets, charts, models, videos (whether purchased or rented), and slides. Lead time is needed to schedule rooms, circulate announcements, and arrange for technical support as well as to obtain supplies (eg, name tags, flip charts, serving supplies, and certificates of completion). Identifying the need for and scheduling appointments with nutrition professionals, physicians, or other health care providers to answer questions should be done in the planning phase.

Incorporating Food Demonstrations into Classes

Food demonstrations and samplings are activities that always rate highly with participants. The resources required for these activities include time to shop for and prepare the food and to clean up after the demonstration; a budget for food and supplies; and facilities for storing, preparing, and serving food as well as for cleaning up. Food safety issues must also be considered.

Samples may be packaged food products or foods prepared by using revised recipes. The size of the samples will depend on the number of foods to be tasted. Generally it is appropriate to have four or five products or recipes to sample. Tasting a product enables individuals to decide whether they would buy it or make the food from scratch.

Participants' reactions to the foods they sample can be compiled to make this activity more structured. The use of a sensory evaluation score sheet, on which participants mark the products they like with a "smiley face," is well accepted. Recipes that receive acceptable ratings can be gathered for a group recipe book and information can be included in newsletters and in future classes.

Cooking demonstrations or classes are another option to consider if facilities are available. In addition to demonstrating heart-healthy meals, these sessions can discuss topics such as measuring techniques and serving sizes. A cooking demonstration can be held in a private home if the kitchen accommodates 10 to 15 people. The appropriateness of any kitchen as a classroom is determined by its size and layout, the kind and number of foods to be prepared, and local health and zoning regulations.

Classes that provide participants with hands-on experience preparing heart-healthy meals are more effective at instilling confidence than are cooking demonstrations. Facilities for a hands-on cooking class might be found in the home economics department of a local high school or at an adult education facility, hospital wellness center, or local church.

Selected recipes should meet nutrition guidelines, create an attractive meal, taste good, and be relatively inexpensive and quick to prepare. It is generally inadvisable to introduce more than one new ingredient (eg, bulgur or tofu) in a recipe. Cooking classes usually require 2 to 3 hours. A short lecture can be given while the food simmers, bakes, or chills. When the food is ready, participants eat, discuss the food, and clean up. The atmosphere in most cooking classes is relaxed and nonthreatening.

Deciding Whether to Refine or Expand an Existing Program

Even if a program is going well, outcomes for participants can be improved, and time should be taken for program assessment. A comprehensive program includes all of the following (32):

- defining measurable objectives for participants,
- pretesting tools,
- incorporating learners' priorities into the educational content,
- providing the minimum amount of information needed to motivate dietary improvement,
- encouraging learners to share successful personal strategies,
- acknowledging and praising learners' efforts, and
- evaluating all sessions.

The most effective nutrition education programs for adults are theory based and use a combination of theories (33). Some programs combine activities that are counterproductive or that violate the principles of a theory. Evaluating a program can determine, in addition to providing information, whether the course helps participants develop critical or creative thinking and problem-solving skills that will enable them to make decisions about their eating patterns.

Promoting a program through newspapers, radio, television, and health care providers will expand the audience for the program. Peer education programs may be a way to reach diverse audiences. Building a community intervention or aligning a program with a community intervention effort is another strategy to consider. Collaboration with the local American Heart Association chapter, medical society, health department, cooperative extension service, or parks and recreation department may be possible if such organizations run smoking-cessation, cholesterol-screening, or related activities that may be beneficial.

Holding focus groups for individuals who stopped coming to class may identify issues that promote or discourage continued attendance. Adding new activities may help decrease the attrition rate. Consumer surveys prepared by the Food Marketing Institute, the American Dietetic Association, and other organizations can help to determine what topics interest the public. Offering heart-healthy door prizes or presenting certificates, pins, a partial refund of the registration fee, or other rewards to people who attend all the classes or who achieve a significant goal may also be ways to improve attendance. Including family members in classes may improve both attendance and compliance with the new eating habits being learned. It may be helpful to have another dietitian attend and evaluate a program or to conduct a needs assessment by polling other heart educators.

Alternative Delivery of Classes

Changes in hospital procedures or staffing may eliminate classes for cardiac inpatients, resulting in a need for new ways to provide nutrition education. Existing programs can be refined for presentation via an in-house television system or used as the basis for a drop-in nutrition education counseling center.

As lifestyles become more complex, nutrition educators must find alternative ways of reaching busy consumers. Home-study and self-study programs via newsletters, television, computer programs, and the Internet and interactions with paraprofessionals or peer educators can be successful in improving knowledge about heart disease and dietary and exercise self-efficacy (34-37). Elements of a self-help kit might include brief illustrated instructions; food- and brand-specific information or shopping guides; a tool for selecting and monitoring goals; colorful, realistic illustrations; items that can be removed, such as recipes, checklists, and shopping cards; and an eating assessment form that uses a simple method of scoring (38, 39).

In many communities, local cable television providers can assist dietitians in preparing and broadcasting classes about heart-healthy nutrition. These programs can also be used in a telecourse, where participants receive an introductory letter and videotapes of the programs; complete quizzes; participate in a dietary analysis project; and communicate with the instructor by mail, telephone, fax, or e-mail.

Some audiences may be attracted to online information. Some patients already communicate with their physician and other health care providers by e-mail. Software is now available that makes it easy to develop World Wide Web sites. A Web-based nutrition course might include audio, video, animations, text, links to other Web sites, and instructor-participant interactions. However, dietitians who are developing and teaching online courses warn that these programs are time-consuming to initiate.

EVALUATION

Careful evaluation should be an integral part of all nutrition education programs and should include a review of educational materials for accuracy, suitability for the intended audience, commercial interest, and educational approach. It may be helpful to have an education specialist evaluate materials and programs.

Forms that participants can use for reactions and feedback are useful. Packaged programs usually include a prepared form that can be adapted as appropriate. Useful questions include

- What would you tell a friend about this class?
- What are the three most important things you learned from this class?
- What knowledge or skills do you still need to make lifelong changes in your diet?
- How do you rate this program on ability to motivate you to change; usefulness of suggestions; accuracy and credibility of leaders' information knowledge; classroom environment (room set up, accessibility, parking); scheduling, registration, and length of sessions; organization of the course; value for money charged; quality of food samples; and cooking demonstrations?
- Which recipes or products will you try?
- What did you like least about the class?
- What specific suggestions do you have for improving the course?
- How would you rate the overall quality of the course?
- How would you rate the instructor (excellent, good, fair, or poor) on knowledge of the subject and effectiveness of teaching methods?

Evaluations that use research protocols to determine the effectiveness of nutrition education may be difficult for participants to complete. Pre- and posttests may help to document the learning that occurred. The evaluation can also be used to assess interest in future classes.

Also important is an evaluation of the program that determines the actual costs and the staff time and resources that were required and investigates whether resources were optimally used.

REFERENCES

1. Wenger NK, Froelicher ES, Smith LK. *Cardiac Rehabilitation as Secondary Prevention.* Clinical Practice Guideline. Quick Reference for Clinicians, No. 17. Rockville, Md: Agency for Health Care Policy and Research; 1995. AHCPR publication 96-0673.

2. Brownson RC, Smith CA, Pratt M, Mack NE, Jackson-Thompson J, Dean CG, Dabney S, Wilkerson JC. Preventing cardiovascular disease through community-based risk reduction: the Bootheel Heart Health Project. *Am J Public Health.* 1996;86:206-213.
3. Curry SJ, Kristal AR, Bowen DJ. An application of the stage model of behavior change to dietary fat reduction. *Health Educ Res.* 1992;7:97-105.
4. Ornish D. *Dr. Dean Ornish's Program for Reversing Heart Disease.* New York, NY: Random House, 1990.
5. Kupka-Schutt L. Heart Smart nutrition education. *J Nutr Educ.* 1992;24:94a.
6. Pelican S. Sane holiday eating. *J Nutr Educ.* 1994;26:166a.
7. Travers KD, Tan M-H, MacCleave AP, Murphy A, Whiting S. Evaluation of a motivational education program for cardiovascular risk reduction: effects on knowledge and behavior. *J Nutr Educ.* 1992;24:109-116.
8. American Heart Association. *Culinary Hearts Kitchen Cooking Course.* American Heart Association. Dallas, Tex; undated.
9. American Association for Retired Persons, American Heart Association. *Eating for HEALTHY Tomorrows.* Washington DC: Healthy Advocacy Services; 1992.
10. Nutri-Smart Inc. *Fat Budgeting the NutriSmart Way.* Penfield, NY: Nutri-Smart; 1993.
11. HealthQuest. *Cholesterol.* Greenville, NC: Pitt County Memorial Hospital; 1996.
12. TVIH Technology Assessment Conference Panel. Methods for voluntary weight loss and control. *Ann Intern Med.* 1992;116:942-949.
13. Parham ES. Nutrition education research in weight management among adults. *J Nutr Educ.* 1993;25:258-267.
14. Pratt C. A conceptual model for studying attrition in weight reduction programs. *J Nutr Educ.* 1990;22:177-182.
15. Gibson C, Nitzke S, Welch C, Thompson M. *Nutrition Education in Small Groups: Developing a Learning Community.* Madison, Wis: Agricultural-Extension; 1992.
16. Balch GI. Nutrition education for adults. *J Nutr Educ.* 1995;27:312-328.
17. Magnus MH. Self-check, group check: congregate meal site nutrition education. *J Nutr Educ.* 1990;33:310d.
18. National Agricultural Library, USDA. Database of food and nutrition software and multimedia programs. Beltsville, Md: Food and Nutrition Information Center.
19. Gans KM, Sundaram SG, McPhillips JB, Hixson ML, Linnan L, Carleton RA. Rate Your Plate: An eating pattern assessment and educational tool used at cholesterol screening and education programs. *J Nutr Educ.* 1993;25:29-36.
20. Sumner NE, Keller B, Diamond L. *Nutrition DISCovery* personalized CD-ROM diet assessment program. *J Nutr Educ.* 1996;28:47c.
21. *Dietary Guidelines and Your Diet.* Hyattsville, Md: USDA, Human Nutrition Information Service; 1992. Home and Garden Bulletins HG-232-1-11.
22. National Center for Nutrition and Dietetics. *Nutrition Fact Sheet. Weight Loss Readiness Quiz.* Chicago, Ill: National Center for Nutrition and Dietetics; undated.
23. American Dietetic Association. *Project Lean Resource Kit: Tips, Tools, and Techniques for Promoting Low-fat Lifestyles.* Chicago, Ill: National Center for Nutrition and Dietetics, 1995.
24. American Heart Association. *Heart at Work.* Dallas, Texas: American Heart Association, 1991.
25. American Heart Association, Virginia Affiliate. *Culinary Hearts Kitchen. Southern Cooking Supplement.* Glen Allen, Va: American Heart Association; undated.
26. Brownell KD. *The LEARN Program for Weight Control.* 6th ed. Dallas, Tex: American Health Publishing Co.; 1994.
27. *Self-Care for a Healthy Heart.* Ft. Collins, Col: Colorado State University Cooperative Extension Service; 1991.
28. *The Heart Care Program.* Minneapolis, Minn: Hall-Foushee Productions Inc.; 1994.
29. *Healthy Dividends: A Plan for Balancing Your Fat Budget.* Oakbrook, Ill: National Dairy Council; 1990.
30. *Low-Fat Express.* Owatonna, Minn: Pineapple Appeal; 1995.
31. Betterly C, Dobson B. Evaluation tools for nutrition education materials. *J Nutr Educ.* 1990;22:140b.
32. Magnus MH. A self-assessment inventory for nutrition educators. *J Nutr Educ.* 1994;26:256a.
33. Contento I, Balch GI, Bronner YL, Lytle LA, Maloney SK, Olson CM, Swadener SS. The effectiveness of nutrition education and implications for nutrition education, policy, programs and research: a review of research. *J Nutr Educ.* 1995;27:277-418.
34. Schaefer N, Falciglia G, Collins R. Adult African-American females learn cooperatively. *J Nutr Educ.* 1990;22:240d.
35. Rose MA. Evaluation of a peer-education program on heart disease prevention with older adults. *Public Health Nurs.* 1992;9:242-247.
36. Krinke UB. Nutrition information topic and format preferences of older adults. *J Nutr Educ.* 1990;22:292-297.
37. Goldberg JP, Gershoff SN, McGandy RB. Appropriate topics for nutrition education for the elderly. *J Nutr Educ.* 1990;22:303-310.
38. Johnston JM, Jansen GR, Anderson J, Kendall P. Comparison of group diet instruction to a self-directed education program for cholesterol reduction. *J Nutr Educ.* 1994;26:140-145.
39. Gans KM, Lovell HJ, Lasater TM, McPhillips JB, Raden M, Carleton RA. Using quantitative and qualitative data to evaluate and refine a self-help kit for lowering fat intake. *J Nutr Educ.* 1996;28:157-163.

RESOURCES

Criteria for listing: produced after 1990, reviewed or listed in the *Journal of Nutrition Education, Journal of American Dietetic Association,* or National Agricultural Library (Food and Nutrition Information Center, US Department of Agriculture).

Division of Health Education, Memorial Hospital of Rhode Island, 111 Brewster St, Pawtucket, RI 02860, 401-729-2369, fax 401-729-2494.

Dodds MP. Change of Heart newsletters for consumers. Reno, NV: University of Nevada School of Medicine, Reno, NV 89520-9913 (702)784-4848.

Heart Memo. National Heart, Lung, and Blood Institute Information Center, PO Box 30105, Bethesda MD 20824-0105. A periodical published by the Office of Prevention, Education and Control providing updates on prevention, education and community activities concerning risk factors for cardiovascular disease. No charge.

Low Fat Life Line Publications, 52 Condolea Ct. Lake Oswego OR 97035.

National Center for Nutrition and Dietetics. 276 West Jackson Blvd. Chicago, IL 60606-6995.

National Cholesterol Education Program, NHLBI, 4733 Bethesda Ave, Suite 530, Bethesda, MD 20814-4820.

Nutrition Counseling Education Services. 1904 East 123rd St., Olathe KS 66061-5886; 1-800-445-5653.

USDA Food and Nutrition Information Center. Visit their information on the World Wide Web. http://www.nal.usda.gov/fnic/pubs/bibs/topics/heart/cvd-ed.html. More than 45 items listed.

The Weight Control Information Network (WIN), 1 WIN WAY, Bethesda MD 20892-3665. WINNIDK@AOL.com.

Packaged Programs

American Dietetic Association. *Project Lean Resource Kit: Tips, Tools, and Techniques for Promoting Low-fat Lifestyles.* National Center for Nutrition and Dietetics, 216 West Jackson Blvd, Chicago, IL 60606-6995. A three-ring binder with background, tips on teaching lower-fat eating patterns, a section on reaching the community, and worksite. Reviewed in *J Nutr Educ,* Sept/Oct 1996 (Reference 23).

American Association for Retired Persons and American Heart Association. *Eating for HEALTHY Tomorrows.* Health Advocacy Services, 601 E Street, NW, Washington, DC, 1992. One-time, two-hour session for older African Americans (Reference 9).

American Heart Association. *Heart at Work* Reviewed in *J Nutr Educ,* Sept/Oct 1991 (Reference 24).

American Heart Association. Virginia Affiliate. *Culinary Hearts Kitchen. Southern Cooking Supplement.* Glen Allen, Va: AHA (Reference 25).

American Heart Association. *Culinary Hearts Kitchen Cooking Course.* American Heart Association. Dallas, Tex (214) 706-1310. Listed in FNIC catalog (Reference 8).

Brownell KD. The LEARN Program for Weight Control. 6th ed. American Health Publishing Co., 1555 W. Mockingbird Lane, Suite 203, Dallas TX 75235. Reviewed in *J Nutr Educ,* 1995;27:153. 16 lessons (Reference 26).

Colorado State University Cooperative Extension Service. *Self-Care for a Healthy Heart.* Ft. Collins, Col, 1991. 303-491-6198. Includes 4 lessons and computer diet analysis protocol (Reference 27).

Hall-Foushee Productions Inc, 1313 5th St, SE, Suite 214B, Minneapolis, MN 55414. *The Heart Care Program.* 4 videotapes, leader's scripts for 4 interactive classes, 14 reproducible handouts, participant booklet, laminated cards. Noted in Practitioner's Bookshelf, *J Am Diet Assoc,* 1994;94:1228 (Reference 28).

National Dairy Council. *Healthy Dividends: A Plan for Balancing Your Fat Budget.* 1990. 10 min video, leader guide, consumer booklet. Reviewed in *J Nutr Educ,* Sept/Oct 1991 (Reference 29).

Nutri-Smart Inc. *Fat Budgeting: The Nutri-Smart Way.* 3-hour workshop kit with leader guide, overheads, participant manual, menu, marketing guide, game. NutriSmart Inc. 2260 Lake Ave, Suite 214, Rochester, NY 14612. Noted in Practitioner's Bookshelf, *J Am Diet Assoc.* 1994;94:116 (Reference 10).

Pineapple Appeal. *Low-Fat Express.* Pineapple Appeal, PO Box 197, Owatonna, MN 55060. A kit with 9 lessons and visual aids, targeted to low-literacy audiences. Reviewed in *J Nutr Educ,* 1996;28:234-235 (Reference 30).

Sample Audiovisual/Handouts

Dahlheimer SS, Scanga DA, Foltz TL. *Heart Wise Nutrition Program Client Handbook.* 1989. Handbook of 23 sections developed for cardiac rehabilitation. Reviewed in *J Am Diet Assoc,* 1990;90:324-325.

Food for Health. *Food for Health* low-fat, low-sodium newsletter. Published 10 times per year. Includes license to reproduce all or part of newsletter. Noted in Practitioner's Bookshelf, *J Am Diet Assoc,* 1995;95:949.

Geiger CJ, Harper PH. *Learning the New Food Labels: An Educator's Slide Kit.* American Dietetic Association, 216 W. Jackson Blvd., Chicago, IL 60606-6995, 1994. 52 color slides, educator's guide and reproducible handouts. Reviewed in *J Nutr Educ,* 1996;28:179-180.

McCann E. *Techniques for Healthy Cooking.* Culinary Institute of America, 433 Albany Post Rd, Hyde Park, NY, 1993. A three-part video series. Reviewed in *J Nutr Educ,* 1994;26:163-164.

National Health Video. Amy Barr, RD, demonstrates low-fat food preparation in 4 13-minute videotapes. National Health Video, 12021 Wilshire Blvd, Suite 550, Los Angeles, CA 90025. Noted in Practitioner's Bookshelf, *J Am Diet Assoc,* 1996;96:92.

NHLBI. *Stay Young at Heart Kit.* Includes recipes, reproducible handouts and graphics. Stock number 017-043-00133-8. Call NHLBI at 202-512-1800. Noted in Practitioner's Bookshelf, *J Am Diet Assoc,* 1995;95:1061.

Parlay International. *Nutrition Kopy Kit.* Parlay International, 5835 Doyle St, #111, Emeryville, CA 94608, 1994. 60 camera ready handouts. Reviewed in *J Nutr Educ,* 1996;28:236-237.

Piazza J, Robinson M, Weiner J, American Heart Association. *Heart and Soul: Foods and Facts for Your Heart.* 7 videos to show African Americans how to prepare typical soul food items with less fat, calories, and sodium. Cleveland, Ohio: Metro Health Clement Center; 1989. Listed in the National Ag Library.

Schwartz C, Schwartz P. *Cholesterol Control: An Eater's Guide.* Emeryville, Calif: Schwartz and Ecker Productions; 1989. 30-minute video on reducing cholesterol through diet alone without feeling deprived. Reviewed in *J Am Diet Assoc,* 1990;90:1024-1025.

Weiss L, O'Neill C. *CNN Healthy Eating Series: Eating Healthy for Life, Eating Healthy for Kids, Eating Healthy for Weight Control, Eating Healthy for Heart Health and Eating Healthy When Eating Out.* Turner Educational Services, 10 N Main St, Yardley, PA 19067. Reviewed in *J Am Diet Assoc,* 1991;91:1486-87.

CHAPTER 16

INTERVENTION STRATEGIES FOR SPECIAL GROUPS

CHERYL ACHTERBERG, PHD; BRENDA EISSENSTAT, MS, RD; AND
SHARON L. PETERSON, PHD, RD

Many nutrition education interventions have facilitated the adoption of healthful food- and nutrition-related behaviors in adults. Nutrition education efforts are usually more effective when they are behaviorally focused and based on appropriate theory and applied research (1). Ways to increase the effectiveness of nutrition education interventions were identified (Box 16-1), and Barnard et al. (2) and others (3-5) identified approaches that help to facilitate compliance with lower fat intake (Box 16-2).

The question remains: can effective intervention strategies be targeted to special population groups? This chapter identifies intervention strategies related to nutrition and heart disease that have been successfully adapted to special groups, including lower-literacy individuals, selected ethnic and cultural groups, women, and the elderly.

Within the vast literature on diet and cardiovascular disease, few studies have reported intervention strategies that were developed specifically for target groups. Much more research is needed to identify the subgroups at risk and to determine the most effective intervention strategies within each group. Practitioners who have achieved success with nutrition interventions for special groups should be encouraged to share their strategies. In general, it is important that dietitians structure nutrition interventions so that recommended changes are compatible with individuals' cultural values and beliefs (6). Suggested additional reading material in this area is listed in the Resources section.

One study of hard-to-reach Americans (defined as white, black, and Mexican American men and women ages 25-64 with 12 or fewer years of education and a family income below the median but above poverty level) identified a deeply held belief that chronic diseases are largely the result of fate and heredity and are therefore beyond individual control (7). An individual's health beliefs, locus of control, and sense of self-efficacy have as great an influence on nutrition-related behaviors as do environmental factors (ie, access to fresh fruits and vegetables, cost, and food cooking and storage facilities) and social factors (ie, cultural food practices, influence of mass media, and family role modeling) (8). An important first step in working with hard-to-reach groups may be to develop and add meaning to the link individuals see between diet and heart disease.

STRATEGIES FOR LOWER-LITERACY AUDIENCES

Distribution of printed materials is a common strategy for disseminating information on reducing heart disease risk. Many dietary guidelines (9,10) and cholesterol education print materials (11,12) are written at the 10th-grade level or above. The 1995 edition of *Dietary Guidelines for Americans* (13) is written at the 13th-grade level. The average reading level of American adults is considered to be 8th grade. Lower-literacy adults, who read at a 5th- to 8th-grade level, comprise up to 20% of the American population (14,15). Thus, most printed materials on nutrition for heart health are inappropriate for most adults and especially inappropriate for lower-literacy adults.

Readability formulas are sometimes used to match health literature with patients' reading levels. However, reading level is but one element that should be considered when developing print materials (16). Although suggestions have been compiled for writing and rewriting printed materials for lower-literacy audiences (Box 16-3), the usefulness of converting existing print materials for lower-literacy audiences has been questioned (17). Rather, new materials should be designed for the needs and interests of lower-literacy audiences, with input from representatives of that audience to improve the materials' effectiveness.

Public-health nutritionists who worked with lower-literacy adults in eight states identified food models, television, videos, posters, verbal explanations, and slides to be among the most effective means of communication. Pamphlets and audiotapes were considered the least effective (18). In other words, visual presentations (preferably using hands-on props) work better than more abstract text-based or audio-only presentations.

BOX 16-1 Ways to Increase Effectiveness of Nutrition Interventions

- Include motivators and reinforcers that have personal meaning for a given group.
- Personalize self-assessment of dietary status or food-related behaviors with feedback in the form of recommendations.
- Use models of change that integrate individual, social, and environmental factors.
- Invite active participation by the target group in the design and implementation of intervention.
- Invite active participation by the target group in the intervention itself.
- Organize mass media health campaigns to increase awareness and improve knowledge.
- Use a systematic behavioral change process.
- Develop interpersonal counseling and education tailored to the specific need group.
- Engender social support from family and peers.
- Use empowerment skills to enhance personal control.
- Use point-of-purchase interventions in grocery stores and restaurants.
- Apply interventions in school meals, work-site cafeterias and vending machines, restaurants, and other community settings.
- Elicit active participation of community leaders.

Source: Adapted from Contento I (1). Reprinted with permission of the *Journal of Nutrition Education.*

BOX 16-2 Ways to Improve Compliance to Lower Fat Intake

- Set limits for total daily fat intake that are lower than the goal. People often underestimate their intake of fat and energy.
- Have nutritionists monitor dietary intake at least monthly. Self-monitoring by occasionally weighing and measuring food and maintaining a food diary is also useful.
- Use family involvement. Include immediate family members, especially the person who purchases and prepares the food.
- Use group support. Monthly meetings can provide support and a forum to introduce new concepts and reinforce new behaviors.
- Provide samples or use packages of recommended foods as teaching tools. These also provide visual cues for patients when shopping.
- Incorporate vegetarian diets, meals, and recipes. Food sampling and introductions to new ingredients can encourage those unfamiliar with vegetarian meals.
- Encourage men to participate in food-related activities. Use real-life experiences such as ordering from a menu or choosing appropriate convenience foods.
- Assess predisposing factors (beliefs, perceived benefits, and motivation).
- Include self-rated diet instruments.
- Review evidence of past success at dietary change and results that can reasonably be anticipated.
- Provide motivation to eat low-fat foods. Be enthusiastic and encouraging. Remind the client of the multiple benefits of dietary change relevant to them.

Source: Adapted from References 2-5.

BOX 16-3 Guidelines for Writing or Rewriting Printed Materials for Lower-Literacy Adults

- Write simply; use familiar and commonly used words.
- Write personally; use "you" rather than "they."
- Use words of two or fewer syllables whenever possible.
- Use active verbs.
- Use simple sentence structure whenever possible.
- Avoid introductory and imbedded phrases and clauses. Limit compound and complex sentences to those where the connecting word (such as "because") clearly shows the relationship between clauses.
- Vary sentence length but avoid sentences with more than 15 words.
- Vary paragraph length but avoid paragraphs with more than 5 sentences.
- Use short headings to introduce paragraphs.
- Write in the active rather than the passive voice.
- Use graphics that are logically linked to the text.
- Use upper- and lowercase letters rather than all capitals.
- Use white or off-white paper and dark blue or black ink.
- Balance the use of text with white space.
- Use an unjustified right margin.
- Avoid excess information.
- Use concrete rather than abstract words or give concrete examples of abstract ideas.
- Apply the content being presented to the reader's personal and cultural experiences.

Source: Institute for the Study of Adult Literacy, College of Education, The Pennsylvania State University.

Participants in focus groups about healthful eating that targeted lower-literacy adults said that they were interested in simple, practical, relevant information about what foods to eat and how to prepare them. Most individuals were interested in recipes, healthful convenience and fast foods, and other foods that they could prepare quickly. Hands-on activities that were enjoyable and encouraged the sharing of ideas and experiences were also valued (19). Trying new recipes and foods as a group was a popular activity. More research is needed to determine effective intervention strategies that target lower-literacy audiences with cardiovascular disease.

STRATEGIES FOR SELECTED ETHNIC AND CULTURAL GROUPS

Developing nutrition interventions that target people from diverse backgrounds presents a variety of challenges. Nutrition educators must recognize the importance of specific foods within cultures and of ethnosocial influences on food choices (20). However, generalizations about food patterns should not be made solely on the basis of race, ethnicity, or geographic origin, because food-choice diversity is common within all cultural and racial groups. Interventions are most effective when nutrition educators focus on each family's unique dietary history and background without making assumptions about food habits on the basis of cultural or racial background (20). Only through in-depth, culturally sensitive interviews can dietitians determine clients' unique dietary practices and health beliefs and begin to tailor meaningful nutrition interventions.

To gain an understanding of relevant food patterns, Hertzler, Stadler, Lawrence, Alleyne, Mattioli, and Majidy (21) suggested using an empowerment approach to stimulate dialogue. For example, ask first about general life concerns, next about general nutrition and food access concerns, and then about family health concerns. Finally, ask the client, "How can I help you with your family eating or nutrition habits?"

Terry (22) suggested doing thorough fieldwork to differentiate between core food habits that are shared by the group and unique food choices that are made by individuals within the group. Effective nutrition education depends on the educator genuinely knowing the client. Ideally, the session should begin in a general way and adopt a more specific, individualized approach when personal rapport has developed.

A rapid assessment tool for food in different cultures is found in Table 16-1. When used as part of a nutrition assessment, this tool may help to identify an individual's food preferences. Box 16-4 contains a list of recommendations for cross-cultural counseling that was developed by the US Departments of Agriculture and Health and Human Services (24).

Little research has been done on the effectiveness of heart disease interventions specifically targeted at African Americans, Asian Americans, Mexican Americans, and American Indians and Alaska Natives. The following sections

TABLE 16-1

Rapid Assessment Tool: Food and Culture

Discuss with client. Check yes or no for each item.

Question	Yes	No
Do you have problems purchasing foods that you want?	_____	_____
Do you prepare foods like Grandma did at least three times per week?	_____	_____
Do you eat fast food more than three times per week?	_____	_____
Do you eat more than three meals per day?	_____	_____
Do you eat more than one snack a day?	_____	_____
Do you prepare most of your meals at home?	_____	_____
Do you eat a special way for religious reasons?	_____	_____
Are you on a special diet?	_____	_____
Do you believe that what you eat can make you healthier?	_____	_____
What is your favorite traditional food?	_____	_____
Do you eat favorite traditional foods?	_____	_____
Do you eat favorite traditional foods daily?	_____	_____
Do you believe children and adults should eat different foods?	_____	_____
Do you use convenience foods daily?	_____	_____
Do you avoid any food because it makes you sick?	_____	_____
Are there certain foods that you don't eat?	_____	_____
Do you eat only certain foods on holidays?	_____	_____

Adapted with permission from Bronner Y (23), *Topics in Clinical Nutrition,* 1994;9(2), © 1994 Aspen Publishers, Inc.

BOX 16-4 Recommendations for Enhancing Cross-Cultural Counseling

- Understand and recognize your own cultural values and biases.
- Acquire basic knowledge of cultural values, health beliefs, and nutrition practices for groups you routinely serve.
- Be respectful of, interested in, and understanding of other cultures without being judgmental.
- Determine level of fluency in English and arrange for an interpreter, if needed.
- Ask clients how they prefer to be addressed.
- Allow clients to choose where they sit so that they are comfortable and you have eye contact with them.
- Avoid body language that may be offensive or misunderstood; for example, do not show the soles of your shoes to Asian clients, who may interpret this as a sign of disrespect.
- Speak directly to clients whether or not an interpreter is present.
- Choose a speech rate and style that promotes understanding and demonstrates respect for the client.
- Avoid slang, technical jargon, and complex sentences.
- Use open-ended questions or questions phrased in several ways to obtain information.
- Determine the client's reading ability before using written materials.
- Build on cultural practices, reinforcing those that are positive and promoting change only in those that are harmful.
- Check for the client's understanding and acceptance of recommendations.
- Be patient and provide counseling in a culturally appropriate environment to promote positive health behavior change.

Source: Adapted from US Depts of Agriculture and Health and Human Services (24).

FIGURE 16-1

African-American foods and the Food Guide Pyramid.

Source: Kittler PG, Sucher K (30). Reprinted with permission from the Penn State Nutrition Center.

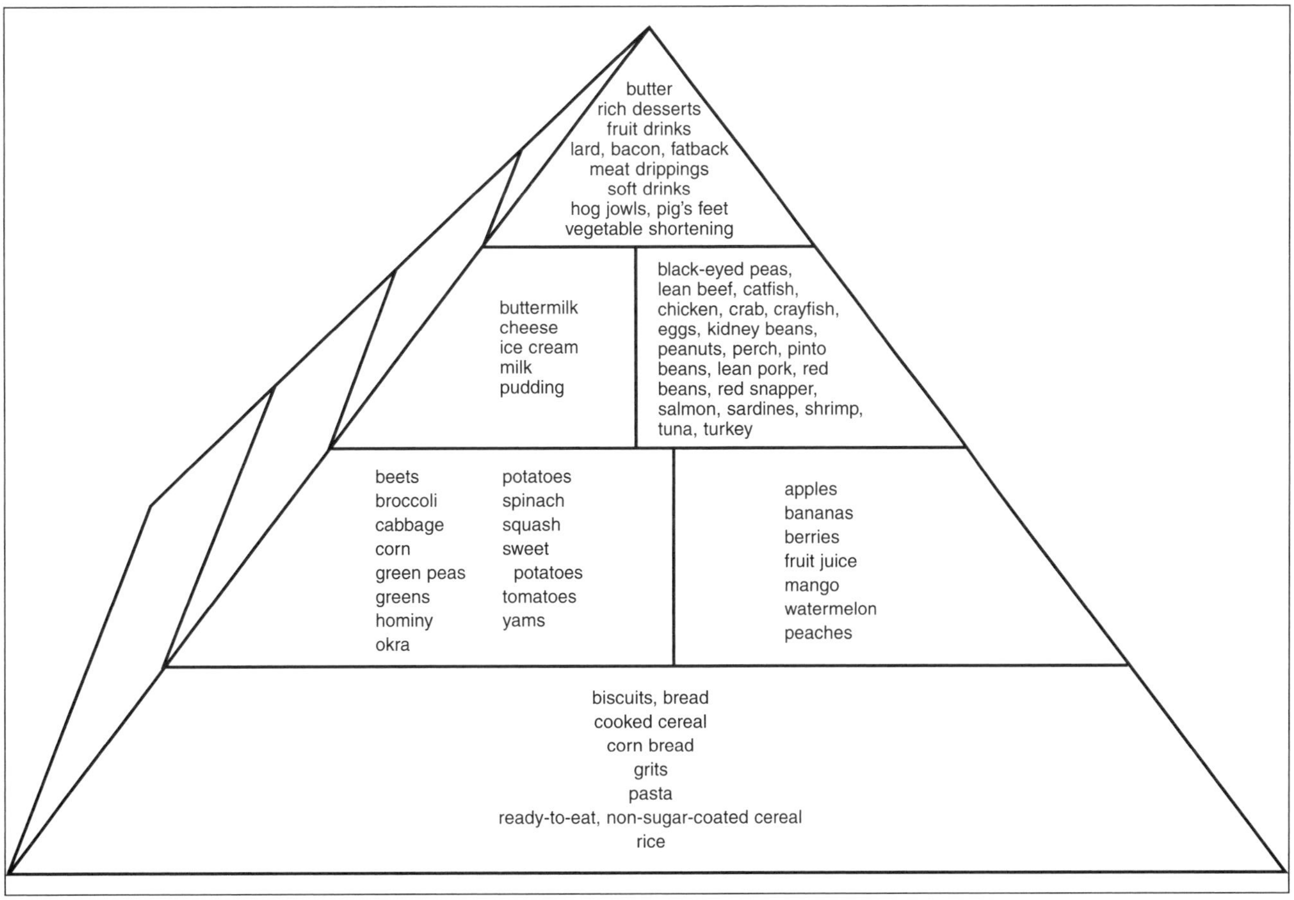

summarize what is known about the effectiveness of interventions in these groups.

African Americans

One nutrition intervention that targeted prevention of cardiovascular disease in African-American families suggested that future efforts be integrated into other ongoing community activities and that intensive diet self-monitoring techniques should be avoided (25). Flack and Wiist (26) suggested the development of church-based cholesterol education programs because churches are a central institution in most African-American communities. Congregations that were screened appeared to have excessive levels of many cardiovascular disease risk factors (26). Community nutrition interventions targeted to church members and their religious leaders may be effective.

African Americans frequently use the term *soul food* to describe the food traditions that developed out of their unique experiences. Soul food combines traditional foods and cooking techniques brought from Africa with foods available in the southern United States and the conditions imposed by slavery. It has taken on added significance as a symbol of African-American identity and African heritage (23,27,28).

The typical diet of a middle-class African-American family may not differ significantly from the conventional diet of other middle-class Americans. In these families, traditional soul food may be served only on holidays or special occasions. Many soul foods, however, are commonly used throughout the southern United States.

Dietitians should be aware of the correlation between a soul-food diet and African Americans' increased risk factors for cardiovascular disease. Traditional soul foods tend to be high in cholesterol, fat, and sodium. A heavy emphasis on vegetables and complex carbohydrates, however, reduces heart disease risk and should be encouraged. Common soul foods and preparation techniques were elaborated by Bronner, Burke, and Joubert (27) and Burke and Raia (29). Burke and Raia (29) also provided a nutrient database for soul foods. Figure 16-1 shows a food pyramid for common soul foods (30).

The cultural significance of soul food can easily be retained when adjustments are made to cooking techniques and ingredient selection to lower fat, cholesterol, and sodium (Box 16-5). Compliance with dietary suggestions is generally higher if people can continue to eat familiar food. The many positive aspects of soul food should be emphasized and its cultural significance respected.

BOX 16-5 **Food Preparation Techniques to Lower Fat, Cholesterol, and Sodium in African-American (or Soul) Foods**

General

- Substitute fat-free mayonnaise in biscuits for regular mayonnaise.
- Serve turkey ham or homemade turkey sausage with sage and seasonings instead of bacon.
- Use "light" or sugar-free syrup or fruit; use egg substitute in pancake, waffle, and biscuit recipes.
- Measure all fats (eg, mayonnaise, margarine, and oil) added to foods.

Frying

- Use nonstick skillet lightly coated with vegetable oil spray for eggs, fish, and vegetables.
- Substitute "low-saturated-fat" oils instead of white shortening or bacon drippings.

Flavoring

- Cook vegetables with smoked but not cured lean meat, such as turkey necks.
- Add flavor without fat or sodium by using liquid smoke sparingly.
- Use low-potassium salt substitute.
- Season with onion, garlic, pepper, or hot sauce to lower the amount of salt.

Source: Adapted with permission from Bronner Y, Burke C, Joubert BJ (27), *Topics in Clinical Nutrition,* 1994;9(2), © Aspen Publishers, Inc.

Asian Americans

A review of the literature located no studies that reported culture-specific nutrition intervention strategies for Asian Americans. This may be due, in part, to the perception that Asian Americans are at lower risk for cardiovascular disease than are other ethnocultural groups. Cachola (31) identified cultural and demographic factors that may influence the effectiveness of interventions among Asian Americans (Box 16-6). Classification issues in survey research also affect Asian Americans, because the term *Asian/Pacific Islander* incorporates people from at least 17 Asian and 8 Pacific nations. Thus, aggregate data cannot discern wide variations in either cultural norms or heart disease risk in different populations of Asians and Pacific Islanders.

Immigration from Asian countries to the United States has taken place for hundreds of years. The first Chinese immigrants arrived in 1782. Two distinct waves of immigration from China occurred with the California gold rush of 1849 to 1924 and from 1965 to 1985 (32). Immigration from the Philippines began in 1899, soon after America took over colonial rule of the islands from Spain. Since 1960 the US Census Bureau has registered over 1 million Filipinos (33). Another large wave of Asian immigrants occurred after the Vietnam conflict. Large Hmong communities are located in California, Wisconsin, and Minnesota. Japanese and Korean immigrants and their descendants are also prevalent across the United States.

As Asian Americans' immigration history and region of origin vary, so does their degree of assimilation within the dominant American culture. Education levels vary widely. Many newly arrived immigrants speak little English and may have had little formal schooling in their homeland. On the other hand, many Asian Americans are highly educated people who are well represented in the health field and in other professions.

When health care professionals counsel Asian-American clients, it is important to be aware of culturally based health beliefs and dietary practices. Figures 16-2 and 16-3 (35, 36) are food pyramids for Chinese- and Vietnamese-American food groups. Box 16-7 suggests strategies for conducting culturally appropriate counseling sessions with Asian Americans. Several excellent references explain traditional health beliefs and dietary practices in different Asian-American populations in the United States (37-39). However, as noted above, it should not be assumed that clients have traditional dietary habits.

Mexican Americans

The Mexican population in America presents a wide variety of food preferences that originate predominantly from the geographic and cultural diversity of Mexico. The Mexican diet combines foods of Spanish and Indian influence. Traditionally the diet was primarily vegetarian, based on corn, beans, and squash. This diet offers many nutritional advantages: it is high in complex carbohydrates, fruits, and vegetables; processed foods are infrequently used; and most meals are nutritionally balanced and simply prepared. (More time-consuming dishes such as tamales and enchiladas are often reserved for holidays and special occasions.)

Dietary habits of concern in the treatment and preven-

BOX 16-6 Factors That Affect Interventions with Asian Americans

- Immigration is a key stress factor because of fragmentation and loss of family members, as well as abrupt adjustments to an unfamiliar culture.
- Health care providers are highly regarded.
- Extended families may take precedence over the nuclear family with regard to health care decisions.
- Elders in the family may be responsible for health care decisions.
- Males may take precedence over females.
- Clients' self-esteem may be based on their ability to please others with their health care decisions.
- Patients may believe in fate more than in medical intervention and may refuse treatment.
- Additional barriers may exist, such as language and the need to migrate to find work.

Source: Adapted from Cachola S (31).

tion of heart disease are the heavy use of added fat, especially lard, and a preference for high-fat meats. High fat and cholesterol intakes have been documented in Mexican-American populations, especially in males (40). Cooking techniques rely heavily on frying and stewing with liberal amounts of oil or lard. The prevalence of obesity, elevated serum triglyceride levels, and diabetes in Mexican-American populations is well documented (41-44). When counseling Mexican-American clients, the positive aspects of the traditional diet should be emphasized and the use of lower-fat cooking techniques and ingredients encouraged.

As a rule, Mexican-American families are proud and private about family problems. Interdependence rather than independence is encouraged. Interdependence and poverty

FIGURE 16-2

Chinese-American foods and the Food Guide Pyramid.

Sources: Kittler PG, Sucher K (30), and Kee MM (34). Reprinted with permission from the Penn State Nutrition Center.

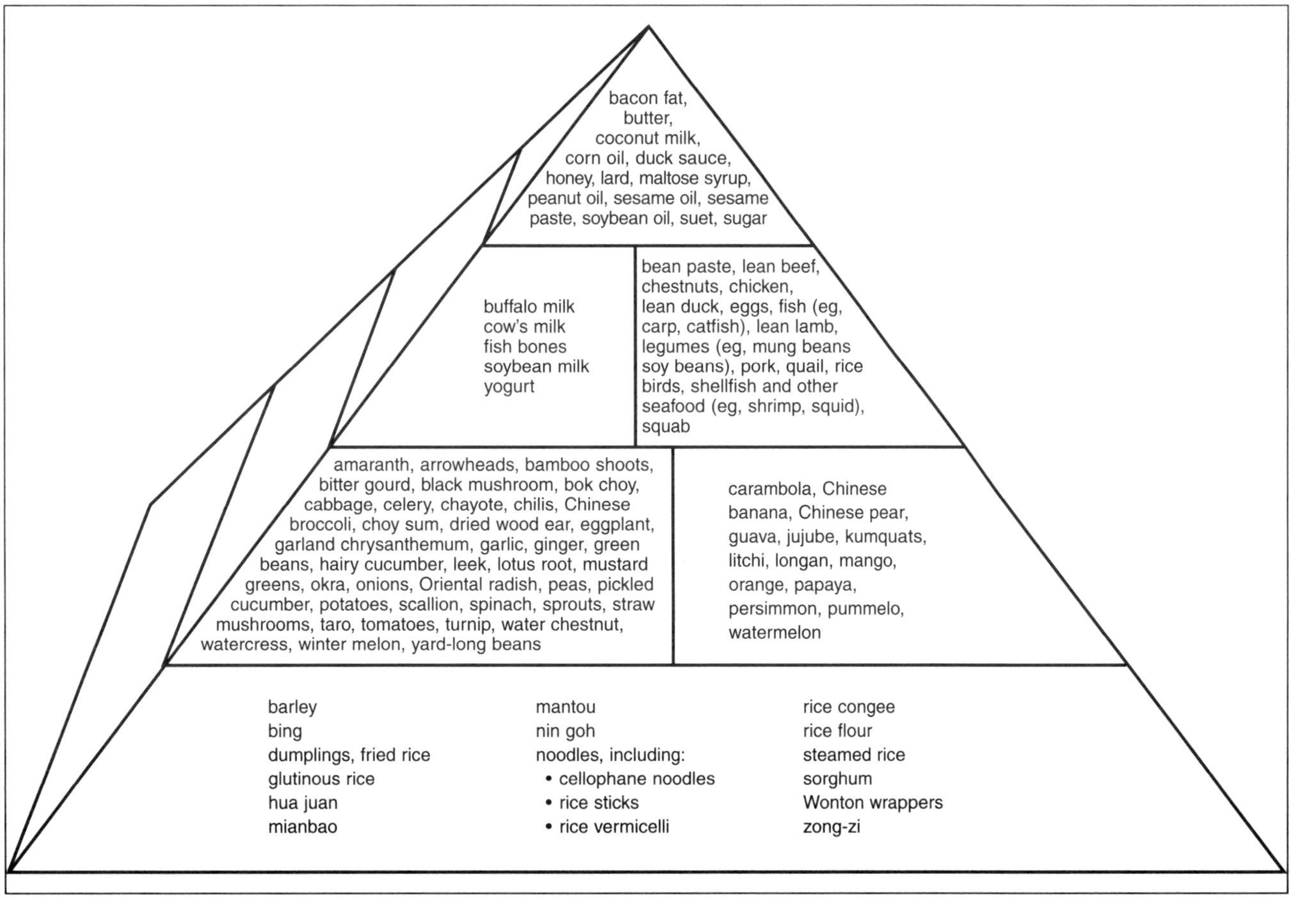

BOX 16-7 Strategies for Culturally Appropriate Nutrition Counseling with Asian Americans

- Dispel myths and misconceptions.
- Take advantage of the cultural concept that certain foods are good for certain organs to teach food groups by their functions, rather than their nutritional properties. For example, tell clients, "These foods are bad for your heart and arteries."
- Encourage consumption of foods that are familiar and culturally acceptable. For example, recommend tofu and green leafy vegetables as food for the bones.
- Use teaching materials such as pictures, food models, and actual packages.
- Discuss portion control in a way that is compatible with communal meal service. Suggest clients place all of their food selections on a separate plate before mealtime. In this way, they can continue to eat with the family while exercising better control over portion sizes.
- Involve the person who cooks the family meals in the counseling session. Conflict and noncompliance may result from lack of general consensus among family members.
- Work with trained interpreters if possible. Family members who interpret may add their own comments or omit certain statements that they believe the client should not tell the dietitian. Children who interpret for their parents or grandparents may not have enough medical vocabulary to communicate effectively.
- Point out mistakes in a way that will not cause clients to lose their self-respect. For example, "Putting your rice into the rice bowl by packing loosely like this is a more accurate way of measuring."

Source: Adapted from Kee MM (34).

FIGURE 16-3

Vietnamese-American foods and the Food Guide Pyramid.

Sources: Passimore J (35), Routhier N (36), Solomon C (37); Laura Le, personal communication, 1996; Tuan Le, personal communication, 1996; and waiter at the Pho Express, personal communication, 1996. Reprinted with permission from the Penn State Nutrition Center.

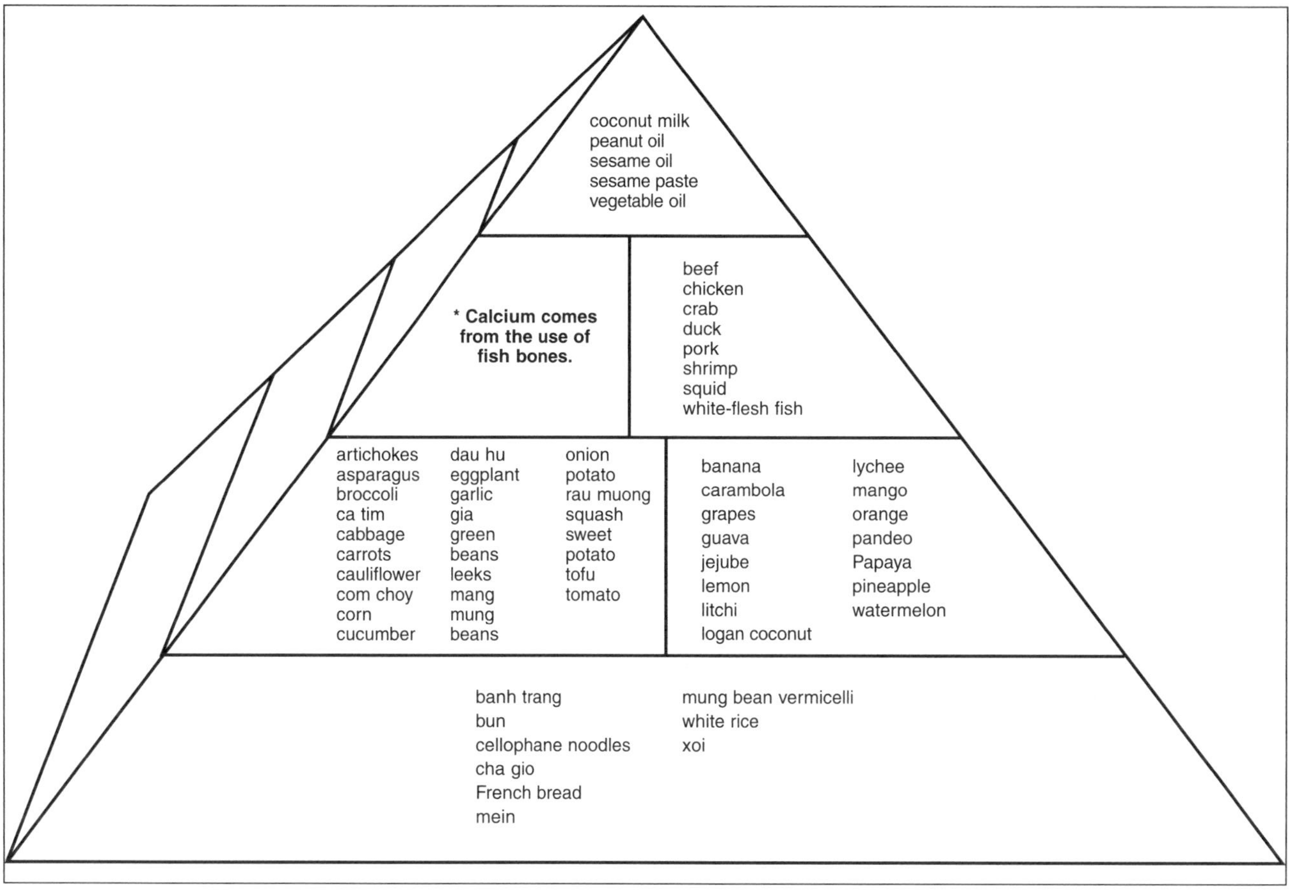

FIGURE 16-4

Mexican-American foods and the Food Guide Pyramid.

Sources: Algert SJ, Ellison EH (47), and Visiting Nurse Association (48). Reprinted with permission from the Penn State Nutrition Center.

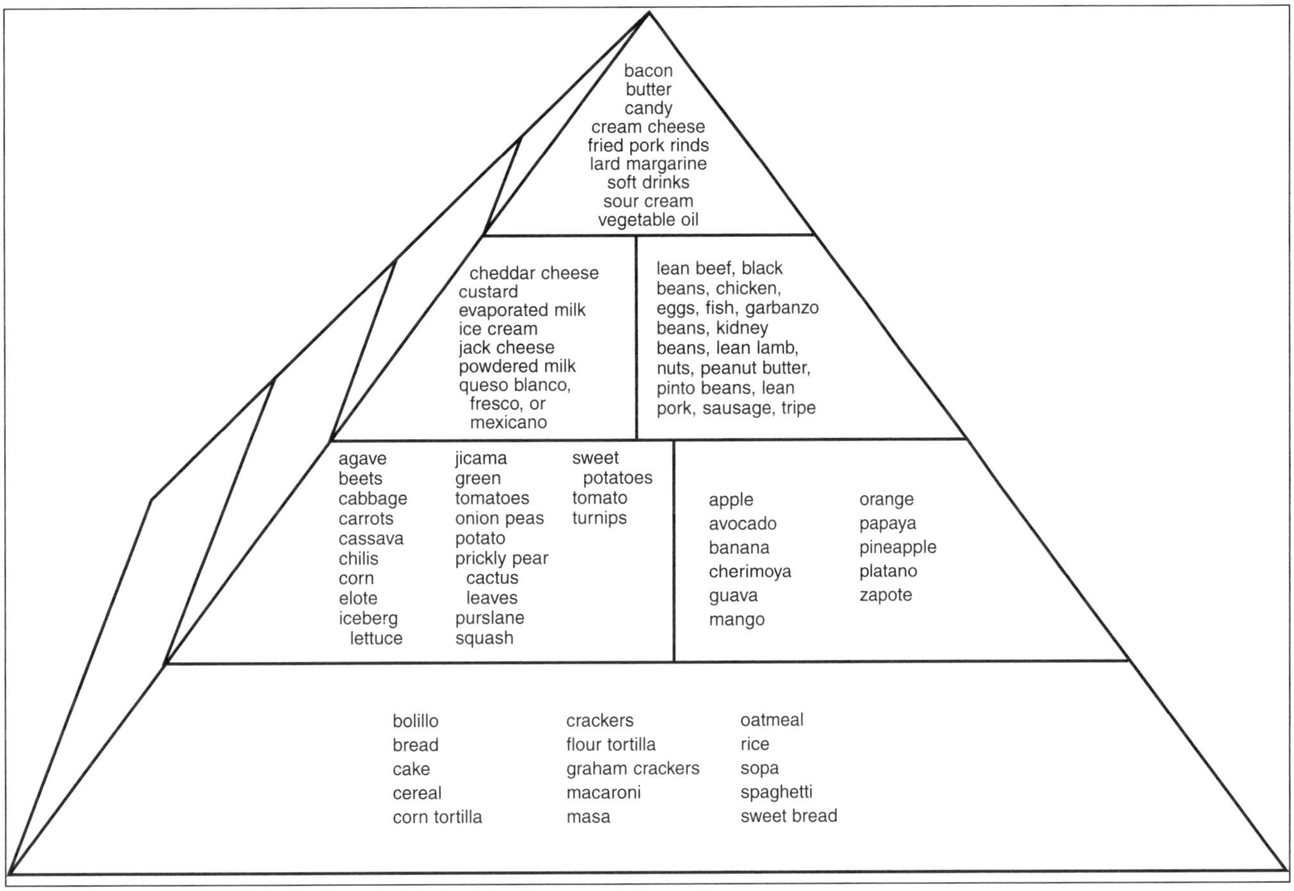

can be barriers to seeking professional health care. However, Mexican Americans may respond favorably to interventions that recognize and support the overriding importance of family and community. Community nutrition programs may be more attractive if advertisements appeal to the good of the family, for example: "Healthful eating will benefit your husband, your children, and your sister." Nutrition intervention efforts should target families and their religious leaders. Other important factors include the use of Spanish-speaking professionals and personal relationships developed over time (45).

Like other ethnic groups, Mexican Americans vary in socioeconomic status and education level. A thorough diet history will include questions about available resources for the purchase and preparation of food. Most Mexican Americans have adopted some US dietary habits. Bilingual children, an increased level of education, and employment are often associated with the introduction of new foods (46). Figure 16-4 is a food guide pyramid for Mexican-American foods.

Several subgroups can usually be identified within any ethnic population. In one study, six unique subgroups were found within the Mexican-American target group. Group members differed significantly along communication, behavioral, psychological, and demographic dimensions as well as in high-density lipoprotein levels and hypertension rates (49).

When numerous subgroups are identified within a population, the intervention program should be more flexible in its approach. Mexican-American subgroups have different needs and experiences that have shaped their attitudes toward health, family, and nutrition. Lack of awareness of and sensitivity to these differences can be a formidable barrier to effective intervention. Diverse strategies may need to be used even when working within an ethnically homogeneous group.

American Indians/Alaska Natives

Lack of understanding of American-Indian and Alaska-Native cultures has been cited as a major barrier for non-Native nutritionists who work with Native-American clients (50). The following 1990 census information documents some important facts and patterns that can help interventionists to better understand this population as a whole, but it also illustrates the impossibility of describing American Indians/Alaska Natives as a homogeneous group.

In 1990, approximately 2 million individuals from more than 500 tribes and villages identified themselves as American Indians or Alaska Natives. Although four tribes (Cherokee, Chippewa, Navajo, and Sioux) each have a population greater than 100,000, most tribes have populations of less than 10,000. More than 50% of the American-Indian/Alaska-Native population lives in six states (Alaska, Arizona, California, New Mexico, Oklahoma, and Washington), but more than 60% lives outside reservations, trust lands, and other tribally or village-designated areas.

Thirty-one percent of American Indians/Alaska Natives have incomes below the poverty level. Thirty-nine percent of the population is under age 20, compared with 29% of the US population as a whole. Although 64% of American-Indian/Alaska-Native households have both a husband and wife present, the proportion of households headed by a single female is 27%, compared with 17% for the US population as a whole (51).

The diversity among American-Indian and Alaska-Native cultures is remarkable and precludes any meaningful statements about typical diets or ways to understand all American Indians and Alaska Natives. Nevertheless, several resources offer valuable insights about cross-cultural work and about promoting health, nutrition, and physical activity specifically in American-Indian and Alaska-Native communities. For example, Eliades and Suitor (20) provide a rich framework for understanding the role of food in many cultures and offer much practical guidance that can assist nutrition educators in learning about cultures different from their own (Box 16-8).

Some specific resources related to American-Indian and Alaska-Native cultures may also be helpful. Researchers with the Strong Heart Study, a three-center, multitribe study of cardiovascular disease risk factors among American Indians in North Dakota, South Dakota, Oklahoma, and Arizona, offered several possible strategies for improving the dietary habits commonly reported by these groups (52). Some of these strategies appear in Box 16-9 along with suggestions offered in print materials developed for American Indians and Alaska Natives by the National Heart, Lung, and Blood Institute and

BOX 16-8 **Ways to Learn About American-Indian and Alaska-Native Communities**

- Become familiar with the community: walk around, go shopping, and read the local newspaper.
- Seek out community leaders.
- Learn about "community markers": visit local restaurants, churches, supermarkets, schools, etc., and locate traditional food sources.
- Check out community groups and informal networks like school and Head Start parent associations and senior citizen groups.
- Attend open community functions like pow-wows and feast days. Browse through craft fairs and flea markets and attend local sports events.
- Find out what people need. Ask questions.

Source: Adapted from Eliades DC, Suitor CW (20).

BOX 16-9 **Examples of Suggestions for Decreasing Heart Disease Risk That Have Been Used with Various American-Indian and Alaska-Native Groups**

- Use traditional food preparation methods like roasting, boiling, broiling, and baking.
- Eat traditional meats like fish, deer, and caribou.
- Choose lean cuts of beef and pork.
- Trim the fat from fresh meat and remove the skin from chicken and other fowl.
- Remove the fat from canned meat.
- Eat beans, vegetables, and fruit.
- Fry foods less often and use vegetable oil instead of lard or shortening for frying.
- Drink low-fat or skim milk.

Source: Adapted from Zephier E (52).

FIGURE 16-5

Current Navajo foods and the Food Guide Pyramid.

Sources: Pelican S, Bachman-Carter K (55) and *Navajo Health and Nutrition Survey,* Navajo Area Indian Health Service, unpublished. Reprinted with permission from the Penn State Nutrition Center.

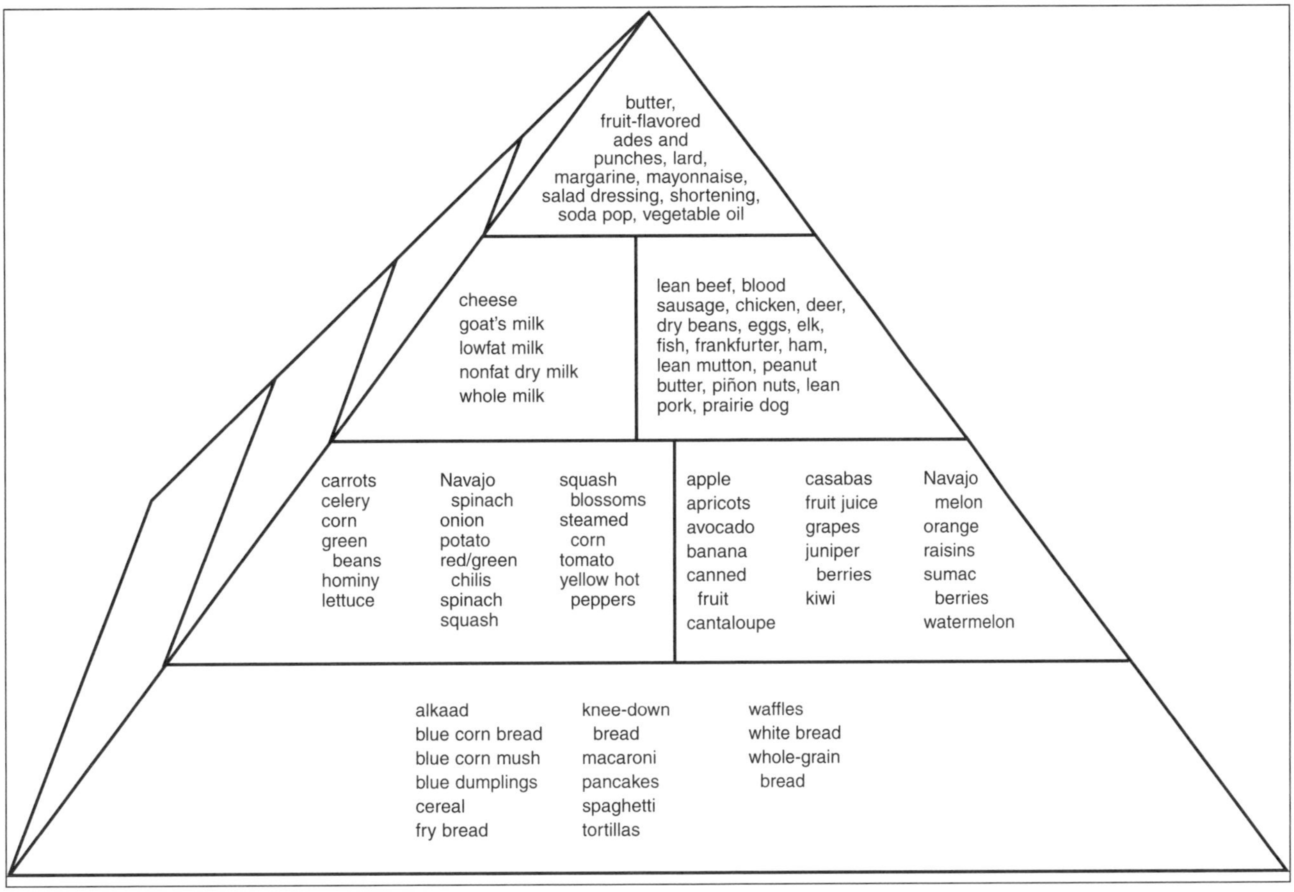

the Indian Health Service (53). Such strategies must be tailored to each client's needs and living situation (eg, accessibility to a supermarket, participation in food assistance programs, and other issues).

The American Dietetic Association's Diabetes Care and Education Practice Group has a monograph series entitled *Ethnic and Regional Food Practices.* The Alaska-Native (54) and Navajo (55) monographs and the soon-to-be-published Plains-Indian monograph provide sample meal patterns that use foods commonly consumed and suggest culturally appealing ways of improving these meals. Figure 16-5 contains a food pyramid for common Navajo foods. Other excellent references provide valuable insights and practical guidance related specifically to helping mobilize American-Indian/Alaska-Native communities to promote and protect their members' health and well-being (56,57).

Wilson, Leonard, Martin, Sterling, and Schmid (58) addressed the culturally appropriate promotion of exercise to reduce heart disease risk. This step-by-step guide is based on physical activity programs that are established in several American-Indian communities. In the Zuni community, for example, running and other endurance exercises are the foundation of a community-based fitness program. In Penobscot, Maine, the local health department revived a traditional 100-mile Sacred Run to encourage running, walking, and canoeing. Other nontraditional sports such as nordic skiing, weightlifting, rowing, and stationary and outdoor bicycling are also popular. Lacrosse was reintroduced in Oneida, Wisconsin. Running was encouraged for Navajo women by reviving a Navajo ceremony that honors a female deity, Changing Woman.

In summary, no hard-and-fast rules apply to working with American Indians and Alaska Natives. On the contrary, to be effective, interventionists need to learn about the specific cultures and lifestyles of the American-Indian and Alaska-Native clients with whom they would like to work. The resources noted above may prove useful as a starting point.

STRATEGIES FOR WOMEN

Researchers with the Women's Health Trial compared the ease of adopting and maintaining five fat-related dietary habits (59). Of these, substitution of specially manufactured low-fat foods and modifications in the purchase and preparation of meat were two easily adopted and maintained habits.

BOX 16-10 Strategies for Enhancing the Effectiveness of Nutrition Intervention in Older Adults

- Use personalized, self-assessment approaches.
- Use a behaviorally oriented approach.
- Use active participation, ie, hands-on experiences.
- Use motivators and reinforcements of behavior.
- Use an empowerment philosophy that includes enhancing personal choice, control, and social support.
- Identify subgroups of older adults and target their specific diet-related problems.
- Be sensitive to age-related physical changes, such as loss of sight and hearing.

Source: Adapted from Contento I (1).

In contrast, avoiding meats, replacing commonly eaten high-fat foods with lower-fat foods, and avoiding fats as flavorings were habits that may require long-term reinforcement strategies to maintain. When avoiding fats as flavorings was adopted, it resulted in the largest decreases in fat intake.

The design of interventions that target leading sources of dietary fat should recognize that sources of fat in women's diets vary by region and ethnicity (60). For example, salad dressing is a predominant source of fat for white women and women in the West and Northeast, whereas frankfurters and bacon are greater sources of fat for African-American women and women in the Midwest and South.

Life stage is another relevant factor. Women's motivations for implementing preventive dietary behavior vary depending on their role within the family (61). Women with young children may be more likely to make changes that target the family's health whereas older women may make changes that target personal health.

STRATEGIES FOR OLDER ADULTS

Several elements have been identified that contribute to the effectiveness of nutrition education interventions for older adults (Box 16-10). Many older adults express an interest in diet and health (62), especially in fat and cholesterol (63,64). It is important to recognize that the most important sources of information about health and nutrition for older adults are physicians and print materials (57,58).

The guidelines suggested earlier for producing print materials for lower-literacy audiences also apply to materials for older adults. Losses in visual acuity are common and reading levels are often low.

Relatively few educational interventions aimed at achieving behavioral change have been empirically tested in this population. Most interventions for older adults are based on group instruction or interaction, often in senior centers or congregate meal programs. These group programs are limited by the fact that the groups are not preexisting or sustainable in the environment beyond the instructional experience. In addition, these groups miss many older adults altogether.

Two studies evaluated the efficacy of nutrition newsletters for older adults (63,64). This approach may be useful for promoting knowledge and attitude change, but its value in behavior change efforts is uncertain. A combination of the strategies presented in Box 16-10 will probably be most effective for achieving behavior change in older adults.

Older adults often feel that they lack control over their environment and they may need a high level of support and follow-up while adopting new behaviors. However, given this support, they may be more receptive to counseling and adopting new behaviors than younger audiences.

CONCLUSION

Much more work is needed to determine the most successful cardiovascular disease intervention strategies for most special groups. Much of the existing data pertain to weight control efforts, but few of these programs have proven successful. It is not clear whether intervention programs designed to decrease weight are fundamentally different from programs designed to decrease risk of heart disease in terms of barriers, expectations, and outcomes.

Transferring methods from one subgroup to another may not be uniformly effective. Audiences should be segmented by key sociodemographic variables so that messages can be tailored effectively. How this segmentation should be done, however, is unclear. It is impractical to divide people into dozens of cells. It would be helpful to establish the relative priority of factors such as age, ethnicity, work status, gender, life stage, and geographic variables in terms of their influence on behavior change.

Researchers and practitioners should make every attempt to report key social and environmental factors that contributed to the success of their programs. They should also specify their target audiences so that a more comprehensive knowledge base can be built and field settings, including inpatient and outpatient clinics, differentiated.

RESOURCES

Bronner Y. Cultural sensitivity and nutrition counseling. *Top Clin Nutr.* 1994;9:13-19.

Bronner Y, Burke C, Joubert BJ. African-American/soul foodways and nutrition counseling. *Top Clin Nutr.* 1994;9:20-27.

Brown LK, Mussell, K. *Ethnic and Regional Foodways in the United States: The Performance of Group Identity.* Knoxville: University of Tennessee Press; 1985.

Burke CB, Raia SP. *Soul and Traditional Southern Food Practices, Customs, and Holidays.* Chicago, Ill: Diabetes Care and Education Practice Group, American Dietetic Association; 1995.

Claudio VS. *Filipino-American Food Practices, Customs and Holidays.* Chicago, Ill: Diabetes Care and Education Dietetic Practice Group, American Dietetic Association; 1994.

Exploring Food, Culture and Nutrition, http://www.fwfs.com. The Four Winds Food Specialists home page contains information on relevant books and other resources (many free) in cultural nutrition. The Web site also contains information on holiday food traditions, recipes, and health data.

Fork, Fingers, and Chopsticks. A quarterly newsletter written for food, nutrition and health professionals working with clients from diverse ethnic, religious, and cultural backgrounds. For ordering information, contact Four Winds Food Specialists, PO Box 70015, Sunnyvale, CA 94086, phone 408-735-8847, or their World Wide Web home page, http://www.fwfs.com.

Hall TA. Designing culturally relevant educational materials for Mexican American clients. *Diabetes Educ.* 1987;13:281-285.

Ikeda JP. *Hmong American Food Practices, Customs, and Holidays.* Chicago, Ill: Diabetes Care and Education Dietetic Practice Group, American Dietetic Association; 1991.

Kee MM. *Chinese American Food Practices, Customs and Holidays.* Chicago, Ill: Diabetes Care and Education Dietetic Practice Group, American Dietetic Association; 1990.

Kittler PG, Sucher KP. *Food and Culture in America: A Nutrition Handbook.* 2nd ed. St Paul, Minn: West/Wadsworth Publishiers; 1997.

Mexican American Food Practices, Customs, and Holidays. Chicago, Ill: Diabetes Care and Education Dietetic Practice Group, American Dietetic Association; 1989.

Romero-Gwynn E, Grivetti L, McDonald R, Stanford G, Turner B, West E, Williamson E. Dietary acculturation among Latinos of Mexican Descent. *Nutr Today.* 1993;28(4):6-12.

Weaver R. *The Soul Food Pyramid.* A colorful patient handout outlining the five major food groups and appropriate serving sizes. To order, contact The Hebni Nutrition Consultants, Inc, 4630 S. Kirkman Road, Suite 201, Orlando, FL 32811, phone/fax 407-345-7999.

REFERENCES

1. Contento I. The effectiveness of nutrition education and implications for nutrition education policy, programs, and research: a review of research. *J Nutr Educ.* 1995;27:279-283, 320-322, 339-346.
2. Barnard AN, Akhtar A, Nicholson A. Factors that facilitate compliance to lower fat intake. *Arch Fam Med.* 1995;4:153-158.
3. Woolcott DM, Sabry JH, Kawash GF. A study of some aspects of food-related behavior among a group of men. *Hum Nutr Appl Nutr.* 1983;37A:199-209.
4. Kristal AR, Patterson RE, Glanz K, Heimendinger J, Hebert JR, Feng Z, Probart C. Psychosocial correlates of healthful diets: baseline results from the Working Well Study. *Prev Med.* 1995;24:221-228.
5. Glanz K, Kristal AR, Sorensen G, Palombo R, Heimendinger J, Probart C. Development and validation of measures of psychosocial factors influencing fat- and fiber-related dietary behavior. *Prev Med.* 1993;22:373-387.
6. Gregory SJ, Clark, PI. The "big three" cardiovascular risk factors among American blacks and Hispanics. *J Holist Nurs.* 1992;10:76-88.
7. White SL, Maloney SK. Promoting healthy diets and active lives to hard-to-reach groups: market research study. *Public Health Rep.* 1990;105:224-231.
8. Bandura A. Self-efficacy: toward a unifying theory or behavior change. *Psychol Rev.* 1977;84:191-215.
9. Glanz K, Rudd J. Readability and content analysis of print cholesterol education materials. *Patient Educ Couns.* 1990;16(2):109-117.
10. Boyd MD, Citro K. Cardiac patient education literature: can patients read what we give them? *J Cardiac Rehab.* 1983;3:513-516.
11. Achterberg C, Bradley E. Bulletin features found most and least appealing to an extension audience. *J Nutr Educ.* 1991;23:244-250.
12. Trenkner LL, Achterberg CL. Use of focus groups in evaluating nutrition education materials. *J Am Diet Assoc.* 1991;91:1577-1581.
13. *Nutrition and Your Health: Dietary Guidelines for Americans.* 4th ed. US Depts of Agriculture and Health and Human Services; 1995. Home and Garden Bulletin No. 232.
14. Hynak-Hankison MT. Literacy crisis: implications for nutrition and dietetic professionals. *Top Clin Nutr.* 1989;4:63-70.
15. Doak C, Doak L, Root J. *Teaching Patients with Low Literacy Skills.* Philadelphia: J B Lippincott, 1985.
16. Meade CD, Smith CF. Readability formulas: cautions and criteria. *Patient Education and Counseling.* 1991;17:153-158.
17. Achterberg CL, Van Horn B, Maretzki A. Evaluation of dietary guideline bulletins revised for a low literate audience. *J Ext.* 1994;32(4).
18. Mettger W. *Communicating Nutrition Information to Low-literacy Individuals: An Assessment of Methods.* Revised final report. American Public Health Association 117th Annual Meeting; October 1989; Chicago, Ill:22.
19. Hartman TJ, McCarthy PR, Park RJ, Schuster E, Kushi LH. Focus group responses of potential participants in a nutrition education program for individuals with limited literacy skills. *J Am Diet Assoc.* 1994;94:744-748.
20. Eliades DC, Suitor CW. *Celebrating Diversity: Approaching Families Through Their Food.* Arlington, Va: National Center

for Education in Maternal and Child Health, 1994.

21. Hertzler AA, Stadler KM, Lawrence R, Alleyne LA, Mattioli LD, Majidy M. Empowerment: a food guidance process for cross-cultural counseling. *J Fam Consumer Sci.* 1995; 87(2):45-50.
22. Terry RD. Discovering and managing cultural food patterns. Presented at the Pennsylvania Dietetic Association Annual Meeting; May 3, 1995. Chicago, Ill.
23. Bronner Y. Cultural sensitivity and nutrition counseling. *Top Clin Nutr.* 1994;9(2):13-19.
24. US Depts of Agriculture and Health and Human Services. *Cross-cultural Counseling: a Guide for Nutrition and Health Counselors.* Alexandria, Va: Food and Nutrition Service, 1986.
25. Baranowski T, Henske J, Simons-Morton B, Palmer J, Tiernan K, Hooks PC, Dunn JK. Dietary change for cardiovascular disease prevention among black-American families. *Health Educ Res.* 1990;5:433-443.
26. Flack JL, Wiist WH. Cardiovascular risk factor prevalence in African-American adult screenees for a church-based cholesterol education program: the Northeast Oklahoma City Cholesterol Education Program. *Ethn Dis.* 1991;1:78-90.
27. Bronner Y, Burke C, Joubert BJ. African-American/soul foodways and nutrition counseling. *Top Clin Nutr.* 1994;9:20-27.
28. Brown LK, Mussell K. *Ethnic and Regional Foodways of the United States: The Performance of Group Identity.* Knoxville: University of Tennessee Press; 1985.
29. Burke CB, Raia SP. *Soul and Traditional Southern Food Practices, Customs, and Holidays.* Chicago, Ill: Diabetes Care and Education Practice Group of the American Dietetic Association; 1995.
30. Kittler PG, Sucher K. *Food and Culture in America.* New York, NY: Van Nostrand Reinhold; 1989.
31. Cachola S. Communication determines success of interventions in Asian Americans. In: *Minority Health Issues for an Emerging Majority.* The 4th National Forum on Cardiovascular Pulmonary Disorders and Blood Resources. June 26-27, 1992; Washington, DC: 69.
32. Tsai SSH. *The Chinese Experience in America.* Bloomington, Ind: Indiana University Press, 1986.
33. Bureau of the Census, US Department of Commerce. *Statistical Abstracts of the USA.* 110th ed. Washington, DC: US Government Printing Office, 1990.
34. Kee MM. *Chinese American Food Practices, Customs and Holidays.* Chicago, Ill: Diabetes Care and Education Dietetic Practice Group of the American Dietetic Association; 1990.
35. Passimore J. *Asia, the Beautiful Cookbook.* San Francisco, Calif: Collins; 1990.
36. Routhier N. *The Foods of Vietnam.* New York, NY: Steward, Taborr and Chang; 1989.
37. Solomon C. *Complete Asian Cookbook.* New York, NY: McGraw Hill, 1982.
38. Claudio VS. *Filipino-American Food Practices, Customs and Holidays.* Chicago, Ill: Diabetes Care and Education Dietetic Practice Group of the American Dietetic Association; 1994.
39. Ikeda JP. *Hmong American Food Practices, Customs, and Holidays.* Chicago, Ill: Diabetes Care and Education Dietetic Practice Group of the American Dietetic Association; 1991.
40. Haffner SM, Knapp JA, Hazuda HP, Stern MP, Young EA. Dietary intakes of macro nutrients among Mexican Americans: the San Antonio Heart Study. *Am J Clin Nutr.* 1985;42:1266-1275.
41. Stern MP, Pugh JA, Gaskill SP, Hazuda HP. Knowledge, attitudes, and behavior related to obesity and dieting in Mexican Americans and Anglos: the San Antonio Heart Study. *Am J Epidemiol.* 1982;115:917-926.
42. Stern MP, Rosenthal M, Haffner SM, Hazuda H, Franco LJ. Sex differences in the effects of sociocultural status on diabetes and cardiovascular risk factors in Mexican Americans: the San Antonio Heart Study. *Am J Epidemiol.* 1984;120:834-851.
43. Hazuda HP, Haffner SM, Stern MP, Eifler CW. Effects of acculturation and socioeconomic status on obesity and diabetes in Mexican Americans: the San Antonio Heart Study. *Am J Epidemiol.* 1988;128:1289-1301.
44. Samet JM, Coultas DB, Howard CA, Skipper BJ, Hanis CL. Diabetes, gallbladder disease, obesity, and hypertension among Hispanics in New Mexico. *Am J Epidemiol.* 1988;128:1302-1311.
45. Viruell EA. Meeting the health care needs of lower income Hispanic communities. In: *Minority Health Issues for an Emerging Majority.* The 4th National Forum on Cardiovascular Health, Pulmonary Disorders and Blood Resources. June 26-27, 1992. Washington, DC:71.
46. Dewey KG, Strode MA, Fitch YR. Dietary change among migrant families in northern California. *Ecol Food Nutr.* 1984:14:11-24.
47. Algert SJ, Ellison EH. *Ethnic and Regional Food Practices.* Chicago, Ill: Diabetes Care and Education Practice Group, American Dietetic Association; 1989.
48. *Spanish Foods in Diabetic Diets.* Milwaukee, Wis: Visiting Nurse Association; 1975.
49. Williams JE, Flora JA. Health behavior segmentation and campaign planning to reduce cardiovascular disease risk among Hispanics. *Health Educ Q.* 1995;22:36-48.
50. Burhansstipanov L. Investigators need to recognize poverty, barriers to access among American Indian women. In: *Minority Health Issues for an Emerging Majority.* The 4th National Forum on Cardiovascular Pulmonary Disorders and Blood Resources. June 26-27, 1992; Washington, DC:44.
51. Bureau of the Census, US Department of Commerce. *We the First Americans.* Washington, DC: U.S. Government Printing Office, 1993.
52. Zephier E. Differences in diet found in communities with higher heart disease rates. In: *Minority Health Issues for an Emerging Majority.* The 4th National Forum on Cardiovascular Pulmonary Disorders and Blood Resources. June 26-27, 1992; Washington, DC:30.
53. Department of Health and Human Services. *Keepers of Wisdom to Strengthen the Hearts.* Bethesda, Md: The National Heart, Lung, and Blood Institute and the Indian Health Service. Fact sheets.
54. Halderson K. *Alaska Native Food Practices, Customs, and Holidays.* Chicago, Ill: Diabetes Care and Education Practice Group of the American Dietetic Association; 1991.
55. Pelican S, Bachman-Carter K. *Navajo Food Practices, Customs, and Holidays.* Chicago, Ill: Diabetes Care and Education Practice group of the American Dietetic Association; 1991.
56. Stanford Center for Research in Disease Prevention. *Restoring Balance: Community-directed Health Promotion for American Indians and Alaska Natives.* Stanford, Calif: Stanford University, 1992.
57. Aberdeen Area Indian Health Service, Health Education and

Epidemiology Program. *Groundswell Towards Health: Resource Manual.* Rapid City, SDak: US Department of Health and Human Services, Public Health Service; 1988.

58. Wilson R, Leonard B, Martin M, Sterling T, Schmid T. *Creating Physical Activity Programs in American Indian Communities.* Atlanta, Ga: U.S. Department of Health and Human Services, Centers for Disease Control and Prevention; 1996.
59. Kristal AR, White E, Shattuck AL, Curry S, Anderson GL, Fowler A, Urban N. Long-term maintenance of a low-fat diet: durability of fat-related dietary habits in the Women's Health Trial. *J Am Diet Assoc.* 1992;92:553-559.
60. Thompson FE, Sowers MF, Frongillo EA, Paria BJ. Sources of fiber and fat in diets of US women aged 19 to 50: implications for nutrition education and policy. *J Public Health.* 1992;82:695-702.
61. Devine CM, Olson CM. Women's dietary prevention motives: life stage influences. *J Nutr Educ.* 1991;23:269-274.
62. Goldberg JP, Gershoff SN, McGandy RB. Appropriate topics for nutrition education for the elderly. *J Nutr Educ.* 1990;22:303-310.
63. Taylor-Davis S. The educational effectiveness of a nutrition newsletter for older adults. University Park, Penn: Pennsylvania State University, 1996. Dissertation.
64. Crockett SJ, Heller ICE, Skauge LH, Merkel JM. Mailed-home nutrition education for rural seniors: a pilot study. *J Nutr Educ.* 1992;24:312-315.

CHAPTER 17

Risk-Factor Management Programs

Jill Metz, PhD, MPH; and James Kenney, PhD, RD

Cardiovascular disease (CVD) risk factor management programs are effective in preventing the development of atherosclerotic disease (primary prevention) and are being used as therapeutic interventions with clients with coronary disease and other clinical atherosclerotic disease (1). The programs reviewed, which can be used as either primary or adjunctive therapy, use lifestyle modification as the primary means of managing risk factors.

The most comprehensive and effective CVD risk reduction programs use a variety of intervention strategies to modify overall CVD risk. This approach is based on the notion that strategies targeting multiple risk factors are more beneficial for the client than are single-intervention strategies, as well as more practical because clients typically have multiple CVD risk factors. In addition to a rigorous diet, effective programs incorporate other behavioral interventions such as stress management, smoking cessation, physical activity, and behavior modification.

These programs usually feature a diet that is very low in fat (less than 10% to 20% energy), low in cholesterol, and high in carbohydrate. Programs that feature such a diet are effective in reducing plasma lipids (1-9), body weight (5,6,9), plasma glucose (2,9), and blood pressure (2,9,10). Significant improvements in well-being and quality of life have also been noted (10,11), in some cases reversing anatomical and functional measures of atherosclerotic disease (4,12,13). Diets slightly higher in total fat (27% energy) but low in saturated fat (8% to 10% energy) retard the overall progression of coronary artery disease in clients referred for angiography (14). It is difficult to judge a program's success by its dietary component alone because weight loss and other behavioral interventions contribute significantly to risk factor modification.

The risk-reduction programs described below are

- the Connor and Connor program,
- the Pritikin program,
- the Ornish program,
- the Cooper Clinic,
- the Duke Center for Living, and
- Intelligent Quisine.SM

Table 17-1 summarizes the components of these programs. Health professionals who are educated about the range of available CVD risk-reduction programs are in the best position to match clients with the most appropriate programs.

Risk-Reduction Programs

See Box 17-1 for contact information for the risk-reduction programs.

Connor and Connor

These investigators' work on the Family Heart Study led to the publication of *The New American Diet* (15) and *The New American Diet System* (16). This self-guided program promotes the progressive adoption of a diet that provides 20% of energy from fat. The program has three phases:

- replacing familiar recipes with lower-fat versions,
- reducing meat intake by experimenting with alternative lunch foods, and
- modifying dinner so that meat is used as a condiment rather than as the primary focus of the meal.

The cholesterol-saturated fat index (CSI) helps individuals make food selections that are low in both cholesterol and saturated fat. Foods with higher CSI scores have greater potential to raise blood cholesterol levels.

The program emphasizes dietary change, although it also addresses physical activity and stress reduction. Its advantages include its family focus, its emphasis on gradual dietary change, its provision of numerous recipes, and its cost-effectiveness. For the motivated client or family, it provides a self-guided approach.

TABLE 17-1

Summary of Components for CVD Risk-Reduction Programs (with the NCEP Diets Provided for Comparison)

Program Component	NCEP		Connor and Connor	Ornish	Pritikin	Cooper Clinic	Duke Center for Living	Intelligent Quisine
	Step I	Step II						
% Fat	≤ 30	≤ 30	20	10	< 10	15-30	15-20	22
% Carbohydrate	>55	>55	65	75	75-80	50-70	65	61
% Protein	15	15	15	15	10-15	10-20	15	17
Cholesterol (mg)	<300	<200	<100	<5 mg	≤ 100	—	<200 mg	120
% Saturated Fat	8-10	<7	5-6	(P/S>1)[a]	—	—	<7%	7
Alcohol	Moderation	Moderation	≤ 3 drinks/week	<2 oz/day	Moderation	Moderation	<2 drinks/day	≤ 3 drinks/week
Smoking cessation	Recommended		Recommended	Recommended	Recommended	Recommended	Recommended	Recommended
Stress management	—		Yes	1 hour/day	Yes	Yes	Yes	Yes
Exercise	Yes		Gradual	3 hours/week	Yes	Major emphasis	Yes	Yes
Behavior modification	Yes		Gradual	Yes	Yes	Yes	Yes	Yes
Program method	• Self-guided or through local classes • Medical nutrition therapy with RD		• Self-guided	• Self-guided • Residential retreat • Outclient	• Self-guided • Residential retreat • Outclient	• Self-guided • Residential retreat • Outclient	• Residential retreat • Outclient	• Self-guided
Other	Step I recommended for primary prevention progressing to step II if needed; step II recommended for secondary prevention			• Social support • Frozen prepared meals available	• Recommend <1600 mg sodium/day			• Program and support available by mail order
Weaknesses	• "Do it yourself"		• "Do it yourself"	• Extreme behavior changes necessary	• Extreme behavior changes necessary	• Efficacy of diet component not yet published	• Efficacy not yet supported by internal research	• "Do it yourself"
Strengths	• Changes attainable for most people • Cost effective • Local affiliates available for referral		• Recipes • Promotes gradual dietary change	• Results in regression of coronary artery disease	• Improves CVD risk factors	• Comprehensive • Focus on fitness • Diet component stresses moderation	• Comprehensive • Personal counselor for ongoing social support	• Convenient • Available by mail order • Support available by phone

[a]Ratio of saturated to unsaturated fatty acids.

The Pritikin Program

This program combines a dietary regimen of 10% fat and less than 1,600 mg sodium with physical activity and stress management to improve CVD risk factors. The program can be self-guided by means of one of the many Pritikin lay publications (17-21), or participants can attend a 7-, 13-, or 26-day residential retreat or a 6-week outpatient program at one of the Pritikin longevity centers, which are located in Santa Monica, California, and Miami Beach, Florida.

Participants in the center programs receive a risk factor-oriented medical evaluation that includes blood-chemistry screening and a treadmill test to determine an appropriate exercise prescription. The diet emphasizes the achievement of ideal body weight through a high intake of vegetables, fruits, whole grains, and nonfat dairy products and, for most people, two or fewer servings of fish per week.

An excellent feature of the program is that it provides many therapeutic modifications that are based on an individual's risk factor profile. An evaluation of the program's nutritional adequacy demonstrated that a sample Pritikin Program dietary plan (1,200 kcal) met or exceeded 100% of the U.S. Recommended Daily Allowance (US RDA) for 13 nutrients, excluding vitamins B-12 (2.4 mg, 40%) and zinc (12.9 mg, 86%) (22). However, the program does not promote energy restriction, and a higher energy intake may meet current age- and sex-specific RDAs for these nutrients (vitamin B12: 2.0 mg; zinc: 12 and 15 mg for women and men, respectively).

Significant improvements in CVD risk factors, including reduced serum lipids, body weight, and plasma glucose and improved myocardial blood flow, were observed in participants with coronary artery disease who adopted the

BOX 17-1 Contact Information for CVD Risk-Reduction Programs

Pritikin Longevity Center 1910 Ocean Front Walk Santa Monica, CA 90405 (800) 421-9911 and 5877 Collins Ave. Miami Beach, FL 33140 (800) 327-4914	Sonja Connor, MS, RD William Connor, MD Division of Endocrinology, Diabetes & Clinical Nutrition Oregon Health Sciences University 3181 SW Sam Jackson Park Rd. Portland, OR 97201 503-494-2001	Gene Erb, RD, LDN Duke Center for Living Sarah W. Stedman Center for Nutritional Studies Duke University Medical Center Box 3487 DUMC Durham, NC 27710 (919) 660-6689
Dean Ornish Preventive Medicine Research Institute 900 Bridgeway, Suite 1 Sausalito, CA 94965 (800) 775-PMRI	Cooper Clinic 12200 Preston Rd. Dallas, TX 75230 (800) 444-5764	Intelligent Quisine[SM] Campbell's Center for Nutrition & Wellness Campbell Place Camden, NJ 08103-1709 (800) 220-0485

Pritikin program (2-4,6-8). The program's main advantage is its rigorous, comprehensive approach to CVD prevention and treatment and its documented improvement of CVD risk factors. However, because of the program's intensity, most clients need extensive behavior modification to successfully adopt it. Consequently, this program may be more appropriate for highly motivated clients who have significant CVD risk factors or who have coronary disease and wish to avoid surgical or drug intervention.

The Ornish Program

The work of Ornish and colleagues in the Lifestyle Heart Trial showed that a very-low-fat (10% fat), nearly vegetarian diet along with smoking cessation, stress management, psychosocial support, and moderate exercise can reverse established coronary atherosclerosis (5,10,12,13). Participants in these studies had documented coronary artery disease and showed significant improvements in CVD risk indexes, including regression of coronary artery stenosis (5,12) and improvement of myocardial perfusion abnormalities (13).

The Ornish diet excludes all animal products except egg whites and one serving daily of nonfat dairy products. Clients who strictly follow this program should be advised to supplement their diets with vitamin B-12 and possibly calcium and vitamin D; in other respects, the diet has been shown to be nutritionally adequate (5).

Ornish and colleagues offer the program at 1-week residential retreats four times each year at the Claremont Resort and Spa in Oakland, California. They also have a multisite demonstration network that offers the program at hospital-based centers across the country. Eligibility is limited to clients who are candidates for bypass surgery or who have undergone a revascularization procedure. The hospital-based program begins with an intensive weekend orientation to introduce participants to the program and the recommended lifestyle changes. This is followed by group meetings three times each week for 3 months and weekly meetings for the rest of the year. Optional long-term support is also available. Demonstration sites include centers in New York, Massachusetts, Florida, Iowa, Nebraska, California, and South Carolina (Box 17-2).

The program can also be self-guided with the use of one of Ornish's books (23-26). As with the Pritikin program, the advantages of the Ornish program are its intensive, comprehensive approach to CVD risk reduction and its documented efficacy. The hospital-based centers make the program available to more people, and participants can expect to receive some insurance reimbursement.

However, as with the Pritikin program, successful adoption of the Ornish program requires intensive lifestyle modification. Although the residential retreats are available to all interested individuals, their high cost restricts their availability to a significant segment of the population at risk for CVD. A limited number of financial scholarships are available through the Preventive Medicine Research Institute. Individuals who pursue this program should be highly motivated.

The Cooper Clinic

The Cooper Aerobics Center, located in Dallas, Texas, provides a variety of preventive medicine programs to individual and corporate clients. The Cooper Clinic, a division of the Cooper Aerobics Center, offers comprehensive preventive medical evaluations, including risk assessment and a lifestyle prescription—an individualized recommendation for preventive nutrition, exercise, and stress management.

Achievement and maintenance of a healthy body weight is the program's primary objective. The diet consists of 15% to 30% fat, 50% to 70% carbohydrate, and 10% to 20% protein daily and includes a prescribed number of servings per day from skim milk products, starches and breads,

BOX 17-2 Hospital-based Providers of the Ornish Program

Alegent Immanuel Medical Center
Alegent Heart Institute
6901 N. 72nd Street
Omaha, NE 68122
Phone: (402) 572-3300
Fax: (402) 572-3305

Beth Israel Medical Center
Phillips Ambulatory Care Center
4th Floor, 10 Union Square East
New York, NY 10003
Phone: (212) 844-6300
Fax: (212) 844-6999

Beth Israel Medical Center
The Wellbridge Center
135 Wells Avenue
Newton, MA 02159
Phone: (617) 667-1333
Fax: (617) 244-6316

Broward General Medical Center
Wellness Center
1625 SE Third Avenue
Fort Lauderdale, FL 33316
Phone: (954) 355-4888
Fax: (954) 355-4347

Mercy Hospital Medical Center
Iowa Heart Center
411 Laurel Street, Suite 1250
Des Moines, IA 50314
Phone: (515) 247-3145
Fax: (515) 288-0840

Mt. Diablo Medical Center
Heart Health Center
2720 Grant Street, Suite 2
Concord, CA 94520
Phone: (510) 674-2200
Fax: (510) 674-2201

Richland Memorial Hospital
Cardiac Ancillary Services
Five Richland Medical Park
Columbia, SC 29203
Phone: (803) 434-3852
Fax: (803) 434-2713

Shiley Sports and Health Center
10820 North Torrey Pines Road
La Jolla, CA 92037
Phone: (619) 554-9282
Fax: (619) 554-4065

fruits, vegetables, and lean meats and substitutes and a limited amount of fats. The program also establishes an exercise program, provides behaviorial strategies, and promotes a lifetime commitment to well-being.

In conjunction with the Cooper Clinic, the Cooper Wellness Program offers 1-day workshops on fitness, stress management, and preventive nutrition and residential retreats of 4, 7, or 13 days.

No studies have been published that document the effectiveness of the comprehensive program. However, Blair, Kohl, Barlow, Paffenbarger, Gibbons, and Macera (27) demonstrated that initially unfit male attendees who increased their physical activity enough to become classified as fit had a 44% reduction in mortality risk. Blair, Kohl, and Barlow (28) also reported that physical fitness in women is inversely associated with all-cause mortality.

The advantages of this program include its focus on physical fitness and the provision of an intensive initial medical evaluation followed by a customized lifestyle prescription for disease prevention. In addition, Kenneth Cooper has published many books (29-37) that allow individuals to follow the program on their own.

Duke Center for Living

The Duke Center for Living (formerly called DUPAC), which is associated with the Sarah W. Stedman Center for Nutritional Studies at Duke University Medical Center in Durham, North Carolina, provides both group and individual educational programs—ranging from outpatient care and classes to residential retreats—for the prevention and treatment of coronary artery disease.

Healing the Heart, the center's secondary prevention and treatment program (for clients with coronary artery disease), is a comprehensive medical and lifestyle management program that is designed to decrease cardiovascular disease indexes. The program begins with a 2-week retreat. Clients receive an initial medical evaluation by a Duke University cardiologist. Skill-development interventions focus on improving diet, managing stress, exercising, learning heart-healthy shopping and cooking techniques, and learning how to dine out healthfully. The diet provides 15% to 20% energy from fat and emphasizes an increase in fruit and vegetable consumption.

The program includes a follow-up component in which clients meet regularly with a personal counselor and ongoing support groups that are designed to optimize long-term compliance. The center offers several other outpatient programs to reduce CVD risk, including a CVD prevention and weight-management program and a comprehensive adult diabetes program. A 2-week diabetes-management retreat is also offered. All programs cater to individual needs and preferences and offer follow-up. No studies have been published on the program's efficacy. However, the program contains components similar to those present in other programs that have documented clinical efficacy.

Intelligent Quisine

This comprehensive meal program developed by the Campbell's Center for Nutrition and Wellness℠ is targeted to individuals with hypertension, dyslipidemia, and diabetes. Its novel approach to nutrient composition and method of implementation provides a unique approach to

CVD risk reduction. The program offers by mail order a diverse line of prepared food products (frozen, canned, and boxed) that meet or exceed 100% of the US RDAs for all essential nutrients while maintaining a nutrient profile that is low in total (22% energy) and saturated fat, cholesterol, sodium, and refined sugar and high in folic acid, calcium, potassium, magnesium, and fiber.

Clients receive an individualized isocaloric diet prescription (based, in part, on the Harris-Benedict equation), that is appropriate for their height, weight, age, sex, and level of physical activity. If the client's body mass index (BMI) is greater than 25, the diet prescription allows for a weekly weight loss of 1 to 2 lb. Each diet prescription includes an Intelligent Quisine breakfast, lunch, and dinner and a prescribed number of snacks, depending on the client's energy needs. Clients are expected to provide one serving each day of a fruit, vegetable, and low-fat dairy product. Additionally, clients are allowed to select from a variety of "free" foods.

The program also includes compliance and support materials for physical activity, stress management, and behavior modification. The results of multicenter clinical trials showed that clients with CVD risk factors who followed the Intelligent Quisine meal plan for 10 weeks could significantly improve their blood pressure, plasma lipids, BMI, glucose metabolism indexes, quality of life, and dietary compliance compared with a control group consuming a self-selected diet (9,11,38).

The primary benefits of this program are the optimal nutrient composition of the food and the preprepared meals, which eliminate the inconvenience of cooking and shopping and which come with instructions on portion control. The cost of participating in the program is approximately $10 per day.

RECOMMENDATIONS FOR PRACTICE

The risk-factor modification programs reviewed here are recommended for primary and secondary prevention of CVD. These programs significantly modify CVD risk factors and affect functional measures of atherosclerotic disease (2-14). However, the efficacy of the more restrictive programs has not been established in healthy individuals. For these individuals the stricter programs may be unnecessarily restrictive.

For individuals with established coronary or other atherosclerotic disease, monitoring progress may help to maintain client motivation. High-risk clients should be monitored at regular intervals by their health care providers and also encouraged to monitor their own progress. Many risk factors can be evaluated at home or through health promotion services offered in the community.

For most individuals the lifestyle modifications taught in these programs are intended to be long term. The benefits of these programs often include improving a client's CVD risk profile while eliminating or reducing the need for medication. When a client's risk profile is improved without drug intervention, the client saves money, avoids drug-related side effects, and may experience improved quality of life and other benefits.

SUMMARY AND CONCLUSIONS

Risk factor management programs are available to assist clients with reducing—in some cases eliminating—their modifiable CVD risk factors. Common features of the programs reviewed here include a low-fat diet and a comprehensive approach to risk reduction. Weight loss is not the primary therapeutic intervention, but achievement and maintenance of a healthy body weight is encouraged along with a low-fat diet, regular physical activity, and stress management.

Most of the reviewed programs offer publications that provide self-guided instruction, and some have multiple treatment sites. Cost of the programs is highly variable, with self-guided instruction being the least expensive. Highly motivated clients may be successful with self-guided instruction, but better results are often obtained through group interaction, which provides a higher level of social support. Unfortunately, the cost of group programs is prohibitive to many clients who seek CVD prevention and treatment. Dietitians should be aware of local risk-reduction programs with similar components that may be more affordable and equally beneficial.

REFERENCES

1. National Cholesterol Education Program. Second report of the Expert Panel on Detection, Evaluation, and Treatment of High Blood Cholesterol in Adults (Adult Treatment Panel II). *Circulation.* 1994;89:1333-1445.
2. Barnard RJ, Jung T, Inkeles SB. Diet and exercise in the treatment of NIDDM: the need for early emphasis. *Diabetes Care.* 1994;17:1469-1472.
3. Beard CM, Barnard RJ, Robbins DC, Ordovas JM, Schaefer EJ. Effects of diet and exercise on qualitative and quantitative measures of LDL and its susceptibility to oxidation. *Arterioscler Thromb Vasc Biol.* 1996;16:201-207.
4. Czernin J, Barnard J, Sun KT, Krivokapich J, Nitzsche E, Dorsey D, Phelps ME, Schelbert HR. Effect of short-term cardiovascular conditioning and low-fat diet on myocardial blood flow and flow reserve. *Circulation.* 1995;92;197-204.
5. Ornish D, Brown SE, Scherwitz LW, Billings JH, Armstrong W, Ports TA, McLanahan SM, Kirkeeide RL, Brand RJ, Gould KL. Can lifestyle changes reverse coronary heart disease? The Lifestyle Heart Trial. *Lancet.* 1990;336:129-133.
6. Barnard RJ, Guzy PM, Rosenberg JM, O'Brien LT. Effects of an intensive exercise and nutrition program on patients with coronary artery disease: five-year follow-up. *J Cardiac Rehab.* 1983;3:183-190.
7. Beard CM, Barnard RJ, Robbins DC, Ordovas JM, Schaefer EJ. Effects of diet and exercise on qualitative and quantitative measures of LDL and its susceptibility to oxidation. *Arterioscler Thromb Vasc Biol.* 1996;16:201-207.
8. Barnard RJ. Effects of life-style modification on serum lipids. *Arch Intern Med.* 1991;151:1389-1394.
9. McCarron DA, Oparil S, Chait A, Haynes RB, Kris-Etherton

P, Stern JS, Resnick LM, Clark S, Morris CD, Hatton DC, Metz JA, McMahon M, Holcomb S, Snyder GW, Pi-Sunyer FX. Nutritional management of cardiovascular risk factors: a randomized clinical trial. *Arch Intern Med.* 1997;157:169-177.
10. Scherwitz L, Ornish D. The impact of major lifestyle changes on coronary stenosis, CHD risk factors, and psychological status: results from the San Francisco Lifestyle Heart Trial. *Homeostasis.* 1994;35:190-204.
11. Hatton DC, Haynes RB, Oparil S, Kris-Etherton P, Pi-Sunyer FX, Resnick LM, Stern JS, Clark S, McMahon M, Morris C, Metz J, Ward A, Holcomb S, McCarron DA. Improved quality of life in patients with generalized cardiovascular metabolic disease on a prepared diet. *Am J Clin Nutr.* 1996; 64:935-943.
12. Gould KL, Ornish D, Kirkeeide R, Brown S, Stuart Y, Buchi M, Billings J, Armstrong W, Ports T, Scherwitz L. Improved stenosis geometry by quantitative coronary arteriography after vigorous risk factor modification. *Am J Cardiol.* 1992;69:845-853.
13. Gould LK, Ornish D, Scherwitz L, Brown S, Edens RP, Hess MJ, Mullani N, Bolomey L, Dobbs F, Armstrong WT, Merritt T, Ports T, Sparler S, Billings J. Changes in myocardial perfusion abnormalities by positron emission tomography after long-term, intense risk factor modification. *JAMA.* 1995;274;894-901.
14. Watts GF, Jackson P, Mandalia S, Brunt JNH, Lewis ES, Coltart DJ, Lewis B. Nutrient intake and progression of coronary artery disease. *Am J Cardiol.* 1994; 73:328-332.
15. Connor SL, Connor WE. *The New American Diet.* New York, NY: Simon and Schuster; 1986.
16. Connor SL, and Connor WE. *The New American Diet System.* New York, NY: Simon and Schuster; 1991.
17. Pritikin R. *The New Pritikin Program. The Easy and Delicious Way to Shed Fat, Lower Your Cholesterol, and Stay Fit.* New York, NY: Simon and Schuster; 1990.
18. Pritikin N. *The Pritikin Promise: 28 Days to a Longer Healthier Life.* New York, NY: Simon and Schuster; 1983.
19. Pritikin N. *The Pritikin Program for Diet and Exercise.* New York, NY: Grosset and Dunlap; 1979.
20. Pritikin N. *The Pritikin Permanent Weight-loss Manual.* New York, NY: Grosset and Dunlap; 1981.
21. Pritikin N. *Diet for Runners.* New York, NY: Simon and Schuster; 1985.
22. Fisher MC, Lachance PA. Nutrition evaluation of published weight-reducing diets. *J Am Diet Assoc.* 1985;85:450-54.
23. Ornish D. *Eat More, Weigh Less: Dr. Dean Ornish's Life Choice Program for Losing Weight Safely While Eating Abundantly.* New York, NY: HarperCollins Publishers; 1993.
24. Ornish D. *Dr. Dean Ornish's Program for Reversing Heart Disease: The Only System Scientifically Proven to Reverse Heart Disease Without Drugs or Surgery.* New York, NY: Random House; 1990.
25. Ornish D. *Stress, Diet, and Your Heart.* New York: Holt, Rinehart & Winston; 1982.
26. Ornish D. *Everyday Cooking with Dr. Dean Ornish: 150 Easy, Low-fat, High-flavor Recipes.* New York, NY: HarperCollins Publishers; 1996.
27. Blair SN, Kohl HW, Barlow CE, Paffenbarger RS, Gibbons LW, Macera CA. Changes in physical fitness and all-cause mortality. A prospective study of healthy and unhealthy men. *JAMA.* 1995;273:1093-1098.
28. Blair SN, Kohl HW, Barlow CE. Physical activity, physical fitness, and all-cause mortality in women: do women need to be active? *J Am Col Nutr.* 1993;12:368-371.
29. Cooper KH. *Preventing Osteoporosis: Dr. Kenneth H. Cooper's Preventive Medicine Program.* New York, NY: Bantam Books; 1989.
30. Cooper KH. *The Aerobics Program for Total Well-Being: Exercise, Diet, Emotional Balance.* New York, NY: M Evans; 1982.
31. Cooper KH. *Controlling Cholesterol: Dr. Kenneth H. Cooper's Preventive Medicine Program.* New York, NY: Bantam Books; 1988.
32. Cooper KH. *Overcoming Hypertension: Dr. Kenneth H. Cooper's Preventive Medicine Program.* New York, NY: Bantam Books; 1990.
33. Cooper KH. *Kid Fitness: a Complete Shape-up Program from Birth Through High School.* New York, NY: Bantam Books; 1991.
34. Cooper KH. *Dr. Kenneth H. Cooper's Antioxidant Revolution.* Nashville, Tenn: T. Nelson Publishers; 1994.
35. Cooper KH. *Running Without Fear: How to Reduce the Risk of Heart Attack and Sudden Death During Aerobic Exercise.* New York, NY: M. Evans; 1995.
36. Cooper KH. *It's Better to Believe.* Nashville, Tenn: Thomas Nelson; 1995.
37. Gordon NF. *The Cooper Clinic Cardiac Rehabilitation Program: Featuring the Unique Heart Points Recovery System.* New York, NY: Simon and Schuster; 1990.
38. Metz JA, Kris-Etherton PM, Morris CD, Mustad VA, Stern JS, Oparil S, Chait A, Haynes RB, Resnick LM, Clark S, Hatton DC, McMahon M, Holcomb S, Snyder GW, Pi-Sunyer FX, McCarron DA. Prepared meal plan improves dietary compliance and cardiovascular risk factors. *Am J Clin Nutr.* 1997; 66:373-385.

APPENDIXES

APPENDIX 1

DIETARY ASSESSMENT RESOURCES

SHARON SUGERMAN, MS, RD, FADA; AND BRENDA EISSENSTAT, MS, RD

This appendix provides listings of data collection and analysis tools as well as assessment tools for special populations. Included are addresses, telephone and fax numbers, e-mail addresses, and World Wide Web sites.

TOOLS FOR DATA COLLECTION AND ANALYSIS

This section contains additional information on computer-related publications, data-collection tools for dietary assessment, computer software for dietary analysis, and sources for external data analysis. A few software products cited in the text are not available for public purchase and therefore are not included in this appendix. Additional information about these products can be obtained from the author cited in the relevant publication. Before any software is purchased, it is advisable to check directly with the manufacturer for demo disks, current pricing, and computer specifications (size, memory, graphics capability, printers needed, and ability to run under Microsoft Windows or Microsoft Windows 95 or on a networked system) because changes are frequent. Software packages usually come with manuals, on-line help screens, or both. Software programs may also have read-me files that contain similar information and can be printed out. Public domain (government) information, software, or shareware instruments can often be downloaded through the Internet or obtained free or at low cost (less than $25). Several companies (indicated in product descriptions) will process food records, recalls, or food frequency questionnaires (FFQs) for a fee.

Byting In

The Grossbauer Group
PO Box 2001
Chesterton, IN 46304-2001
(219) 926-2883 (phone); (219) 929-1502 (fax)
http://www.grossbauer-group.com (World Wide Web)

A bimonthly newsletter for food and nutrition professionals (yearly subscription: $65). Topics include nutritional analysis tools, counseling aids, food service management packages, brief software reviews, and information on World Wide Web sites of interest. Byting In's biannual review, Software Buyer's Guide, is also available.

Cancer Research Center of Hawaii Diet Questionnaire

Cancer Research Center of Hawaii
Cancer Etiology Program
Epidemiology Section
1236 Lauhala Street
Honolulu, HA 96813
(808) 586-2985 (phone); (808) 586-2982 (fax)

An extensive (16-page) questionnaire used in the Hawaii-Los Angeles Multiethnic Cohort Study, this quantitative FFQ includes many Asian and Hispanic items, as well as standard American foods. Serving size is both described and for some items photographically illustrated in three portion sizes. Current price for printing and analysis of one questionnaire is $10. The diet questionnaire plus additional demographic and cancer risk factor questions are available in both English and Spanish as the Hawaii Cancer Research Survey.

Carotenoids

See USDA-NCI Carotenoid Food Composition Data Base.

CBORD Diet Analyzer and CBORD Professional Diet Analyzer

The CBORD Group, Inc
61 Brown Road
Ithaca, NY 14850
Client Services Department: (607) 257-3991 (phone); (607) 257-1902 (fax)

The CBORD Master Nutrient Database is designed for use with the Professional Diet Analyzer. It contains more than 19,000 foods, approximately 200 national brands, and up to 97 nutrients and includes recalls, recipes, a quantified FFQ, menu planning, and recipe analysis with a retention-factor option. A low-cost subset of the database, containing approximately 2,800 food items and 30 nutrients, can be used with Diet Analyzer (includes recalls and recipes).

The CBORD Group's major software efforts are in health care food service administration, but its nutrient analysis component is available as a stand-alone option. The best feature of this component is an on-screen nutrient spreadsheet that can be viewed while the user enters data. CBORD provides excellent technical support. Additional foods can be added to the database and for a fee CBORD will assist in adding larger numbers of items from other databases.

Computrition Nutritional Analysis

Computrition, Inc
PO Box 4689
Chatsworth, CA 91313-4689
Marketing: Marty Adrick (800) 200-4459

The program includes a database of approximately 20,000 food items and 24 nutrients and has many hospital food and nutrition service applications. Additional foods can be added and a variety of options are available. The basic nutrient analysis program for diets, menus, and recipes is approximately $300 and includes toll-free telephone support.

Dine Healthy and Pyramid Challenge

DINE Systems, Inc
586 North French Road
Amherst, NY 14228
(800) 688-1848 (phone); (716) 688-2505 (fax)

Dine Healthy (approximately $199) includes a database of nearly 10,000 foods and 26 nutrients; analyzes food records and recalls, recipes, physical exercise and activity, and percent body fat; and calculates a DINE "healthy eating" score (a consumer-friendly summary report with valuable messages about the importance of each nutrient). For additional information see *Byting In*, August 31, 1996 (review), or Dennison D, Dennison K, and Frank G. The DINE System: improving food choices of the public. *J Nutr Educ*. 1994;94:87-92.

Pyramid Challenge is an interactive MS-DOS or CD-ROM program that is an effective screening and assessment tool for school-age children, low-literacy populations, or community groups.

Food Intake Analysis System (FIAS)

Human Nutrition Center
University of Texas Health Science Center at Houston
School of Public Health
Box 20186
Houston, TX 77225
(713) 792-4533

This system contains a database with approximately 7,300 foods and 30 nutrients and can analyze food records, recalls, and recipes. The recipe feature clearly documents ingredients assumed for mixed dishes and can be customized, including calculation of retention factor values (eg, for flour, grains, moisture loss, fat, cooking method, and more). An excellent feature is a standardized default quantity assumption for when a respondent cannot describe serving size.

The Food Processor Plus and Genesis R&D

ESHA Research
PO Box 13028
Salem, OR 97309
(800) 659-3742
http://www.esha.com (World Wide Web)

The Food Processor Plus (approximately $549) analyzes food recalls, records, and recipes. Its database includes more than 16,000 foods and 114 nutrients and dietary constituents. The analysis can be formatted to display any subset of desired nutrients. The system is user-friendly and includes an excellent demo disk and tutorial; additionally, the manufacturer provides good customer service. Foods can be entered as raw or cooked, trimmed or untrimmed; conversion calculations are made automatically. Report features include diabetic exchanges, Food Guide Pyramid servings, and the ability to export information to word processors and spreadsheets. Transferring data from a laptop computer to a hard drive can be complicated, however, because data are saved as a related series of files. Reports can be incomplete for some nutrients and exchanges because for some items ESHA uses imputed data to enhance information provided by manufacturers and chain restaurants. For additional information see *Byting In*, October 31, 1995 (review).

Genesis R&D ($2,500) is a more powerful program that can produce Nutrition Facts labels and make adjustments for dairy and meat fat factors and includes many commercial ingredient items in its database. Its user-friendly interface is similar to Food Processor Plus.

Food Models, 3-D Lifelike Representations

NASCO
901 Janesville Avenue
Fort Atkinson, WI 53538-0901
(800) 558-9595

See also Nutrition Consulting Enterprises, Nutrient Data System, and Professional Nutrition Systems for two-dimensional and abstract geometric three-dimensional models.

Food and Nutrition Information Center (FNIC) Software and Multimedia Programs Database

Food and Nutrition Information Center
USDA National Agricultural Library

10301 Baltimore Boulevard, Room 304
Beltsville, MD 20705-2351
(301) 504-5719 (phone); (301) 504-6409 (fax)
fnic@nalusda.gov (e-mail)

The FNIC provides a descriptive listing of nutrition software for diet analysis and nutrition education. The information is available electronically on the US Department of Agriculture (USDA) World Wide Web site (http://www.nal.usda.gov/fnic). Custom database searches and printed reports for selected topics (available quarterly) can be obtained at no charge.

Harvard Semiquantitative Food Frequency Questionnaire

Laura Sampson, MS, RD
Harvard School of Public Health Nutrition Department
665 Huntington Avenue
Boston, MA 02115
(617) 432-2435
nhlas@gauss.bwh.harvard.edu (e-mail)

More commonly known as the Willett FFQ, this questionnaire is available as a PC analysis program in DOS that is used either with scanned data or on-line. Investigators can also purchase blank forms for $0.25 per copy and request analysis at $9 or $11 per FFQ, depending on the type of form selected. For $30, data will be returned on disk. Many validation and calibration studies have been done with this questionnaire; versions have been used with diverse populations and with children. See Thompson FE, Byer T. Dietary assessment resource manual. *J Nutr*. 1994;124S: 2296S-2298S.

HHHQ-DIETSYS Analysis Software Package and User's Guide: Health Habits and History Questionnaire

For scientific information:
Block Dietary Data System
2634 Laconte Ave.
Berkeley, CA 94709
(510) 704-8514 (phone or fax)
For computer software assistance:
DIETSYS Update
Information Management Services, Inc
12501 Prosperity Drive, Suite 200
Silver Spring, MD 20904
dietsys@nih.gov (e-mail)

Also known as the Block FFQ, this dietary analysis system was developed by the National Cancer Institute, Information Management Services, Inc, Bethesda, MD, and Block Dietary Data Systems. To receive information about obtaining current or new versions at no charge, contact http://www.Nutritionquest.com or write to Information Management Services. To receive software and documentation contact the NCI DIETSYS home page, http://www.seerims.nci.nih.gov/ScientificSystem/DIETSYS. To subscribe to the electronic mailing list for the exchange of ideas, send an e-mail message saying "subscribe diet-epi [your full e-mail address] [your real name]" to majordomo@sph.berkeley.edu.

The Block FFQ includes a 98-item food list with two portion size options and specifics for sex and age. A briefer version containing 60 items is also available. The database has room for 207 food items and was recently updated to simplify modifications for use in special populations or with specific foods and nutrients of interest. It is vital to read Chapter 10 of the *User's Manual*, "Developing Your Own Questionnaire," and to enter at least one practice questionnaire before field testing a final instrument. The FFQ can be used alone or with additional cancer or chronic disease health risk questions. Data entry is easy. For a fee, DIETSYS will analyze food records for you. The HFFQ, a Hispanic version based on 24-hour recall foods eaten by Hispanic HANES participants (Mexican, Puerto Rican, and Cuban) was developed recently. Contact Block Dietary Data Systems for ordering information.

See also Nutrition DISCovery CD-ROM Program.

Interactive Design and Development

Mary Guy Miller, President
1700 Kraft Drive, Suite 1000
Virginia Tech Corporate Research Center
Blacksburg, VA 24060
(540) 231-2627 (phone); (540) 231-2628 (fax)
mmiller@vt.edu (e-mail)

Interactive Design and Development is a producer of innovative interactive computer programs for assessment of dietary data.

See also Nutrition DISCovery CD-ROM Program.

Journal of Food Composition and Analysis

The *Journal of Food Composition and Analysis*, Kent K Stewart, editor, is an official publication of the United Nations University International Network of Food Data Systems.

Nutrition Consulting Enterprises (NCE) Food Portion Visual

Nutrition Consulting Enterprises
PO Box 1255, Route 30 Station
Framingham, MA 01701
(508) 875-6220

The NCE *Food Portion Visual* is a validated, fold-out pictorial representation of two-dimensional geometric shapes that can be used to describe food portion sizes. NCE also offers related such as training of recall interviewers and data coders; consultation on research design, methods, and nutrient databases; and nutrient analysis of recalls.

NutriBase Professional Nutrition Manager and NutriBase Personal Nutrition Manager, 1996

CyberSoft, Inc
3851 East Thunderhill Place

Phoenix, AZ 85044
800-959-4849 (phone), 602-759-4079 (fax)

NutriBase Professional Nutrition Manager (approximately $130) is an excellent value and a cost-effective interface for the USDA Nutrient Data Base for Standard Reference foods. Its database includes 95 nutrients and 45,000 food items and has an extensive listing of restaurant and brand name items (70 restaurants, approximately 3,000 items). Nutrients for some items, especially the brand name and restaurant items, however, are incomplete. The program analyzes food records, recalls, and recipes and accommodates 200 clients. Additional features include on-line documentation of nutrient sources for each item; the ability to build a separate, personally selected frequent food minidatabase to speed data entry; a glossary of food and cooking terms; and text appropriate for enhancing client reports.

NutriBase Personal Nutrition Manager (approximately $70) is a consumer version with 10 nutrients (similar to Nutrition Facts nutrients) and a limit of 5 consumers. The program is especially useful for clients who frequently eat at chain restaurants. The database has been well checked for integrity but is relatively new and has not been cited in the literature. Reviewed in *Byting In*, August 31, 1996.

Nutrient Data System (NDS)

The Nutrition Coordinating Center (NCC)
University of Minnesota, Division of Epidemiology
1300 South Second Street, Suite 300
Minneapolis, MN 55454-1015
(612) 626-9450 (phone); (612) 626-9444 (fax)
webmaster@keystone.ncc.umn.edu (e-mail)
http://www.ncc.umn.edu (World Wide Web)

NDS analyzes food recalls, records, and recipes. Several versions are available: NDS 93 (93 nutrients, approximately $8,000 initial copy), NDS 32 (32 nutrients, approximately $2,550), Counseling NDS (approximately $595, same nutrients as NDS 32 but cannot produce summary files for export of data for statistical analysis), and Data Collection NDS (for which you collect the data and the NCC analyzes it at a cost per record or recall). A new Windows-based version, Research Version 4.0, was targeted for release in fall 1997. Key features of Research NDS 4.0 include the ability to customize data collection, add additional foods, and sort foods by food groups for export analysis. A modified version of NDS was used for NHANES III.

NDS has sequential, hierarchical screen data entry (first choose food item, such as broccoli; then type kind [fresh or frozen]; then cooking method; and then fat or salt added). The database is complete with few missing values and includes range checks for portion sizes that are questionably high. NDS is a good choice for multisite studies when standardized data collection and default assumptions are needed and when fatty acid or sodium content is a variable of interest. Additional foods currently cannot be added to the database, but NCC will assist in determining how to code "missing" foods, which are often foods new to the marketplace. NCC will also assist in customizing the database for a fee. The current database includes many Hispanic foods taken from the Nationwide Food Consumption Survey, release 7, 1991. Nutrients of special interest include beta carotene, fatty acids, many sugars, three types of fiber, olestra, and phytic acid. It is anticipated that carotenoids will be added in the fall 1997 release; *trans* fatty acids are scheduled to be added to the spring 1998 release or as soon as the data become available.

NCC also provides interviewer training and certification and sells two- and three-dimensional abstract food models, record-keeping data forms, and booklets. For additional information see Sievert YA, Schakel SF, Buzzard IM. Maintenance of a nutrient database for clinical trials. *Control Clin Trials*. 1989;10:416-25.

Nutrient Databank Directory

Nutrient Databank Directory, 9th edition (approximately $17), University of Delaware, Newark, Jack L Smith, editor, 1993

Order from: University of Delaware
Department of Nutrition and Dietetics, Alison Hall
Newark, DE 19715-3360

Nutrition DISCovery CD-ROM Program

Mead Johnson and Company, Mead Johnson Nutritionals
PO Box 14676
Baltimore, MD 21298-9057

Nutrition DISCovery (approximately $6.95) is a CD-ROM version created in 1995 of the diet interview portion of the Block FFQ including chronic disease–related health risk factors and physical activity. The Read-me file contains a thorough reference list of data sources and other FFQ methodologic issues. This cutting-edge tool has interesting potential. For further information see Sumner NE, Keller B, Diamond L. Nutrition DISCovery™ Personalized CD-ROM Diet Assessment Program. *J Nutr Educ*. 1996;28:47C.

See also Interactive Design and Development.

Nutritionist IV Diet Analysis

First Databank, Inc
1111 Bayhill Drive
San Bruno, CA 94066
(800) 633-3453 (phone); (415) 588-5454 (phone); (415) 588-4003 (fax)
info@firstdatabank.com (e-mail)
http://www.firstdatabank.com (World Wide Web)

Nutritionist IV analyzes food records and recalls, recipes, food product formulations, and energy expenditure from activity. Its database contains more than 15,500 foods and 74 nutrients (including US, Canadian, and Malaysian databases). It is one of the best choices for analyzing Asian foods. Special features include a helpful quick search with a "display more" option; a data entry screen that shows food item, amount, portion, and your choice of four nutrients with subtotals for meals; and an on-screen preview of nutrient values that change concurrently with serving amount changes. Many customized queries and reports are possible. Program weaknesses have been noted during attempts to remedy omissions such as adding meals or reassigning days.

PicSort

Kristin Tomey
University of Illinois at Chicago
Department of Human Nutrition and Dietetics
1919 West Taylor Street, Room 650 (M/C 517)
Chicago, IL 60612
(312) 355-0340 (phone); (312) 413-0319 (fax)

An interesting pictorial FFQ based on the National Cancer Institute questionnaire, PicSort consists of 99 laminated cards with a full-color illustration on one side and a serving size sketch on the other. Also included is a set of general instructions, sample data recording formats, and a printed list of the 99 foods. Cost is $55 per set. Particularly appropriate for less literate respondents. This FFQ was most recently cited in Kumanyika SK, Tell GS, Shemanski L, Martel J, Chinchilli VM. Dietary assessment using a picture-sort approach. *Am J Clin Nutr*. 1997;65(suppl):1123S-1129S.

Portion Photos of Popular Foods

The American Dietetic Association
216 W. Jackson Boulevard
Chicago, IL 60606-6995
(800) 877-1600 ext 5000 (phone); (312) 899-4899 (fax)

Portion Photos of Popular Foods, edited by Mary Abbott Hess, contains actual-size, full-color photos of more than 100 of the most frequently consumed foods in the US in 3 portion sizes. Nutrition Facts label, USDA Pyramid, and diabetic exchange portions are coded for the educator's ease in nutrition assessment and counseling sessions. Cost is $129.95 for ADA members, $150 for nonmembers.

Professional Nutrition Systems, Inc

Westwood Plaza Tower
1900 West 47th Place, Suite 110
Westwood, KS 66205
(913) 432-3329 (phone); (913) 432-3395 (fax)

Professional Nutrition Systems offers data collection instruments and provides related services such as training recall interviewers, consulting on research design and methodology, and performing nutrient analysis of recalls. A video entitled *Keeping Your Food Diary* (running time: 14:45) is available for purchase to educators to use with students, patients, or study participants (cost of less than $20; Hoffman-LaRoche). Other products available are a diet diary and realistic pictorial two-dimensional food models of common serving sizes of muffins, meats, measuring utensils, pizza, dessert foods, and circles that come in a format that fits, folded, into a business-sized envelope. Professional Nutrition Systems has done extensive work with clinical lipid-lowering trials.

Quick Check for Diet Progress, Quick Check for Fat and Cholesterol (English and Spanish versions), Quick Check for Fat

Nutrition Scientific
1510 Oxley Street, Suite F
South Pasadena, CA 91030
(818) 441-0021 (phone); (213) 962-5582 (fax)
To purchase, contact Neal DeWitt, Marketing Director.
For scientific questions, contact Robert Selzer, President.

Nutrition Scientific provides analysis of 26- to 46-item limited-nutrient semiquantitative FFQs most appropriate for health screening ($100 to $135 for 100 tests). The tools provide pictorial food portions to simplify measuring and improve accuracy for individuals not accustomed to using measuring tools. Nutrition Scientific provides personalized service and for a fee will customize your database. Programs are bar-coded and data can be entered with a low-cost scanning pen or can be quickly entered into a computer. A major drawback is that foods or nutrients cannot be added to the database.

Also available is the 3-Day Cholesterol Control Reporter, a quantitative standardized food record incorporating the same bar-code scanning and pictorial portion sizes as the Quick Check programs. The 26-page, food record workbooks are $6 each; analysis software is $595 (free with an order of 100 books or more) or Nutrition Scientific will analyze the records ($25 per record). Also available in Spanish.

trans Fatty Acids

See USDA Special Purpose Table #1.

USDA-NCI (National Cancer Institute) Carotenoid Food Composition Data Base

Michele Forman
National Cancer Institute
Bethesda, MD 20892
(301) 496-8559

The USDA-NCI Carotenoid Food Composition Data Base, version 1, 1993, is a free, public-domain ASCII file database with documentation. It contains alpha and beta carotene, lutein, cryptoxanthin, and lycopene values for all fruits and vegetables and many mixed dishes. The database can be imported as a spreadsheet with some editing.

USDA Nutrient Data Base for Standard Reference and USDA Special Purpose Table #1

Nutrient Data Laboratory
Agricultural Research Service, USDA
4700 River Road, Unit #89

Riverdale, MD 20737

(301) 734-8491 (phone); (301) 734-5643 (fax)

For electronic access: Nutrient Data Laboratory Bulletin Board (301) 734-5078

http://www.nal.usda.gov/fnic/foodcomp (World Wide Web)

ndlinfo@rbhnrc.usda.gov (e-mail)

The USDA Nutrient Data Base for Standard Reference, release 11, is a public domain, on-line version of *Agricultural Handbook* No. 8. It can be downloaded at no cost from http://www.nal.usda.gov/fnic/foodcomp. For a fee, diskettes can be ordered from the National Technical Information Service, Springfield, VA 22161; (703) 487-4650. Data sets are available on 3½" and 5½" diskettes in ASCII or DBF relational file formats. The database includes more than 5,600 food items, 22 food categories, and 70 food components. Costs vary with specific version needed (update, all nutrients, or abbreviated), but are approximately $200 to $300. A coding manual comes with the database and update files are available with each new release.

USDA's Special Purpose Table #1 is a public domain database containing information on *trans* fatty acids and related lipid constituents.

Westat

1650 Research Boulevard

Rockville, MD 20850

(301) 251-1500

Dee Schofield, Marketing Director

Westat is a major provider of research and technical assistance to social service and nutrition surveys, including NHANES, the Continuing Survey of Food Intake by Individuals, and the NCI Polyp Prevention Trial (nutrition data) and Prostate, Lung, Colorectal and Ovarian Cancer Screening Trial (overall coordination). Services available include data collection, coordination and analysis for general or nutrition data only, quality control, and training of survey staff.

World Food

Office of Technology Licensing

2150 Shattuck Avenue, Suite 510

University of California, Berkeley, CA 94707-1315

(510) 643-7201 (phone); (510) 642-4566 (fax)

World Food (approximately $300 to investigators from developed countries; less than $75 to those from developing nations) is helpful as an ancillary database for Latin American, African, Middle Eastern, and Southeast Asian foods. Nutrients are based on major ingredient components and similarities between foods rather than exact values. For scientific issues contact Suzanne P Murphy, PhD, RD, (510) 642-5572 (phone), (510) 642-0535 (fax). For additional information see *Byting In*, February 29, 1996.

DIETARY ASSESSMENT FOR SPECIAL POPULATIONS

Multicultural General or Multiracial, Including Regional US Food Practices

1. American Dietetic Association, American Diabetes Association. *Ethnic and Regional Food Practices: A Series.* Chicago, Ill: American Dietetic Association, American Diabetes Association; 1989-present. [Individual 23- to 36-page books on food practices, customs, and holidays; order through the American Dietetic Association Catalog of Products and Services, ADA Customer Service Publications Department, (800) 877-1600, extension 5000 (phone); (312) 899-4899 (fax). Existing titles in the series include the following:
   Cajun-Creole, 40 pp, 1996
   Indian-Pakistani, 32 pp, 1996
   Soul and Traditional Southern, 29 pp, 1995
   Filipino American, 38 pp, 1994
   Alaska Native, 24 pp, 1993
   Hmong American, 24 pp, 1992
   Navajo, 26 pp, 1992
   Chinese American, 36 pp, 1989
   Jewish, 23 pp, 1989
   Mexican American, 26 pp, 1989
2. Borrud LG, Pillow PC, Allen PK, McPherson RS, Nichaman MZ, Newell GR. Food group contributions to nutrient intake in whites, blacks, and Mexican Americans in Texas. *J Am Diet Assoc.* 1989;89:1061-1069.
3. Bronner Y. Cultural sensitivity and nutrition counseling. *Top Clin Nutr*. 1994;9:20-27.
4. Buzzard IM, Willett WC, eds. Dietary Assessment Methods: Proceedings of the First International Conference on Dietary Assessment Methods: Assessing Diets to Improve World Health. *Am J Clin Nutr*. 1994;59(suppl):143S-306S.
5. Kittler PG, Sucher K. *Food and Culture in America*. 2nd ed. St. Paul, Minn: West/Wadsworth; 1997.
6. McDowell MA, Briefel RR, Alaimo K, Bischof AM, Caughman CR, Carroll MD, Loria CM, Johnson CL. *Energy and Macronutrient Intakes of Persons Ages 2 Months and Over in the United States: Third National Health and Nutrition Examination Survey, Phase 1, 1988-91. Advance Data From Vital and Health Statistics.* No. 255. Hyattsville, Md: National Center for Health Statistics; 1994. (Includes description of methodology for NHANES III.)
7. Serdula M, Coates, R, Byers T, Mokdad A, Jewell S, Chavez N, Mares-Perlman J, Newcomb P, Ritenbaugh C, Treiber F, Block G. Evaluation of a brief telephone questionnaire to estimate fruit and vegetable consumption in diverse study populations. *Epidemiology*. 1993;4:455-463.
8. Stern J, Stern M. *Real American Food*. New York, NY: Alfred A Knopf; 1986. (ISBN 0-394-53953-2.)
9. Von Welanetz D, Von Welanetz P. *The Von Welanetz Guide to Ethnic Ingredients*. New York, NY: Warner Books; 1982. (ISBN 0-446-38420-8; soft-cover.)
10. Willett WC, Sampson L. Dietary Assessment Methods: Proceedings of the Second International Conference on Dietary Assessment Methods. *Am J Clin Nutr.* 1997;65(suppl):1097S-1368S.
11. Coates RJ, Monteith CP. Assessments of food-frequency questionnaires in minority populations. *Am J Clin Nutr*. 1997;65 (suppl);1108S-1115S.

12. Consider attending the conference Well-Controlled Studies of Diet and Lipid Metabolism in Humans, held annually at the Pennington Biomedical Research Center, 6400 Perkins Road, Baton Rouge, LA 70808-4124; contact Marlene Windhauser, PhD, RD (windhamm@mhs.pbrc.edu).

Low Literacy, Regardless of Ethnicity

1. Kumanyika S, Tell GS, Fried L, Martel J, Chinchilli VM. Picture-sort method for administering a food frequency questionnaire to older adults. *J Am Diet Assoc.* 1996;96:137-144.
2. Kumanyika SK, Tell GS, Shemanski L, Martel J, Chinchilli VM. Dietary assessment using a picture-sort approach. *Am J Clin Nutr.* 1996;65(suppl):1123S-1129S.
3. Doak CC, Doak LG, Root JH. Testing patient comprehension (chapter 3) and Testing readability of written materials (chapter 4). In: Doak CC, Doak LG, Root JH. *Teaching Patients with Low Literacy Skills.* Philadelphia, Pa: JB Lippincott Company; 1985.

African American and Traditional Southern Food Practices

1. American Dietetic Association, American Diabetes Association. *Ethnic and Regional Food Practices: Soul and Traditional Southern.* Chicago, Ill: American Dietetic Association, American Diabetes Association. (See reference 1 in the Multicultural section for publication year and number of pages.)
2. Ammerman AS, Haines PS, DeVellis RF, Strogatz DS, Keyserling TC, Simpson RJ, Siscovik DJ. A brief dietary assessment to guide cholesterol reduction in low-income individuals: design and validation. *J Am Diet Assoc.* 1991;91: 1385-1390. (For Southern US, low-income populations, includes Dietary Risk Assessment Instrument.)
3. Armstrong JE, Larson B. Dietary practices and concerns of adult urban black men of high socioeconomic status. *J Am Diet Assoc.* 1990;90:1716-1717.
4. Bronner Y, Burke C, Joubert BJ. African-American/soul foodways and nutrition counseling. *Top Clin Nutr.* 1994;9:20-27.
5. Campbell MK, Polhamus B, McClelland JW, Bennett K, Kalsbeek WK, Coole D, Jackson B, Demark-Wahnefried W. Assessing fruit and vegetable consumption in a 5-a-Day study targeting rural blacks: the issue of portion size. *J Am Diet Assoc.* 1996;96:1040-1041.
6. Coates RJ, Eley JW, Block G, Gunter EW, Sowell AL, Grossman C, Greenberg RS. An evaluation of a food frequency questionnaire for assessing dietary intake of specific carotenoids and vitamin E among low-income black women. *Am J Epidemiol.* 1991;134:658-671.
7. Croft JB, Temple SP, Lankenau B, Heath GW, Macera CA, Eaker ED, Wheeler FC. Community intervention and trends in dietary fat consumption among black and white adults. *J Am Diet Assoc.* 1994;94:1284-1290.
8. Liu K, Slattery M, Jacobs D Jr. Is dietary recall the method of choice in black populations? *Ethn Dis.* 1994;4:12-14.

Asian and Asian American

1. American Dietetic Association, American Diabetes Association. *Ethnic and Regional Food Practices: Chinese American, Hmong American, Indian-Pakistani, Filipino American.* Chicago, Ill: American Dietetic Association, American Diabetes Association. (See reference 1 in the Multicultural section for publication years and numbers of pages.)
2. Chinese Food Composition Tables. Published as a special issue of *J Food Comp Anal.* 1990;3.
3. Dignan CA, et al. *The Pacific Island Food Composition Tables.* Palmerston North, New Zealand: SPC, INFOODS, and Crop & Food Research; 1994. [To purchase contact Ruth Broie (brodier@crop.cri.nz), Crop & Food Research, Private Bag 11030, Palmerston North, New Zealand; 64-6-356-8300 (phone), 64-6-351-7050 (fax). Cost is US $35.00.]
4. Food and Agriculture Organization of the United Nations, US Department of Agriculture. *Food Composition Tables for the Near East.* Rome, Italy: FAO; 1982.
5. Gopalan C, Rama Sastri BV, Balasubramanian SC. *Nutritive Value of Indian Foods.* Hyderabad, India: National Institute of Nutrition, Indian Council of Medical Research; 1984;204 pp. (In English.)
6. Hankin JH, Wilkens LR, Kolonel LN, Yoshizawa CN. Validation of a quantitative diet history method in Hawaii. *Am J Epidemiol.* 1991;133:616-628. [Men and women, Japanese, Caucasian, Chinese, Filipino, and Hawaiian.]
7. Kollipara UK, Brittin HC. Increased iron content of some Indian foods due to cookware. *J Am Diet Assoc.* 1996;96:508-509.
8. Pan WH, Wang JL, Chang SC, Chen ML. Cooking oil absorption by foods during Chinese stir-frying: implications for estimating dietary fat intake. *J Am Diet Assoc.* 1993;93: 1442-1444.
9. Sridaran G, Kolhatkar RR. Ethnic food practices of Asian Indians. *Top Clin Nutr.* 1994;9:45-48.
10. Wu-Jung CJ. Understanding food habits of Chinese Americans. *Top Clin Nutr.* 1994;9:20-27.

Children

1. *Journal of School Health*, entire May 1991 issue, volume 61, is devoted to assessment of diet and physical activity in children.
2. Young Children's Diet Assessment Questionnaire (see figure showing questionnaire on p. 2303S in Thompson FE, Byer T. Dietary assessment resource manual. *J Nutr.* 1994;124S: 2296S-2298S), Dennison et al, Mary Imogene Bassett Hospital Research Institute.
3. Baranowski T, Dworkin R, Henske JC, Clearman DR, Dunn JK, Nader PR, Hooks PC. The accuracy of children's self-reports of diet: Family Health Project. *J Am Diet Assoc.* 1986;86:1381-1385.
4. Byers T, Trieber F, Gunter E, Coates R, Sowell A, Leonard S, Mokdad A, Jewell S, Miller D, Serdula M, Chavez N, Maref-Perlman J, Newcomb P, Ritenbaugh C, Triber F, Block G. The accuracy of parental reports of their children's intake of fruits and vegetables: validation of a food frequency questionnaire with serum levels of carotenoids and vitamins C, A and E. *Epidemiology.* 1993;4:350-355.
5. Domel SB, Thompson WO, Baranowski T, Smith AF. How children remember what they have eaten. *J Am Diet Assoc.* 1994;94:1267-1272.
6. Eck LH, Klesges RC, Hanson CL. Recall of a child's intake from one meal: are parents accurate? *J Am Diet Assoc.* 1989;89:784-789.
7. Hammond J, Nelson M, Chinn S, Rona RJ. Validation of a food frequency questionnaire for assessing dietary intake in a

study of coronary heart disease risk factors in children. *Eur J Clin Nutr*. 1993;47:242-250.

8. Hertzler AA, Bowens J, Hull S. Preschoolers' reporting of food habits. *J Am Diet Assoc*. 1993;93:1159-1161.
9. Mack KA, Blair J, Presser HB. Measuring and improving data quality in children's report of dietary intake. In: Warnecke RB, ed. *Health Survey Research Methods Conference Proceedings*. Hyattsville, Md: US Department of Health and Human Services; 1996. PHS 96-1013.
10. Rockett HRH, Wolf AM, Colditz GA. Development and reproducibility of a food frequency questionnaire to assess diets of older children and adolescents. *J Am Diet Assoc*. 1995;95:336-340.
11. Treiber FA, Leonard SB, Frank G, Musante L, Davis H, Strong WB, Levy M. Dietary assessment instruments for preschool children: reliability of parental responses to the 24-hour recall and a food frequency questionnaire. *J Am Diet Assoc*. 1990;90:814-820.
12. Van Horn L, Stumbo P, Moag-Stahlberg A, Obarzanek E, Hartmuller G, Farris R, Kimm YS, Frederick M, Snetselaar L, Liu K. The Dietary Intervention Study in Children (DISC): dietary assessment methods for 8-10 year olds. *J Am Diet Assoc*. 1993;93:1396-1403.

European and European American Immigrants

Note for dietary assessment: metric measures are typically used and food described in terms of gram weight, not volume. This is also common in African, Asian, and Hispanic populations.

1. Souci SW, Fachmann W, Kraut H. *Food Composition and Nutrition Tables 1989/90*. Deutsche Forschungsanstalt fur Lebensmittelchemie, Garching b. Munchen, 4th ed. Stuttgart, Germany: Wissenschaftliche Verlagsgesellschaft mbH; 1989. (Table in English, German, and French.)

Hispanic and Hispanic American

1. American Dietetic Association, American Diabetes Association. *Ethnic and Regional Food Practices: Mexican American*. Chicago, Ill: American Dietetic Association, American Diabetes Association. (See reference 1 in the Multicultural section for publication year and number of pages.)
2. Abrams B, Guendelman S. Nutrient intake of Mexican-American and non-Hispanic white women by reproductive status: Results of two national studies. *J Am Diet Assoc*. 1995;95:926-918. (Mexican participants in the Hispanic Health and Nutrition Examination Survey [HHANES], 24-hour recall.)
3. Ballew C, Sugerman SB. High-risk nutrient intakes among low-income Mexican women in Chicago, Illinois. *J Am Diet Assoc*. 1995;95:1409-1413. (Chicago population, 24-hour recall.)
4. Block G, Norris JC, Mandel RM, DiSogra C. Sources of energy and six nutrients in diets of low-income Hispanic-American women and their children: quantitative data from HHANES, 1982-1984. *J Am Diet Assoc*. 1995;95:195-208. (HHANES women aged 17 to 34 years and their children aged 1 to 5 years; 24-hour recall.)
5. Chavez N, Sha L, Persky V, Langenberg P, Pestano-Binghay E. Effect of length of US residence on food group intake in Mexican and Puerto Rican women. *J Nutr Educ*. 1994;26:79-86. (Chicago population, FFQs.)
6. Frank GC, Zive M, Nelson J, Broyles SL, Nader PR. Fat and cholesterol avoidance among Mexican-American and Anglo preschool children and parents. *J Am Diet Assoc*. 1991;91:954-958.
7. Knapp JA, Hazuda HP, Haffner SM, Young EA, Stern MP. A saturated fat/cholesterol avoidance scale: sex and ethnic differences in a biethnic population. *J Am Diet Assoc*. 1988;88:172-177. (San Antonio, Texas; mixed income population; brief instrument.)
8. Kuczmarski MF, Kuczmarski RJ, Najjar M. Food usage among Mexican-American, Cuban and Puerto Rican adults: findings from Hispanic HANES. *Nutr Today*. 1995;30:30-37. (All HHANES participants, FFQ and 24-hour recall.)
9. Loria CM, McDowell MA, Johnson CL, Woteki CE. Nutrient data for Mexican-American foods: are current data adequate? *J Am Diet Assoc*. 1991;91:919.
10. Lyons GK, Woodruff SI, Candelaria JI, Rupp JW, Elder JP. Development of a protocol to assess dietary intake among Hispanics who have low literacy skills in English. *J Am Diet Assoc*. 1996;96:1276-1279. (California, 24-hour recall; use of NDS software.)
11. McDowell M, Loria CM. Cultural considerations in analyzing dietary data from the Hispanic Health and Nutrition Examination Survey. Proceedings of the 14th National Nutrient Databank Conference, Ithaca, NY. Cebord Group. 1990. 43-46.
12. Murphy SP, Castillo RO, Martorell R, Mendoza FS. An evaluation of food group intakes by Mexican-American children. *J Am Diet Assoc*. 1990;90:338-393. (HHANES children and teens, FFQ.)
13. National Center for Health Statistics. *Plan and Operation of the Hispanic Health and Nutrition Examination Survey, 1982-84*. Washington, DC: US Government Printing Office, Vital and Health Statistics. DHHS publication (PHS) 85-1321. (Includes public domain bilingual FFQ.)
14. Rodriguez JC. Diet, nutrition and the Hispanic client. *Top Clin Nutr*. 1994;9:28-39.
15. Romero-Gwynn E, Gwynn D, Grivetti L, McDonald R, Stanford G, Turner B, West E, Williamson E. Dietary acculturation among Latinos of Mexican descent. *Nutr Today*. 1993;28:6-12. (Low-income women of Mexican heritage living in California, nonquantitative FFQ.)
16. Shalhoub J, Murray C. *Clinical Spanish for Dietitians*. Redondo Beach, Calif: Plycon Press; 1977.
17. Zive MM, Taras HL, Broyles SL, Frank-Spohrer G, Nader PR. Vitamin and mineral intakes of Anglo-American and Mexican-American preschoolers. *J Am Diet Assoc*. 1995;95:329-335. (Study of Children's Activity and Nutrition; San Diego area low- to middle-income preschool children. Two 24-hour modified recalls, including direct observation of lunch and dinner plus interview with parent for breakfast and snacks.)
18. Food frequency, modified from NCI HHHQ: Tufts Elderly Health and Nutrition Study. Contact Katherine Tucker, PhD, Epidemiology Program, USDA Human Nutrition Research Center on Aging at Tufts University, 711 Washington Street, Boston, MA 02111, (617) 556-3351, tucker@hnrc.tufts.edu. Questionnaire (118-item) includes fat-modified foods and foods of importance to Puerto Rican elderly.
19. Food frequency, not modeled on NCI instrument: Southwestern United States (copyright protected by

University of Arizona Questionnaires). Contact Douglas L Taren, PhD, Associate Professor; University of Arizona Health Sciences Center; Department of Family and Community Medicine, Tucson, AZ 85724 (602) 626-7863, nutrisec@arizvax.ccit.arizona.edu. Bilingual Spanish questionnaire with English translation.

20. Food Intake and Growth of Hispanic Children in Hartford. A comprehensive questionnaire that includes: recall, FFQ, food habits, and the Radimer/Cornell Hunger Scale (developed by researchers at the Nutrition Science Dept. at Cornell University and translated into Spanish by Dr. Perez-Escamilla). The questionnaire was developed by the University of Connecticut Family Nutrition Program and the Hispanic Health Council. The target Hispanic population is mostly Puerto Rican low-income parents responding for children; Separate English and Spanish versions. Contact: Dr. David Hinnelgreen, Hispanic Health, 175 Main St, Hartford, CN 06106. (860) 527-0856 or Rafael Perez-Escamilla Dept of Nutr Sci., Univ of Connecticut, Stores, CN 06269. (860) 486-5073.
21. See also Cancer Research Center of Hawaii Diet Questionnaire and Nutrition Scientific (listed under Quick Check for Diet Progress) and HHHQ-DIETSYS in the Tools for Data Collection and Analysis section.

Native American

1. American Dietetic Association, American Diabetic Association. *Ethnic and Regional Food Practices: Alaska Native and Navajo.* Chicago, Ill: American Dietetic Association, American Diabetes Association. (See reference 1 in the Multicultural section for publication years and numbers of pages.)
2. Aspenland A, Pelican S. Traditional food practices of contemporary Taos Pueblo. *Nutr Today.* 1992;27:6-12.
3. Shelley G. Seminole Indian food traditions. In: Lieberman LS, Bobroff LB, eds. *Cultural Food Patterns of Florida: A Handbook.* Gainesville, Fla: Florida Cooperative Extension Service, University of Florida; 1990.
4. Smith CJ, Schakel SF, Nelson RG. Selected traditional and contemporary foods currently used by the Pima Indians. *J Am Diet Assoc.* 1991;91:338-341.
5. Wolfe WS, Weber CW, Arviso KD. Use and nutrient composition of traditional Navajo foods. *Ecol Food Nutr.* 1985;17:323-344.

Older Adults

1. Kumanyika S, Tell GS, Shemanski L, Polak J, Savage PJ. Eating patterns of community-dwelling older adults: the cardiovascular health study. *Ann Epidemiol.* 1994;4:404-415.
2. Murphy SP, Everett DF, Dresser CM. Food group consumption reported by the elderly during the NHANES I epidemiologic follow-up study. *J Nutr Educ.* 1989;21:214-220.
3. Patterson RE, Kristal AR, Coates RJ, Tylavsky FA, Ritenbaugh C, VanHorn L, Caggiula AW, Snetselaar L. Low-fat diet practices of older women: prevalence and implications for dietary assessment. *J Am Diet Assoc.* 1996;96:670-679.
4. Garry PJ, Chumlea WC, eds. Epidemiologic and Methodologic Problems in Determining Nutritional Status of Older Persons: Conference Proceedings. Am *J Clin Nutr.* 1989;50(suppl):1121S-1234S. (Supplement includes four articles pertaining to dietary assessment.)
5. Hankin JH, Yoshizawa CN, Kolonel LN. Reproducibility of a diet history in older men in Hawaii. *Nutr Cancer.* 1990;13:129-140.

APPENDIX 2

Examples of Modified Foods Available in US Grocery Stores

BRENDA EISSENSTAT, MS, RD

Food Item	Modification (if any)	kcal	Fat (g)	Saturated fat (g)	% kcal (fat)	Na+ (mg)	Cholesterol (mg)
Meat							
Bologna, beef 1 oz	Regular	90	8	4	80	300	15
	Light 50% <fat	60	4.5	1.5	68	310	15
	Fat free	20	0	0	0	280	5
Hot dogs, beef 1 hot dog ~ 56 g	Regular	180	16	7	83	670	35
	Light	110	8	2	65	710	10
	Low fat	60	1.5	0.5	25	430	20
	Fat free	50	0	0	0	470	15
Bacon, 2 slices ~25 g	Regular	80	7	3	75	340	15
	25% less fat	60	4.5	1	67	260	15
	Low sodium	100	8	1.5	70	220	10
Ground turkey, cooked ~ 4 oz	Regular	280	23	7	35	95	95
	Lean	190	10	3	47	75	75
	75% less fat	170	9	3	47	65	110
	99% fat free	110	1	0	9	40	50
Chicken							
Breast Tenders, breaded 85-90 g	Regular	240	15	3.5	58	480	30
	Fat free	130	0	0	0	480	30
Breast 2 oz	with skin	170	10	3	53	230	65
	without skin	110	1	0	9	350	55
Dairy or Refrigerated Foods							
Eggs	1 large	70	4	1.5	50	55	215
Egg substitute ¼ cup	Cholesterol free	30	0	0	0	100	0
Butter 1 Tbsp	Regular	100	11	8	100	85	30
	Light	50	6	4	100	70	20
Margarine 1 Tbsp	Regular	90	10	1.5	100	65	0
	Light	45	4	1	78	70	0
	70% less fat	30	3.5	0	100	55	0
	Fat free	5	0	0	0	90	0
Cheese 1 oz	Regular	70	5	3.5	64	290	15
	⅓ less fat	50	3	2	60	330	10
	Fat free	30	0	0	0	290	<5

Food Item	Modification (if any)	kcal	Fat (g)	Saturated fat (g)	% kcal (fat)	Na+ (mg)	Cholesterol (mg)
Cookie dough ~ 32 g	Regular	140	6	2.5	43	110	10
1 or 2 cookies	50% less fat	110	3	1.5	23	85	<5
Refrigerator biscuits	Regular	200	9	3	42	550	0
1 biscuit ~ 61 g	Reduced fat	190	7	2	38	620	0
Pudding ½ cup	Regular	170	6	1.5	9	160	0
	Fat free	100	0	0	0	240	0
Cream cheese 2 Tbsp	Regular	100	10	6	90	90	30
	⅓ less fat	70	6	4	86	120	20
	Fat free	25	0	0	0	135	<5
Sour cream 2 Tbsp	Regular	60	5	3.5	83	30	15
	Light	35	2	1.5	43	30	10
	Fat free	30	0	0	0	25	<5
Yogurt 8 oz	Low fat	240	3	1.5	10	135	15
	Light or fat free	100	0	0	0	120	5
Cottage cheese ½ cup	Regular	120	5	3	37	470	25
	Low fat	90	2.5	1.5	22	380	15
	Fat free	80	0	0	0	430	5
Nondairy creamer 1 Tbsp	Regular	20	1.5	0	2	5	0
	Fat free	10	0	0	0	0	0
Milk 8 oz	3.25% fat (whole)	150	8	5	47	120	35
	2% fat (reduced-fat)	120	4.5	3	33	120	20
	1% fat (low-fat)	100	2.5	1.5	20	130	10
	Skim (nonfat)	90	0	0	0	125	5
Whipped topping 2 Tbsp	Regular	20	2	1	75	0	<5
	Fat free	5	0	0	0	0	0
Frozen Foods							
TV dinners ~270 g	Meat loaf and potatoes	390	24	8	55	910	80
	Low fat	250	7	2	25	570	45
Pizza, pepperoni	Regular	450	28	10	56	890	40
⅓ pizza ~148 g	Low fat	390	12	4	34	650	45
Fruit pie, apple	Regular	270	11	2	37	300	0
⅙ pie ~ 123 g	Reduced fat, no sugar	210	8	1.5	33	290	0
Ice cream ½ cup	Regular	160	8	6	45	30	30
	Light, no sugar	90	4	2.5	39	35	20
	Fat free	110	0	0	0	50	0
Frozen yogurt ½ cup	Regular	170	6	2	32	100	5
	Low fat	130	2.5	1.5	17	50	10
	Fat free	110	0	0	0	80	<5
Cool Whip 2 Tbsp	Regular	25	1.5	1.5	60	0	0
	Light	20	1	1	50	0	0
	Fat free	15	0	0	0	0	0
Waffles or pancakes	Regular	200	7	0	30	580	15
2 waffles ~ 72 g	Low fat	160	1	.5	6	540	0
Snacks							
Potato chips 1 oz	Regular	160	10	3	56	180	0
	Low fat, baked	140	6.7	1	43	130	0
	Lightly salted	150	10	3	60	85	0
	Fat free, baked	110	0	0	0	190	0
Peanuts 1 oz	Regular	160	14	2.5	75	110	0
	Unsalted	160	14	2	75	0	0

Food Item	Modification (if any)	kcal	Fat (g)	Saturated fat (g)	% kcal (fat)	Na+ (mg)	Cholesterol (mg)
Snacks (cont'd)							
Popcorn, microwave	Buttered	170	13	2.5	69	390	0
1 pkg ~5.5 cup popped	Low fat	90	2	0	22	280	0
	Salt free	170	12	2.5	63	0	0
	94% fat free	120	5	0	37	380	0
Chocolate 37 g	Regular	200	12	7	55	30	10
18 g	33% less fat	80	3.5	2	38	40	5
20 g	45% less fat	80	2.5	1.5	31	30	0
43 g	Sugar free	230	17	11	70	60	5
Beverages							
Hot chocolate 28 g	Regular mix	110	1.5	0	9	150	0
	No sugar added	50	0	0	0	160	0
	Fat or sugar free	25	0	0	0	135	0
Evaporated milk ½ c	Regular	130	3	1	23	40	10
	Low fat	120	1.5	0	12	40	5
	Fat free	110	0	0	0	40	<5
Iced tea 1 cup	Regular	100	0	0	0	10	0
	Diet	0	0	0	0	25	0
Cola 8 fl oz	Regular	100	0	0	0	25	0
	Diet	0	0	0	0	25	0
Crackers							
Soda crackers (5)	Regular	60	2	0	33	180	0
	50% less salt	60	2	0	33	35	0
	Fat free	60	0	0	0	180	0
	Whole wheat	60	1.5	0	17	130	0
Seasoning							
Salt ¼ tsp	Table salt	0	0	0	0	590	0
	33% <sodium	0	0	0	0	390	0
	Salt free	0	0	0	0	0	0
Desserts							
Cookies (1)	Chocolate chip	80	4.5	1.5	50	60	0
	Reduced fat	70	3	1	43	70	0
Muffins, blueberry		170	5	1	29	220	20
1 muffin ~ ¼ cup mix	Fat free	120	0	0	0	190	0
Cake, prepared from mix	White	230	9	2.5	35	290	0
1/12 pkg (43 g)	Reduced fat	220	6	1.5	25	290	0
Icing 2 Tbsp	Regular	140	5	1.5	32	20	0
	Reduced fat	130	2.5	1	15	30	0
Brownie, prepared from	Regular	190	2	0	42	110	0
mix 1/20 pkg	Reduced fat	170	0	0	0	400	0
Gelatin desserts ½ c	Regular	90	0	0	0	10	0
	Light	60	0	0	0	10	0
	Sugar free	0	0	0	0	10	0
Vegetable Oil or Shortening							
Vegetable oil 1 T	Regular	120	14	1.5	100	0	0
Light olive oil 1 T	Regular	120	14	2	100	0	0
Shortening 1 T	Solid	110	12	3	100	0	0
Light Bake 1 T	Fat free	35	0	0	0	5	0
Spray oils		0	0	0	0	0	0
Bread and Cereals							
Dry cereal, granola ½ cup	Low fat	220	3	1	13	150	0
	Fat free	110	0	0	0	240	0
Danish pastry, (1)	Regular	220	11	3	45	170	20

Food Item	Modification (if any)	kcal	Fat (g)	Saturated fat (g)	% kcal (fat)	Na+ (mg)	Cholesterol (mg)
Bread and Cereals (cont'd)							
Danish	Fat free	130	0	0	0	130	0
Wheat bread	Regular	120	1.5	0	12	230	0
2 slices	Light	80	1	0	6	210	0
Toaster pastries (1)	Regular	200	5	1.5	25	180	0
	Low-fat	190	3	0.5	13	160	0
Granola bar (1)	Regular	100	3	0	27	85	0
	Low-fat	110	2	0	13	80	0
Soup							
Cream of chicken	Regular	120	8	2.5	60	860	15
½ cup condensed	98% fat-free, 33% less sodium	80	2.5	1	28	480	15
Chicken vegetable, ½ cup condensed	Regular	80	2	0.5	22	940	10
1 cup (ready to serve)	98% fat-free	100	1.5	0	14	660	0
Rice-noodle mix, ½ cup	Regular	240	1	4	0	980	0
	⅓ less salt	240	1	4	0	640	0
Miscellaneous							
Croutons (6)	Regular	35	1.5	0	33	90	0
	Fat free	30	0	0	0	80	0
Salad dressing,	Regular	170	18	3	95	280	0
Ranch 2 Tbsp	⅓ less fat	100	11	2	99	310	10
	Fat free	50	0	0	0	350	0
Mayonnaise 1 Tbsp	Regular	100	11	2	100	75	5
	Light	50	5	1	90	90	5
	Fat free	10	0	0	0	130	0
Ketchup 1 Tbsp	Regular	15	0	0	0	190	0
	⅓ less sugar	10	0	0	0	100	0
Gravy ¼ cup	Regular	45	4	0	78	270	5
	Fat free	10	0	0	0	300	0
Peanut butter 2 Tbsp	Regular	190	16	3	76	130	0
	Low sodium	200	18	2.5	81	10	0
	25% less fat	190	12	2.5	58	250	0
	30% less fat	180	11	2	55	150	0
Jelly 1 Tbsp	Regular	50	0	0	0	0	0
	Low sugar	25	0	0	0	0	0
	Light	10	0	0	0	0	0
Syrup ¼ cup	Regular	200	0	0	0	135	0
	Light	100	0	0	0	160	0
	Sugar free	35	0	0	0	135	0
Canned Vegetables							
Baked beans ½ cup	with pork	170	3	1	15	490	5
	Vegetarian	140	.5	0	0	480	0
Green peas ½ cup	Regular	60	0	0	0	390	0
	½ sodium	60	0	0	0	195	0
	No salt added	60	0	0	0	10	0
Whole tomatoes ½ cup	Regular	25	0	0	0	220	0
	No salt added	25	0	0	0	0	0
Spaghetti sauce ½ cup	Regular	80	3	1	31	480	0
	Low-fat	50	1	0	20	390	0
	Fat-free	50	0	0	0	390	0

APPENDIX 3

Resources About Nutrition and Cardiovascular Disease and Low-Fat Eating

NATALIE UPDEGROVE PARTRIDGE, MS, RD; AND LYNNE M DEMOOR, MS, RD

The purpose of this appendix is to help health professionals locate resources consistent with current recommendations for nutrition for the prevention and treatment of cardiovascular disease. Also included are materials for consumers.

Price information is not listed because of the many variables that affect price, such as tax for certain states, shipping and handling charges, discounts for multiple copies, and discounts for certain organizations. Please contact each organization for price information before ordering. There is a charge for most items listed.

You can find many of the books listed at local bookstores and libraries. For most books, the publisher's address and phone number are provided. For those books without an address and phone number, contact your local library or bookstore for assistance. Some publishers do not sell directly to consumers; others, including some for which we have provided an address and phone number, prefer that you go to your bookstore or library first.

Because of the number of materials available about nutrition and cardiovascular disease and low-fat eating, this is not a comprehensive list and should be used as a starting point for locating materials. Health care professionals should review all materials to be sure they are consistent with the guidelines and philosophy of their institution's program or organization.

The materials are divided into several sections. Organizations to Contact for More Information includes information about organizations that either provide information about heart disease or assist the public with obtaining information about a variety of nutrition topics, including heart disease and low-fat eating. Materials for Consumers includes lists of brochures and handouts, books, newsletters and magazines, audiovisuals, and curriculum guides and other teaching materials suitable for use by or with consumers. Materials for Children and Adolescents includes descriptions of materials for children, parents, and professionals. Materials for Health Professionals includes listings of books, reports, and manuals; audiovisuals; meetings and conferences, and journals and newsletters.

Organizations to Contact for More Information

American Association of Cardiovascular and Pulmonary Rehabilitation (AACVPR)

7611 Elmwood Avenue, Suite 201
Middleton, WI 53562
(608) 831-6989 (phone); (608)831-5122 (fax)
aacvpr@tmahq.com (e-mail)

The AACVPR is a professional multidisciplinary organization that provides education for health care professionals. Publications include *Journal of Cardiopulmonary Rehabilitation* (bimonthly), *News and Views of AACVPR* (quarterly newsletter), *Guidelines for Cardiac Rehabilitation Programs, Guidelines for Pulmonary Rehabilitation Programs, Outcomes Resource Manual,* Cardiac and Pulmonary Rehabilitation Weeks Media Kits, and the following position papers: "Cardiac Rehabilitation Services: A Scientific Evaluation," "Efficacy of Risk Factor Intervention and Psychosocial Aspects of Cardiac Rehabilitation," and "Scientific Basis of Pulmonary Rehabilitation."

The American Dietetic Association's National Center for Nutrition and Dietetics (NCND)

216 West Jackson Boulevard
Chicago, IL 60606-6995
(800) 366-1655 (Consumer Nutrition Hot Line)
(312) 899-0040, ext 4653 (general information)
(312) 899-0040, ext 4774 (library services)
(800) 877-1600, ext 4853 (for ADA members)
(312) 899-1739 (fax)
http://www.eatright.org (World Wide Web)

The NCND is the public education center for The American Dietetic Association. NCND promotes optimal nutrition, health, and well-being for the public through a variety of programs and services including a consumer nutrition hot line, written nutrition materials (in English and Spanish), and national public awareness campaigns: Project LEAN (Low-fat Eating for America Now) and the Eat Right America Campaign, which are celebrated each March during National Nutrition Month. For the health professional, NCND staffs a resource library and provides educational materials to support client counseling.

American Heart Association (AHA)

National Center
7272 Greenville Avenue
Dallas, TX 75231-4596
(800) AHA-USA-1 or (214) 373-6300
http://www.amhrt.org (World Wide Web)
(888) MY-HEART (Each One Reach One campaign to increase awareness of heart disease and strokes in women)

The American Heart Association is a nonprofit, voluntary health organization supported by private funds. Its mission is to reduce disability and death caused by cardiovascular diseases and stroke. The AHA educates health care professionals about new ways to prevent, diagnose, and treat heart disease and stroke. The AHA provides journals and publications, brochures, scientific statements, videos, and training packages.

Food and Nutrition Information Center (FNIC)

US Department of Agriculture
National Agricultural Library
Room 304, 10301 Baltimore Boulevard
Beltsville, MD 20705-2351
(301) 504-5719 (phone); (301) 504-6409 (fax)
fnic@nalusda.gov (e-mail)
http://www.nal.usda.gov/fnic/ (World Wide Web)

FNIC provides technical assistance to professionals looking for nutrition information. The FNIC staff can help you locate research, resources, and answers to clients' questions about cardiovascular disease and related topics. Resources, such as audiovisuals, can be borrowed from FNIC's collection at the National Agricultural Library through an interlibrary loan. FNIC publishes a peer-reviewed resource list called *Nutrition and Cardiovascular Disease Nutri-Topics.* FNIC publications are available from FNIC's Gopher and World Wide Web sites on the Internet.

International Society on Hypertension in Blacks (ISHIB)

2045 Manchester Street, NE
Atlanta, GA 30324
(404) 875-6263 (phone); (404) 875-6334 (fax)

ISHIB is a nonprofit membership organization devoted to ethnicity and disease. ISHIB was founded to respond to the problem of high blood pressure among blacks and to bridge the black-white disease gap. The organizational scope has been expanded to include renal disease, diabetes, stroke, and lipid disorders. ISHIB's objectives are to stimulate research and clinical investigation, disseminate scientific findings, educate the public about harmful effects and prevention of hypertension and its concomitant diseases, and develop health-related programs that improve the quality of life. ISHIB publishes a quarterly medical journal, *Ethnicity & Disease.*

National Heart, Lung and Blood Institute (NHLBI) Information Center

PO Box 30105
Bethesda, MD 20824-0105
(301) 251-1222 (phone); (301) 251-1223 (fax)
(800) 575-WELL (recorded messages for consumers)
nhlbiic@dgs.dgsys.com (e-mail)
fido.nhlbi.nih.gov (Gopher)
gopher://gopher.nhlbi.nih.gov (World Wide Web)

The NHLBI Information Center provides information about diet and cardiovascular disease, including hypertension, to consumers and professionals. The NHLBI Information Center staff can answer questions about diet and cardiovascular disease and provide information about NHLBI programs. Materials for professionals include *HeartMemo*, a quarterly newsletter; Stay Young at Heart kit for worksite nutrition education; and reports summarizing current recommendations. Materials for consumers include one-page quizzes, materials for clients with low literacy levels, posters, booklets, and fact sheets. The NHLBI Information Center is funded by the National Institutes of Health under the Department of Health and Human Services. The NHLBI coordinates the National Cholesterol Education Program.

Sports, Cardiovascular, and Wellness Nutritionists (SCAN)

Dietetic Practice Group of The American Dietetic Association
7730 East Belleview, G-6
Englewood, CO 80111
(303) 779-1950 (phone); (303) 771-8737 (fax)

SCAN sponsors an annual symposium and regional workshops. Products and services available to SCAN members and nonmembers include SCAN's PULSE (quarterly newsletter), SCAN's *Annual Guide to Books and Organizations, SCAN's Innovative Product Catalogue of Nutrition and Health Education Materials,* and SCAN's Member Locator Service.

Materials for Consumers

Brochures and Handouts

The following organizations produce consumer-level brochures and handouts. Selected titles available at the time of publication of this manual are listed under each organization. Please contact the organization for current prices and to verify availability of titles.

The American Dietetic Association

216 West Jackson Boulevard
Chicago, IL 60606-6995
(800) 877-1600, ext 5000 (phone); (312) 899-4899 (fax)

The New Cholesterol Countdown. Revised 1995. 12 panels. (Spanish title: *Un Plan Excelente Para Reducir El Alto Colesterol)*

Lowfat Living: A Guide to Enjoying a Healthy Diet. 1993. 12 panels.

The Sodium Story. 1991. 12 panels.

National Center for Nutrition and Dietetics Nutrition Fact Sheet series (camera-ready handouts) include the following:

ABC's of Fats, Oils, and Cholesterol. 1995. (also available in Spanish)

Facts About Sodium and Healthy Blood Pressure. 1995.

Triglycerides. 1992.

American Heart Association

See AHA listing on page 286 for address and telephone information.

The American Heart Association Diet: An Eating Plan for Healthy Americans. 1991. 18 pp. 51-1031.

Dining Out: A Guide to Restaurant Dining. 1992. 15 pp. 50-067-A.

Easy Food Tips For Heart-Healthy Living. 1994. 9 pp. 51-1090. (Spanish title: *Consejos prácticos para el Corazón y la alimentación Saludables.* 51-1092.)

Eat Well, But Wisely. Not dated. 4 panels. 51-0002. (Spanish title: *Coma Bien, Pero Con Cuidado.* 51-0003.)

How to Choose a Nutrition Counselor for Cardiovascular Health: A Consumer Guide. Not dated. 12 pp. 50-1034.

How to Have Your Cake and Eat It Too. 1994. 6 panels. 64-9536.

How to Read the New Food Label. Not dated. 8 panels. 51-1052. (Spanish title: *Cómo leer la Nueva Etiqueta De Los Alimentos.* 51-1054.)

Making Mexican Food 'Heart Healthy.' 1992. 8 panels. (Spanish title: *Cómo Hacer Comida Mexicana 'Saludable para el Corazón.'* 64-8075.)

Now You're Cookin': Healthful Recipes to Help Control High Blood Pressure. 1993. 28 pp. 50-1050.

Nutritious Nibbles: A Guide to Healthy Snacking. 1990. 8 pp. 51-054-A.

Recipes for Low-Fat, Low-Cholesterol Meals. 1992. 48 pp. 50-1042.

Save Food Dollars and Your Heart. Not dated. 8 pp. 50-1057.

Savor the Flavors: How to Choose Healthful Meals When Dining Out. 1995. 19 pp. 50-1080.

Step by Step: Eating to Lower Your High Blood Cholesterol. 1994. 99 pp. 64-4001. (also available from the National Heart, Lung and Blood Institute)

Tips for Eating Out. 1995. 6 panels. 50-1073.

American Heart Association San Francisco Division

120 Montgomery Street, Suite 1650
San Francisco, CA 94104
(415) 433-2273 (phone); (415) 362-8035 (fax)

Doctors Answer Your Questions About Blood Pressure. Not dated. 12 pp.

Eat Heart Smart. Not dated. 12 panels. (Chinese)

Eating Heart Smart Filipino Style. Not dated. 12 panels.

Eating Heart Smart Chinese Style. 1991. 12 panels. (English and Chinese)

Eating Heart Smart With Soul. Not dated. 12 panels.

Your Heart and Cholesterol. Not dated. 8 pp. (Chinese)

American Medical Association

Healthy Heart Series
c/o Milner-Fenwick, Inc
2125 Greenspring Drive
Timonium, MD 21093
(800) 432-8433 (phone); (410) 252-6316 (fax)

Guide to Controlling Your Cholesterol. 1994. 16 pp. MB-03.

Guide to Your Healthy Heart. 1994. 16 pp. MB-01.

California Project LEAN

California Department of Health Services
PO Box 942732, MS-675
Sacramento, CA 94234-7320
(916) 322-6851 (phone); (916) 324-7763 (fax)

California Chefs Cook Lean. 1994. 41 pp. (spiral-bound cookbook)

Celebrate Health with a Lowfat Fiesta. Not dated. 8 panels.

Compre, Cocine, & Cene Con Poca Grasa. 1995. 8 panels. (In Spanish and for low-literacy audiences. English title: *Shop, Cook, & Eat Lean.)*

Eat Lean Mexican Cuisine. Not dated. 8 panels.

Shop, Cook, & Dine Lean. 1994. 8 panels.

Shop, Cook, & Eat Lean. 1995. 8 panels. (for low-literacy audiences)

Food and Drug Administration (FDA)

5600 Fishers Lane, Room 15A19, HFI-40*
Rockville, MD 20857
(301) 443-9057 (fax)

A Consumer's Guide to Fats. 1994. 5 pp. FDA 95-2286. (originally appeared in FDA Consumer in May 1994)

The New Food Label: Help in Preventing Heart Disease. 1995. 6 pp. FDA 95-2290. (originally appeared in *FDA Consumer* in December 1994)

The New Food Label: Scouting for Sodium and Other Nutrients Important to Blood Pressure. 1995. 5 pp. FDA 95-2284. (originally appeared in *FDA Consumer* in September 1994)

Food and Nutrition Information Center

See FNIC listing on page 286 for address and telephone information.

Nutrition and Cardiovascular Disease Nutri-Topics. 1995. 5 pp. (resource list for consumers)

---

*Use HFI-40 code behind street address for multiple copies; for single copies use code HFE-88.

Health Promotion Council of Southeastern Pennsylvania, Inc

311 South Juniper Street, Suite 308
Philadelphia, PA 19107-5803
(215) 546-1276 (phone); (215) 545-1395 (fax)
hlphpc@libertynet.org (e-mail)

Mr. Bates Learns About Cholesterol. Not dated. 4 pp. (for low-literacy clients)

Health Trend Publishing

PO Box 17420
Encino, CA 91416
(818) 906-7120

Cholesterol Control. 1994. 32 pp.

International Food Information Council (IFIC)

1100 Connecticut Avenue, NW
Suite 430
Washington, DC 20036
(202) 296-6540

Sorting Out the Facts About Fat. 1995. 8 pp. (IFIC Review)

KRAMES Communications

1100 Grundy Lane
San Bruno, CA 94066-3030
(800) 333-3032 (phone); (415) 244-4512 (fax)

Healthy Cooking. 1995. 6 panels.

Low-Fat Eating. 1995. 6 panels.

You Can Control Your Cholesterol: A Guide to Low-Cholesterol Living. 1993. 16 pp. (also available in Spanish)

National Cancer Institute (NCI)

Office of Cancer Communications
Building 31, Room 10A-24
9000 Rockville Pike
Bethesda, MD 20892
(800) 4-CANCER
In Alaska: (800) 638-6070
In Hawaii: (800) 524-1234

Celebre la Cocina Hispana (Celebrate Hispanic Cooking): *Healthy Hispanic Recipes.* 1995. 44 pp. NIH publication 95-3906(s). (Introduction in Spanish; recipes in both Spanish and English.)

Down Home Healthy Cookin': Recipes and Healthy Cooking Tips. 1995. 16 pp. NIH publication 95-340SSV. (For African-Americans; a longer version of this booklet with four-color photographs is available from the US Government Printing Office. See *Down Home Healthy: Family Recipes of Black American Chefs* on page 289.)

National Heart, Lung and Blood Institute (NHLBI) Information Center

For single copies and information on ordering multiple copies and black-and-white reproducibles, when available, use address and telephone information under NHLBI entry in the organizations section.

Are You at Risk? 1994. 4 pp. Facts About Heart Disease and Women Series. NIH publication 94-3654.

Check Your Cholesterol and Heart Disease I.Q. 1995. 2 pp. NIH publication 95-3794.

Check Your High Blood Pressure Prevention I.Q. 1994. 2 pp. NIH publication 94-3671.

Eat Right to Help Lower Your High Blood Pressure. 1992. 30 pp. NIH publication 92-3289. (for low-literacy clients; 5th-grade reading level)

Eat Right to Lower Your High Blood Cholesterol. Reprinted 1992. 14 pp. NIH publication 92-2972. (for low-literacy clients; 5th-grade reading level)

Facts About Blood Cholesterol. Revised 1994. 28 pp. NIH publication 94-2696.

Facts About How to Prevent High Blood Pressure. 1994. 20 pp. NIH publication 94-3281.

Getting Physical. 1994. 4 pp. Facts About Heart Disease and Women Series. NIH publication 94-3656.

High Blood Pressure & What You Can Do About It. Revised 1994. 31 pp. NIH publication 55-222A.

High Blood Pressure: Treat It for Life. 1994. 30 pp. NIH publication 94-3312.

Preventing and Controlling High Blood Pressure. 1994. 4 pp. Facts About Heart Disease and Women Series. NIH publication 94-3655.

Reducing High Blood Cholesterol. 1994. 4 pp. Facts About Heart Disease and Women Series. NIH publication 94-3658.

So You Have Heart Disease. 1995. 4 pp. Facts About Heart Disease and Women Series. NIH publication 95-2645.

So You Have High Blood Cholesterol. Revised 1993. 34 pp. NIH publication 93-2922.

Step By Step: Eating To Lower Your High Blood Cholesterol. Revised 1994. 100 pp. NIH publication 94-2920.

National Institute on Aging

National Institutes of Health
PO Box 8057
Gaithersburg, MD 20898-8057
(800) 222-2225

Be Sensible About Salt. AGE PAGE. 1991. 2 pp.

University of Connecticut Cooperative Extension System

3624 Horsebarn Road Extension
Storrs, CT 06269-4017
(203) 486-1783 (phone); (203) 486-3674 (fax)

How Much Fat? Developed by the University of Connecticut Cooperative Extension System and the American Cancer Society. 1991. 4 pp. 91-38.

Shopping to Lower Your Fats. Developed by the University of Connecticut Cooperative Extension System and the American Cancer Society. 1992. 3 pp. 91-62.

University of Georgia Cooperative Extension

Extension Editor
Hoke Smith Building, UGA
Athens, GA 30602
(706) 542-8944 (phone); (706) 542-2162 (fax)
cnimmons@uga.cc.uga.edu (e-mail)

Cut Your Fat...For the Health of It. 1990. 2 pp. Circular 761-14. (for low-literacy audiences)

Cut Your Salt...For the Health of It. 1990. 2 pp. Circular 761-17. (for low-literacy audiences)

Less Fat...For the Health of It. 1990. 6 pp. Circular 761-6.

The Vegetarian Resource Group

PO Box 1463
Baltimore, MD 21203
(410) 366-8343

Heart Healthy Eating Tips: The Vegetarian Way. Not dated. 8 panels.

Washington State Apple Commission

PO Box 18
Wenatchee, WA 98807
(509) 663-9600 (phone); (509) 662-5824 (fax)

Healthy Choices for People with High Blood Pressure. 1990. 8 panels.

Washington State Department of Health

Heart Health Program
PO Box 47836
Olympia, WA 98504-7836
(360) 664-8578 (phone); (361) 586-5440 (fax)

Check It Out! Heart Health Client Education Information Sheets. 1995 (Eight 8½" by 11" camera-ready sheets; English on one side; Spanish on the other; available in camera-ready format only. Topics include risk factors, smoking, physical activity, stress, cholesterol, weight control, hypertension, and children with high blood cholesterol.)

Check It Out! Wallet Card. 1991. 4-panel wallet card. Available in camera-ready format only.

Cookbooks

American Heart Association Cookbook. 5th ed. New York, NY: Times Books; 1991. 643 pp. Available from Random House, 400 Hahn Road, Westminster, MD 21157, (800)793-2665.

American Heart Association Low-Salt Cookbook. New York, NY: Times Books; 1990. 349 pp. Available from Random House, 400 Hahn Road, Westminster, MD 21157, (800) 793-2665.

American Heart Association Quick & Easy Cookbook. New York, NY: Times Books; 1994. 274 pp. Available from Random House, 400 Hahn Road, Westminster, MD 21157, (800) 793-2665.

Baggett N, Glick R. *100% Pleasure: From Appetizers to Desserts, the Low-Fat Cookbook for People Who Love to Eat.* Emmaus, Pa: Rodale Press, Inc; 1994. 370 pp. Available from Rodale Books, 33 East Minor Street, Emmaus, PA 18098, (800) 848-4735 or (610) 967-5171.

Bielunski M, Lamb Parenti S, Yeh I. *Skinny Beef.* Chicago, Ill: Surrey Books; 1993. 208 pp. Available from the National Cattleman's Beef Association, Education Department, 444 North Michigan Avenue, Chicago, IL 60611-9909, (800) 368-3138, fax: (312) 670-9440, fax: (800) 368-3136, or Surrey Books, Inc, 230 East Ohio Street, Suite 120, Chicago, IL 60611, (800) 326-4430.

Burt L, Mercer N. *High Fit-Low Fat.* Memphis, Tenn: Favorite Recipes Press; 1993. 160 pp. Available from M-Fit Supermarket Program, 24 Frank Lloyd Wright Drive, Ann Arbor, MI 48106-0363, (313) 998-7645.

Chase L, Rivers J. *Down Home Healthy: Family Recipes of Black American Chefs.* Bethesda, Md: National Cancer Institute, National Institutes of Health; 1993. 44 pp. Available from Superintendent of Documents, US Government Printing Office, Washington, DC 20402, (202) 512-1800, fax: (202) 512-2250.

Clark Grogan B. *The (Almost) No Fat Cookbook: Everyday Vegetarian Recipes.* Summertown, Tenn: Book Publishing Company; 1994. 192 pp. Available from Book Publishing Company, PO Box 99, Summertown, TN 38483, (800) 695-2241.

Cook Healthy Cook Quick. Birmingham, Ala: Oxmoor House; 1994. 240 pp. Available from Oxmoor House, PO Box 1862, Birmingham, AL 35201, (800) 633-4910.

Cooking Light 199x. (annual cookbook) Birmingham, Ala: Oxmoor House. Available from Oxmoor House, PO Box 1862, Birmingham, AL 35201, (800) 633-4910.

Daley R. *In the Kitchen With Rosie.* New York, NY: Alfred A Knopf, Inc; 1994. 129 pp.

Dewitt D, Wilan MJ, Stock MT. *Hot, Spicy, & Meatless: Over 150 Delicious, Fiery, and Healthful Recipes.* Rocklin, Calif: Prima Publishing; 1994. 262 pp. Available from Prima Publishing, PO Box 1260, Rocklin, CA 95677-1260, (800) 632-8676 or 916-632-4400.

Donkersloot M. *The Fast Food Diet: Quick and Healthy Eating at Home and On the Go.* New York, NY: Simon and Schuster; 1991. 269 pp. Available from Simon and Schuster, 200 Old Tappan Road, Old Tappan, NY 07675, (800) 223-2336.

Hachfeld L, Eykyn, B. *Cooking A La Heart.* 2nd ed. Mankato, Minn: Appletree Press; 1992. 455 pp. Available from Appletree Press, Inc, 151 Good Counsel Drive, Suite 125, Mankato, MN 56001-3198, (800) 322-5679.

Harsila J, Hansen E. *Seafood: A Collection of Heart-Healthy Recipes.* Richmond Beach, Wash: National Seafood Educators; 1990. 276 pp. Available from National Seafood Educators, PO Box 60006, Richmond Beach, WA 98160, (800) 348-0010 or in the Seattle area 546-6410.

The Healthy Heart Cookbook. Birmingham, Ala: Oxmoor House; 1992. 256 pp. Available from Oxmoor House, PO Box 1862, Birmingham, AL 35201, (800) 633-4910.

Hinman B. *Burgers 'N Fries 'N Cinnamon Buns: Low-fat, Meatless Versions of Fast Food Favorites.* Summertown, Tenn: The Book Publishing Company; 1993. 76 pp. Available from The Vegetarian Resource Group, PO Box

1463, Baltimore, MD 21203, (410) 366-8343.

Hinman B. *The Meatless Gourmet: Favorite Recipes from Around the World.* Rocklin, Calif: Prima Publishing. 1995. 488 pp. Available from Prima Publishing, PO Box 1260, Rocklin, CA 95677-1260, (800) 632-8676 or (916) 632-4400.

Hinman B, Snider M. *Lean and Luscious and Meatless.* Rocklin, Calif: Prima Publishing; 1992. 463 pp. Available from Prima Publishing, PO Box 1260, Rocklin, CA 95677-1260, (800) 632-8676 or (916) 632-4400.

The Low-Fat Way to Cook. Birmingham, Ala: Oxmoor House; 1993. 256 pp. Available from Oxmoor House, PO Box 1862, Birmingham, AL 35201, (800) 633-4910.

Magida P, Grunes B. *Skinny Chocolate: Over 100 Sinfully Delicious-Yet Low-Fat-Recipes for Cakes, Cookies, Savories and Chocoholic Treats.* Chicago: Surrey Books; 1994. 200 pp. Available from Surrey Books, Inc, 230 East Ohio Street, Suite 120, Chicago, IL 60611, (800) 326-4430.

Moquette-Magee E. *The Fight Fat & Win* Cookbook. Minnetonka, Minn: Chronimed Publishing Co; 1995. 210 pp. Available from Chronimed Publishing Co, 13911 Ridgedale Drive, Suite 250, Minnetonka, MN 55305, (800) 876-6540.

Ponichtera BJ. *Quick and Healthy Volume II: More Help for People Who Say They Don't Have Time to Cook Healthy Meals.* The Dalles, Oreg: ScaleDown; 1995. 263 pp. Available from ScaleDown, 1519 Hermits Way, The Dalles, OR 97058, (503) 296-5859.

Ponichtera BJ. *Quick and Healthy: Recipes and Ideas for People Who Say They Don't Have Time to Cook Healthy Meals.* The Dalles, Oreg: ScaleDown; 1991. 261 pp. Available from ScaleDown, 1519 Hermits Way, The Dalles, OR 97058, (503) 296-5859.

Smith MA. *366 Low-Fat, Brand-Name Recipes in Minutes.* Minneapolis, Minn: Chronimed Publishing Company; 1995. 360 pp. Available from Chronimed Publishing Co, 13911 Ridgedale Drive, Suite 250, Minnetonka, MN 55305, (800) 876-6540.

Smith MJ. *60 Days of Lowfat, Low-Cost Meals in Minutes.* Minnetonka, Minn: Chronimed Publishing Company; 1992. 296 pp. Available from Chronimed Publishing Co, 13911 Ridgedale Drive, Suite 250, Minnetonka, MN 55305, (800) 876-6540.

Wasserman D. *The Lowfat Jewish Vegetarian Cookbook: Healthy Traditions from Around the World.* Baltimore, Md: The Vegetarian Resource Group; 1994. 224 pp. Available from The Vegetarian Resource Group, PO Box 1463, Baltimore, MD 21203, (410) 366-8343.

What's Cooking at the Cooper Clinic: Our Best Recipes for Your Best Health. Dallas, Tex: The Nutrition Department of the Cooper Clinic; 1992. 228 pp. Available from Nutrition Department, Cooper Clinic, 12200 Preston Road, Dallas, TX 75230, (800) 444-5764.

Woodruff S. *Secrets of Fat-Free Cooking.* Garden City Park, NY: Avery Publishing Group; 1995. 184 pp. Available from Avery Publishing Group, 120 Old Broadway, Garden City Park, NY 11040, (800) 548-5757.

Woodruff S. *Secrets of Fat-Free Baking.* Garden City Park, NY: Avery Publishing Group; 1994. 232 pp. Available from Avery Publishing Group, 120 Old Broadway, Garden City Park, NY 11040, (800) 548-5757.

Other Books

The American Dietetic Association staff. *Cut the Fat!: More Than 500 Easy and Enjoyable Ways to Reduce Fat From Every Meal.* New York, NY: HarperCollins. 1996. 211 pp. Available from The American Dietetic Association; *see* page 287.

American Heart Association. *6 Weeks to Get Out the Fat.* New York, NY: Times Books; in press. Available from Random House, 400 Hahn Road, Westminster, MD 21157, (800) 793-2665.

American Heart Association Brand Name Fat & Cholesterol Counter. 2nd ed. New York, NY: Times Books; 1995. 429 pp. Available from Random House, 400 Hahn Road, Westminster, MD 21157, (800) 793-2665.

American Heart Association's Your Heart: An Owner's Manual. New York, NY: Prentice Hall; 1995. 368 pp. Available from Prentice Hall, Box 11071, Des Moines, IA 50336, (800) 947-7700.

Connor S, Connor W. *The New American Diet System.* New York, NY: Simon & Schuster; 1991. 574 pp. Available from Simon & Schuster, 200 Old Tappan Road, Old Tappan, NJ 07675, (800) 223-2336.

DeBakey ME. *The New Living Heart Diet.* New York, NY: Simon & Schuster; 1996. Available from Simon & Schuster, 200 Old Tappan Road, Old Tappan, NJ 07675, (800) 223-2336.

DeBakey M, Gotto A, Scott L. *The Living Heart Guide to Dining Out.* New York, NY: Master Media; 1993. 170 pp. Available from Master Media, 1205 O'Neill Highway, Dunmore, PA 18512, (800) 334-8232.

DeBakey M, Gotto A, Scott L, Foreyt J. *The Living Heart Brand Name Shopper's Guide.* New York, NY: Master Media; 1993. 430 pp. Available from Master Media Limited, 1205 O'Neill Highway, Dunmore, PA 18512, (800) 334-8232.

Franz M. *Fast Food Facts.* 4th ed. Minnetonka, Minn: Chronimed Publishing; 1994. 112 pp. Available from Chronimed Publishing Co, 13911 Ridgedale Drive, Suite 250, Minnetonka, MN 55305, (800) 876-6540.

Goor R, Goor N. *Eater's Choice: A Food Lover's Guide to Lower Cholesterol.* 3rd ed. New York, NY: Houghton Mifflin Co; 1992. 571 pp. Available from Houghton Mifflin Co, 215 Park Avenue South, New York, NY 10003, (800) 225-3362.

Harlan TJ. *It's Heartly Fare: A Food Book That Makes Sense of Fat, Cholesterol, and Salt.* Atlanta, Ga: Pritchett & Hull Associates, Inc; 1993. 60 pp. Available from Pritchett & Hull Associates, Inc, 3440 Oakcliff Road, NE, Suite 110, Atlanta, GA 30340-3079, (800) 241-4925 or 770-451-0602, fax: (800) 752-0510 or (770) 454-7130. Includes 8-page practice supplement; 14-page staff teaching guide available.

Kwiterovich P, Lipid Research Clinic Staff. *The Johns Hopkins Complete Guide for Preventing and Reversing Heart Disease.* Rocklin, Calif: Prima Publishing; 1993. 395 pp. Available from Prima Publishing, PO Box 1260, Rocklin, CA 95677-1260, (800) 632-8676 or (916) 632-4400.

Lapchick JM, Mo R. *The Brand-Name Guide to Low-Fat and Fat-Free Foods.* Minneapolis, Minn: Chronimed Publishing Co; 1995. 160 pp. Available from Chronimed Publishing Co, 13911 Ridgedale Drive, Suite 250, Minnetonka, MN 55305, (800) 876-6540.

Moquette-Magee E. *Fight Fat and Win.* Updated and revised edition. Minnetonka, Minn: Chronimed Publishing; 1994. 330 pp. Available from Chronimed Publishing Co, 13911 Ridgedale Drive, Suite 250, Minnetonka, MN 55305, (800) 876-6540.

Mosca L, Rubenfire M, Rock C. *The M-Fit Grocery Shopping Guide: Your Guide to Healthier Choices.* Memphis, Tenn: Favorite Recipes Press; 1995. 400 pp. Available from M-Fit Supermarket Program, 24 Frank Lloyd Wright Drive, Ann Arbor, MI 48106-0363, (313) 998-7645.

Ornish D. *Dr. Dean Ornish's Program for Reversing Heart Disease.* New York, NY: Random House, Inc; 1990. 631 pp. Available from Random House, Inc, 201 East 50th Street, New York, NY 10022, (800) 733-3000.

Piscatella JC. *Controlling Your Fat Tooth.* New York, NY: Workman; 1991. 526 pp.

Schwartz Wennik R. *Drawing the Line on Fat and Cholesterol.* Lynnwood, Wash: Labyrinth Publishing Works; 1992. 176 pp. Available from Labyrinth Publishing Works, PO Box 83, Lynnwood, WA 98046, (206) 778-1340.

Skim the Fat: A Practical & Up-To-Date Food Guide. The American Dietetic Association. Minnetonka, Minn: Chronimed Publishing; 1995. 218 pp. Available from The American Dietetic Association [*see* page 287] or Chronimed Publishing Co, 13911 Ridgedale Drive, Suite 250, Minnetonka, MN 55305, (800) 876-6540.

Warshaw HS. *The Restaurant Companion.* 2nd ed. Chicago, Ill: Surrey Books; 1995. 360 pp. Available from Surrey Books, Inc, 230 East Ohio Street, Suite 120, Chicago, IL 60611, (800) 326-4430.

Newsletters and Magazines

Change of Heart. University of Nevada/Washoe County Cooperative Extension Service, PO Box 11130, Reno, NV 85920-9913, (702) 784-4848. (series of newsletters for professionals to use with consumers)

Cooking Light. Southern Living, Inc, PO Box C-549, Birmingham, AL 35282-9990, (800) 336-0125.

Eating Well: The Magazine of Food and Health. PO Box 1001, Charlotte, VT 06446, (800) 344-3350.

FDA Consumer. Superintendent of Documents, Government Printing Office, PO Box 371954, Pittsburgh, PA 15250-7954, (202) 512-1800, fax: (202) 512-2233.

Food For Health. 15084 North 92nd Place, Scottsdale, AZ 85260-2824, (800) 484-9513 (code 1000), fax: (602) 451-7642.

Hope Health Letter. Seattle, Wash: The Hope Heart Institute. For subscription information: International Health Awareness Center, Inc, 350 East Michigan Avenue, Suite 301, Kalamazoo, MI 49007-3851, (616) 343-0770. (group subscriptions available)

Lipid Clinic News. Oregon Health Sciences University, L-465 Department of Medicine, 3181 SW Sam Jackson Park Road, Portland, OR 97201-3098, (503) 494-7775.

Nutrition Action Health Letter. Center for Science in the Public Interest (CSPI), 1875 Connecticut Avenue, NW, Suite 300, Washington, DC 20009-5728, (202) 332-9110.

The Peanut Institute Newsletter. PO Box 70157, Albany, GA 31708, (888) 8-PEANUT. Provides information on nutritional composition of peanuts and the role peanuts play in a healthful diet.

Tufts University Diet and Nutrition Letter. PO Box 57857, Boulder, CO 80322-7857, (800) 274-7581 or (303) 447-9330.

Audiovisuals

American Medical Association. *AMA Healthy Heart Series.* Timonium, Md: Milner-Fenwick; 1994. Includes four videocassettes: *Guide to Controlling Your Cholesterol* (13 minutes), *Guide to High Blood Pressure Control* (10 minutes), *Guide to Your Healthy Heart* (16 minutes), and *Guide to Stop Smoking.* Each video has an accompanying client booklet. Available from Milner-Fenwick, Inc, 2125 Greenspring Drive, Timonium, MD 21093, (800) 432-8433 or (410) 252-1700, fax: (410) 252-6316.

Cardiovascular Disease: Prevention and Control. Houston, Tex: InforMed, Inc; 1993. Includes 20-minute videocassette. Available from Educational Video Network, Inc, 1401 19th Street, Huntsville, TX 77340, (800) 3-INFORM or (409) 95-5767.

Cholesterol Control. Beaverton, Oreg: Mosby Great Performance; 1995. Includes 9-minute, 48-second videocassette and an activity booklet. Available from Mosby Great Performance, Order Department, 11830 Westline Industrial Drive, St. Louis, MO 63146, (800) 433-3803 or (503) 690-9181, fax: (800) 535-9935.

Controlling Cholesterol. Princeton, NJ: Films for the Humanities & Sciences, Inc; 1991. Includes 28-minute videocassette. Available from Films for the Humanities & Sciences, Inc, PO Box 2053, Princeton, NJ 08543, (609) 452-1128.

The HeartCare Program: Dietary Management of Cholesterol. Revised ed. Minneapolis, Minn: Hall-Foushee Productions, Inc; 1994. Includes four 12-minute videocassettes, curriculum guide, audiotape, camera-ready masters, brochures, and shopping cards. Available from Hall-Foushee Productions, Inc, 1313 Fifth Street, SE, Suite 214B, Minneapolis, MN 55414, (800) 478-3829, (612) 379-3829, fax: (612) 379-3829.

High Blood Pressure: A Lifestyle and Medical Approach to Hypertension. Beaverton, Oreg: Mosby Great Performance; 1995. Includes 10-minute videocassette and booklets. Available from Mosby Great Performance, Order Department, 11830 Westline Industrial Drive, St. Louis, MO 63146, (800) 433-3803 or (503) 690-9181, fax: (800) 535-9935.

How to Read the New Food Label for Persons With Heart Disease. Los Angeles, Calif: National Health Video; 1994. Includes 12-minute video. Available from National Health Video, 12021 Wilshire Boulevard, Los Angeles, CA 90025, (800) 543-6803.

Lean Life Foods Slide Set. Shingle Springs, Calif: NutriVisuals, 1993. Includes 80 slides, script, and recipes. Also available with audiotape. Available from NutriVisuals, PO Box 1367, Shingle Springs, CA 95682, (916) 677-1969.

Lean 'n Easy: Preparing Meat with Less Fat and More Taste. Chicago, Ill: The American Dietetic Association and the National Cattlemen's Beef Association; 1994. Includes 25-minute videocassette, leader's guide, and 17 camera-ready masters. Available from The American Dietetic Association [*see* page 287] or the National Live Stock and Meat Board, Education Department, 444 North Michigan Avenue, Chicago, IL 60611-9909, (800) 368-3138, (312) 670-9440, fax: (800) 368-3136.

The New Lean Life Foods. Shingle Springs, Calif: NutriVisuals; 1995. Includes 31-minute videocassette. Available from NutriVisuals, PO Box 1367, Shingle Springs, CA 95682, (916) 677-1969.

Northeast Network for Food, Agriculture, and Health Policy Education. *A Heart Healthy Diet: Who Makes the Choices?* Ithaca, NY: Cornell University. Includes 10-minute videocassette, camera-ready masters, leader's guide, and poster. Available from Cornell University Resource Center, 7 Cornell Business and Technology Park, Ithaca, NY 14850, (607) 255-2080, fax: (607) 255-9946; order no. 305HHD.)

Put Away Your Frying Pan. Philadelphia, Penn: Health Promotion Council of Southeastern Pennsylvania, Inc; not dated. For African Americans; includes 10-minute videocassette. Available from Health Promotion Council of Southeastern Pennsylvania; *see* page 288.

Put the Fat Back: Smart Shoppers Take Control. Philadelphia, Penn: Health Promotion Council of Southeastern Pennsylvania, Inc; 1991. For African-Americans; includes 16-minute videocassette. Available from Health Promotion Council of Southeastern PA; *see* page 288.

Quick and Easy Low-fat Cooking. Chicago, Ill: The American Dietetic Association; 1995. Trainer's kit; includes 12-minute video, manual, eight transparencies, and sample consumer booklet. Additional booklets and companion poster also available. Available from The American Dietetic Association; *see* page 287.

Recreating Taste in Low Fat Cooking. Chicago, Ill: The American Dietetic Association and the National Cattlemen's Beef Association; 1994. Includes 25-minute videocassette, 1 poster, and 10 camera-ready masters. Available from The American Dietetic Association [*see* page 287] or the National Cattlemen's Beef Association, Education Department, 444 North Michigan Avenue, Chicago, IL 60611-9909, (800) 368-3138, (312) 670-9440, fax: (800) 368-3136.

Curriculum Guides and Other Teaching Materials

Beans, Beans, Good for Your Heart. Bethesda, Md: National Heart, Lung and Blood Institute; 1993. Order No. 55-591. Includes one poster. Available from NHLBI Information Center; *see* page 286.

Buhr SE. *How Much Fat? Teaching Test Tubes.* Includes 10 test tubes representing the amount of fat in foods and a teaching pamphlet. Available from Nutrition Counseling Education Services [NCES], 1904 East 123rd Street, Olathe, KS 66061-5886, (800) 445-5653, fax: (800) 251-9349.

A Change of Plate. Chicago, Ill: National Cattleman's Beef Association (formerly National Live Stock and Meat Board); 1991. Includes leader's guide, eight camera-ready masters, flip chart, and three food models. Available from National Cattleman's Beef Association, Education Department, 444 North Michigan Avenue, Chicago, IL 60611-9909, (800) 368-3138, (312) 670-9440, fax: (800) 368-3136.

Choose Lean Meats Poster. Chicago, Ill: National Cattleman's Beef Association (formerly National Live Stock and Meat Board); not dated. Includes one poster. Available from National Cattleman's Beef Association, Education Department, 444 North Michigan Avenue, Chicago, IL 60611-9909, (800) 368-3138, (312) 670-9440, fax: (800) 368-3136.

Do You Know Your Cholesterol Numbers? Bethesda, Md: National Heart, Lung and Blood Institute; 1995. Order No. 55-693. Includes one poster. Available from NHLBI Information Center; *see* page 286.

Eating for Pleasure and Health: How to Buy and Fix Good Food with Less Fat. (Spanish title: *Comiendo Por Placer Y Salud.)* Madison, Wis: University of Wisconsin-Extension Food and Nutrition Education Program (EFNEP); 1993. For consumers with low literacy skills. Includes workbook with lessons and handouts. Available from Cooperative Extension Publications, 30 North Murray Street, Room 245, Madison, WI 53715, (608) 262-3346.

High Blood Pressure Doesn't Have to Kill You to Take Away Your Life. Bethesda, Md: National Heart, Lung and Blood Institute; 1993. Includes one poster. Order No. 55-587. Available from NHLBI Information Center; *see* page 286.

In Matters of the Heart, Be Choosy. Bethesda, Md: National Heart, Lung and Blood Institute; reprinted 1995. Includes one poster. Order No. 55-542. Available from NHLBI Information Center; *see* page 286.

Keeping the Pressure Down: A Wellness Approach to Blood Pressure. Washington, DC: National Council on the Aging (NOA); 1992. For older adults. Includes one flip chart, one program leader's manual, personal health record booklets, and multiple copies of four brochures. Available from NOA, 409 Third Street, SW, Washington, DC 20024, (202) 479-1200, fax: (202) 479-0735.

Logan R, Benedict M. *Heart Bingo.* 1993. Includes game for up to 25 players. Available from Lowfat Lifeline, 234 Cass Street, Port Townsend, WA 98368, (800) 294-9801 or (360) 379-9724, fax: (360) 385-6835.

Low-Fat Express. Owatonna, Minn: Pineapple Appeal; 1995. Includes nine-lesson curriculum with full-color food photographs, fat model, artery model, 32 tubes of fat, cookbook, food guide, handouts, and kitchen gadgets. For consumers with low literacy skills. Available from Pineapple Appeal, RR #1, Highway 14W, PO Box 197, Owatonna, MN 55060, (800) 321-3041 or (507) 455-3041, fax: (507) 455-2307.

National Cholesterol Education Month Kit. Bethesda, Md: National Heart, Lung and Blood Institute (NHLBI). Annual kit. Includes materials, such as sample handouts, camera-ready masters, boiler plate article, and ideas to use to promote and conduct activities for National Cholesterol Education Month. Available from NHLBI Information Center; *see* page 284.

Project LEAN Resource Kit: Tips, Tools, and Techniques for Promoting Low-Fat Lifestyles. Chicago, Ill: The American Dietetic Association; 1995. Includes binder with information about fat, teaching about low-fat eating, physical activity, reaching the community, and teaching at the worksite. Includes 20 camera-ready masters and two 1996 updates. Available from The American Dietetic Association; *see* page 287.

Riley G. *Lipo-Visuals Teaching Kit.* Includes 36 test tubes and 5 color-coded flash cards. Available from Nutrition Counseling Education Services [NCES], 1904 East 123rd Street, Olathe, KS 66061-5886, (800) 445-5653, fax: (800) 251-9349.

Self-Care for a Healthy Heart. Fort Collins, Colo: Colorado State University Cooperative Extension; 1991. Includes lessons for consumers. Available from Cheri Pineda, CSU Cooperative Extension, 200 Gifford Building, Fort Collins, CO 80523-1571, (970) 491-1305; fax: (970) 491-7252.

Stay Young at Heart. Bethesda, Md: National Heart Lung and Blood Institute; 1995. NIH publication 94-3648. Includes nutrition education program to use in worksites, cafeterias, and other settings with manual, 50 quantity and consumer recipes, and camera-ready masters. Available from Government Printing Office, Superintendent of Documents, PO Box 371954, Pittsburgh, PA 15250-7954, (202) 512-1800, fax: (202) 512-2250.

MATERIALS FOR CHILDREN AND ADOLESCENTS

Brochures and Handouts

The American Dietetic Association

See page 287.

Heart Healthy Eating for Children. 1997. 12 panels.

Growing Up Healthy: Fat, Cholesterol, and More. 1991. 8 panels.

Egg Nutrition Center

1819 H Street, NW, Suite 520
Washington, DC 20009
(202) 833-8850
eggnutr@aol.com (e-mail)

Children and Cholesterol: Counseling Parents on a Responsible Diet and Lifestyle. 1993. 8 panels.

A Dozen Heart-Healthy Habits for Kids (...and their parents). 1993. 12 panels. (inside is a fold-out poster)

National Heart, Lung and Blood Institute (NHLBI)

For single copies and information on ordering multiple copies, use address and telephone information under NHLBI entry in the organizations section.

Eating With Your Heart In Mind. 1992. 36 pp. NIH publication 92-3100. (for 7- to 10-year-olds)

Heart Health...Your Choice. 1992. 39 pp. NIH publication 92-3101. (for 11- to 14-year-olds)

Hearty Habits: Don't Eat Your Heart Out. 1993. 57 pp. NIH publication 93-3102. (for 15- to 18-year-olds)

Parents' Guide. Cholesterol in Children: Healthy Eating is a Family Affair. 1992. 52 pp. NIH publication 92-3099.

Washington State Department of Health Heart Health Program

See page 289.

To Parents with High Cholesterol. 1995. 2 pp. (part of set of eight camera-ready handouts; English on one side, Spanish on the other)

Books and Cookbooks for Consumers

Moquette-Magee E. *200 Kid-Tested Ways to Lower Fat in Your Child's Favorite Foods.* Minneapolis, Minn: Chronimed Publishing; 1993. 319 pp. Available from Chronimed Publishing, PO Box 59032, Minneapolis, MN 55459-9686, (800) 848-2793.

Reiman R, Hanc J. *Combating Your Child's Cholesterol: A Pediatrician Shows You How.* New York, NY: Plenum Press; 1993. 316 pp. Available from Plenum Press, 233 Spring Street, New York, NY 10013, (212) 620-8000.

Snyder AH, Adams LB. *The SPIN Cookbook: A Collection of Heart Healthy, Low Fat, and Low Cholesterol Recipes.* 2nd ed. San Francisco, Calif: The J. David Gladstone Institutes; 1994. Available from Gladstone Institute of Cardiovascular Disease, 2550 23rd Street, PO Box 419100, San Francisco, CA 94141-9100, (415) 826-7500.

Winston M, Holub J. *American Heart Association Kids' Cookbook.* 1st ed. New York, NY: Times Books; 1993. 127 pp. Available from Random House, 400 Hahn Road, Westminster, MD 21157, (800) 793-2665.

Audiovisuals

Cut the Fat from Your Diet: Using the Food Guide Pyramid (for teens). Huntsville, Tex: Educational Video Network; 1994. Includes 30-minute videocassette and one reproducible handout. Available from Educational Video Network, 1401 19th Street, Huntsville, TX 77340, (409) 295-5767, fax: (409) 294-0233.

Ralphie's Class Presents a Healthy Heart. Niles, Ill: United Learning; 1993. For grades 2-4. Includes 13-minute videocassette, teacher's guide, and four reproducible handouts. Available from United Learning, 6633 West Howard Street, PO Box 48718, Niles, IL 60714-0718, (800) 424-0362.

Termineater. Scottsdale, Ariz: Dream Street Films; 1993. For elementary-aged children. Includes 16-minute videocassette and instructor's guide. Available from Dream Street Films, (602) 970-1952.

Curriculum Guides and Other Teaching Materials

The CATCH (Child and Adolescent Trial for Cardiovascular Health) Intervention Program Materials. Bethesda, Md: National Heart, Lung and Blood Institute; 1996. Available from NHLBI Information Center; *see* page 286. Materials include

- *Go for Health 4: Taking Off.* For 4th grade. Includes 24 40-minute lessons on nutrition and physical activity and 6 activity packets to promote family involvement.
- *Go for Health 5: Breaking Through Barriers.* For 5th grade. Includes 16 40- to 50-minute lessons on nutrition and physical activity and 4 activity packets to promote family involvement.
- *Hearty Heart & Friends.* For 3rd grade. Includes 15 30-minute sessions about healthy eating patterns, 9 video episodes, and 5 activity packets to promote family involvement.
- See also Chapter 10, Resources.

Cholesterol in School Age Children. Mendham, NJ: Infinity Impressions, Ltd; 1990. Includes 1 manual and 19 transparencies. Available from Infinity Impressions, Ltd, 88 East Main Street, Suite 500, Mendham, NJ 07945, (800) 926-7696, fax: (201) 543-9231.

Eating Smart for Your Heart. University Park, Penn: The Pennsylvania State University; 1993. For families of 4- to 10-year-olds. Includes story books with audiotapes, activity book, and parent guide. Available at 3 levels: level 1 for ages 4-5, level 2 for ages 6-8, and level 3 for ages 9-10. Available from Penn State Nutrition Center, 5 Henderson Building, University Park, PA 16801-5663, (814) 865-6323.

Fat: A Balancing Act. Seattle, Wash: Washington State Dairy Council; 1993. For grades 7-12. Includes poster, brochure, six duplicating masters, and three lesson plans. Available from Washington State Dairy Council, 4201 198th Street, SW, Suite 102, Lynnwood, WA 98036, (206) 744-1616, fax: (800) 470-1222 or (206) 670-1222.

Heart-Healthy Lessons for Children. Phoenix, Ariz: Arizona Heart Institute and Foundation; 1991. For grades K-6. Includes different lessons for lower and upper elementary grades on the heart, cholesterol and fats, high blood pressure and sodium, exercise, and smoking. Includes 21 camera-ready masters and 8 transparencies. Available from Arizona Heart Institute and Foundation, 2632 North 20th Street, Phoenix, AZ 85006, (602) 266-2200.

HeartPower! Dallas, Tex: The American Heart Association; 1996. For grades K-8. Includes five different kits for preschool through grade 1 in Spanish, preschool, kindergarten through grade 2, grades 3 through 5, and middle school. Available from your local American Heart Association chapter or (800) AHA-USA-1.

Logan R, Benedict M. *Heart Bingo.* 1993. For ages 15 and up. Includes game for up to 25 players. Available from Lowfat Lifeline, 234 Cass Street, Port Townsend, WA 98368, (800) 294-9801 or (360) 379-9724, fax: (360) 385-6835.

Books and Reports for Professionals

Eat Smart. Bethesda, Md: National Heart, Lung and Blood Institute (CATCH Program); 1996. Manual for school food service directors and cooks for reducing fat, saturated fat, and cholesterol in school meals; includes recipes. Available from NHLBI Information Center; *see* page 286.

Filer LJ Jr, Lauer RM, Leupker RV. *Prevention of Atherosclerosis and Hypertension Beginning in Youth.* Philadelphia, Penn: Lea & Febiger; 1994. 293 pp. Available from Lea & Febiger, 200 Chester Field Parkway, Malvern, PA 19355, (215) 251-2230.

Highlights of the NCEP Report on Blood Cholesterol Levels in Children and Adolescents. Bethesda, Md: National Institutes of Health; 1991. 11 pp. NIH publication 91-2731. Available from NHLBI Information Center; *see* page 286.

National Cholesterol Education Program: Report of the Expert Panel on Blood Cholesterol Levels in Children and Adolescents. Bethesda, Md: National Institutes of Health; 1991. 119 pp. NIH publication 91-2732. Available from NHLBI Information Center; *see* page 286.

MATERIALS FOR HEALTH PROFESSIONALS

Books, Reports, and Manuals

Byrne KP. *Understanding and Managing Cholesterol: A Guide for Wellness Professionals.* Champaign, Ill: Human Kinetics Publishers; 1991. 344 pp. Available from Human Kinetics Publishers, Box 5076, Champaign, IL 60825-5076, (800) 747-4457.

The Cardiovascular Health of Women. HeartMemo Special Issue. Bethesda, Md: National Heart, Lung and Blood Institute; 1994. 28 pp. NIH publication 55-653.

Available from NHLBI Information Center; *see* page 286.

Cardiovascular Patient Education Resource Manual. Frederick, Md: Aspen Publishers, Inc; 1994. 500 pp. Available from Aspen Publishers, Inc, 7201 McKinney Circle, Frederick, MD 21701, (800) 638-8437.

Chef's Handbook: Low-fat Quantity Food Preparation. Chicago, Ill: The American Dietetic Association; 1993. Binder with 108 loose-leaf sheets and recipe cards. Available from The American Dietetic Association; *see* page 287.

Coleman E. *Cardiovascular Nutrition & Fitness.* San Marcos, Calif: Nutrition Dimension; 1995. 160 pp. Continuing education course. Available from Nutrition Dimension, PO Box 1478, San Marcos, CA 92079, (619) 598-1709.

A Communication Strategy for Public Information: The National Cholesterol Education Program. Bethesda, Md: National Heart, Lung and Blood Institute; 1994. 26 pp. NIH publication 94-3292. Available from NHLBI Information Center; *see* page 286.

Declining Serum Total Cholesterol Levels Among U.S. Adults: The National Health and Nutrition Examination Surveys. Bethesda, Md: National Heart, Lung and Blood Institute; 1993. 8 pp. Order No. 55-609. Available from NHLBI Information Center; *see* page 286.

Eating Less Fat: A Progress Report on Improving America's Diet. Washington, DC: Institute for Science in Society (ISIS); 1992. 67 pp. Available from ISIS, 1850 M Street, NW, Suite 275, Washington, DC 20036, (202) 331-0613.

Fifth Report of the Joint National Committee on Detection, Evaluation, and Treatment of High Blood Pressure. National High Blood Pressure Education Program. Bethesda, Md: National Heart, Lung and Blood Institute; 1993; reprinted 1995. 51 pp. NIH publication 95-1088. Available from NHLBI Information Center; *see* page 286.

Kritchevsky D, Carroll KK. *Nutrition and Disease Update: Heart Disease.* Champaign, Ill: AOCS Press; 1994. 279 pp. Available from AOCS Press, PO Box 3489, Champaign, IL 61826-3489, (217) 359-2344.

Margolis S, Goldschmidt-Clermont PJ. *Coronary Heart Disease: The Johns Hopkins White Papers.* Baltimore, Md: Johns Hopkins Medical Institutions; 1995. 59 pp. Available from Johns Hopkins Medical Institutions, PO Box 420083, Palm Coast, FL 32142-9064, (800) 829-9170 or (904) 446-4675.

Margolis S, Klag MJ. *Hypertension: The Johns Hopkins White Papers.* Baltimore, Md: Johns Hopkins Medical Institutions; 1995. 45 pp. Available from Johns Hopkins Medical Institutions, PO Box 420083, Palm Coast, FL 32142-9064, (800) 829-9170 or (904) 446-4675.

NHBPEP Coordinating Committee Statement on Salt. Bethesda, Md: National Heart, Lung and Blood Institute; 1995. 2 pp. Order No. 55-683. Available from NHLBI Information Center; *see* page 286.

Nutrition and Cardiovascular Disease Nutri-Topics. Educator and Health Professional/Researcher Levels. 1995. 12 pp and 15 pp. Resource lists. Available from Food and Nutrition Information Center; *see* page 286.

Prevalence of High Blood Cholesterol Among US Adults: An Update Based on Guidelines from the Second Report of the National Cholesterol Education Program Adult Treatment Panel. Bethesda, Md: National Heart, Lung and Blood Institute; 1993. 6 pp. Order No. 55-649. Available from NHLBI Information Center; *see* page 286.

Redmond GP, ed. *Lipids and Women's Health.* New York, NY: Springer-Verlag; 1991. 260 pp.

Report of the Expert Panel on Population Strategies for Blood Cholesterol Reduction. Bethesda, Md: National Heart, Lung and Blood Institute; 1990, reprinted 1993. 139 pp. NIH publication 93-3046. (36-page executive summary also available [NIH publication 93-3047]) Available from NHLBI Information Center; *see* page 286.

Rifkind B, ed. *Lowering Cholesterol in High Risk Individuals and Populations.* New York, NY: Marcel Dekker, Inc; 1995. 392 pp. Available from Marcel Dekker, Inc, PO Box 5019, Monticello, NY 12701, (800) 228-1160.

Second Report of the Expert Panel on Detection, Evaluation, and Treatment of High Blood Cholesterol in Adults (Adult Treatment Panel II). National Cholesterol Education Program. Bethesda, Md: National Heart, Lung and Blood Institute; 1993. 180 pp. NIH publication 93-3095. (28-page executive summary also available [NIH publication 93-3096]) Available from NHLBI Information Center; *see* page 286.

Spiller GA, ed. *Handbook of Lipids in Human Nutrition.* Boca Raton, Fla: CRC Press, Inc; 1996. 233 pp. Available from CRC Press, 2000 Corporate Boulevard, NW, Boca Raton, FL 33431, (407) 994-0555.

Trends in the Prevalence, Awareness, Treatment, and Control of Hypertension in the Adult U.S. Population. Data from the Health Examination Surveys—1960 to 1991. Bethesda, Md: National Heart, Lung and Blood Institute; 1995. 10 pp. NIH publication 95-3791. Available from NHLBI Information Center; *see* page 286.

Triglyceride, High Density Lipoprotein, and Coronary Heart Disease. NIH Consensus Development Conference February 26-28, 1992. NIH Consens Statement. 1992;10(2):28 pp. Available from NIH Consensus Program Information Service, PO Box 2577, Kensington, MD 20891, (800) NIH-OMAR [644-6627], fax: (301) 816-2494, http://text.nlm.nih.gov [World Wide Web], gopher://gopher.nih.gov/Health and Clinical Information [Gopher])

Washington State Heart Disease and Stroke Prevention Plan. Olympia, Wash: Washington State Department of Health. 1995. 43 pp. Available from Community & Family Health, Noninfectious Disease and Injury Prevention, Heart Health Program, Airdustrial Park, Building 10, PO Box 47835, Olympia, WA 98504-7835, (360) 753-4311, fax: (360) 753-9100.

Working Group Report on Hypertension in Diabetes. Bethesda, Md: National Heart, Lung and Blood Institute; reprinted 1995. 32 pp. NIH Publication 95-3530. Available from NHLBI Information Center; *see* page 286.

Working Group Report on Hypertension in the Elderly. Bethesda, Md: National Heart, Lung and Blood Institute; 1995. 20 pp. NIH Publication 94-3527. Available from NHLBI Information Center; *see* page 286.

Working Group Report on the Primary Prevention of Hypertension. Bethesda, Md: National, Heart, Lung and Blood Institute; 1993. 49 pp. NIH publication 93-2669. Available from NHLBI Information Center; *see* page 286.

Zaret BL, Moser M, Cohen LS . *Yale University School of Medicine Heart Book.* New York, NY: William Morrow & Co, Inc; 1992. 432 pp. Also appropriate for educated and motivated consumers.

Audiovisuals

Chef's Creating LEAN: A Nutrition Course for Food Professionals. Chicago, Ill: The American Dietetic Association; 1994. Includes 132 color slides, 24 reproducible masters, and a manual. Available from The American Dietetic Association; *see* page 287.

Cholesterol Lowering in the Management of Coronary Heart Disease. National Cholesterol Education Program. Bethesda, Md: Medical Communications Resources, Inc, and the National Heart Lung and Blood Institute in cooperation with the American Heart Association; 1995. Order No. 55-657. For practicing physicians and others who treat cardiovascular patients. Includes 38-minute videocassette. Available from NHLBI Information Center; *see* page 286.

Second Report of the Expert Panel on Detection, Evaluation, and Treatment of High Blood Cholesterol in Adults. Bethesda, Md: National Heart Lung and Blood Institute; 1993. Order No. 55-589. Includes 30-minute videocassette. Available from NHLBI Information Center; *see* page 286.

Journals and Newsletters for Health Professionals

American Journal of Cardiology

Box 173306
Denver, CO 80217-3306
(800) 662-7776

American Journal of Clinical Nutrition

9650 Rockville Pike, L-2130
Bethesda, MD 20814-3998
(301) 530-7026 or 7038 (phone); (301) 571-8303 (fax)

American Journal of Epidemiology

The Johns Hopkins University School of Hygiene and Public Health
111 Market Place, Suite 840
Baltimore, MD 21202-6709
(410) 955-3441 (phone); (410) 955-0344 (fax)

American Journal of Hypertension

Elsevier Science, Inc
655 Avenue of the Americas
New York, NY 10010
(212) 989-5800 (phone); (212) 633-3990 (fax)

American Journal of Preventive Medicine

Oxford Journals Fulfillment
2001 Evans Road
Cary, NC 27513
(919) 677-0977 (phone); (919) 677-1714 (fax)

American Journal of Public Health

American Public Health Association
1015 15th Street, SW
Washington, DC 20005
(202) 789-5600

Annals of Epidemiology

Elsevier Science, Inc
655 Avenue of the Americas
New York, NY 10010
(212) 989-5800 (phone); (212) 633-3990 (fax)

Annals of the New York Academy of Sciences

The New York Academy of Sciences
2 East 63rd Street
New York, NY 10021
(800) 843-6927 or (212) 838-0230 (phone);
(212) 888-2894 (fax)

Arteriosclerosis, Thrombosis, and Vascular Biology

Scientific Publishing
American Heart Association
7272 Greenville Avenue
Dallas, TX 75231-4596
(214) 706-1310 (phone); (214) 691-6342 (fax)
pubcust@amhrt.org (e-mail)

British Journal of Nutrition

Cambridge University Press, Journals Department
40 West 20th Street
New York, NY 10011-4211
(212) 924-3900 (phone); (212) 691-3239 (fax)

British Medical Journal

British Medical Association
c/o Mercury Airfreight International Ltd, Inc
2323 Randolph Avenue
Avenel, NJ 07001
or
BMA House, Tavistock Square
London WC1H 9JR England
(44) 171 387 4499 (phone); (44) 171 383 6418 (fax)
Editor@bmjedit.demon.co.uk (e-mail)
http://www.bmj.com/bmj/ (World Wide Web)

Circulation

Scientific Publishing
American Heart Association
7272 Greenville Avenue
Dallas, TX 75231-4596
(214) 706-1201 (phone); (214) 691-6342 (fax)
pubcust@amhrt.org (e-mail)

Environmental Nutrition

PO Box 420451
Palm Coast, FL 32142-0451
(800) 829-5384
76521.2250@compuserve.com (e-mail)

Ethnicity and Disease

International Society on Hypertension in Blacks
69 Butler Street, SE
Atlanta, GA 30303
(708) 216-4117 (fax)

European Journal of Clinical Nutrition

The Subscription Department, Macmillan Press Ltd
Houndmills, Basingstoke
Hampshire, RG21 2XS United Kingdom
(44) 0 1256 29242 (phone); (44) 0 1256 810526 (fax)

HeartMemo

National Heart, Lung and Blood Institute (*see* page 286)

Hypertension

Scientific Publishing, American Heart Association
7272 Greenville Avenue
Dallas, TX 75231-4596
(214) 706-1310 (phone); (214) 691-6342 (fax)
pubcust@amhrt.org (e-mail)

Journal of the American College of Cardiology

Elsevier Science, Inc
655 Avenue of the Americas
New York, NY 10010
(212) 989-5800 (phone); (212) 633-3990 (fax)

Journal of the American College of Nutrition

PO Box 3000
Denville, NJ 07834
(800) 875-2997 or (201) 627-2997

Journal of The American Dietetic Association

The American Dietetic Association (*see* page 287)
(800) 745-0775, extension 5000, or (312) 899-0040, extension 5000

Journal of the American Medical Association (JAMA)

Subscriber Services, American Medical Association
PO Box 10945, Chicago, IL 60610
(800) 262-2350 (phone); (312) 464-5831 (fax)

Journal of Cardiovascular Risk

Current Sciences
20 North Third Street
Philadelphia, PA 19106-2199
(215) 577-2210 (phone); (215) 574-3533 (fax)
info@phl.cursci.com (e-mail)

The Journal of Nutrition

Subscriptions Department
American Society of Nutritional Sciences
9650 Rockville Pike
Bethesda, MD 20814-3990
(301) 530-7103

Journal of Nutrition Education

Decker Periodicals
One James Street South, 11th Floor
Hamilton, Ontario, L8P 4R5 Canada
(800) 568-7281 or (905) 522-7017 (phone);
(905) 522-7839 (fax)

The Lancet

655 Avenue of the Americas
New York, NY 10010
(212) 633-3800 (phone); (212) 633-3850 (fax)

Medical Clinics of North America

Periodicals Fulfillment, WB Saunders Company
6277 Sea Harbor Drive, 4th Floor
Orlando, FL 32891-4800
(800) 654-2452 (phone); (800) 874-6418 (fax)

The New England Journal of Medicine

NEJM Customer Service Department
PO Box 803
Waltham, MA 02254-0803
(800) THE-NEJM

Nutrition & the M.D.

Lippincott-Raven Publishers, Department 1B
1185 Avenue of the Americas
New York, NY 10036
(800) 853-2478 (phone); (212) 869-3495 (fax)

Nutrition Close-Up

Egg Nutrition Center
1819 H Street, Suite 520
Washington, DC 20006
(202) 833-8850

Nutrition Today

Williams & Wilkins
428 East Preston Street
Baltimore, MD 21202
(800) 638-6423 or (410) 528-4105

Pediatrics

American Academy of Pediatrics
PO Box 927
Elk Grove Village, IL 60009-0927
(708) 228-5005

Preventive Medicine

Academic Press Inc, Office of the Publishers
6277 Sea Harbor Drive
Orlando, FL 32887-4900
(619) 230-1840 (phone); (619) 699-6800 (fax)

SCAN's PULSE

Sports, Cardiovascular, and Wellness Nutritionists (SCAN) Dietetic Practice Group (*see* page 286)

The Soy Connection

PO Box 20421
Kansas City, MO 64195-0421
(800) TALK-SOY (800-825-5769) (8:00 am to 4:00 pm CST)

SUPERMARKET SAVVY

PO Box 666
Herndon, VA 22070-0666
(800) 657-2889 or (703) 742-3364 (phone);
(703) 742-3316 (fax)
ssavvy@aol.com (e-mail)

World Review of Nutrition and Dietetics

S Karger Publishers, Inc
26 West Avon Road
PO Box 529
Farmington, CT 06085
(203) 675-7834 (phone); (203) 675-7302 (fax)

Meetings and Conferences

American Association of Cardiovascular and Pulmonary Rehabilitation holds its annual national convention for professionals in the fall. For more information, contact the organization (*see* page 285).

American Dietetic Association (*see* page 287) holds its annual meeting in October.

American College of Sports Medicine (ACSM) holds its annual meeting during the last week in May. For more information call ACSM at (317) 637-9200.

American Heart Association (AHA) sponsors Scientific Sessions, the world's largest meeting on cardiovascular disease. Held annually in November. For more information call (214) 706-1100.

American Public Health Association (APHA) holds its annual meeting in October or November. For more information call (202) 789-5600.

Federation for American Societies in Experimental Biology (FASEB). Various societies participating in FASEB sponsor the annual Experimental Biology Conference in April. For more information call (301) 530-7010.

International Society of Behavioral Medicine holds its annual meeting in March to April. The topics cover a wide range of areas in behavioral medicine, including cardiovascular disease, obesity, and women's health. For more information call (301) 251-2790.

International Society on Hypertension in Blacks (ISHIB) holds an annual international interdisciplinary conference for health care professionals. The focus is on the research of hypertension and its concomitant diseases. The conference location usually alternates between the United States and other parts of the world. For more information call (404) 875-6263.

Sports, Cardiovascular, and Wellness Nutritionists (SCAN) Annual Symposium. Held annually in April. Cardiovascular disease is the focus of the meeting every fourth year, but cardiovascular topics are presented annually. Contact SCAN office, 90 S Cascade Ave, Suite 1190, Colorado Springs, CO 80903, (719) 475-7751 (phone); (719) 475-8748 (fax).

INDEX

D

E